Mosby's
QUESTIONS &
ANSWERS for
NCLEX-PN

Mosby's QUESTIONS & ANSWERS for NCLEX-PN

MARY O. EYLES, MA, RN

Director of Education
Kessler Medical Rehabilitation Research and Education Corporation
West Orange, New Jersey

Associate, Department of Physical Medicine and Rehabilitation
University of Medicine and Dentistry of New Jersey–New Jersey Medical School
Newark, New Jersey

Former Director of Continuing Education
National Association for Practical Nurse Education and Service, Inc.

SECOND EDITION

 Mosby

St. Louis   Baltimore   Boston   Carlsbad   Chicago   Minneapolis   New York   Philadelphia   Portland
London   Milan   Sydney   Tokyo   Toronto

Mosby

Dedicated to Publishing Excellence

A Times Mirror
Company

Senior Editor: Loren S. Wilson
Editorial Assistant: Laura Nettler
Project Manager: Patricia Tannian
Project Specialist: Ann E. Rogers
Book Design Manager: Gail Morey Hudson
Manufacturing Manager: Don Carlisle
Cover Design: Teresa Breckwoldt

SECOND EDITION

Printed in the United States of America

Composition by The Clarinda Company
Printing/binding by Maple-Vail Book Mfg. Group

Mosby, Inc.
11830 Westline Industrial Drive
St. Louis, Missouri 63146

International Standard Book Number
0-3230-0151-3

98 99 00 01 02 / 9 8 7 6 5 4 3 2 1

Contributors

ASSOCIATE EDITOR

Mary Jo Candido, MS, RN
Coordinator
Northern New Jersey Robert J. Kennedy Stroke Association
Kessler Medical Rehabilitation Research and Education
Corporation
West Orange, New Jersey

Former Adjunct Instructor
Union County College of Nursing
Elizabeth, New Jersey

CONTRIBUTORS

Kim Inman Smith, BSN, MA, MSN
Instructor, Shelton State Community College
Tuscaloosa, Alabama

Lajuana B. Jordan, MSN, RN
Program Director, Danville Community College
Danville, Virginia

Mary C. Kishman, MSN, RN
Night Nursing Supervisor, Shriners Burns Institute
Cincinnati, Ohio

Sharon Powell-Laney, RN, MSN
Coordinator, Indian County Area Vocational Technical School
Indiana, Pennsylvania

Cheryl Pratt, MSN, BSN
Instructor, South Central Technical College
North Mankato, Minnesota

Kay Swartzwelder, RN, BSN, CNOR
Instructor
South Point, Ohio

REVIEWER PANEL

Lois Harrion, RN, BA, MS
Ernestine M. Johnson, ASN, BSN, MSA
Shirley Kallen, RNC, BS
Joann E. Peuterbaugh, MSN
Ann M. Porter, ADN, BSN
Sharon A. Roberts, ARNP, MS
Shirley Stamford, RN, BSN
Helene Thomas-Taylor, RN, BSN, CNOR

Preface

This newly revised review tool from Mosby was developed to help you prepare for the NCLEX-PN examination in the United States and the Practical Nurse/Nursing Assistant Registration/Licensure examination in Canada. Two thousand questions provide ample experience in answering questions. The broad scope of content covered enables you to evaluate your knowledge of nursing and your readiness for the NCLEX-PN. Answers with rationales promote understanding and help you learn from your mistakes.

The questions in this text were developed by experienced educators and practitioners. All questions follow the stand-alone, multiple-choice format used in the computerized NCLEX examination. The content covered by the questions was selected from the areas identified in the Test Plan for the NCLEX-PN.

Chapter 1 discusses the NCLEX examination—what it will test and how. Study techniques and test-taking tips are provided to help you make the best use of your time and abilities.

Chapters 2, 3, and 4 include 1350 questions covering medical/surgical, psychiatric/mental health, and maternal/child nursing. Questions in each of these chapters are grouped by subtopic to enable you to review and evaluate specific content areas.

Chapter 5 provides two comprehensive practice examinations (250 questions each) that reflect the scope of the NCLEX examination. Use these practice tests to evaluate your overall knowledge and to help you learn to pace yourself for the actual examination.

Chapters 6 and 7 include the answers and rationales for all of the questions, and they are tabbed for easy location and removal. Rationales explain why the correct answers are right and why each of the other options is wrong. Rationales also indicate the cognitive level, step of the nursing process, client needs category, and level of difficulty for each question. Use this information to determine your specific areas of strength and weakness.

A computer disk at the back of the book contains 150 additional questions that provide experience with computerized testing.

This text is a logical companion to *Mosby's PN AssessTest* and *Mosby's Comprehensive Review of Practical Nursing*. These three components make up a complete review and study package for any student preparing for the NCLEX-PN.

I would like to take this opportunity to thank my colleagues for their efforts, which have culminated in the development of this text. My appreciation also extends to the professionals who have served on the editorial review panel. In addition, I would like to thank those at Mosby for assisting in the development of this review book, especially Susan Epstein, Loren Wilson, Laura Nettler, Ann Rogers, and Gail Hudson. And of course, thanks and gratitude to Mary Jo Candido, Associate Editor, and to my family, especially my husband Robert, all of whom have been extremely supportive throughout the duration of this entire project.

To all who are about to become LP/VNs, our best wishes for a successful examination and a rewarding career.

Mary Eyles

Contents

3 Maternal-Child Health Nursing Review Questions, 57

6 Answers and Rationales for Review Questions, 148

7 Answers and Rationales for Comprehensive Examinations, 243

Mosby's
QUESTIONS &
ANSWERS for
NCLEX-PN

CHAPTER 1

Preparing for the NCLEX-PN Examination

> *The practice of nursing is regulated by law for the principal purpose of public protection. The respective State Boards of Nursing are charged with the responsibility of upholding the regulation of such law. The National Council Licensure Examination for Practical Nurses (NCLEX-PN) covers all areas of the practical/vocational nursing curriculum and has been further designed to test nursing knowledge, including the ability to apply principles of that knowledge to individual clinical situations in a safe and effective manner.*

NCLEX-PN

THE NCLEX-PN was developed by the National Council of State Boards of Nursing (NCSBN). The examination is based on a test plan that is designed to evaluate entry-level performance while incorporating the nursing process and identified patient needs. As stated in the actual test plan, "the Practical Nurse Test Plan is distinguished from the Registered Nurse Test Plan by the scope of practice as defined by member jurisdictions, by the practical nurse job analyses, and by the tested levels of cognitive abilities."

In April 1994 the National Council began administering the NCLEX-PN examination via computerized adaptive testing (CAT), a change from the traditional paper-and-pencil method of testing. The number of questions per individual will vary on the CAT and will be based on the candidate's performance, which measures knowledge, skills, and abilities. All successful candidates will answer no fewer than 75 questions and a maximum of approximately 195 questions within a 5-hour time frame. Rest periods (one mandatory after the first 2 hours of testing and one optional following the next 90 minutes of testing) and a computer tutorial are included within the 5-hour testing session. Tests are scored to determine the number of correct answers (raw score). The raw score is then measured against the set standard, which is the minimum score set to guarantee that the test taker is competent in the nursing knowledge and skills being tested. Scores reflect the "pass" or "fail" status of the candidate, with the majority of the boards using the same pass/fail score as determined by the Angoff method, a criterion-referenced, standard-setting technique commonly used by the NCSBN.

A candidate who fails the examination will receive a diagnostic profile that will assist in focusing further study efforts for retaking the examination.

The examination has been developed with the basic knowledge necessary for the practice of practical/vocational nursing and contains test items reflecting the cognitive levels of knowledge, comprehension, and application.

The two major components of the test plan are (1) the phases of the nursing process and (2) patient needs.* Keep in mind that the elements of accountability, nutrition, anatomy and physiology, growth and development, documentation, communication, fundamentals, and patient education are found throughout the examination.

The percentage of test items on the examination relative to the *phases of the nursing process* as set forth in the test plan are as follows:*

1. Data Collection (assessment) 27-33%: The collection of data in patients with predictable outcomes, which contributes to a database and assists in the formulation of a nursing diagnosis.
   - Gathers information relative to the patient from various sources—patient, family members, records, other team members
   - Communicates information relative to the patient through accurate documentation and reporting
   - Contributes to the formulation of nursing diagnoses by assisting with the organization and determination of significant relationships between collected data and identified patient needs and/or problems
2. Planning 17-23%: Participates in setting goals, both short term and long term for meeting patient needs and ways in which to best achieve those goals.
   - Contributes to the development of nursing interventions necessary to achieve set goals
   - Communicates patient needs that may indicate an alteration of goals
   - Assists in developing the plan of care in cooperation with the patient and other health care team members
   - Participates in the development of a plan of care that provides for patient safety and comfort while ensuring maintenance of optimal functioning
3. Implementation 27-33%: Initiate and complete nursing actions necessary to accomplish set goals by performing ba-

---

*Adapted from NCLEX-PN Test Plan for National Council Licensure Examination for Practical Nurses, 1995.

sic therapeutic and preventative nursing measures in a safe and effective care environment.
- Carry out the established plan of care
- Participate in patient care conferences
- Prepare patients for procedures
- Observe for and initiate appropriate nursing interventions to compensate for adverse responses to care and/or treatment
- Initiate life-saving interventions when appropriate in emergency situations
- Involve the patient in care, taking into consideration needs and preferences
- Reinforce patient teaching relative to the diagnosis and treatment regimen for maintenance and promotion of health
- Monitor care given to patients by unlicensed nursing personnel
- Document all information accurately relative to patient responses to implementation of care, and report same to other members of the health care team

4. Evaluation 17-23%: Participates in determining the extent to which goals have been achieved and interventions have been successful.
- Participates in evaluating effectiveness of nursing interventions
- Assists in evaluating patient response to nursing care
- Assists in identifying factors that may interfere with the patient's ability to fully comply with the plan of care
- Assists in determining the extent to which planned outcomes have been achieved
- Documents where appropriate and reports to other members of the health care team the patient's response to care, therapy, and/or teaching

Percentage of items on the examination relative to *patient needs* as set forth in the test plan are as follows:

1. Safe, Effective Care Environment 16-22%: Includes coordinated care, environmental safety, and safe and effective treatments and procedures. Examples of the *essential* knowledge, skills, and abilities for this category of patient needs are as follows:
   - Advance directives, Communication skills, Confidentiality, Continuity of care, Environment and personal safety, Expected outcomes of various treatments, General and specific protective interventions, Informed consent, Knowledge and use of equipment used to provide nursing care, Legal accountability, Quality assurance, Patient rights, and Team participation

2. Physiologic Integrity 49-55%: Includes physiologic adaptation, reduction of risk potential, and provision of basic care. Examples of the *essential* knowledge, skills, and abilities for this category of patient needs are as follows:
   - Activities of daily living, Basic pathophysiology, Body mechanics, Comfort interventions, Effects of immobility, Emergency interventions, Expected response to therapies, Fluid balance, Invasive procedures, Medication administration, Normal body structure and function, Nutritional therapies, Pharmacologic actions, Skin and wound care, and Use of special equipment

3. Psychosocial Integrity 8-14%: Includes psychosocial adaptation and coping and/or adaptation skills. Examples of the

essential knowledge, skills, and abilities for this category of patient needs are as follows:
   - Behavior norms; Chemical dependency; Common treatment modalities; Cultural, religious, and spiritual influences on health; Mental health concepts; and Therapeutic communication

4. Health Promotion and Maintenance 15-21%: Includes growth and development through the life span, self-care and support systems, and prevention and early treatment of disease. Examples of the *essential* knowledge, skills and abilities for this category of patient needs are as follows:
   - Community resources, Concepts of wellness, Death and dying, Disease prevention, Growth and development through the life span, Human sexuality, Parenting, Principles of immunity, and Teaching appropriate to the scope of practice.

Please note that the NCLEX-PN examination contains several test items that are being validated for use in future NCLEX-PN examinations. These questions are not identifiable, and whether answered correctly or not, the test taker neither gains nor loses points.

REVIEW AND PREPARATION FOR NCLEX-PN

The key to effective review and preparation for the examination lies solely with YOU and the goals you have set for yourself. Review is necessary in order to become familiar with the extent of your nursing knowledge, allowing you to identify your areas of strength as well as those areas in which you need additional study. Review texts, such as *Mosby's Comprehensive Review of Practical Nursing* and *Mosby's PN Assess Test,* will give you the added benefit of increasing your familiarity with and ability to respond to test questions similar to those presented in the NCLEX-PN examination.

How, what, when, and where you study are entirely up to you; however, being practical and using common sense are vital to the study process. The following suggestions will be helpful to you when devising a study plan that is right for *you:*
- Begin with a *positive attitude!*
- Establish the priority of the study plan as a means of accomplishing the ultimate goal—passing the NCLEX-PN examination.
- Develop a realistic study-time schedule that is somewhat flexible to accommodate what needs to be done within the time available; follow the schedule as closely as possible, revising the schedule if necessary; pinpoint a study time that is convenient for you rather than for someone else; specify the amount of time you will need for study; be prepared for the unexpected; and provide for free time in the overall schedule.
- Improve your organizational ability by developing a checklist for the study plan and schedule you have designed for yourself.
- Improve your ability to remember through repetition, visualization, associating facts and concepts with use of the senses (touch, smell, hearing), and creating a cue system that will serve to jog your memory on more difficult or complicated concepts.
- Choose a quiet study environment where the possibility of interruptions will be minimal or eliminated completely.

- Plan to study in an upright position by sitting in a chair at a desk or a table; refrain from using a comfortable overstuffed chair or studying in bed.
- Include a few quick stretch breaks in each block of study time.

What and how to study must be included in the study plan. Most nursing professionals would agree that whether you decide to study by yourself, with a friend, or as part of a group, you will need to allow a solid 6 to 8 weeks or more of study prior to sitting for NCLEX-PN. Cramming is *not* recommended. You may also wish to consider taking a review course that provides for more study structure and in most cases incorporates a review book such as *Mosby's Comprehensive Review of Practical Nursing.* Use of a review text is recommended because the most important and vital areas of the practical/vocational nursing curriculum are usually presented in an outline format that allows for a much quicker yet thorough review of the topic. Also included are questions and comprehensive examinations similar to NCLEX-PN. The review text thus increases students' familiarity and self-confidence with multiple-choice questions and the format of NCLEX-PN.

Review of material and exposure to questions relevant to that material provide a means to identify strengths and weaknesses, thus allowing for quality study time on weaker areas of comprehension. Once weaker areas have been identified, it may be necessary to refer to nursing school texts, handouts, class notes, or nursing journals for further study in those particular areas of content.

Whichever way you decide to study, do not simply read through the material looking only for facts and hoping you will be able to recall what you've read. It will be necessary to think in-depth as you read, looking for main and associated ideas. Review what you've read, repeating important information in the context of larger ideas as a means of retaining what you've just learned.

This text contains two examinations, each having two parts. Each part contains 125 questions, with a recommended completion time of 2 hours. Although time may no longer be a major concern during the actual examination, which in a way decreases the anxiety of taking a timed test, becoming more proficient in time-management skills will only be to your advantage during the actual examination. In addition, this text also comes with a computer disk containing 125 questions similar to those on NCLEX-PN, which will facilitate and enhance your ability, as well as comfort, with a computerized testing format.

TEST-TAKING SKILLS: STRATEGIES FOR SUCCESS

No matter how many tests you have taken, preparation for a licensing examination creates a bit more anxiety than usual. Being prepared and becoming more comfortable and familiar with the testing format will help decrease your anxiety level. A certain amount of anxiety will always be present, however, serving to sharpen your senses and make you more alert to the realities of the testing procedure and content.

While in school, you were most likely exposed to several methods of testing. The NCLEX-PN examination deals only with the objective method and more specifically with the objective multiple-choice form of testing. Each question contains a stem (the main intent of the question), followed by four possible options/answers that either complete a statement or answer the question presented. Only *one* of the four choices is the best or most appropriate answer; the remaining three options are known as *distractors,* so named because they are written in such a way that they *could* be correct and so distract you to a certain degree. Knowing that your nursing knowledge is being subtly tested, your strength in that knowledge will lead you to the correct response.

Although this form of testing may be familiar to you, consider the following in an attempt to avoid some of the more common test-taking errors:

- **Answer the question that is being asked.** To do so you need to *read,* not scan, the situation and the question carefully, looking for key words or phrases. Do not read anything into the question or apply what you did in a similar situation during one of your clinical experiences. Instead, think about what the question is *really* asking. Reflect back on your nursing knowledge, asking yourself how you would handle the situation in an ideal setting. Then choose what you feel to be the *best* or *most appropriate* response.
- **Identify key words or phrases.** Key words or phrases in the stem of the question, such as *first, only, primary, early, best,* or *most appropriate* are essential when determining the intent of the question. Words such as *only, always, never,* and *all* in the options will frequently be evidence of an incorrect response. There are no absolutes in nursing, as there are none in life. Of course, there are exceptions to every rule, so answer with care.
- **Identify option parts (components) as being correct or incorrect.** If for instance each option contained three supposed side effects of a given drug, you would be wise to consider each side effect individually as being correct or not for the drug in question. If even one of the three in any given option is incorrect, then the option itself is not the correct answer.
- **Identify and eliminate options that you know are definitely incorrect.** By doing so you will have increased your chances of selecting the correct answer, in addition to having more time to focus on the true nature of the question.
- **Identify options that are similar in nature.** If three of the options all share a direct relationship to one another, then the fourth option (not necessarily in that order) will most likely be the correct answer, as it is this option that will either include the other three or totally exclude them from the situation. If neither is the case, then the question is not written properly.
- **Identify words in options that are identical, similar in nature, or closely related to those in the stem.** Such similarities can provide clues to the correct response.
- **Be alert to grammatical inconsistencies.** If the response, which is intended to complete the stem (presented as an incomplete sentence), makes no grammatical sense, it can be considered to be a distractor rather than the correct answer. Likewise, if the stem phrase indicates a singular in the response and several of the options provide responses that are plural, one can safely eliminate those as the correct answer.

- **Answering questions.** You have at least a 25% chance of selecting the correct answer. Wild guesses should be avoided at all costs. Should you feel insecure about a question, try to eliminate the options you feel are definitely incorrect by calling on your nursing knowledge and one or more of the methods listed. This will increase your chances of making an educated guess at the correct answer. *Remember,* although there is no penalty for guessing on the examination, the subsequent question will, to an extent, be based on the response to a given question. That is, if you answer incorrectly, the computer will formulate the next question accordingly based on your knowledge/skill performance on the examination up to that point.

- **At times, the correct answer may be the longest option given.** Although the longest answer option may be correct in some cases, don't consider it foolproof. Test developers are very much aware of this technique and may include wordy options that are incorrect as a way of testing your knowledge. In most cases, test developers take great care in making all options the same length.

- **Avoid looking for an answer pattern or code.** Often four or five consecutive questions will have the same letter or number for the correct answer.

- **Have confidence in your initial response.** It will probably be the correct answer. Serious consideration should be given before recording a response, because once a response has been entered, another question will appear on the screen. On the CAT test, skipping questions or going back to review and/or change responses is not possible.

- **Budget your time wisely.** Remember, although time is not a factor, don't spend too much time on any one question. One minute is the recommended time that should be allotted to a single question. Not all questions will consume a full minute; some may take only 15 or 20 seconds to read and answer.

- **Answer those questions that you know first.** *During practice study sessions* in which the more traditional paper-and-pencil method of testing is used, it is recommended that you answer those questions that you know first, returning to the more difficult questions at a later time, as this is an excellent way to build confidence in preparation for the actual examination. As already noted, skipping and/or returning to change a response is not possible on the CAT test.

The night before the examination you may wish to review some material; but then relax and get a good night's sleep. Make sure to set your alarm or arrange to have someone call you. In the morning allow yourself plenty of time to dress, have breakfast, and arrive at the testing site at least 15 to 30 minutes before the start of the test. Be sure you know where to park and where the test will be given (room location). In addition, remember to take eyeglasses (if needed), your admission card, and a second form of identification. Once seated in the testing center, listen to the examiner carefully. All candidates will be given a short training session that includes a keyboard tutorial complete with a practice session. No prior computer experience is necessary. Failure to listen to the directions thoroughly may lead to an error that could cost considerable points. Should you have any question about these instructions, ask the examiner for further explanations. By doing so, you will be able to control your stress level and proceed confidently.

One final note: no two candidates will be given the same questions to answer, because the examination is individualized according to the candidate's knowledge and skills while meeting test plan requirements.

Above all, approach the examination with a *positive attitude* about yourself, your nursing knowledge, and your test-taking abilities.

CHAPTER 2

Medical-Surgical Nursing Review Questions

1. A patient with rheumatoid arthritis is seen in the clinic. The nurse knows that her assessment of the patient will most likely reveal the following:
   ① Pain more severe in the late evening, less severe in the morning
   ② Low-grade fever only during the night
   ③ Pain and stiffness more severe in the morning
   ④ Constant bone pain, with a history of fractures

2. For the most effective decrease in pain and stiffness, the nurse will instruct the patient with rheumatoid arthritis to:
   ① Take a cool bath or shower on rising in the morning
   ② Actively exercise all joints using weights
   ③ Take aspirin 20 minutes before rising in the morning
   ④ Perform aerobic exercises for 30 minutes three times a week

3. To prevent flexion deformities in a patient with rheumatoid arthritis, the nurse should include which of the following positions in the turning schedule?
   ① High Fowler's
   ② Prone
   ③ Sims'
   ④ Trendelenburg's

4. The nurse who is caring for a patient with increasing disability due to rheumatoid arthritis will:
   ① Provide complete bed rest with range of motion exercises
   ② Limit the patient's activities
   ③ Keep the patient's joints immobilized
   ④ Prevent contractures and maintain range of motion in all the joints

5. To relieve pain and inflammation in a patient with rheumatoid arthritis, the nurse will administer an antiinflammatory agent:
   ① Between meals
   ② With meals
   ③ At bedtime
   ④ On a limited basis

6. The nurse knows that rheumatoid arthritis differs from osteoarthritis because it is characterized by:
   ① Degeneration of the joint
   ② Chronic inflammatory reaction in the synovial membrane
   ③ Porous and brittle bones
   ④ Inflammation of the bone

7. Rehabilitation for a patient with rheumatoid arthritis is directed toward:
   ① Bed rest
   ② Feeding her meals
   ③ Total care
   ④ Adaptation to physical limitations

8. A patient tells the nurse that she has heard of a new cure for her condition, rheumatoid arthritis, and is seeking information on it. The nurse's response should be:
   ① "That's great! You should be happy that this is really happening."
   ② "You should talk to your physician about this."
   ③ "Tell me about it, and we can let your physician know."
   ④ "You have to be careful about these cures. They are just a lot of empty promises that are quite costly."

9. When planning nursing care for a patient with gout, the nurse remembers that the pathologic cause of gout is:
   ① The body's inability to metabolize purines
   ② The body's inability to produce insulin
   ③ Inflammation in a joint
   ④ Inflammation of the large intestine

10. When assessing a patient with a diagnosis of gouty arthritis, the nurse is aware that the most common subjective complaint is:
    ① Limited range of motion of all joints
    ② Sweating of hands and feet
    ③ Acute pain in the great toe
    ④ Morning stiffness

11. When teaching dietary restrictions to a patient with gout, the nurse will tell the patient to avoid:
    ① Cheese, milk, and dairy products
    ② Marbled hamburger, lean steaks, and pork
    ③ Potatoes, breads, and sugar
    ④ Liver, kidney, and sardines

12. For a patient with gout, which of the following drugs would most likely be on the drug profile?
    ① Allopurinol
    ② Corticosteroids
    ③ Acetaminophen
    ④ Estrogen replacement

13. The signs and symptoms the nurse would most expect during the initial assessment of a patient with a herniated disc at L5-S1 is:
    ① Acute pain in the lower back, pain radiating across the buttock, and sciatic leg pain
    ② Pain aggravated by motion, edema, and crepitus
    ③ Subjective pain, limited motion, and localized swelling
    ④ Bone pain, progressive weakness, and anemia

14. The nurse knows that the tests that will be done to confirm an initial diagnosis of a herniated intervertebral disk at L5-S1 are:
    ① Health history, blood chemistries, and x-ray examination
    ② Computed tomography, magnetic resonance imaging, and physical examination
    ③ Bone scan, x-ray examination, and bone biopsy
    ④ Bone scan, arthroscopy, and x-ray examination

15. The nurse will explain to the patient who is scheduled for a laminectomy that the surgical procedure involves:
    ① Removing only the extruding disk material
    ② Usually fusing several disks together to stabilize the spine
    ③ Removing the arch of the vertebrae and then removing the disk
    ④ Guiding a needle into the nucleus pulposus to inject chymopapain, performed using a local anesthetic

16. The nurse knows that postoperative laminectomy care involves:
    ① Maintaining bed rest, providing complete care, anticipating needs by leaving the call bell within reach, and establishing means of communication
    ② Frequent observation of respiratory and neurologic functioning, maintaining spinal alignment at all times, and instituting active and passive range-of-motion exercises as soon as prescribed
    ③ Not turning the patient on the side, observing for signs of hemorrhage, observing for swelling, notifying the physician if necessary, and administering analgesics judiciously
    ④ Assessing the incision for signs of infection, monitoring intake and output, encouraging sitting in a straight-back chair for a limited period, and monitoring for respiratory distress

17. Upon discharge, the nurse will instruct the patient who has had a lamenectomy:
    ① Not to drive until permitted by the surgeon, to avoid twisting motions of the trunk, and not to lift anything weighing more than 5 lb
    ② To practice environmental safety, including use of grab bars in the bathroom, rubber mats in the shower or tub, and a side rail on the bed
    ③ To carefully monitor intake and output, to wear thigh-high antiembolism stockings, and to do isometric exercises
    ④ To eat only a soft diet, to work toward independence in hygiene and dressing, and to exercise daily as tolerated

18. Which of the following factors places a person at higher risk for the development of osteoporosis?
    ① Male gender
    ② Hispanic origin
    ③ African-American heritage
    ④ Caucasian heritage

19. The nurse explains to the patient that osteoporosis is caused by:
    ① Having small bones
    ② Increased estrogen levels
    ③ A loss of bone density
    ④ Taking 1600 mg of calcium daily

20. The patient is admitted to the hospital with acute low back pain. She is scheduled for a myelogram in the morning. The nurse knows that the first intervention(s) in the management of pain relief may be:
    ① Administer the prn narcotic analgesia
    ② Provide a back massage in a dimly lit room with soft music playing
    ③ Tell the patient to "hold on" until morning, as the pain should be gone after the procedure
    ④ Have her ambulate as soon as possible to relieve the back pressure from lying in the bed

21. While working at a construction site the patient experienced severe back pain and numbness down his left leg. He asks the nurse's advice on what he could do to eliminate the pain. The nurse will make the following suggestion:
    ① Bed rest for 48 to 72 hours
    ② Apply ice packs to the area for the next 2 days
    ③ Call the doctor or go to the emergency room
    ④ Apply a heating pad to the area for 72 hours

22. Which position is most tolerable for low back pain?
    ① Supine with knees elevated
    ② Prone with feet elevated
    ③ Sims' with left knee flexed
    ④ Lithotomy with knees elevated

23. The patient who has fractured her right hip has been placed in Buck's traction with 10 pounds of weight until she can be prepared for surgery. The nurse checks and documents neurovascular status:
    ① Once a day
    ② Once per shift
    ③ Every 4 hours
    ④ Every 15 minutes

24. The patient has returned from surgery for a left total hip arthroplasty. The blood supply to the head of his femur was interrupted in a car accident. The nurse monitors his vital signs frequently immediately postoperatively because:
    ① Osteomyelitis may occur
    ② Rejection of the new hip joint may occur
    ③ Patients who have hip replacements get confused
    ④ Hypovolemic shock is common with this surgery

25. The nurse observes which of the following precautions to prevent dislocating the new prosthesis of a patient who has had a replacement of the left hip?
    ① Instruct the patient to cross her legs only at the ankles
    ② Turn the patient every 2 hours
    ③ Elevate the head of the bed only to 60 degrees
    ④ Place an abductor pillow between the patient's legs

26. Identify the best site for administration of heparin to a patient who has fractured both femurs.
    ① Deltoid muscle
    ② Gluteus medius muscle
    ③ Abdomen within 2 inches of the umbilicus
    ④ Abdomen except within 2 inches of the umbilicus

27. The patient has come to the doctor's office for a check-up after treatment for temporomandibular joint (TMJ) syndrome. Which of the following statements would make the nurse believe more teaching is necessary?
    ① "I try to avoid grinding my teeth at night."
    ② "I've considered getting braces."
    ③ "I have been limiting exercise."
    ④ "I have tried several stress relievers."

28. The nurse that is caring for a patient with a fracture of the tibia knows that the tibia is:
    ① The main weight-bearing bone of the leg
    ② Located at the upper aspect of the leg
    ③ Surrounded by little muscular tissue
    ④ Connected to the lateral malleolus

29. The nurse knows that the diagnosis on x-ray of a complete fracture of the tibia means:
    ① It is a torsion fracture
    ② The bone is splintered into three or more fragments
    ③ It is a telescoped fracture
    ④ The fracture line extends entirely through the bone

30. A patient who recently suffered a fractured leg during a skiing accident asks the nurse if he will be able to ski again. The nurse's most appropriate response is:
    ① "Of course. You'll be on skis again in no time!"
    ② "A fractured bone never heals completely, and it leaves the bone weak. You should hang up your skis."
    ③ "It is a bit early to determine this, but it usually doesn't affect future skiing. What kinds of concerns do you have?"
    ④ "You should ask your physician when he comes in."

31. When caring for a patient in a full leg cast, the nurse's main goal is:
    ① Application of support to prevent further injury
    ② Immobilization of the leg to promote healing
    ③ Ensuring comfort and pain relief
    ④ Prevention of hemorrhage and shock

32. When placing a patient with a full leg cast on a bedpan, the nurse should:
    ① Support the cast with pillows
    ② Protect the edge of the cast with plastic
    ③ Elevate the head of the bed
    ④ Ask the patient to lift himself

33. To clean debris and drainage from an open wound, the nurse would:
    ① Use a sterile 4 × 4 pad, move from the outer edge of the wound to the center
    ② Use a sterile 4 × 4 pad, move from the center of the wound outward
    ③ Use a sterile 4 × 4 pad, move from the center of the wound outward in a circular motion
    ④ Use a new sterile 4 × 4 pad for each area cleaned, move from the center of the wound outward

34. The main consideration of the nurse when doing wound care is:
    ① Preparing supplies
    ② Checking drainage tubes
    ③ Giving attention to the patient's needs
    ④ Reducing the transfer of microorganisms

35. The nurse is to apply a roller bandage to a patient's arm. The arm should be wrapped starting at:
    ① The wrist, wrapping toward the hand
    ② The wrist, wrapping toward the elbow
    ③ The elbow, wrapping toward the wrist
    ④ The fingers, wrapping toward the wrist

36. To prevent complications during the first 24 hours after application of a cast, the nurse knows that the casted area should be assessed:
    ① Every 15 minutes
    ② Every hour
    ③ Every 3 hours
    ④ Every 4 hours

37. The nurse prepares to petal a patient's cast. The primary purpose of petaling a cast is to help prevent:
    ① The cast from becoming wet
    ② The cast from becoming too tight
    ③ Debris from getting under the cast
    ④ The cast from irritating the patient's skin

38. Surgical reduction of the fracture and insertion of an Austin-Moore prosthesis is done. In planning nursing care for the patient, it is important that the leg with the hip prosthesis be kept slightly:
    ① Abducted
    ② Adducted
    ③ Flexed
    ④ Prone

39. When turning a patient with a hip prosthesis, the nurse will:
    ① Place the patient on the affected side
    ② Place the patient on the unaffected side
    ③ Maintain the patient's head at a 90-degree angle
    ④ Maintain the patient's head at a 45-degree angle

40. To plan postoperative nursing care for a patient with a hip prosthesis, the nurse knows that the patient:
    ① Will be getting up the next day after surgery
    ② Is not allowed to have full weight bearing until 3 days after surgery
    ③ Will be allowed partial weight bearing in 7 to 10 days and can use crutches in 3 to 6 months
    ④ Will be allowed partial weight bearing in 10 to 14 days and full weight bearing in about 4 weeks

41. A patient with a hip prosthesis has become depressed and says, "I'm never going to walk right again, am I?" The nurse's best response will be:
    ① "What makes you think you will never walk right again?"
    ② "Of course you will, it is just going to take time!"
    ③ "You will be up and walking before you know it."
    ④ "Why don't we see if there is something good on television?"

42. A patient is admitted to the floor preoperatively for preparations for a below-the-knee amputation (BKA) to be done in the morning. Which of the following would be the most appropriate nursing diagnosis?
    ① Disturbance in self-esteem
    ② Impaired skin integrity
    ③ Altered tissue perfusion
    ④ Disturbance in body image

43. Following surgery for a below-the-knee amputation, the patient tells the nurse, "It hurts so much." Before administering medication for pain relief, the nurse will make which initial assessment?
    ① Where is his discomfort?
    ② Does he have a pulse deficit?
    ③ Is his urine output adequate?
    ④ Does he have active bowel sounds?

44. A patient with a below-the-knee amputation has a compression bandage applied. The compression bandage would be achieving the desired effect on the residual limb if which of these observations were made by the nurse?
    ① The incision is well approximated
    ② The wound is free of drainage
    ③ There is no evidence of edema
    ④ The skin edges are pink

45. Following his below-the-knee amputation, the patient received instructions about care of the residual limb. Which of these comments by the patient indicates the need for further teaching?
    ① "I'll rub my residual limb with alcohol twice a day."
    ② "I'll press my residual limb against a pillow when the wound is healed."
    ③ "I'll bathe my residual limb with soap and water every day."
    ④ "I'll be sure to exercise the joints above and below my residual limb every day."

46. A patient with a below-the-knee amputation is being taught to walk with crutches. Which basic principle of crutch walking should the nurse emphasize for this patient?
    ① When ascending stairs, the crutch and the residual limb should go up first
    ② The major part of the body weight is maintained by the patient's axilla
    ③ The patient should continually check his foot position when walking with crutches
    ④ Before starting to walk, the patient begins the gait in the tripod position

47. A patient with severe arteriosclerosis is scheduled for a left midthigh amputation. Preoperative teaching should include making the patient aware:
    ① Of the adjustment period needed when using an artificial limb
    ② Of the need to turn frequently
    ③ That he will not experience phantom limb pain
    ④ Of the need to lie on his back without too much movement

48. Preoperative care for a patient scheduled in surgery for a left midthigh amputation should include:
    ① Elevation of the affected leg to decrease the need for blood to circulate to the area
    ② Repeated blood work to determine the amount of blood flow to the lower extremity
    ③ Bed rest to decrease movement of the affected leg
    ④ Palpation of bilateral pedal pulses

49. In caring for a patient immediately following a left midthigh amputation and for the first 48 hours following surgery, the nurse should:
    ① Keep the residual limb lowered in the bed to promote circulation to the operative site
    ② Elevate the residual limb on pillows
    ③ Observe for signs of bleeding under the dressing
    ④ Place bed boards under the mattress for firm support under the residual limb

50. The most common postoperative complication that the nurse should watch for following a midthigh amputation is:
    ① Contractions of hip flexors and abductor muscles
    ② Hemorrhage at the operative site
    ③ Infection at the operative site
    ④ Embolism caused by decreased mobility

51. Following a midthigh amputation, application of elastic wraps to the residual limb is necessary primarily to:
    ① Decrease the chance of hemorrhage at the operative site
    ② Shrink and reshape the residual limb
    ③ Decrease the chance of edema at the operative site
    ④ Decrease the chance of infection at the operative site

52. The immediate action of the nurse for a patient with profuse epistaxis would be to:
    ① Obtain the patient's medical history and available insurance
    ② Decrease the patient's level of anxiety, if present
    ③ Apply pressure on the bridge of the nose
    ④ Assess the patient's vital signs every 15 minutes

53. When caring for a patient with an epistaxis, the nurse should place the patient in:
    ① Supine position with the head tilted backward
    ② Supine position with the head leaning forward
    ③ Fowler's position with the head leaning forward
    ④ Fowler's position with the head tilted backward

54. A total laryngectomy and radical neck dissection is planned for a patient with cancer of the larynx. The patient asks the nurse about the effect the surgery will have on his breathing. The nurse's response is based on the fact that the patient will breathe through:
    ① His nose
    ② His mouth
    ③ A temporary tracheostomy
    ④ A permanent tracheostomy

55. When suctioning secretions of a patient with a tracheostomy, the nurse will turn off the suction as the catheter is inserted to prevent:
    ① Irritation of the lining of the trachea and loss of additional oxygen
    ② Blocking of the catheter with mucus
    ③ Infection of the oral cavity
    ④ "Kinking" of the catheter

56. Following a total laryngectomy, which of the following findings during the nurse's assessment indicates a need to suction the patient's laryngectomy tube?
    ① Decreased pulse and decreased respiratory rate
    ② Moisture on the neck dressing and increased swallowing
    ③ Increasing respirations and use of accessory muscles
    ④ Chest pain and a dry, hacking cough

57. Nursing actions during suctioning of a laryngectomy tube would include:
    ① Continuous suctioning while withdrawing the catheter
    ② Suctioning limited to no more than 10 seconds
    ③ Applying suction while inserting the catheter
    ④ Positioning the patient supine

58. When a patient is first admitted to the postanesthesia unit (recovery room) following a laryngectomy, the patient should be positioned:
    ① In a supine position
    ② In a side-lying position
    ③ With the head down
    ④ In a sitting position

59. As part of discharge planning for the patient who has a total laryngectomy, the nurse would include teaching about which of the following daily activities that would require modification?
    ① Bathing
    ② Walking
    ③ Sleeping
    ④ Exercising

60. The patient has been diagnosed with chronic obstructive pulmonary disease (COPD) and is a long-time smoker. The nurse will expect the patient's primary symptoms to be:
    ① Joint pain, peripheral edema, and cough
    ② Dyspnea and heart irregularities
    ③ Shortness of breath and dyspnea on exertion
    ④ Heart irregularities and cyanosis

61. The patient is admitted with chronic obstructive pulmonary disease (COPD). She is experiencing dyspnea and has cyanotic nail beds. Which of the following nursing actions are most important initially?
    ① Apply oxygen at 6-8 liters/min
    ② Give narcotics as ordered
    ③ Raise the head of the bed 20 degrees
    ④ Apply oxygen at 2 liters/min

62. Chest pain is a common symptom in a patient with pneumonia, usually occurring on the affected side. When it does occur, the nurse should encourage the patient to:
    ① Breathe deeply to relieve the pain
    ② Lie on the affected side to cough
    ③ Cough frequently
    ④ Lie on the unaffected side to cough

63. The main purpose of forcing fluids by mouth in an elderly patient with pneumonia is to:
    ① Help rid the body of waste products
    ② Maintain proper nutrition
    ③ Dilute the toxins in the body
    ④ Lower the body temperature

64. Which of the following diagnostic tests will be ordered to determine the causative agent in a patient with pneumonia?
    ① X-ray examination
    ② Gastric lavage
    ③ Blood and sputum tests
    ④ Bronchoscopy

65. When evaluating the response of a patient with pneumonia to the administration of acetaminophen (Tylenol), the nurse is aware that acetaminophen is used specifically to aid in:
    ① Kidney function
    ② Sputum reduction
    ③ Fever reduction
    ④ Fluid retention

66. In the assessment of a patient with pneumonia, the nurse will know that oxygen shortage is occurring by all of the following except:
    ① Cyanosis
    ② Dyspnea
    ③ Increased respiratory rate
    ④ Decreased pulse rate

67. Which of the following signs and symptoms would the nurse expect to find in a patient with spontaneous right pneumothorax?
    ① Breathing that is not symmetric
    ② Harsh productive cough
    ③ Pain that is increased by sitting up
    ④ Audible wheezing or rhonchi

68. A 30-year-old male comes to the clinic with sharp chest pain, difficulty breathing, and a dry, hacking cough. The doctor scheduled in the clinic for the day will not arrive for at least 2 more hours. Which of the following would be the best action by the nurse?
    ① Prepare the patient to be taken to the emergency room immediately
    ② Advise the patient to go home and rest
    ③ Make the patient comfortable and have him wait for the doctor
    ④ Order a chest x-ray and angiograms

69. Which of the following statements by a patient with a chest tube connected to an underwater drainage system indicates the patient's understanding of the system?
    ① "I'll empty the drainage container and record the results."
    ② "I'll lie on my right side while the drainage system is in place."
    ③ "I'll keep the drainage system below the level of my chest."
    ④ "I will remain in bed until the drainage system is removed."

70. While bathing a patient with a chest tube connected to an underwater-seal drainage system, the nurse observes that the chest tube has fallen out. Which of these actions should the nurse perform *first?*
    ① Seal off the wound
    ② Call the team leader
    ③ Prepare for CPR
    ④ Reinsert the tube

71. A patient with multiple knife wounds to the chest is diagnosed in the emergency room as having a sucking chest wound. This condition is also known as:
    ① Pneumothorax
    ② Pneumonia
    ③ Epistaxis
    ④ Hemothorax

72. Which of the following observations by the nurse would most likely indicate that a lung has been punctured?
    ① White, frothy sputum from the mouth
    ② Bright-red, frothy sputum from the mouth
    ③ Thick, purulent drainage from the mouth
    ④ Copious, dark red drainage from the mouth

73. When caring for a patient with an underwater-seal drainage system, the nurse knows that the chest tubes are inserted into the
    ① Thoracic cavity
    ② Punctured lung
    ③ Pleural space
    ④ Visceral space

74. In planning nursing care for a patient with underwater-seal drainage, the nurse should remember that the primary goal for using this procedure is to:
    ① Allow expansion of the affected lung by draining secretions and air by gravitation
    ② Restore the negative pressure within the thoracic cavity
    ③ Restore the atmospheric pressure within the thoracic cavity
    ④ Equalize the pressure within the thoracic cavity by allowing expansion of both lungs

75. When caring for a patient with an underwater-seal drainage system, the nurse must know that the bottle closest to the patient:
    ① Provides drainage of secretions by suction
    ② Provides drainage of secretions via gravity
    ③ Measures the patient's inspiration
    ④ Measures the patient's expiration

76. When caring for a patient with an underwater-seal drainage system, the nurse should make sure the system remains:
    ① Higher than the patient
    ② Lower than the patient
    ③ At the same level as the patient's chest
    ④ The level of the bottles is not important

77. The nurse's prime responsibility when caring for a patient with underwater-seal drainage is to:
    ① Keep the drainage system at eye level
    ② Monitor the patient's weight daily
    ③ Empty the drainage system every hour
    ④ Observe the patient and drainage system every hour

78. If a bottle in the underwater-seal drainage system breaks, which action should the nurse carry out *first?*
    ① Call for help
    ② Observe for respiratory distress
    ③ Raise the head of the bed and check vital signs
    ④ Clamp the chest tubes immediately

79. When assessing a patient for possible pneumothorax, the nurse is most likely to observe symptoms of:
    ① Shortness of breath and sharp pain on the affected side
    ② Sharp pain that is relieved by leaning forward
    ③ Increased breath sounds on the affected side
    ④ Absence of breath sounds on the unaffected side

80. When moving a patient with a chest tube from the stretcher to the bed, the *most* appropriate action is to:
    ① "Strip" the tube to enhance drainage
    ② Mark the time of measurement and the fluid level
    ③ Raise the bottle to chest height to check for air bubbles
    ④ Place the drainage system at the foot of the bed

81. The nurse assesses the water-seal chamber of the drainage system. Which finding indicates that the system is working effectively?
    ① No fluctuation is observed in the water-seal chamber
    ② Continuous and constant bubbling is noted in the water seal
    ③ Fluctuations are observed rising with inspirations and falling with expirations
    ④ The fluctuation of the fluid in the water-seal chamber increases during the first 24 hours

82. The physician is preparing to remove a chest tube. The nurse should instruct the patient to:
    ① Take several rapid, shallow breaths
    ② Inhale deeply and hold her breath
    ③ Perform a Valsalva's maneuver
    ④ Do pursed-lip breathing

83. The nurse would expect a patient with tuberculosis to report:
    ① Expectoration of thick, rust-colored sputum
    ② Consistent high fever
    ③ Development of dependent edema
    ④ Generalized skin rash

84. While collecting a sputum specimen for acid-fast bacillus testing, the nurse will instruct the patient to:
    ① Do abdominal breathing while coughing
    ② Cleanse her mouth with hydrogen peroxide before taking the specimen
    ③ Take a deep breath and cough from the diaphragm
    ④ Sit in semi-Fowler's position

85. A patient with tuberculosis is placed on isoniazid (INH) and pyrazinamide (Tebrazid). The nurse would expect the patient to have:
    ① Negative sputum tests in 1 week
    ② A return of energy in 2 to 3 days
    ③ Absence of a cough in 1 week
    ④ A normal temperature in 3 weeks

86. When teaching a patient with tuberculosis who is taking rifampin on an outpatient basis, the nurse should instruct her to:
    ① Double the next dose if a dose is missed
    ② Weigh herself once a week
    ③ Expect urine color to be dark orange
    ④ Decrease the dose if anorexia and nausea develop

87. A patient who is exhibiting signs and symptoms that suggest tuberculosis is given a Mantoux test. The nurse knows that a positive reading indicates that the patient has:
    1. Been exposed to the disease but does not necessarily have it
    2. An active case of TB
    3. No active case of TB at this time
    4. Been exposed to the disease and has it

88. When planning to collect sputum from a patient with tuberculosis, the nurse knows that sputum specimens must be obtained in the early morning because:
    1. It is easier for the night nurse to collect the specimen
    2. Coughing up sputum does not occur during the day hours
    3. An arbitrary assignment of time has been given
    4. Secretions pool overnight and are less likely to be contaminated

89. The nurse has identified that the primary patient teaching for a patient with tuberculosis would be:
    1. Strict isolation technique, avoiding family and friends
    2. Proper disposal and handwashing techniques related to coughing and sneezing
    3. Proper diet to gain weight
    4. Rest to regain his strength

90. The main pharmacologic treatment for tuberculosis (TB) includes isoniazid (INH) and *para*-aminosalicylate sodium (PAS). In planning care for a patient receiving these medications, the nurse is aware that they are used:
    1. To prevent the TB organisms from multiplying
    2. For 6 to 8 weeks
    3. To destroy the TB organisms
    4. For the rest of the patient's life

91. A patient with a diagnosis of tuberculosis (TB) asks the nurse the main purpose of drug therapy. The nurse's best response is that drug therapy is used:
    1. To cure him of the disease
    2. To prevent recurrence of the disease
    3. To arrest the disease
    4. To develop immunity to the TB organism

92. When performing a history and physical examination on a patient with tuberculosis, the nurse will expect the patient to have:
    1. Expiratory wheeze
    2. Confusion
    3. Night sweats
    4. Hemothorax

93. The nurse knows that the sputum test for AFB is done on a patient with tuberculosis to identify the causative organism known as:
    1. *Shigella* bacillus
    2. Gas bacillus
    3. Koch's bacillus
    4. Epstein-Barr virus

94. When administering a tuberculin skin test, the nurse would insert the needle at an angle of:
    1. 15 degrees
    2. 25 degrees
    3. 45 degrees
    4. 90 degrees

95. After administering a tuberculin skin test, it is important for the nurse to:
    1. Massage the area with firm strokes
    2. Massage the area with gentle strokes
    3. Refrain from massaging the site of injection
    4. Rub the site with an alcohol swab

96. The relative of a patient with tuberculosis expresses concern about a positive result to the tuberculin skin test. The nurse explains that the positive skin test indicates that:
    1. The relative also has TB and needs to be admitted to the hospital
    2. The relative has been exposed to the TB organism; further tests may be required
    3. The relative has an immunity to the TB organism and does not need to worry
    4. The relative has had an allergic reaction to the skin test and should not take it again

97. The nurse knows that asthma is:
    1. A chronic, progressive condition that involves destruction of the elastic tissues of the alveolar walls
    2. A chronic dilation of a bronchus or bronchi, with secretions of large amounts of purulent sputum
    3. A respiratory disorder characterized by recurring episodes of labored breathing with wheezing on expiration
    4. An infectious disease caused by a tubercle bacillus

98. Which of the following risk factors will the nurse identify as the primary cause of emphysema?
    1. Recent history of pneumonia
    2. Smoking two packs of cigarettes a day
    3. Living in an industrial area
    4. High-fat and high-cholesterol diet

99. Theophylline (Theo-Dur) therapy was started for a patient with emphysema. The main pharmacologic action of this drug is:
    1. Relaxation of bronchial smooth muscle
    2. Bronchial constriction
    3. Liquefying and thinning secretions
    4. Vasoconstriction of major vessels

100. A patient with emphysema is receiving aminophylline intravenously. The most common side effect that the nurse must observe for is:
    1. Bradycardia
    2. Hypotension
    3. Lethargy
    4. Weight gain

101. When doing a physical assessment on a patient with emphysema, which of the following will the nurse expect to find?
    1. Thin body build and pigeon chest
    2. Cyanotic skin color and dry, sparse hair
    3. Peripheral edema and moist, shiny skin
    4. Barreled chest and clubbing of the fingers

102. Which of the following drugs will the nurse most likely give to the patient who is in respiratory distress?
    ① Morphine
    ② Isuprel
    ③ Inderal
    ④ Mannitol

103. After a bronchoscopy is performed on a patient with suspected lung cancer, the nurse knows that the most important postprocedural order is to:
    ① Save all sputum
    ② Observe the neck dressing for drainage
    ③ Keep NPO until the gag reflex has returned
    ④ Whisper rather than talk for at least 1 week

104. Which of the following is the most important immediate postop nursing action after a bronchoscopy?
    ① Keep on bed rest 4-6 hours after bronchoscopy
    ② Keep NPO for 1-2 hours after bronchoscopy
    ③ Give only fluids 1-2 hours after bronchoscopy
    ④ Give only bland diet for 2 days after bronchoscopy

105. A localized lesion was observed during a bronchoscopy, and the patient is scheduled for a pneumonectomy. In this surgical procedure:
    ① The localized, diseased portion is removed
    ② Segments of diseased lung are removed
    ③ One lobe of the lung is removed
    ④ An entire lung is removed

106. Nursing interventions during the postoperative period following a pneumonectomy will *most likely* include:
    ① Monitoring closed chest drainage
    ② Placing the patient in semi-Fowler's position
    ③ Administering anticoagulant medications
    ④ Positioning the patient in the supine position for the first 24 hours

107. A chest x-ray that confirms a diagnosis of pulmonary edema will show:
    ① Thickened bronchial margins
    ② Widened intercostal spaces
    ③ Enlarged main pulmonary artery
    ④ Increased fluid in the pleural space and an enlarged heart

108. Pulmonary edema is caused by the:
    ① Increase of fluid in the circulating blood
    ② Decrease of fluid in the bronchi
    ③ Increase of fluid in the bronchi
    ④ Decrease of fluid in the circulating blood

109. After administration of a STAT order for Lasix 40 mg PO, the nurse will evaluate the effects of the medication by:
    ① Monitoring intake and output and checking for facial edema
    ② Recording daily weights and monitoring intake and output
    ③ Limiting fluid intake and checking for pedal edema
    ④ Checking for pedal and facial edema

110. A patient with pulmonary edema tells the nurse she is frightened by her difficult breathing. She says she feels she is suffocating. The nurse's response would be to:
    ① Have her take some deep breaths to relax, and report the condition to the charge nurse
    ② Tell her that there is medication she can have that will help her breathing
    ③ Tell her that she is too anxious over this and that the anxiety is making her worse
    ④ Report this condition to the charge nurse

111. Which device will be recommended for oxygen administration for a patient with pulmonary edema who is discharged to home?
    ① Face mask
    ② Oxygen tent
    ③ Nasal catheter
    ④ Nasal cannula

112. Diuril is given to expel fluid from the body and prevent pulmonary edema. When evaluating patient response to the drug, the nurse should also observe for:
    ① Hematuria
    ② Nausea and vomiting
    ③ Diarrhea
    ④ Muscular weakness and cramping

113. The nurse knows which of the following factors increases the risk of coronary artery disease for the patient?
    ① An active lifestyle
    ② The patient's father died at age 50 of lung cancer
    ③ The patient's cholesterol level is 176 mg/dl
    ④ The patient has diabetes mellitus

114. Venous blood is pumped from the right atrium into the right ventricle through the:
    ① Tricuspid valve
    ② Biscuspid valve
    ③ Aortic valve
    ④ Mitral valve

115. The patient who has had a heart attack informs the nurse that she smokes only a few cigarettes a day and she doesn't really think she needs to quit. The nurse provides her with which of the following pieces of information?
    ① Smoking causes about one half of the heart attacks in women
    ② Smoking any amount of cigarettes per day increases the risk of a cardiac event
    ③ Smoking has a higher risk factor for men than it does for women
    ④ Smoking cessation now will reduce the risk of a cardiac event within 2 months

116. The nurse knows that prevention strategies relevant to the cardiovascular system to include in a plan of care to prevent adverse effects of immobility are:
    ① Appropriate exercises, frequent turning, proper positioning, and increased fluid intake
    ② Getting the patient out of the bed once per day and decreasing kilocalories and fluid intake
    ③ Forbidding strenuous exercise, placing the patient in a supine position, and performing continuous hemodynamic monitoring
    ④ Placing the patient on complete bed rest and limiting the number of visitors allowed

117. The patient has just returned from a cardiac catheterization. What assessment would justify the nurse calling the physician?
    ① Bruising at the catheter insertion site
    ② Redness at the catheter insertion site
    ③ Absence of a pulse distal to the insertion site
    ④ Pain at the insertion site

118. The cardiac patient asks about cardiac enzyme tests (CK, LDH, AST) that have been ordered by the physician. The nurse explains that cardiac enzymes are:
    ① Proteins found specifically in heart muscle that measure the amount of damage
    ② Released from the heart tissue as a result of damage
    ③ Required for the electrical impulses to form
    ④ Indicators for the amount of damage to the valves of the heart

119. Before his test, the patient states he doesn't understand what an echocardiogram is. The nurse explains that the test examines the:
    ① Arteries of the heart
    ② Veins of the heart
    ③ Electrical activity of the heart
    ④ Walls of the heart

120. The sinoatrial node is located in the:
    ① Left atrium
    ② Right atrium
    ③ Left ventricle
    ④ Right ventricle

121. When planning the nursing care for a patient with angina pectoris, the nurse understands that this condition results from:
    ① Arteries that harden, thicken, and lose their elasticity
    ② Obstruction of a coronary artery or one of its branches
    ③ Failure of the heart to pump sufficient blood through the body
    ④ Insufficient oxygenated blood to the myocardial tissue

122. The nurse understands that the factor distinguishing angina pectoris from myocardial infarction is that the pain:
    ① Usually lasts longer than 15 minutes
    ② Usually occurs during periods of exertion
    ③ Is accompanied by diaphoresis and tachycardia
    ④ Does not radiate to the upper extremities

123. The patient who is having anginal pain will describe it to the nurse as a:
    ① Mild midepigastric pain
    ② Sharp, burning, substernal pain
    ③ Severe, crushing chest pain
    ④ Dull, ache-like pain in the arm

124. Which of these statements made by a patient with angina would indicate the need for further teaching about nitroglycerin therapy?
    ① "I will take one nitroglycerin tablet before engaging in strenuous activity."
    ② "I will store the nitroglycerin tablets in a dark container."
    ③ "I will discard nitroglycerin tablets that cause a burning sensation under my tongue."
    ④ "I can take three nitroglycerin tablets 5 minutes apart to control chest pain."

125. The nurse knows that the outstanding symptom of angina pectoris is:
    ① Acute pain that is often mistaken for indigestion
    ② Severe cyanosis
    ③ Elevation of blood pressure
    ④ Chest pain that radiates down the left arm

126. If the nurse leaves a supply of nitroglycerin tablets at the patient's bedside, she should:
    ① Check on the number of tablets left in the bottle and record the amount taken by the patient each time
    ② Check the patient's blood pressure q6h and record
    ③ Discourage the patient from taking too many pills, which could lead to drug dependency
    ④ Realize that she has no responsibility for the patient regarding nitroglycerin

127. If a patient has an angina attack, the nurse should record:
    ① Onset, duration, and intensity of the pain
    ② Activity, vital signs, and intensity of the pain
    ③ Onset, duration of pain, vital signs, and activity
    ④ Duration, intensity of the pain, and activity

128. A patient with angina pectoris is being discharged to go home. Nursing instructions for the patient and family members regarding continuity of care would include:
    ① Diet, activity, drug therapy, and avoiding risk factors
    ② Avoiding emotions of anxiety and avoiding exercise
    ③ Exercise, eating heavy meals, and extreme temperature changes
    ④ Diagnostic tests, exercise, and dietary modifications

129. The patient has a diagnosis of angina pectoris. This condition is best described by which of the following?
    ① An area of necrosis of the myocardium
    ② Rubbing of an enlarged epicardium against the pericardial sac
    ③ Inability of the coronary arteries to meet the oxygen needs of the myocardium
    ④ Generalized vasospasm throughout the endocardium and surrounding structures

130. Which is the most significant factor for a patient with essential hypertension?
    ① The patient has two small children
    ② The patient has been losing weight lately
    ③ The patient has lost both parents because of the disease
    ④ The patient has a cousin with the disease

131. The patient has a history of hypertension. The nurse is alert for which of the following symptoms?
    ① Epistaxis
    ② Red, swollen gums
    ③ Stiff neck
    ④ Inflamed eyes

132. The nurse knows that it is not unusual for the patient with hypertension to stop taking the prescribed medication. The usual reason for this is:
    ① The medications are too expensive
    ② All the symptoms of hypertension disappear
    ③ The patient did not receive adequate instructions
    ④ The patient finds the side effects too bothersome

133. The dietitian has instructed a patient with essential hypertension to moderate caffeine intake. The nurse understands the reason for this is that caffeine acts in the body to:
    ① Constrict blood vessels
    ② Increase cholesterol in the blood levels
    ③ Harden the blood vessels
    ④ Dilate the blood vessels

134. A patient with a blood pressure of 140/88 exercises very little and smokes at least one pack of cigarettes a day. The nurse would recommend which of the following as a priority in his health teaching?
    ① He should get 10 to 12 hours of sleep
    ② He should give up smoking
    ③ He should consider early retirement
    ④ Additional exercise is not appropriate for the patient at this time

135. In assessing a patient with hypertension, the nurse is aware that a sign of primary hypertension, as opposed to other types of hypertension, is an elevation of:
    ① Atrioventricular pressure
    ② Diastolic pressure
    ③ Systolic pressure
    ④ Pulse pressure

136. The nurse is discussing the appropriate diet for a patient with hypertension. One of the snacks the patient should avoid is:
    ① Carrots
    ② Pretzels
    ③ Oranges
    ④ Jello

137. In planning care for patients with hypertension, the nurse knows that the treatment is usually directed toward:
    ① Preventing further damage to the blood vessels
    ② Increasing the urine output
    ③ Lowering the blood pressure below normal level
    ④ Repairing the damaged blood vessels

138. Which of the following health care suggestions made by the nurse would be most helpful to a patient who has a history of hypertension, weighs 250 pounds, and is 5 feet, 8 inches tall?
    ① Enroll in a quick weight-loss program
    ② A gradual weight loss is best
    ③ Use a vegetarian diet
    ④ Count calories but do not exceed 1000 calories per day

139. Which of the following indicates that a diabetic patient understands his high risk for developing atherosclerosis?
    ① "The high blood sugars damage the lining of the blood vessels."
    ② "My high uric acid levels cause blockage of my blood vessels."
    ③ "My tingling feet are the result of damaged muscles."
    ④ "Keeping my blood sugar low will prevent heart damage."

140. While doing a health history, the nurse is looking for risk factors that may contribute to cardiovascular disease. Which of the following would be the best indicators of possible cardiovascular disease?
    ① Under 40 years old, no relatives with CVD, blood pressure of 150/86
    ② Over 40 years old, diabetic, cholesterol level of 280
    ③ Over 40 years old, minimal exercise, nonsmoker
    ④ Over 40, normal blood pressure, diabetic

141. As part of his preoperative care, the nurse explains to the patient the rationale for wearing thromboembolic stockings as:
    ① They facilitate return of blood to the heart
    ② They prevent clots from forming in the arteries
    ③ They promote arterial blood flow to the legs
    ④ They provide support to the muscles of the legs

142. A patient complains of pain in the lower extremities, tingling and numbness of the toes, and cramping of the calf muscles. The nurse knows that this is commonly called intermittent claudication and is caused by:
    ① Poor circulation
    ② Tight clothing
    ③ Poor diet
    ④ Inadequate rest

143. The nurse recognizes that the most frequent initial indication of coronary artery disease in women is:
    ① Mitral valve prolapse
    ② Endocarditis
    ③ Angina
    ④ Myocardial infarction

144. A patient has been hospitalized with an anterolateral myocardial infarction and she has many medical problems including diabetes, hypertension, and obesity. Her parents both died while in their fifties of cardiovascular disease. She smokes half a pack of cigarettes daily, and she drinks two beers per day. Of the following combinations of risk factors, which is most dire for this patient?
    ① Diabetes and hypertension
    ② Obesity and family history
    ③ Smoking and alcohol use
    ④ Gender and age

145. The nurse will explain myocardial infarction to the patient as:
    ① A blockage in the heart muscle
    ② A scarring of the valves
    ③ Oxygen deprivation to the heart muscle
    ④ The heart's inability to pump fluid

Medical-Surgical Nursing Review Questions **15**

146. The patient has been taking Reserpine for 12 weeks to treat hypertension. His blood pressure today is 150/92. During the assessment the patient says he has become impotent. He is disturbed and asks what he can do. Which of the following is the *best* nursing response?
① Refer the patient to a psychologist
② Set up a meeting with the wife and husband
③ Refer the patient to his physician
④ Refer the patient to a discussion group

147. A patient suddenly grabs his chest and says that he is having chest pain, as well as pain radiating down both arms. His lips are cyanotic, and he is perspiring heavily. The patient's symptoms most likely indicate:
① Angina pectoris
② Myocardial infarction
③ Anxiety attack
④ Indigestion

148. Nursing assessment for a patient with a myocardial infarction includes collecting subjective and objective data. Subjective data include noting the patient's:
① Dyspnea, vertigo, and weakness
② Behavior and pulse abnormalities
③ Vital signs and skin color
④ Dyspnea, pallor, and diaphoresis

149. A primary nursing goal in caring for a patient with a myocardial infarction is to:
① Reduce stress and anxiety level
② Allow gradual increase in activities
③ Provide diversional activities
④ Provide complete bed rest

150. The *most important* aspect of the nursing care for a patient with chest pain would be to:
① Elevate the legs and note the degree of pitting edema
② Note the color, character, and amount of sputum
③ Monitor intake and output and weigh daily
④ Evaluate/record onset, duration, and intensity of chest pain

151. When the patient who has had a myocardial infarction is transferred to the intermediate care unit from the cardiac intensive care unit, the nurse prepares to provide health teaching. With which of the following will the nurse begin her teaching?
① Nutritional counseling, because it is the easiest for the patient to understand
② Assessing the patient's knowledge about coronary artery disease and myocardial infarctions
③ Medication therapy, because it is the most essential
④ Asking the patient what he would like to know about his illness

152. A patient's serum cholesterol level is 260 mg/dl. Which of the following recommendations by the nurse is the *best* nutritional counseling for this patient?
① Eat only foods low in cholesterol
② Eat a soft, high-protein diet
③ Maintain a low-fat diet
④ Eat only easily digestible foods

153. The nurse knows the diet for a patient with a diagnosis of hypertension would most likely be:
① Bland
② Low sodium
③ High fat
④ High cholesterol

154. The nurse will teach the patient who has been ordered to take nitroglycerin tablets as needed to:
① Place the tablet under the tongue
② Drink with plenty of water or juice
③ Always take with meals
④ Always take before bedtime

155. The pain associated with a myocardial infarction differs from that of angina in that the pain is:
① Relieved with rest
② Not relieved by rest
③ Considerably less severe
④ Quickly relieved with nitroglycerin

156. A patient who has been admitted with an acute myocardial infarction becomes restless and experiences a rapid drop in blood pressure. He develops sudden dyspnea; productive coughing of pink-tinged, frothy sputum; and orthopnea. Crackles in the lungs and a respiratory rate of 32 are noted. These symptoms *most likely* indicate:
① Pulmonary edema
② Cardiogenic shock
③ Pulmonary embolus
④ Right-sided failure

157. Appropriate nursing measures to promote oxygenation for the patient with dyspnea include positioning the patient:
① Upright to decrease venous return
② In the supine position to encourage rest
③ With the legs elevated to promote venous return
④ With the head down to facilitate drainage of the upper respiratory tract

158. The diagnostic test *most* often ordered to evaluate the presence and scope of valvular heart disease is:
① Chest x-ray examination
② Electrocardiogram (ECG)
③ Serial blood cultures
④ Echocardiogram

159. In planning nursing care for a patient with congestive heart failure (CHF), the nurse will:
① Encourage interaction with others; get the patient out of bed and the room; and have the patient do short, focused activities
② Limit activities while providing and maintaining periods of rest; instruct the patient to avoid smoking or use of nicotine products; and induce analgesia and sedation as ordered
③ Avoid having the patient sit for prolonged periods of time; auscultate the abdomen for bowel sounds; and assess the skin and mucous membranes
④ Reinforce the importance of daily planning activities to conserve energy; encourage self-care as tolerated; and provide small, frequent feedings

160. A patient who has congestive heart failure (CHF) asks the nurse why he is short of breath. The nurse will explain that shortness of breath is primarily caused by:
    ① Increased anxiety and feelings of helplessness
    ② Pulmonary embolism
    ③ Acute bronchitis
    ④ Decreased cardiac output

161. The nurse knows that early signs of congestive heart failure (CHF) are:
    ① Shallow, rapid, dyspneic respirations
    ② Paroxysmal nocturnal dyspnea and dyspnea on exertion
    ③ Dyspnea on exertion, cerebral anoxia, and chronic cough
    ④ Malaise, elevation of temperature, and night sweats

162. In planning care for a patient with congestive heart failure, the nurse should know that the condition is:
    ① An occlusion of a major coronary artery or one its branches
    ② An infection or inflammation of the inner membranous lining of the heart, particularly the valves
    ③ A decrease of blood flow through the heart and great vessels
    ④ An enlargement or ballooning of an artery

163. When auscultating respirations of a patient with congestive heart failure, the types of sounds the nurse would expect to hear are:
    ① Diminished or absent breath sounds
    ② Crackling
    ③ Expiratory wheezing
    ④ Inspiratory sounds louder than expiratory sounds

164. A patient has fallen and bruised his right lower leg. In assessing the injury, the nurse must distinguish the body's response. The process of the body's reaction to injury or irritation is called:
    ① Inflammation
    ② Allergy
    ③ Infection
    ④ Immunity

165. The nurse teaches the patient with congestive heart failure (CHF) that it is important to do mild exercises of the legs and wear antiembolitic stockings because they:
    ① Reduce circulation to the legs and ease the workload of the heart
    ② Prevent abdominal edema
    ③ Prevent clot formation in the lower extremities
    ④ Reduce edema of the extremities

166. For a patient with cardiac disease, a low-salt diet is prescribed. Which of the following foods contain the least amount of sodium?
    ① Baking soda
    ② Citrus fruits
    ③ Milk and cheese
    ④ Canned meats

167. The nurse is to administer digitalis to a patient. This drug is classified as a(n):
    ① Antianxiety agent
    ② Coagulant
    ③ Respiratory stimulant
    ④ Cardiotonic

168. A major complication of congestive heart failure is pulmonary edema. Some of the findings that suggest a patient has pulmonary edema are:
    ① Dyspnea on exertion, nausea, and vomiting
    ② Orthopnea and angina
    ③ Thick, tenacious sputum and anxiety
    ④ Dyspnea and frothy, pink-tinged sputum

169. The purpose of weighing a patient with congestive heart failure (CHF) daily is to determine loss of:
    ① Blood volume
    ② Tissue fluid
    ③ Body fat
    ④ Appetite

170. The nurse knows that congestive heart failure (CHF) occurs most often because of:
    ① Incomplete emptying of the left ventricle
    ② Incomplete emptying of the right ventricle
    ③ Rapid emptying of the left ventricle
    ④ Rapid emptying of the right ventricle

171. In planning care for a patient with congestive heart failure, the nurse should observe for which of the following signs and symptoms?
    ① Fatigue
    ② Restlessness
    ③ Excessive thirst
    ④ Respiratory difficulty

172. When developing the nursing care plan for a patient with a diagnosis of congestive heart failure, which of the following should be an important consideration?
    ① Prevention of infection
    ② Early ambulation
    ③ Skin integrity
    ④ Increased fluid intake

173. Fluid and electrolyte balance need to be maintained for patients with congestive heart failure by which of the following?
    ① Maintaining strict input and output and daily levels
    ② Limiting fluid intake and maintaining daily levels
    ③ Limiting activity and maintaining a salt-free diet
    ④ Limiting activity and maintaining a low-sodium diet

174. The nurse is teaching a patient with endocarditis who is about to be discharged. The nurse will focus on:
    ① The need for a sedentary lifestyle
    ② Forcing fluids to prevent dehydration
    ③ Prophylactic antibiotic therapy for dental procedures
    ④ The need for wearing a mask in crowds to prevent upper respiratory tract infections

175. In planning care for a patient with endocarditis, the nurse knows that this is:
    ① An enlargement or ballooning of an artery
    ② A decrease of blood flow through the heart
    ③ An occlusion of a major artery or one of its branches
    ④ An infection or inflammation of the inner membranous lining of the heart, particularly the valves

176. In setting up a care plan, the nurse is aware that rheumatic fever is:
    ① A disease of adults
    ② More prevalent in males
    ③ More prevalent in females
    ④ More prevalent in children

177. In preparing a patient for a cardiac catheterization the nurse should explain that the patient will:
① Experience a great deal of pain
② Be able to see the catheter pass through the superior vena cava on the monitor
③ Have her meals held for 24 hours before the examination
④ Not have blood samples taken

178. The nurse knows that the P wave in an electrocardiogram is:
① The impulse from the sinoatrial node
② The ventricular contractions
③ Helpful in diagnosing myocardial infarction
④ Helpful in diagnosing valvular lesions

179. When taking a blood pressure, the nurse is aware that the period of relaxation of the heart muscle is called:
① Refractory period
② Systole
③ Diastole
④ Atrial systole

180. Chronic valvular disorders develop when healing occurs in rheumatic fever. The heart valves frequently affected are the:
① Mitral and aortic
② Tricuspid and mitral
③ Aortic and pulmonary
④ Pulmonary and semilunar

181. The nurse caring for a patient with arteriosclerotic heart disease knows that delayed treatment of the disease may result in:
① Myocardial infarction
② Pulmonary edema
③ Congestive heart failure
④ Endocarditis

182. A patient with rheumatic heart disease has orders that blood pressure be checked q4h. When taking blood pressure, the nurse is aware that the best site to use is the:
① Radial artery
② Popliteal artery
③ Femoral artery
④ Brachial artery

183. In caring for a patient with rheumatic heart disease, the primary nursing intervention that the nurse will implement includes:
① A low-sodium diet
② Bed rest
③ Steroid therapy
④ Sublingual nitroglycerin

184. When planning nursing care for a patient with coronary occlusion, the nurse knows this diagnosis means:
① A seizure
② A spasm of the muscles
③ A stationary blood clot
④ An obstruction or cutting-off

185. A coronary artery bypass graft is performed on a patient with a diagnosis of coronary artery disease. In planning postoperative care for this patient, the nurse is aware that this procedure is done:
① To bypass occluded vessels in the neck
② To bypass occluded vessels in the heart
③ To insert a pacemaker
④ To remove the lining of the artery

186. The most common use of cardiac catheterization is to determine the:
① Amount of blood entering the right atrium
② Degree of blockage of the coronary arteries
③ Pressure in the left ventricle
④ Strength of ventricular contraction

187. Patients requiring cardiac diagnostic studies that involve the use of a contrast medium are questioned before the study about their:
① Dietary intake of foods high in fat
② Use of an antihistamine in the past week
③ Recent gain or loss of weight
④ Allergies, especially to seafood and iodine

188. A patient has a cardiac catheterization. Which of the following nursing interventions is *most* important during the first 4 to 6 hours after the procedure?
① Assess circulation to the extremity used for catheter insertion
② Maintain the extremity used for the procedure in a flexed position
③ Keep the extremity elevated on at least two pillows
④ Limit the intake of fluids

189. A patient with arteriosclerosis of the lower extremities asks the nurse why the physician has told him to stop smoking. The nurse replies:
① "There is no connection between smoking and your condition."
② "Smoking dulls your appetite and prevents healing of your legs."
③ "The physician is afraid your condition might spread to your lungs."
④ "Nicotine is a drug present in cigarettes that narrows the blood vessels and makes your condition worse."

190. While doing an assessment of a patient with arterial insufficiency of the left foot related to arteriosclerosis, the nurse would make the following observation:
① Loss of hair on the extremity
② Enlarged blood vessels in the leg
③ Warm, moist skin on the affected extremity
④ Swelling of the feet at the end of the day

191. A patient with peripheral vascular disease suddenly develops pain in his left foot. Which of these assessments of the patient's foot would the nurse report immediately to the team leader?
① Numbness and tingling
② Warm to the touch
③ Brisk capillary refill
④ Absent pedal pulse

192. A femoral/popliteal bypass is performed on the patient's left extremity. In the immediate postoperative period, which of these measures would be the most important indication that blood supply to the leg was improving?
    ① Obtaining his vital signs q4h
    ② Checking the temperature of his leg
    ③ Monitoring his urine output q1h
    ④ Encouraging a high fluid intake

193. The nurse would assess a patient for signs of thrombophlebitis in a lower extremity by noting:
    ① An elevated platelet count
    ② A positive Chvostek's sign
    ③ A positive Homans' sign
    ④ Decreased hemoglobin level

194. The nurse must recognize that the primary symptoms of superficial thrombophlebitis include:
    ① Fever, nausea, and vomiting
    ② Pain, heat, and redness
    ③ Diarrhea or constipation, and abdominal discomfort
    ④ Anorexia, and pain when walking

195. When explaining the diagnosis of thrombophlebitis to a patient who has been on bed rest for several weeks, the nurse's best statement would be that thrombophlebitis is:
    ① An ulcer that becomes infected
    ② A traumatic inflammation of blood vessels
    ③ An inflammation of a vein with clot formation
    ④ An inflammation of an artery with clot formation

196. The nurse should observe the patient with deep-vein thrombosis for the possibility of an embolism, as indicated by:
    ① Pain at the site
    ② Warm affected areas
    ③ Bradycardia
    ④ Decreased respirations

197. While caring for a patient with deep-vein thrombosis, the nurse is aware of the possibility of an embolism, which is defined as:
    ① A stationary blood clot
    ② A blood clot in the arteries
    ③ A blood clot that lodges in the brain only
    ④ A clot circulating in the blood

198. The nurse is caring for a patient on the first postoperative day. Knowing that immobility is one of the causes of thrombophlebitis, the nurse is aware that this complication is best prevented by:
    ① Taking vitamin C daily
    ② Early ambulation to increase circulation
    ③ Massaging the extremities
    ④ Restricting activity, even in bed

199. The nurse is bathing a patient. She knows that which of the following is contraindicated with a diagnosis of thrombophlebitis?
    ① Massaging the legs
    ② Rubbing the neck
    ③ Turning in bed as necessary
    ④ Elevating the head of the bed

200. The nurse is instructing a patient with arteriosclerosis of his lower extremities on proper care of his feet and legs. Which of the following would the nurse include in her teaching program?
    ① To be careful applying heat to the feet and legs
    ② To wear snug shoes
    ③ To allow the legs to hang/dangle independently at all times
    ④ That it is all right to go out in extremely cold weather

201. A 76-year-old man has been hospitalized with bed rest prescribed for a week. The nurse assists the patient out of bed for the first time. As he begins to walk, he complains of pain in his right leg. To establish the basis of this patient's complaint, which of these assessments should the nurse carry out *first?*
    ① Ask him to describe the pain
    ② Inspect his leg for evidence of trauma
    ③ Test for Homans' sign
    ④ Check his pedal pulses

202. If a patient's diagnosis is thrombophlebitis, what other signs or symptoms might the nurse expect to find?
    ① Decreased pedal pulses on the affected leg
    ② Ecchymosis on the area that has pain
    ③ Dry, flaky skin, particularly on the foot
    ④ Redness and edema of the affected leg

203. Nursing interventions on the care plan of a patient with thrombophlebitis would most likely include:
    ① Increasing foods containing vitamin C
    ② Range-of-motion exercises to all extremities
    ③ Bed cradle and cold compresses to the extremities
    ④ Continual use of elastic stockings

204. A patient is discharged on a regimen of warfarin sodium (Coumadin). Which food, if avoided by the patient, would indicate that he understands his teaching plan about vitamin K?
    ① Milk
    ② Oranges
    ③ Spinach
    ④ Bran cereal

205. A condition that makes a person more susceptible to the development of varicose veins is:
    ① Repeated bacterial infection in the veins
    ② Improper functioning of the valves that control the flow of blood through the veins
    ③ Congenital malformation of the lower extremities in which there is improper circulation
    ④ Deposits of material along the wall of the veins

206. In planning care for a patient who has varicose veins of the lower extremities, the nurse knows that varicose veins are those that have become:
    ① Enlarged and engorged with blood
    ② Hardened, with narrowed openings
    ③ Atrophied because of blood vessel constriction
    ④ Infected by invasion of bacteria

207. In preparing to administer a drug used to treat a patient with an embolism, the nurse knows the classification of the drug is:
    ① Antibiotics
    ② Vitamins
    ③ Thrombolytic agents
    ④ Antineoplastic agents

208. A patient is receiving a blood transfusion. As the nurse is doing AM care, the patient begins to complain of itching. The nurse notices a red rash beginning on the patient's right arm above the IV site. What would be the best action by the nurse?
  ① Stop the blood transfusion and call the doctor
  ② Slow the blood transfusion and call the doctor
  ③ Smooth Benadryl cream over the area and watch closely
  ④ Finish AM care, then report the incident to the charge nurse

209. A 28-year-old patient has pallor of the mucous membranes and nail beds. She has a history of fatigue and exertional dyspnea. Her hemoglobin level is 8 g/dl. A diagnosis of iron deficiency anemia is made. What is the *most likely* physiologic reason for the assessment findings?
  ① Impaired production of red blood cells
  ② Decreased production of white blood cells
  ③ Platelet destruction and internal bleeding
  ④ Reduced oxygen-carrying capacity of hemoglobin

210. Which nursing assessment is *most* appropriate for the patient with iron deficiency anemia?
  ① Pain
  ② Anxiety
  ③ Fluid volume deficit
  ④ Activity intolerance

211. A specific nursing intervention for the patient with iron-deficiency anemia would be:
  ① Absolute bed rest
  ② Increased use of vitamins
  ③ Increased periods of exercise
  ④ Short work sessions with rest periods

212. Which of the following statements by a patient with anemia indicates understanding of the dietary teaching by the nurse?
  ① "I won't drink tea or coffee with my meals."
  ② "I will include eggs in my diet daily."
  ③ "I'll drink a quart of milk every day."
  ④ "I'll include green leafy vegetables every day."

213. To provide appropriate nursing care for a patient in sickle cell crisis, the nurse is aware that sickle cell anemia is caused by:
  ① The herpes virus
  ② *Staphylococcus* bacteria
  ③ Repeated blood transfusions
  ④ An abnormal heredity trait

214. What will the nurse expect the laboratory reports of a patient with leukemia to indicate?
  ① Large numbers of immature white blood cells
  ② Decreased number of T-lymphocytes
  ③ Marked increase in hematocrit
  ④ Low level of hemoglobin

215. The nurse will caution a patient with thrombocytopenia against which of the following?
  ① Sharing his room with another patient
  ② Using a disposable razor
  ③ Engaging in activity
  ④ Having visitors

216. A patient receiving an intensive course of chemotherapy for acute leukemia has developed leukopenia. His temperature, taken orally, is 100.8° F. What nursing action is *most* warranted?
  ① Take future temperatures rectally
  ② Look for a source of infection
  ③ Monitor for bleeding
  ④ Force fluids

217. While caring for a patient with leukemia, the nurse is concerned about controlling possible complications. An example of good medical asepsis to follow in *all* situations is:
  ① Changing a dressing with nonsterile gloves
  ② Slowing the IV when the site is red and warm to touch
  ③ Cleansing the rubber stopper on the penicillin before drawing up the medication
  ④ Wearing the same isolation gown for each day of the patient's care

218. The nurse knows that AIDS is a disease caused by:
  ① Epstein-Barr virus
  ② Herpes simplex virus
  ③ Human immunodeficiency virus (HIV)
  ④ Hepatitis B virus

219. Universal precautions used in caring for a patient with AIDS include:
  ① Blood and body fluid precautions
  ② Private room with door closed
  ③ Use of disposable utensils, dishes, and trays
  ④ Full isolation technique

220. The patient is immunocompromised as a result of AIDS. He is concerned whether he should receive vaccines to help prevent some contagious diseases. The nurse recognizes which of the following vaccines are contraindicated for the patient?
  ① Tetanus, diphtheria
  ② Diphtheria, pertussis
  ③ Oral poliovirus
  ④ Inactivated poliovirus

221. The nurse knows the three major routes of transmission of AIDS are:
  ① Breast milk, sexual intercourse, and lacrimal secretions
  ② Cerebrospinal fluid, sexual intercourse, and blood
  ③ Saliva, lacrimal secretions, and urine
  ④ Sexual intercourse, blood, and transplacental (perinatal)

222. The diagnostic test enzyme-linked immunosorbent assay (ELISA) is used for diagnosis of which of the following?
  ① Kaposi's sarcoma
  ② AIDS
  ③ Cytomegalovarus
  ④ Herpes simplex virus type II

223. What assessment will the nurse most likely make on a male patient diagnosed with AIDS?
  ① A history of constipation
  ② A red, itchy rash on his legs
  ③ A subnormal temperature in the late afternoon
  ④ The presence of purplish lesions on his trunk

224. A patient with AIDS has candidiasis. Which information given on the assessment would most likely indicate this condition?
① "I have pain in my legs at night."
② "My skin is very dry."
③ "My throat is sore."
④ "I have difficulty digesting fats."

225. When caring for a patient with AIDS, the nurse would include which of following in the treatment plan?
① Have visitors and staff wear cap, mask, and gown
② Isolate blood pressure equipment and thermometer
③ Be sure the patient has his or her own bathroom
④ Wash spilled body fluid with chlorine bleach

226. The patient is to receive 200 ml of formula diluted to half strength every 2 hours through a gastric feeding tube. Before the nurse administers the formula, she withdraws 160 ml of gastric contents. What should the nurse do next?
① Discard the withdrawn fluid and continue with the tube feeding
② Return the fluid and continue with the tube feeding
③ Return the fluid and withhold feeding
④ Discard the fluid and withhold the feeding

227. A hernia in which the blood supply has been cut off is termed:
① Incarcerated
② Incisional
③ Strangulated
④ Umbilical

228. The patient who is scheduled for a barium enema will be prepared by the nurse to expect to:
① Have coffee and toast the morning of the test
② Take radiographic dye tablets
③ Have a needle inserted in the liver area
④ Be NPO after midnight and receive enemas until clear

229. When preparing a patient for an endoscopy procedure, the nurse should:
① Administer radiographic dye tablets as prescribed
② Monitor the patient for bleeding or bile leakage
③ Obtain a signed consent form
④ Know there are no specific preparations

230. After a patient returns from having an endoscopy, he asks for a drink of water and something to eat. The appropriate nursing action would be to:
① Offer a drink of water and order the prescribed diet
② Explain that the patient needs to wait until his gag reflex is functional
③ Explain to the patient that solid food or drink is not allowed for 24 hours
④ Instruct the patient to take small sips of water until the meal trays are served

231. A patient is admitted to the hospital for a gastric ulcer work-up. While obtaining the admission history, which of the following complaints would suggest to the nurse that the patient has a gastric ulcer?
① Pain experienced 3 hours after meals, relieved by food
② Pain experienced before meals, not relieved by vomiting
③ Pain 1 hour after eating, increased by food
④ Pain experienced only during the night

232. Which of the following signs and symptoms would alert the nurse to a possible perforated gastric ulcer?
① Gradual decrease in body temperature
② Epigastric fullness and regurgitation
③ Blood-tinged drainage in the vomitus
④ Persistent and intense abdominal pain

233. Following a subtotal gastrectomy, the nurse will be prepared to implement the following physician's order:
① Start clear fluids as soon as bowel sounds are heard
② Irrigate the nasogastric tube per order with sterile water
③ Connect the nasogastric tube to low intermittent suction
④ Advance the tube hourly as ordered by the physician

234. The nurse is teaching a postgastrectomy patient about dumping syndrome. The patient would indicate the need for further instruction when which of the following statements is made?
① "I will lie down after eating a meal."
② "I will eat smaller portions of food, more frequently."
③ "I will not drink liquids when I eat."
④ "I will avoid fats and increase carbohydrates."

235. The nurse notices that a patient's urine specimen collected for culture and sensitivity has not been delivered to the laboratory. The nurse would be concerned because the specimen:
① Should be warm when it arrives in the laboratory
② May accidentally spill and require another collection
③ Sitting on the counter for a long period could result in growth of microorganisms
④ Sitting on the counter for a long period could result in the microorganisms dying and producing a false report

236. In preparing the patient for a fiberoptic endoscopy, the nurse will instruct the patient to:
① Not take anything by mouth after midnight
② Take a cleansing enema the night before
③ Take a cleansing enema the morning of the examination
④ Take a laxative the night before the examination

237. The primary medical treatment for a patient with duodenal ulcers is:
① Promote healing by diet therapy
② Reduce the signs and symptoms with drug therapy
③ A diet low in fat and carbohydrates
④ A diet high in protein and milk products

238. After a trial of medical management for duodenal ulcers, the patient's vomiting and abdominal distention became worse. He was admitted for a vagotomy. In planning postoperative care for the patient, the nurse knows that this type of surgery is performed to remove:
① The gastric-producing portion of the lower stomach
② The scar tissue lining the stomach
③ The vagal innervation to the fundus of the stomach
④ The entire stomach

239. The complication known as dumping syndrome occurs after gastroenterostomy surgery. In planning care for this type of patient, the nurse knows that this syndrome is caused by:
① Decreased intestinal mobility
② Increased hydrochloric acid in the stomach
③ Decreased hydrochloric acid in the stomach
④ A rapid gastric emptying

240. The nurse would instruct a patient with dumping syndrome to:
① Recline for 1 hour after meals
② Recline for 1 hour before meals
③ Drink a lot of fluids during meals
④ Increase the intake of carbohydrate foods

241. When interviewing a patient with ulcerative colitis, which of the following symptoms will the nurse expect to be reported?
① Anorexia and constipation
② Liquid, tarry stools
③ Epigastric pain after meals
④ Frequent bloody diarrhea

242. Which breakfast food selection by a patient with ulcerative colitis indicates that further instruction is needed?
① Oatmeal, orange slices, and milk
② Soft-cooked egg, toast, and herb tea
③ Apple juice, English muffin, and jelly
④ Cream of rice cereal, white toast, and marmalade

243. The nurse would expect the drainage from an ileostomy to have which of these characteristics?
① Semiliquid consistency with mucus
② Semiformed consistency with blood
③ Formed stool, brown in color
④ Tarry and soft consistency

244. In preparing a patient for a gastric analysis, the nurse must know that the drug used to stimulate the flow of gastric juices is:
① Histamine
② Belladonna
③ Atropine
④ Opium tincture (Paregoric)

245. The nurse will include which of the following in her care plan for a patient with ulcerative colitis?
① Bed rest with bedside commode privileges
② A restriction of visitors or phone calls
③ Teaching the patient how to manage the disease at home
④ Semiprivate room, bedside commode, and restriction of visitors

246. The nurse will expect the first bowel movement after a transverse loop colostomy to be:
① Mostly bloody, with small clots mixed with liquid stool
② Liquid, light-brown stool
③ Semisolid, brown stool
④ Solid, brown stool, with a small amount of blood

247. An expected outcome of treatment for a patient with ulcerative colitis would be:
① Fewer stools, better formed with no mucus, blood, or pus in them
② A softening of the hard and constipated stools
③ No change in the formed, soft, brown stools
④ A decrease in the watery, brown stools

248. Following a transverse loop colostomy, the stoma appears mostly pink with some purple discoloration at the lower border. Which of the following is an appropriate action by the nurse?
① Clean the area around the stoma and record the observation in the nurses' notes
② Carefully place a clean pouch over the stoma to prevent any further bruising
③ Cover the stoma with a petrolatum gauze dressing to prevent any further irritation to the stoma
④ Apply a clean dressing and pouch, and notify the physician about the discoloration

249. The nurse knows that symptoms of a partial intestinal obstruction with the passage of "pencil-shaped" stools are characteristic of cancer of the:
① Sigmoid
② Cecum
③ Transverse colon
④ Descending colon

250. To prepare the patient for a sigmoidoscopy, the nurse will:
① Administer a cathartic the evening before the procedure
② Administer an enema the morning before the procedure
③ Explain to the patient that she will drink a chalk-like fluid
④ Administer a cathartic and enema the evening before the procedure and an enema the morning of the procedure

251. A diagnosis of cancer of the descending colon with rectal involvement is made. In planning care for this patient, the nurse knows that the surgical procedure most likely to be done would be a:
① Sigmoid colostomy
② Ileostomy
③ Colectomy
④ Right hemicolectomy

252. If a patient complains of cramping during a colostomy irrigation, the nurse should:
① Lower the container of fluid
② Discontinue the irrigation
③ Advance the catheter 2 more inches
④ Stop the flow until the cramping subsides

253. When doing an irrigation of a sigmoid colostomy, the nurse knows that the cone should be inserted into the stoma opening no more than:
① 2 inches
② 4 inches
③ 10 inches
④ 12 inches

254. Which of the following behaviors exhibited by a patient with a colostomy just before discharge should be of concern to the nurse and reported to the charge nurse?
① Not eating the food sent at each meal
② Refusing to care for the colostomy
③ Wearing loose-fitting clothing
④ Having periods of anger over why this happened

255. To plan appropriate nursing care, the nurse will understand that cholelithiasis is the medical term for:
    ① Presence of gallstones in the gallbladder or biliary tree
    ② An inflammation of the gallbladder
    ③ Presence of renal calculi in one or both kidneys
    ④ An inflammation of the nephrons of the kidneys

256. In caring for a patient with cholelithiasis, the nurse will observe for which of the two following characteristic symptoms?
    ① Jaundice and liver tenderness
    ② Abdominal rigidity and paralytic ileus
    ③ Liver enlargement and bleeding disorders
    ④ Indigestion after a high-fat meal and jaundice

257. A patient is scheduled for surgery with a common bile duct exploration. The nurse would expect the patient to return from surgery with:
    ① An underwater-seal drainage
    ② A T-tube
    ③ A Penrose drain
    ④ A tracheotomy

258. A low-fat diet has been ordered for a patient with cholelithiasis. Which of the following food sources would be most appropriate?
    ① Ground sausage, vegetables, and fruits
    ② Ground turkey, avocados, and fruits
    ③ Marbled hamburger, lean steak, and vegetables
    ④ Skinless chicken, vegetables, and fruits

259. A patient is admitted to the emergency room with a primary diagnosis of cholecystitis. The nurse will carefully observe for which of the following symptoms?
    ① Voiding large amounts of light yellow urine
    ② Sensation of nausea and bloating after eating fried food
    ③ Stool becoming dark, which may be evidence of blood
    ④ Abdominal pain after eating a diet high in carbohydrates

260. Postoperative care for a patient who has had a cholecystectomy with a nasogastric tube in place will include:
    ① Irrigating the nasogastric tube with normal saline every 6 hours
    ② Wrapping the open end of the tube with sterile gauze
    ③ Obtaining a clear-liquid diet for the patient
    ④ Attaching the nasogastric tube to low, intermittent suction

261. Which of the following measures for a patient with a T-tube in place following a common bile duct exploration with a cholecystectomy would be most appropriate?
    ① Complete a sterile dressing change as necessary
    ② Reinforce the dressing as often as needed
    ③ Encourage the patient to lie as still as possible
    ④ Keep the patient sedated as long as the T-tube is in place

262. The patient is to be discharged with the T-tube and drainage system in place. Which of the following discharge instructions are correctly given by the nurse?
    ① Wear snug clothing, or a binder, to prevent any movement of the T-tube
    ② Soak in the bathtub for 20 minutes twice a day to clean the incision site
    ③ Tape the drainage tubing to the abdomen below the level of the T-tube
    ④ Expect a certain amount of redness and tenderness around the incision site

263. The nurse explains to the patient that hepatitis A is spread:
    ① Through the oral-fecal route
    ② Through sexual intercourse
    ③ Through intravenous drug use
    ④ By unknown routes

264. The nurse knows that jaundice in a patient with hepatitis is caused by:
    ① A poorly functioning pancreas
    ② Intestinal obstruction
    ③ Large amounts of bile pigment in the blood
    ④ An unknown factor

265. In developing a care plan for a patient with hepatitis, the nurse will include:
    ① Universal precautions and disinfection of body fluids and secretions
    ② Monitoring antibiotic intravenous administration
    ③ Bed rest with bathroom privileges
    ④ Restrictive fluid intake

266. Changes in the liver caused by viral hepatitis affect certain laboratory test results. In planning care for these patients, the nurse is aware that the laboratory results would most likely show:
    ① Elevated hemoglobin and hematocrit levels
    ② Elevated direct bilirubin and AST levels
    ③ Increased serum albumin and AST levels
    ④ Decreased serum albumin and elevated hemoglobin levels

267. In planning care for a patient with a diagnosis of hepatitis B, the nurse knows that treatment considerations include:
    ① A high-fat diet
    ② Bed rest for several weeks
    ③ No specific dietary regimen
    ④ A moderate exercise regimen

268. Monitoring stools of a patient with hepatitis A is important. The nurse caring for such a patient would expect that the stools will be:
    ① Dark brown
    ② Black
    ③ Clay-colored
    ④ Green

269. The patient is admitted for hepatitis B infection. She is experiencing nausea and pain in the upper right quadrant of the abdomen. She reports lack of appetite for the past 4 days. Nursing intervention(s) will include the following:
① Teach ways hepatitis B is transmitted
② Provide six small meals and high-calorie snacks in between
③ Administer vitamin K as prescribed
④ Monitor for signs of bleeding

270. The patient has advanced cirrhosis of the liver. When discussing medication administration, the nurse will consider the following:
① The liver is the least important organ in drug metabolism
② The liver does not play any role in drug metabolism
③ The liver is the most important organ in drug metabolism
④ The heart is the most important organ in drug metabolism

271. The husband of a patient diagnosed with cirrhosis of the liver has frequently called his wife's employer to say she was sick when she was actually intoxicated. He has exhibited what type of behavior?
① Caring
② Codependent
③ Confrontational
④ Realistic

272. The patient with a diagnosis of acute pancreatitis has been experiencing epigastric pain and episodes of vomiting. Other signs or symptoms of acute pancreatitis most likely include:
① Soft abdomen
② Bloody urine
③ Elevated serum amylase level
④ Elevated serum creatinine level

273. Discharge teaching for a patient with pancreatitis included information about a low-fat diet. Which of the following meals selected by the patient would best indicate an understanding of patient teaching?
① A tuna salad sandwich and tea
② Hamburger, roll, and decaffeinated coffee
③ Steamed vegetables and skimmed milk
④ Grilled cheese sandwich and ginger ale

274. What laboratory results would the nurse expect that would confirm the diagnosis of appendicitis?
① Agranulocytosis
② Leukopenia
③ Leukocytosis
④ Aplastic anemia

275. The nurse will watch for signs and symptoms of which of the following complications of a ruptured appendix?
① Peritonitis
② Ileitus
③ Colitis
④ Diverticulitis

276. Before surgery, until laboratory results are returned, the nurse can expect the physician to order which of the following for a patient exhibiting symptoms of appendicitis?
① Narcotics for pain relief
② Heat applied to the abdomen
③ Cleansing enema
④ Ice bag applied to the abdomen

277. The nurse knows that the cause of acute appendicitis is:
① Unknown
② Overeating
③ Infection
④ Overexertion

278. Immediate postoperative teaching that is imperative for a patient who has undergone an appendectomy includes:
① The fact that he or she will be able to play sports again
② The fact that he or she will no longer have pain
③ What he or she is to expect and why it is done
④ That he or she doesn't need his appendix for any specific body function

279. A patient comes to the doctor's office following treatment for carpal tunnel syndrome. Which of the following would indicate that the patient understood instructions on the treatment?
① The patient has avoided working on the computer
② The patient has avoided exercise
③ The patient has limited calcium intake
④ The patient has avoided rich foods such as gravies and sauces

280. Which of the following interventions should be included in teaching a diabetic patient who is experiencing difficulty with peripheral neuropathy?
① Get out of bed slowly in the morning
② Examine the feet each day
③ Soak the feet daily in warm water
④ Remove calluses promptly with a file

281. Then nurse knows that the purpose of administering metoclopramide (Reglan) to a patient with autonomic neuropathy is to:
① Prevent postural hypotension
② Facilitate gastric emptying
③ Regenerate nervous tissue
④ Heighten sensation in the periphery

282. The patient has been taking Inderal but is still experiencing occasional migraine headaches. She is requesting information on health changes that may eliminate the headaches. The nurse's best response will include which of the following?
① Avoid chocolate and citrus fruits
② Increase caffeine-containing beverages
③ Begin strenuous exercise at the first sign of an attack
④ Limit sleep to 4 to 5 hours per night

283. When assessing for the earliest sign of increased intracranial pressure, the nurse observes for changes in which of the following?
① Level of responsiveness
② Intensity of a headache
③ Pupillary status
④ Vital signs

284. A patient fell and struck his left temporal area. He denies loss of consciousness and is alert and oriented. The nurse instructs him to return to see the physician immediately if which one of the following were to occur?
① A lump on the head
② Complaints of headache
③ Blackened left eye
④ Forceful vomiting

285. Which of the following is the position of choice when caring for a patient with increased intracranial pressure (ICP)?
① Supine, with the bed flat
② Prone, with the head of the bed flat
③ Sims' position, with foot of the bed elevated 30 degrees
④ Supine, with the head of the bed elevated 30 degrees

286. When assessing vital-sign changes in a patient with increased intracranial pressure, the nurse observes for which of the following?
① Bradycardia, hypertension, and subnormal temperature
② Fever and hypertension
③ Bradycardia, hypertension, and fever
④ Tachycardia and normal temperature

287. The Glasgow Coma Scale is used to determine a patient's level of consciousness. The nurse has completed her assessment and finds the numerical value totals 14. This means the patient is:
① Neurologically impaired
② Not neurologically impaired
③ Comatose
④ Disoriented

288. When the nurse collects subjective data from a patient with a head injury, which of the following would apply?
① Vertigo, diplopia, and headache
② Results of diagnostic tests such as brain scan
③ Pupillary reaction to light
④ Cerebrospinal drainage from the ears and/or nose

289. While observing a patient for signs of increased intracranial pressure, the nurse notes that the blood pressure changes from 110/70 to 130/60, and the pulse rate is now 120. What would be the appropriate nursing action?
① Report the vital-sign changes to the physician when he makes rounds
② Recheck vital signs and report immediately to the charge nurse
③ Wait 1 hour, recheck vital signs, and document immediately
④ These changes are not necessary to report because they are insignificant

290. When caring for a patient with increased intracranial pressure, the nurse knows to *avoid* which of the following positions?
① Semi Fowler's
② Lateral
③ Supine
④ Trendelenburg's

291. The nurse will explain preoperative and postoperative procedures to the patient scheduled for a craniotomy to reduce fear of:
① Increased intracranial pressure
② Hair loss
③ Loss of self-esteem
④ The unknown

292. When assessing a patient after a craniotomy, the nurse knows that which of the following signs is the *most* critical?
① Dilated and fixed pupils
② Decreasing pulse pressure
③ Motor response is flaccid
④ Vital signs are blood pressure 140/82, pulse rate 72, and respirations 20

293. Which of the following signs indicates the patient is at risk for developing a complication common to a craniotomy?
① Glucose in the urine
② Clear discharge from the nose
③ Ecchymotic areas around the eyes
④ Abdominal pain and diarrhea

294. A nurse notices a patient having a seizure. Which of the following should the nurse do first?
① Check the patient's respirations
② Place the patient in the supine position
③ Apply ice to the patient's axillae and groin
④ Call for assistance

295. A patient has a grand mal seizure. A priority nursing intervention for the patient during a seizure is to:
① Loosen constrictive clothing and monitor vital signs
② Open the patient's jaw and insert a seizure stick
③ Position the patient on his or her side and suction the patient's mouth
④ Provide for privacy and a safe environment

296. After receiving patient teaching about phenytoin (Dilantin), a patient with epilepsy would indicate understanding of the teaching plan if he or she made which of the following statements?
① "I will expect to gain weight on Dilantin."
② "I will notify my physician if my gums bleed."
③ "I will stop the Dilantin if my urine turns pink."
④ "I can drive a car now that I'm on Dilantin."

297. The nurse observes the patient with a seizure disorder behaving as if he were partially unconscious and aimlessly picking at his clothing. The nurse knows these are symptoms of which characteristic seizure activity?
① Psychomotor
② Akinetic
③ Jacksonian
④ Myoclonic

298. What nursing assessment is most valuable in establishing the medical diagnosis of a patient with a history of two seizures a day for the last 3 days?
① A complete skull series of examinations
② A neurologic examination
③ Developmental health history
④ Complete blood cell count

299. An epileptic patient has a seizure, during which recurrent, generalized seizure activity is observed by the nurse. The nurse knows that this type of seizure is called:
① Grand mal
② Psychomotor
③ Petit mal
④ Status epilepticus

300. The nurse observes a patient having several seizures. The patient does not regain consciousness between the seizures. A primary nursing goal would be prevention of:
① Toxic disturbances
② Metabolic problems
③ Hypertension
④ Brain damage

301. A patient reporting increased epileptic seizure activity is concerned about driving a car. The nurse will inform the patient that most laws require:
① Driving only during daylight hours
② Evidence that seizures occur no more frequently than every 6 months
③ Evidence that seizures are under medical control
④ That the patient carry a medical identification card at all times

302. The nurse is teaching a patient with a seizure disorder about auras that are sometimes associated with seizures. The nurse will describe an aura as:
① Postseizure amnesia state
② Generalized feeling of relaxation
③ Hallucination during a seizure
④ Warning of impending seizure

303. The nurse knows that a typical postictal response after epileptic seizure activity is:
① Status epilepticus
② Headache
③ Reduced blood pressure
④ Kidney failure

304. Anticonvulsants are used in treating seizure disorders and are considered:
① Cholinergic blocking agents
② Central nervous system (CNS) stimulants
③ Antispasmodics
④ CNS depressants

305. Which of the following individuals is at greatest risk for a cerebrovascular accident (CVA)?
① 40-year-old male schoolteacher
② 35-year-old sedentary male manager
③ 55-year-old female with hypertension
④ 80-year-old female with renal disease

306. A patient states that early this morning his left leg became numb and he couldn't control it. He states that he feels fine now. He chews snuff regularly. He watches his blood pressure and his average pressure is 134/78. He likes to work in his garden. The nurse recognizes that the patient has which of the following treatable risk factors for a stroke?
① High blood pressure
② History of transient ischemic attack
③ Cigarette smoking
④ Sedentary lifestyle

307. A patient is being discharged from the hospital after recovering from a cerebrovascular accident (CVA). He ambulates with a walker and continues to exhibit an unsteady gait. Discharge considerations should include making a home environmental assessment of the following factors:
① Ability to reach cooking appliances, perform household tasks, and call 911
② Condition of automobile, presence of handicap tags, height of vehicle, and personal assistance when going out
③ Availability of community resources, volunteer help from church, and presence of significant others to assist in care
④ Poorly placed extension cords, presence of throw rugs, clutter, and width of hallways and doors

308. A patient has had an acute onset of seizure activity. What diagnostic test would the nurse expect to be performed first?
① Electroencephalogram (EEG)
② Electrocardiogram (ECG)
③ Magnetic resonance imaging (MRI)
④ Computed tomography (CT) scan

309. A stroke survivor is unable to walk because his gait is so unsteady and clumsy. The nurse recognizes this as:
① Otic
② Ataxic
③ Apneic
④ Aphasic

310. The patient has been hospitalized with a stroke. His entire left side has been affected. The nurse notes when she is removing his dinner tray that he did not eat any of the food on the left side of his tray. How can the nurse assist the patient with his tray?
① Remind him to eat all of the food on the tray
② Feed him the food on his tray
③ Move the food to the right side of the tray
④ Tell him what types of food are on the tray

311. To provide appropriate nursing care for a patient with multiple sclerosis, the nurse understands that this disease is characterized by:
① Seizures that last longer than 15 minutes
② Progressive degeneration of nerve cells caused by insufficient dopamine
③ Progressive degeneration of the myelin sheath of the brain and spinal cord
④ Attacks of vertigo and tinnitus with progressive hearing loss

312. Which of the following are included in a neurologic check using the Glasgow Coma Scale?
① Rate pain on a scale of 1 to 10
② Rate the ability to follow commands
③ Rate the changes in vital signs
④ Rate the level of orientation

313. When observing a patient with interference of motor nerve impulses, the nurse would note:
① Premonition or sign (aura) and a seizure lasting 1 to 2 minutes
② Loss of muscle tone, slurred speech, and paresthesia
③ Disorientation and drainage of cerebrospinal fluid from the ears and nose
④ Tremor and fingers having a "pill-rolling" movement

314. In planning the nursing care for a patient with multiple sclerosis, the nurse should encourage the patient to:
① Remain as active as possible without becoming fatigued
② Exercise all joints several times a day
③ Adapt to complete bed rest and antibiotic therapy
④ Maintain a low-calorie, low-protein, and low-fat diet

315. Nursing interventions for a patient hospitalized with multiple sclerosis should be directed toward:
① Assisting the patient with social and occupational activities
② Encouraging the patient to seek treatment that promises a cure
③ Increasing the patient's independence in self-care
④ Providing complete bed rest and breathing exercises twice a day

316. When teaching the patient and family members about multiple sclerosis, the nurse should include all of the following *except:*
① Drugs that stop the degenerative process
② Facts about the disease process
③ Ways to conserve energy and avoid fatigue
④ Drugs that the patient is taking to treat symptoms

317. To promote optimal functioning of a patient with Parkinson's disease, the nurse will recommend the following:
① Discussing current events with neighbors
② Building model airplanes
③ Playing bridge
④ Planting a vegetable garden

318. Which of the following goals are most appropriate and realistic in planning nursing care for a patient with Parkinson's disease?
① Preparing for terminal care
② Stopping progression of the disease
③ Maintaining optimal body functioning
④ Curing the disease

319. Nursing diagnoses for a patient with Parkinson's disease would include all of the following *except:*
① Alteration in comfort, resulting from the disease process
② Impaired physical mobility related to neuromuscular deterioration
③ Alteration in self-care ability: feeding, hygiene, and toileting
④ Knowledge deficit regarding the disease process

320. The medical term for hypersecretion of the growth hormone in adults is:
① Simmonds' disease
② Graves' disease
③ Gigantism
④ Acromegaly

321. When caring for a patient with hypersecretion of the growth hormone, the nurse should observe for which of the following?
① Coarse facial features; broad hands, fingers, and feet
② Headache, weakness, and visual disturbances
③ Symmetric overgrowth of the long bones of the body
④ Increased height (8 to 9 feet tall)

322. The primary nursing intervention in treating adult patients who have increased growth hormone is to:
① Observe for tetany: tingling of hands and feet, facial muscle spasms, and muscle twitching
② Explain the need for a diet high in calcium but low in phosphorus; instruct the patient to avoid milk, cheese, and egg yolks
③ Observe for adrenal crisis: falling blood pressure, tachycardia, elevated temperature, convulsions, and coma
④ Assist the patient to accept his altered body image by emphasizing his value as an individual

323. During the initial assessment of a patient with hyperthyroidism, the nurse will expect the patient to exhibit:
① Excitability
② Lethargy
③ Intolerance to cold
④ Anorexia

324. A patient has a subtotal thyroidectomy. In the immediate postoperative period, the patient should be kept in which of these positions?
① Flat in bed, without a pillow
② Side-lying, with the head of the bed elevated 15 degrees
③ Semi-Fowler's, with the head on a small pillow
④ Prone, with a small pillow under the head

325. In the postoperative room of the thyroidectomy patient, the most important thing the nurse should be sure to have at the bedside is a:
① Warmed blanket
② Padded tongue blade
③ Foley catheter setup
④ Tracheostomy set

326. When teaching a thyroidectomy patient about taking an iodine preparation at home, the nurse instructs the patient:
① To take it at bedtime
② To take it with a straw
③ To take it without diluting it
④ To take it first thing in the morning

327. The nurse knows that the following will be found in a patient with hyperthyroidism:
① A bruit in the carotid arteries
② A bruit over the thyroid
③ A low T_3 resin uptake
④ A high blood sugar level

328. A patient is admitted with hyperthyroidism. She is 30 pounds underweight even though she reports a "ravenous appetite." Her vital signs are pulse 136, respirations 32, blood pressure 190/96, and temperature of 100.2° F. An appropriate nursing diagnosis for the patient is:
① Alteration in nutrition: less than body requirements related to increased metabolic rate
② Alteration in nutrition: more than body requirements related to increased metabolic rate
③ Alteration in nutrition: less than body requirements related to decreased metabolic rate
④ Alteration in nutrition: more than body requirements related to decreased metabolic rate

329. In the early postoperative period, a thyroidectomy patient should be given which of these instructions?
① "Expectorate your saliva until you are able to swallow."
② "Range-of-motion exercises will prevent contractures."
③ "Do not turn your head from side to side."
④ "Deep breathe and cough every hour to avoid respiratory complications."

330. A patient has had a thyroidectomy. The nurse caring for this patient must remember that postoperatively the patient is:
① Restricted to fluid intake
② Cautioned not to cough
③ Placed in a prone position
④ Administered morphine frequently

331. After a thyroidectomy, a patient should be carefully observed for decreases in calcium levels. A sign of this would be:
① Muscle pain
② Dependent edema
③ Cold intolerance
④ Involuntary tremors

332. When caring for a patient with hyperthyroidism, the nurse is aware that the principal action of the iodine preparation just administered is to:
① Reduce the activity of the thyroid gland
② Increase production of thyroxin
③ Increase the activity of the thyroid gland
④ Increase the activity of the pancreas

333. In teaching a patient about hyperthyroidism, the nurse should also inform the patient that the condition is also known as:
① Myxedema
② Cretinism
③ Colloid goiter
④ Graves' disease

334. The nurse knows that the diagnostic test for T_3 resin uptake measures the functioning of which of the following glands?
① Parotid
② Parathyroid
③ Thyroid
④ Pituitary

335. In planning care for a patient with hyperthyroidism, the nurse knows hyperthyroidism exists when:
① The patient is lethargic
② Thyroxin blood level is high
③ Thyroxin blood level is low
④ Amount of thyroid hormone is unchanged

336. When caring for a thyroidectomy patient, the nurse should observe for which major complication associated with this type of surgery?
① Urinary retention
② Tetany
③ Shrill voice
④ Dehydration

337. When preparing an iodine preparation for oral administration to a thyroidectomy patient, the nurse should:
① Dilute it well
② Give it at bedtime
③ Give it whenever necessary
④ Give it the first thing in the morning

338. One of the major complications for the thyroidectomy patient is thyroid crisis. A major nursing priority would be to observe for:
① Increased pulse rate
② Decreased pulse rate
③ Slowed respirations
④ Subnormal temperature

339. When giving regular insulin, the nurse knows:
① Food must be taken at least 2 to 3 hours after the injection
② Regular insulin must be taken at least 1 hour after meals
③ Food must be taken approximately ½ hour after the injection
④ Regular insulin peaks in 8 hours; food must be taken at that time

340. The nurse knows that included in a self-care teaching plan for diabetics with the flu, cold, or minor gastrointestinal upsets would be the following recommendations:
① Self-care interventions are necessary only if vomiting and/or abdominal pain are present
② If you are not able to eat the usual foods, replace the foods with carbohydrates in the form of liquids or soft foods
③ Call your physician immediately
④ Hold your insulin and eat whatever you can keep in your stomach

341. Meal plans for the diabetic patient are generally made up of:
① 75% complex carbohydrates, 15% protein, and 35% fat; concentrated sweets are avoided
② 50% carbohydrates, 25% protein, and 20% fat; concentrated sweets are avoided
③ 55% to 65% carbohydrates, 12% to 15% protein, and 20% to 30% fats; concentrated sweets are avoided
④ 80% complex carbohydrates, 10% fats, and 12% protein; concentrated sweets are encouraged

342. The nurse will assess the patient with diabetic ketoacidosis for:
    ① Profuse diaphoresis
    ② Lethargy
    ③ Tremors
    ④ Tachycardia

343. A diabetic patient has seen his ophthalmologist, who has recommended laser surgery for his left eye. The nurse explains that laser surgery is frequently performed on patients with diabetes in order to:
    ① Reattach the retina
    ② Prevent the rupture of blood vessels
    ③ Increase the level of glucose in the vitreous humor
    ④ Restore color vision to the rods and cones

344. A diabetic patient has been experiencing problems with autonomic neuropathy. Which of the following would be associated with autonomic neuropathy in a diabetic?
    ① Anemia
    ② Hypokalemia
    ③ Impotence
    ④ Muscle cramps

345. The nurse explains to a patient who has been an insulin-dependent diabetic for more than 5 years that he should see an ophthalmologist:
    ① Quarterly
    ② Semi-annually
    ③ Yearly
    ④ Once every 5 years

346. The nurse will tell the diabetic patient that the signs of early diabetic peripheral neuropathy include:
    ① Color changes when the feet are dependent
    ② Numbness and tingling in the feet
    ③ Complaints of itching
    ④ Loss of fine motor skills

347. The diabetic patient is beginning to have problems with her eyes. The nurse recognizes that a late symptom of persistent hyperglycemia is:
    ① Blind spots
    ② Continual tearing
    ③ Eye pain
    ④ Blindness

348. The patient's health history includes insulin-dependent diabetes and mild hypertension. The patient's husband had always administered her insulin injection. She calls the office and asks the nurse, "What will I do now that my husband has died and can no longer give me insulin?" The best reply would be:
    ① "Don't you have another family member who could give you the insulin?"
    ② "You will need to come into the office for a check-up."
    ③ "I will come to your home this afternoon and show you how to self-administer the insulin."
    ④ "I'll try to find someone who might be able to help; I'll call tomorrow."

349. Which of the following instructions should be taught to the patient with diabetic proliferative retinopathy?
    ① Avoid the Valsalva maneuver
    ② Perform range-of-motion exercises on the eye daily
    ③ Use only hypoallergenic makeup
    ④ Wear sunglasses when outdoors

350. The patient who is taking insulin will be taught to check his blood glucose level:
    ① After strenuous activity
    ② Two hours after meals
    ③ Before his lunch
    ④ Before strenuous activity

351. The nurse will teach the patient with diabetes that an early symptom of hypoglycemia is:
    ① Flushed face
    ② Diploplia
    ③ Slurred speech
    ④ Hunger

352. The nurse will know that teaching has been effective when the patient states the primary organ involved in diabetes is the:
    ① Liver
    ② Ileum
    ③ Stomach
    ④ Pancreas

353. A patient states that he is afraid he will lose his job as a laborer because of his diabetes. The nurse's *best* response should be:
    ① "Don't worry about that now; there's time later to think about it."
    ② "Being a laborer is stressful. You'll have to get another job."
    ③ "You're surely eligible for unemployment benefits. Why not sit back and collect what is due you?"
    ④ "You seem concerned about your job. Do you want to talk about it?"

354. Diabetic education is an important aspect of patient care, and the nurse must remember to:
    ① Have answers to anticipated questions written out so she can read them to the patient
    ② Involve the patient in decision making concerning his or her care
    ③ Identify community resources available to the patient
    ④ Encourage involvement of family and significant others

355. The nurse would know that the patient understood how to use the diabetic food exchange list if which of the following foods was substituted for a serving of peanut butter?
    ① Fruit salad
    ② Hamburger
    ③ Tomato soup
    ④ Corn muffin

356. The patient has signs of early renal failure as a result of his diabetes and has enrolled in an exercise program to help maintain his weight. What effect does exercise have on renal functioning?
    ① It accelerates destruction of the renal cortex
    ② It reverses minor abnormalities in the kidney
    ③ It increases pressure within the nephron
    ④ It decelerates blood flow to the kidneys

357. Which of these statements, made by a patient with diabetes, indicates understanding of the relationship between exercise and insulin requirements?
① "When I exercise, I may need less insulin."
② "When I exercise more, I need more insulin."
③ "There is no change in the insulin requirement when exercise is increased."
④ "If I eat enough, I don't need to exercise or adjust my insulin."

358. A patient will be taking NPH insulin in the morning before breakfast and another smaller dose of NPH insulin at bedtime. The nurse should teach this patient that on this regimen, the most common times for a hypoglycemic reaction would be:
① Before breakfast and 1 hour after lunch
② Between 4 and 5 PM and during the night
③ 1 hour after breakfast and 1 hour after dinner
④ 1 hour after lunch and during the night

359. The nurse knows that the development of type II diabetes mellitus in middle-aged people is most directly related to which of these risk factors?
① A history of obesity
② Eating many sweets
③ An infection that doesn't heal
④ A history of polyria

360. The patient who has type II diabetes and takes glyburide (Micronase) 2.5 mg daily should be instructed to:
① Adjust glyburide according to her capillary blood glucose levels
② Exercise immediately following the ingestion of glyburide
③ Take glyburide in the morning after breakfast
④ Avoid drinking alcohol with the drug

361. The nurse is teaching a type II diabetic patient about the mechanism of action of oral hypoglycemic agents. Which of the following statements made by the patient would indicate understanding of the teaching plan?
① "The medication will replace my insulin."
② "The medication will help me digest glucose better."
③ "The medication will help me lose weight."
④ "The medication will help my pancreas produce more insulin."

362. The patient has been switched from oral diabetic agents to insulin once a day. She has cataracts and has difficulty reading the dosages on the syringe. Which of the following nursing interventions would help her avoid injecting an incorrect insulin dosage?
① Teach the patients's granddaughter how to administer the insulin
② Arrange to have the syringes pre-filled by the public health nurse
③ Advise the patient never to mix insulin
④ Advise the patient to continue to try to get an accurate dose

363. A patient is admitted to the floor with a nonhealing ulcer on her right foot. Laboratory studies reveal a blood sugar of 300. The nurse does the initial assessment and begins planning the nursing care. Which of the following would be the most important nursing diagnosis for this patient?
① Adjustment, impaired
② Activity intolerance
③ Skin integrity, impaired
④ Gas exchange, impaired

364. To control type II diabetes, the patient's priority goal would be to:
① Participate in a trial of insulin injections
② Achieve and maintain ideal body weight
③ Avoid carbohydrate-containing foods
④ Test her capillary blood sugar four times a day

365. When planning care for a patient with diabetes mellitus, the nurse knows that this condition:
① Interferes with the absorption of minerals
② Interferes with the absorption of vitamins
③ Involves a disorder in carbohydrate metabolism
④ Involves the pituitary gland

366. The nurse knows that a normal blood glucose level is:
① 50 to 75 mg/100 ml of blood
② 70 to 160 mg/100 ml of blood
③ 100 to 200 mg/100 ml of blood
④ 60 to 110 mg/100 ml of blood

367. In preparing to teach the diabetic patient about the drug tolbutamide (Orinase), the nurse knows that it is:
① An oral insulin
② A drug that does not have to be taken regularly
③ A hypoglycemic agent that lowers the blood sugar
④ A drug that can be given to all diabetic patients

368. The nurse knows that signs and symptoms of diabetic coma include:
① Cool, moist skin
② Rapid, shallow respirations
③ Increased blood pressure
④ Fruity odor to the breath

369. The nurse is teaching a patient with adult-onset diabetes. She tells him that:
① Diet, exercise, and oral hypoglycemic agents are indicated in adult-onset diabetes
② Diet, exercise, and insulin injections are needed
③ Insulin injections replace what the body doesn't produce
④ Major weight loss is necessary

370. The nurse will be alert for acidosis in the diabetic patient that is caused by:
① Too much insulin
② Too little insulin
③ The absence of ketone bodies
④ Overeating

371. The nurse should know that the two outstanding characteristic symptoms of diabetes mellitus are:
① Hypoglycemia and glycosuria
② Hyperglycemia and glycosuria
③ Hypoglycemia and hypokalemia
④ Hyperglycemia and glycogen

372. When a patient is diagnosed with diabetes mellitus, the nurse should observe for symptoms of impending diabetic coma. These symptoms include:
    ① Skin moist and pale, and extreme thirst
    ② Skin dry and pale, and extreme hunger
    ③ Skin dry and flushed, and extreme thirst
    ④ Skin flushed and moist, and anorexia

373. The nurse should understand that diabetic acidosis may occur as a complication of diabetes mellitus. This is caused by:
    ① Increased amounts of glucose in the blood
    ② Decreased amounts of glucose in the blood
    ③ The pancreas producing an excessive amount of insulin
    ④ The pancreas producing an excessive amount of pancreatic juices

374. If diabetic acidosis is left untreated, the nurse should expect which of the following symptoms to occur?
    ① Trembling sensation and profuse perspiration
    ② Decreased blood pressure and a fruity odor to the breath
    ③ Generalized muscle weakness and blurred vision
    ④ Tingling sensation of the lips or tongue, and headaches

375. The nurse who is caring for a diabetic patient knows that increased metabolism of fats and proteins caused by accumulated glucose and waste products would most likely manifest in the condition known as:
    ① Insulin reaction
    ② Hypoglycemia
    ③ Diabetic retinopathy
    ④ Ketoacidosis

376. Nursing assessment of a patient with Cushing's syndrome will include looking for signs of:
    ① Weight loss
    ② Skin breakdown
    ③ Low blood pressure
    ④ Hypoglycemia

377. One of the primary goals of nursing care of a patient with Cushing's syndrome should be that the patient:
    ① Consumes a high-carbohydrate, low-fat diet
    ② Increases fluids to 3 liters per day
    ③ Experiences increased mental stability
    ④ Gains weight of 2 pounds within 1 week

378. Discharge teaching for a patient with Cushing's syndrome includes:
    ① Avoiding foods with a high sodium content
    ② Maintaining a high-protein, low-calcium diet
    ③ Frequently shaving skin to prevent infection
    ④ Frequently monitoring urine and blood glucose levels

379. The nurse knows that Cushing's syndrome is caused by:
    ① Increased production of ACTH
    ② Decreased production of ACTH
    ③ Decreased production of insulin
    ④ Increased production of thyroid hormone

380. When assessing a patient with Cushing's syndrome, the nurse will expect to find:
    ① Hypotension and weight loss
    ② Anorexia and muscle weakness
    ③ Muscle weakness and osteoporosis
    ④ Moon face and hypotension

381. In planning care for a patient with Cushing's syndrome, the nurse's primary concern will be:
    ① Accurately recording intake and output
    ② Protecting her from infection
    ③ Testing the urine for sugar
    ④ Preparing her for surgery

382. The nurse knows that the adrenocorticotropic hormone (ACTH):
    ① Is secreted by the adrenal glands
    ② Is a factor that influences growth
    ③ Influences the activity of the cortex of the adrenal glands
    ④ Diminishes the function of the medulla of the adrenal glands

383. The priority postoperative nursing measure for a patient with an adrenalectomy is to:
    ① Observe for hemorrhage
    ② Prevent hypertension
    ③ Encourage fluid intake
    ④ Accurately record intake and output

384. In caring for a patient with an adrenalectomy, the nurse knows that an unavoidable sequela after surgery is:
    ① Addison's disease
    ② Hypoparathyroidism
    ③ Hyperparathyroidism
    ④ Simple goiter condition

385. For a patient with an adrenalectomy, discharge planning should include the recommendation to:
    ① Increase salt intake
    ② Avoid stress
    ③ Restrict activity
    ④ Administer insulin

386. When preparing the patient for a cystoscopic examination, the nurse explains that the purpose of the exam is to:
    ① Determine the size, shape, and location of the kidneys
    ② Visualize the prostate gland
    ③ Visualize the size of the ureters
    ④ Visualize the inside of the bladder

387. The nurse is teaching the patient with a neurogenic bladder as the result of insulin-dependent diabetes. Which of the following interventions should the nurse include in teaching the patient to manage her neurogenic bladder?
    ① Void at least every 4 hours
    ② Increase fluid intake to a gallon per day
    ③ Avoid eating spicy foods
    ④ Wear incontinence pads during the night

388. Which of the following types of diet should the patient with diabetic renal adenopathy be instructed on?
    ① A low-fat diet
    ② A low-sodium diet
    ③ A high-protein, low-carbohydrate diet
    ④ A low-protein, high-carbohydrate diet

389. The nurse anticipates that the physician will order which of the following diagnostic examinations to confirm that a renal calculus is lodged in a ureter?
① KUB
② Cystourethrogram
③ Cystometry
④ Proctoscopy

390. The patient has been treated for cystitis and is receiving the following medications: Bactrim, Pyridium, and oral contraceptives. The nurse collects a urine specimen for culture and sensitivity and notes that the urine has a reddish-orange color. Which of the following is the most appropriate nursing action?
① Report the finding to the doctor immediately
② Send the urine to the hospital for a more thorough study
③ Be unconcerned about the color
④ Check the specific gravity

391. The nurse knows that urine culture and sensitivity studies are done to:
① Analyze the elements present in the urine
② Determine if the urine contains evidence of malignant cells
③ Identify the organism causing the infection in the urinary tract
④ Localize the site of the inflammatory process in the urinary tract

392. The patient was admitted with urinary calculi and has an order to strain all urine. The nurse knows the urine is being strained so that:
① It can be tested for sugar
② It can be examined for bacteria
③ Minute stones and blood clots can be detected
④ The amount can be accurately measured

393. The nurse tells the patient the purpose of a cystoscopic exam is to:
① Catheterize the patient
② Visualize the inside of the bladder
③ Determine the location of the kidneys
④ Visualize the prostate

394. Following a cystoscopic examination, the nurse should examine the patient for:
① Level of consciousness
② Blood in the urine
③ Nausea and vomiting
④ Constipation

395. When preparing the patient for an intravenous pyelogram, what question is essential for the nurse to ask?
① Have you had this test before?
② Have you had a bowel movement today?
③ Do you have any allergies?
④ When did you last eat?

396. What should the nurse include in her discharge teaching to a patient who has had a transurethral prostatectomy (TURP)?
① Decrease your dietary fiber for the next 2 weeks
② Avoid sitting in hot tubs
③ Decrease your fluid intake for the next 2 weeks
④ Avoid vigorous exercise for the next 2 weeks

397. The doctor prescribed amitriptyline (Elavil) for the patient and cautioned her that this drug may cause her bladder to become overdistended and not empty completely. The patient spoke with her public health nurse regarding her recent tendency to dribble urine. The nurse explains to the patient that she is experiencing which type of incontinence?
① Functional incontinence
② Overflow incontinence
③ Stress incontinence
④ Urge incontinence

398. The patient is on the telephone when she suddenly has the urge to void. She abruptly concludes the phone call and begins the trip to the bathroom when she loses control of her bladder. This type of urinary incontinence is known as:
① Functional incontinence
② Stress incontinence
③ Overflow incontinence
④ Urge incontinence

399. The patient has had six children. When she feels the urge to sneeze, she quickly crosses her legs to prevent incontinence. Which type of incontinence is the patient experiencing?
① Functional incontinence
② Overflow incontinence
③ Stress incontinence
④ Urge incontinence

400. To obtain a 24-hour urine specimen, a patient should be given which of these instructions?
① Collect each voiding in separate containers for the next 24 hours
② For the next 24 hours, retain a 30-ml specimen of each voiding after recording the amount voided
③ Keep a record of the time and amount of each voiding for 24 hours
④ Discard the first voided specimen and then collect the total volume of each voiding for 24 hours

401. The most common x-ray examination procedure used to visualize the kidney and related structures is a(n):
① Cholecystography
② Cystography
③ Intravenous pyelogram
④ Retrograde pyelography

402. The nurse knows that the symptoms of renal calculi include:
① Dribbling at the end of urination and pyuria
② Severe flank pain and hematuria
③ Frequency of urination and dysuria
④ Urgent, uncontrollable urination and polyuria

403. If a patient is admitted with a diagnosis of renal calculi, which of the following should the nurse assess for during the admission procedure?
① Flank pain radiating to the testes
② Polyuria and thirst
③ Burning and frequency of urination
④ Painless hematuria

404. The nurse knows that the pain from renal calculi is referred to as:
① Floating kidney
② Nephrosclerosis
③ Hydronephrosis
④ Renal colic

405. When a patient is admitted with renal calculi, the nursing care plan should include:
① Limiting fluid intake
② Straining the urine
③ Limiting food intake
④ Maintaining bed rest

406. The physician orders hydromorphone (Dilaudid) 5 mg intramuscularly for pain for a patient with renal calculi. The nurse is preparing the medication and finds a multiple-dose vial that indicates hydromorphone 2 mg/ml for intramuscular use. How much hydromorphone should the nurse administer to the patient?
① 1.5 ml
② 2 ml
③ 2.5 ml
④ 5 ml

407. When caring for a postoperative patient, the nurse knows that the determining factor for advancing a diet from clear liquids to solid foods is:
① Recovering from the anesthesia
② Return of peristalsis
③ Discontinuing the IV
④ Absence of abdominal pain

408. When initiating dietary teaching for the patient with kidney stones, the nurse should advise limiting intake of which of the following foods?
① Meat, fish, and poultry
② Eggs, cheese, and milk
③ Plums, prunes, and cranberries
④ Vegetables, fruits, and carbohydrates

409. A patient must restrict calcium in his diet because of the development of calcium stones. He would demonstrate understanding of his dietary plan if he selected which of the following foods for lunch?
① Macaroni and cheese, green salad, and tea
② Broiled hamburger, roll, and steamed carrots
③ Yogurt, mixed fruit, and broccoli
④ Baked fish, spinach, and skim milk

410. The most common early symptom of a malignant bladder tumor is:
① Suprapubic pain
② Elevation of temperature
③ Painless hematuria
④ Dysuria

411. What symptom will the nurse expect the patient with an enlarged prostate to present with?
① Spasms of the bladder
② Abdominal tenderness
③ Flank pain
④ Urinary retention

412. The nurse would expect the patient with benign hypertrophy of the prostate gland to have:
① Hematuria with associated pain
② A persistent low-grade temperature
③ Perineal tenderness during bowel movements
④ Complaints of inability to void

413. The nurse is calculating urine output on a patient with a three-way urethral catheter attached to a continuous bladder irrigation system. The patient's intake is IV fluids 800 ml, irrigating solution 2000 ml, and amount of drainage in the Foley bag 3800 ml. His urine output should be documented as:
① 3800 ml
② 1800 ml
③ 1000 ml
④ 800 ml

414. A patient has had a transurethral prostatic resection (TURP). During a continuous bladder irrigation, the patient states that he feels like he has to void. The nurse's *first action* should be to:
① Explain to him that this is a normal sensation
② Manually irrigate the Foley catheter with 100 ml of irrigant
③ Palpate the bladder above the symphysis pubis
④ Report this to the team leader immediately

415. Following a transuretheral prostatectomy (TURP), the patient has a three-way Foley catheter with continuous bladder irrigations. He complains of pressure in his bladder and a need to urinate. What would the nurse do first?
① Check the patency of the catheter
② Irrigate the catheter
③ Empty the GU bag
④ Provide the patient a urinal

416. Several days after a TURP, the patient's urethral catheter is removed. To help the patient regain bladder control, the nurse will instruct the patient to:
① Drink 1500 ml of fluid daily
② Take a sitz bath twice a day
③ Do leg-raising exercises three times a day
④ Contract and relax the perineal muscles

417. The major problem experienced by a patient with a neoplasm of the prostate is:
① Urgency
② Frequency
③ Difficulty in urinating
④ Burning on urination

418. The nurse knows that neoplasm of the prostate most often occurs in men who:
① Have a high incidence of infection
② Are over 55 years of age
③ Have sedentary jobs
④ Are sexually inactive

419. A patient has had a suprapubic prostatectomy. In planning postoperative care for this patient, the nurse knows that the incision is made:
① Through the perineum
② In the urethra
③ Under the bladder
④ Over the bladder

420. Following a patient's surgery for a suprapubic prostatectomy, the nurse notes a suprapubic catheter was left in place. The nurse's *major* responsibility in caring for this patient is:
① Administering analgesics because this procedure is painful
② Limiting fluid intake to decrease output and facilitate healing
③ Frequently checking the amount, color, and consistency of urine from the catheter
④ Administering antibiotics

421. The nurse will plan to irrigate a suprapubic catheter when:
① The flow of urine decreases and there are blood clots in the tubing
② There are a few blood clots flowing through the tubing
③ Her judgment, with no specific times or indications, deems it to be appropriate
④ The patient asks for pain medication, which indicates problems with the catheter

422. After a suprapubic prostatectomy, the dressing must be changed frequently, because it becomes saturated with urine during a bladder spasm and the urine doesn't flow through the catheter. Because there is urine in the wound, the nurse should:
① Change the dressing without following clean technique
② Change the dressing following sterile technique
③ Leave the wound open and put an emesis basin by his side to catch the urine
④ Give him analgesics frequently to stop the spasm and flow of urine onto the abdomen

423. After a bilateral inguinal herniorrhaphy with a mesh graft reinforcement, the patient asks when he can eat. What is the *best response* by the nurse?
① "When you are able to 'pass gas.' "
② "The day after surgery."
③ "When bowel sounds are present in all four quadrants of your abdomen."
④ "When the IV fluids the physician ordered are finished."

424. A patient has not been able to void for 8 hours after his surgery. What is the *best* nursing intervention?
① Help him stand beside the bed to void
② Apply pressure over the bladder area (Credé's maneuver)
③ Catheterize him with a small catheter
④ Notify the physician

425. Which of the following instructions should the nurse include in the discharge teaching of a patient after his surgery for repair of bilateral inguinal hernias?
① Return to work after a 4- to 6-week recuperation period
② Remain on a soft diet, low in roughage, for 2 weeks
③ Avoid lifting objects heavier than a book for 4 to 6 weeks
④ Avoid bathing or showering until seeing the physician for a checkup

426. When the nurse takes the vital signs of a patient who has developed acute renal failure, she expects to find:
① A weak, thready pulse
② A low body temperature
③ Shallow respirations
④ An elevated blood pressure

427. A patient tells the nurse that he is having trouble breathing. The nurse should take which of these actions *first?*
① Determine the pulse rate
② Report this to the team leader
③ Elevate the head of the bed to high-Fowler's position
④ Instruct to breathe deeply

428. An external shunt is inserted into the left arm of a patient scheduled to have hemodialysis. The nurse should assess the patient for which of the following to ensure proper functioning of the external shunt?
① There is no bleeding at the site
② The arm is not edematous
③ A radial pulse is palpable
④ A bruit is audible

429. The nurse teaches a patient with renal failure about his low-protein diet. The patient would demonstrate an understanding of the protein content of food if he selected which of these desserts?
① Baked custard with caramel sugar
② Yogurt with fruit
③ Applesauce with raisins
④ Gelatin with whipped cream

430. A patient complains about dysuria and a purulent discharge from the penis. The physician suspects gonorrhea. To establish a diagnosis, the nurse knows the physician will order which of the following tests?
① Blood test
② Anal culture
③ Throat culture
④ Culture of penal discharge

431. When a 54-year-old patient asks the nurse how often a Pap test should be done, the nurse will respond:
① "Whenever you have irregular menstrual periods."
② "Annually for someone your age."
③ "Every 5 years until you are 40 years old."
④ "Every 3 years until you are 40 years old."

432. During a routine gynecologic examination, which of the following is the position of choice for a pelvic examination?
① Sims'
② Lithotomy
③ Trendelenburg's
④ Dorsal recumbent

433. The most effective nursing intervention in the prevention of the spread of infectious agents is:
① Wearing gloves for all patient contact
② Meticulous handwashing
③ Wearing a fluid-resistant cover gown
④ Maintaining strict surgical asepsis for all patient contact

434. When preparing a patient for a gynecologic examination, the nurse should:
    ① Have the patient empty her bladder
    ② Withhold meals before the examination
    ③ Restrict fluid intake for 24 hours before the examination
    ④ Encourage the patient to drink 500 to 1000 ml of fluid before the examination

435. A nurse is preparing to assist the physician in a gynecologic examination. The patient is 29 years old and has been taking birth control pills since she was 18. It is important for the nurse to know that a Pap test is done to:
    ① Determine ovarian functioning
    ② Measure the length of the cervix
    ③ Test the acidity level of vaginal secretions
    ④ Detect the presence of cervical cancer early

436. Which body organ is the most important for sexual arousal?
    ① Penis
    ② Female genitalia
    ③ Ovaries
    ④ Brain

437. The patient is describing extremely heavy bleeding during her menstrual period. Which of the following symptoms should the nurse document as part of an initial patient assessment?
    ① Amenorrhea
    ② Menorrhagia
    ③ Metrorrhagia
    ④ Dysmenorrhea

438. After a hysterectomy for uterine cancer, which will be followed by chemotherapy, the patient appears anxious and asks, "How will my husband feel about me now that I am half a woman and will soon have no hair?" Which of the following responses by the nurse is the *most appropriate?*
    ① "I wouldn't really worry about it. He's your husband, and I'm sure he loves you very much."
    ② "Would you like to discuss this matter with your physician?"
    ③ "Would you like me to sit for a while so we could talk about how you feel?"
    ④ "I can recommend a fine store that will design a wig for you."

439. Which of the following will the nurse include in a teaching plan for a patient being discharged after a radical hysterectomy?
    ① It is okay to resume normal sexual activity within 2 weeks
    ② It is recommended to resume all previous activities, even jogging
    ③ Physical activity should be limited to that which avoids strain
    ④ Heavy lifting is to be avoided for at least 12 months

440. A patient has symptoms of metrorrhagia and dyspareunia. A physical examination by the physician indicates endometrial-like cells growing elsewhere in the pelvic cavity. The nurse knows this condition is called:
    ① Endometritis
    ② Endometriosis
    ③ Endophthalmitis
    ④ Endamoebiasis

441. The patient who is preparing for her annual gynecologic examination tells the nurse that she is nervous and wants a nurse present during the examination. The *most appropriate* response by the nurse would be:
    ① "It is not necessary because the physician can be trusted."
    ② "I will stay with you during the examination."
    ③ "If you are nervous, you should ask your husband to stay with you."
    ④ "If you are nervous, you should see a therapist about your fears."

442. Early postoperative nursing care for a patient who has had a posterior colporrhaphy includes:
    ① Low-Fowler's position
    ② A regular diet
    ③ A stool softener
    ④ Enemas

443. The nurse's best explanation of cervical cancer, stage I would be:
    ① The cancer extends beyond the cervix but not beyond the pelvic wall
    ② The cancer is confined to the epithelium of the cervix
    ③ The cancer is completely confined to the cervix
    ④ The cancer involves the bladder and the rectum

444. The patient with toxic shock syndrome (TSS) has a temperature of 102° F, hypotension, diarrhea, impaired renal function, and hyperemia of the conjunctivae. Which of the following expected patient outcomes should the nurse consider a *priority* in planning care for this patient?
    ① Activity tolerance with a pulse rate increase of no more than 60
    ② Describes methods of practicing safe sex
    ③ Urine output returns to normal limits
    ④ Demonstrates increased knowledge of condition

445. Which of the following descriptions of the vaginal discharge is the nurse most likely to document for the possible diagnosis of candidiasis?
    ① White
    ② Grayish white
    ③ Thick, white, curdlike
    ④ Copious, frothy, greenish yellow

446. A patient's initial diagnosis is *Chlamydia trachomatis* infection, which is later confirmed by a culture. The patient is ordered to receive tetracycline and sees the nurse for counseling. While counseling this patient, the nurse should:
    ① Discuss infertility with the patient
    ② Suggest she share her medication with her partner
    ③ Explain the life-threatening aspects of the condition
    ④ Include information on prevention of recurrence of the infection

447. Which of the following recommendations by the nurse is vital in early detection of breast cancer?
    ① Ultrasonography
    ② Yearly mammogram
    ③ Breast self-examinations
    ④ Annual examinations by the physician

448. Following a radical mastectomy, the affected arm is elevated to facilitate circulation and prevent edema. When preparing the patient's environment, it is vital the nurse:
① Ensure complete privacy
② Maintain a dimly lighted room
③ Place the telephone on the side of the unaffected arm
④ Indicate that no injections or blood tests be done on the affected arm

449. After a modified radical mastectomy, the patient has a dressing over the surgical area. When checking the dressing for hemorrhage it will be necessary for the nurse to:
① Remove the uppermost layers of the dressing and observe for drainage
② Turn the patient q4h to check the dressing
③ Remove the entire dressing to observe the operative site
④ Feel with the hand under the patient's side and turn the patient to check for drainage

450. To facilitate proper positioning of the patient's arm after a modified radical mastectomy, the nurse will take which of these actions?
① Flex her left arm across her chest while she is in a semi-Fowler's position
② Abduct her left arm at least 8 inches and suspend it from a trapeze or IV pole
③ Place her left arm on pillows with her elbow higher than her shoulders and her wrist higher than her elbow
④ Keep her in high-Fowler's position with her hand on one pillow

451. As the nurse prepares to change a mastectomy patient's dressing for the first time, the patient begins to cry and says, "I can't bear to look at my ugly body." The nurse's *best* response would be:
① "Even though you feel disfigured now, you can always have reconstructive surgery."
② Say nothing, and change the dressing
③ "Everyone feels that way after a mastectomy. You'll get used to it."
④ "You're having a difficult time right now."

452. Discharge teaching is begun for a postmastectomy patient. Which of these instructions is important to include?
① Eat a diet that is high in carbohydrates and vitamin C
② Exercise the affected arm once a day
③ Avoid having blood pressure taken in the affected arm
④ Take frequent rest periods throughout the day

453. A patient had a positive mammogram and was referred to a surgeon for a biopsy. She did not keep her appointment. What defense mechanism is she using?
① Fantasy
② Rationalization
③ Denial
④ Projection

454. A nurse is teaching a patient how to do a breast self-examination. On return demonstration, which action by the patient would indicate understanding of the instructions?
① Raising her arms above her head and inspecting her breasts
② Putting a small pillow under her left shoulder when she examines her right breast
③ Lying on her side while she examines the breast
④ Keeping her right arm at her side while examining her right breast

455. The nurse knows that to promote healing of a decubitus ulcer, the proper intervention plan involves:
① Maintaining proper body alignment, supine position, with the bed in low the position
② Placing the patient in a wheelchair 4 hours each shift while assessing for discomfort frequently
③ Frequently changing position, keeping bed linens dry, gently massaging the affected area, and providing adequate nutrition
④ Preventing friction when moving, decreasing protein in the diet, and maintaining strict bed rest

456. During the physical assessment examination the nurse identifies a sacral decubitus that appears blistered and cracked. The lesion is correctly identified as a decubitus in which stage?
① Stage I
② Stage III
③ Stage IV
④ Stage II

457. The nurse is assessing a patient with severe burns. Most of her chest is burned, as well as her hands and the upper inner parts of her arms. On the basis of the rule of nines, what percentage of her body surface is involved?
① 26%
② 27%
③ 45%
④ 54%

458. An IV of 1000 ml Ringer's lactate was started on a patient with severe burns. The amount of Ringer's lactate solution the patient will receive will be based on:
① The percentage of body surface area that is burned relative to body weight
② The total amount of fluid the patient usually drinks in a 24-hour period
③ A standard amount of 4000 ml, which is given to all burn patients
④ The percentage of body surface that is burned

459. The primary reason for inserting a Foley catheter in a patient with severe burns is to:
① Avoid using the bedpan
② Avoid urinary incontinence
③ Measure the amount of urine in the bladder
④ Measure urine output hourly

460. A burn patient was placed on "reverse precautions." When the patient asks the nurse why this is necessary, the nurse's *most appropriate* response would be:
① "To prevent the spread of microorganisms to other patients"
② "To prevent potential exposure of microorganisms to hospital personnel"
③ "To protect visitors from exposure to microorganisms"
④ "To protect you from the transmission of microorganisms that may be present in the hospital"

461. The patient with severe burns is placed in isolation. Which of the following isolation techniques should the nurse be prepared to observe in the patient's hospital environment?
① Enteric precaution
② Drainage precaution
③ Protective isolation
④ Respiratory isolation

462. The nurse notes that a patient is to have a homograft. This type of skin graft is used primarily to help:
① Decrease pain at the burn sites
② Improve circulation at the burn sites
③ Prevent fluid loss from the burn sites
④ Stimulate growth of tissue at the burn sites

463. Meperidine hydrochloride (Demerol) was prescribed for a patient with second-degree burns. The nurse should know that the primary reason for this drug is to:
① Reduce anxiety
② Prevent nausea
③ Promote sleep
④ Relieve discomfort

464. Of the following combinations of foods, which has the highest protein content?
① Cheese cubes and peanuts
② Cheese spread and potato chips
③ Jello with cream, and a glass of milk
④ Popcorn with butter, and pretzels

465. The most common complication and cause of death in burn patients after the first 72 hours is:
① Heart failure
② Infection
③ Renal failure
④ Contractures

466. A team conference is held to discuss a burn patient's readiness for discharge. Major considerations for the patient should include:
① The degree of healing and scarring of the burns, as well as emotional and physical well-being
② The fact that the patient has pledged not to smoke in bed
③ The degree of return demonstration the patient exhibits changing the dressing
④ The degree of family involvement in patient care

467. The nurse knows that melanoma may be caused from exposure to which of the following types of radiation?
① Ionizing
② De-ionizing
③ Ultraviolet
④ Superviolet

468. The nurse has received an order from the physician to administer saline gtts ou q15″ × 8 doses to the patient. Where should the nurse apply the gtts?
① Right eye
② Left ear
③ Both eyes
④ Mouth

469. The diabetic patient has undergone laser surgery to prevent a hemorrhage into the left eye. As part of her discharge teaching, the nurse will tell the patient to:
① "Avoid getting anything in your eye."
② "Be careful climbing stairs."
③ "Avoid being near anyone with pinkeye."
④ "Avoid driving at night."

470. The physician has ordered the patient's left eye to be irrigated with normal saline. The nurse flushes the irrigant:
① From inner canthus to outer
② From outer canthus to inner
③ From upper lid to lower
④ From lower lid to upper

471. Which of the following eye problems is related to acute serum glucose changes?
① Cataracts
② Blurry vision
③ Conjunctivitis
④ Diplopia

472. Which of the following instruments will be used to examine the patient's ears?
① Ophthalmoscope
② Laryngeal mirror
③ Otoscope
④ Pomeroy syringe

473. As the physician prepares to examine the patient's throat, the nurse should have which of the following instruments ready for use?
① Schiøtz tonometer
② Laryngeal mirror
③ Ophthalmoscope
④ Otoscope

474. The patient tells the nurse that her vision has been blurry in the left eye and it seems to be getting progressively worse. She says, "It's like a film over my eye that I've had for 3 months, and I can't wipe it away." The nurse realizes this could be indicative of:
① Refractive errors
② Glaucoma
③ Retinal detachment
④ Cataracts

475. The nurse should recommend that patients having eye problems make an appointment to have their eyes examined. The most appropriate eye care professional should be a(n):
① Ophthalmologist
② Optometrist
③ Optician
④ Neurologist

476. When a patient under the age of 40 develops a cataract, the most probable causative factor is:
① Trauma
② Age
③ Weight
④ Job related

477. Which of the following will the nurse observe as signs and symptoms of an impending complication of cataract extraction?
① Nausea and vomiting
② Blurred vision and diplopia
③ Myopia and purulent drainage
④ Spots (floaters) and flashes of light

478. The patient with cataracts has difficulty seeing because the cataract is caused by:
① Increased intraocular pressure
② An opacity and clouding of the lens
③ A contagious infection of the eye
④ Retinal detachment

479. In postoperative teaching of the patient after cataract surgery the nurse will:
① Emphasize the need for bed rest for 3 months
② Emphasize the need to wear dark glasses at all times
③ Demonstrate how to instill eye drops
④ Demonstrate how to apply warm, wet compresses

480. The patient who is scheduled for cataract surgery tells the nurse that she is too old to go through a surgical procedure and hesitates to learn about her postoperative care. The nurse's response should be:
① "Oh, you're not too old! There's not that much to learn."
② "You'll be surprised how well you will do!"
③ "The physician and nursing staff will assist you!"
④ "You seem concerned about your surgery and your postoperative care. Do you want to talk about it?"

481. During cataract surgery for a 72-year-old woman, the surgeon implanted an intraocular lens in her right eye. The nurse should caution the patient to notify her or the physician of any complications such as:
① Sudden pain, erythema, drainage, or sudden visual change
② Flash of light, increase in "floaters," or blurred vision
③ A drooping eyelid
④ Blurred vision

482. During the admission process for a patient scheduled for cataract surgery, which of the following interventions is *not* necessary?
① Orient the patient to the room
② Speak in a louder voice than normal
③ Ask the patient what assistance he or she will need
④ Place the call light where the patient can find it

483. The patient had cataract surgery with a local anesthetic and sedation. Which of the following is an appropriate postoperative nursing action?
① Encourage coughing and deep-breathing exercises
② Not move the patient in bed. This patient should have complete bed rest
③ Administer medication promptly if nausea occurs
④ Not allow visitors in the room because they may disturb the patient's rest

484. How can the nurse best help the patient at mealtime following his return to the unit after cataract surgery?
① Feed him his meal
② Chop his food into small pieces
③ Allow him to manage the meal by himself
④ Orient him to where the food is on the plate

485. Which of the following *best* describes a glaucoma screening program?
① Color blindness evaluation
② Acuity testing with a Snellen chart
③ Tonometer used to detect increasing intraocular pressure
④ Obtaining a specimen for culture and sensitivity studies

486. The patient is being prepared for cataract surgery. The nurse should instill the eye drops:
① In the center of the eye
② Near the tear duct
③ On the upper conjunctiva
④ In the center of the lower lid

487. The nurse knows that the following will be used to check refraction errors in the eye:
① Ophthalmoscope
② Snellen chart
③ Otoscope
④ Tonometer

488. The nurse will identify glaucoma as the physiologic result of a(n):
① Increase in the vitreous humor fluid
② Increase in the intraocular pressure
③ Decrease in the aqueous fluid
④ Decrease in the intraocular pressure

489. The nurse knows that another name for closed-angle glaucoma is:
① "The sneak thief" glaucoma
② Preglaucoma
③ Acute glaucoma
④ Chronic glaucoma

490. The nurse knows that the occurrence of glaucoma is most often related to:
① Height
② Weight
③ Race
④ Age

491. The nurse is to prepare the patient for a glaucoma test. The instrument used to test for glaucoma is the:
① Ophthalmoscope
② Snellen chart
③ Otoscope
④ Tonometer

492. Which of the following statements made by the patient would indicate a symptom of open-angle glaucoma?
① "I have a greenish discharge from my eye."
② "I bump into people I don't see walking alongside of me."
③ "Sometimes I have pain in my eyes."
④ "My eyes have a reddened appearance sometimes."

493. A patient with glaucoma asks the nurse why he has to take the timolol maleate (Timoptic) eyedrops. The nurse will inform him that the medicine acts by:
① Dilating the pupil
② Promoting production of aqueous humor
③ Reducing muscle contractions of the eye
④ Decreasing the formation of aqueous humor

494. A glaucoma patient is taking timolol maleate (Timoptic) eyedrops and acetazolamide (Diamox). The two *most important* assessments for this patient would be:
① Blood pressure and electrolyte readings
② Apical pulse and serum drug levels
③ Urinalysis and blood pressure readings
④ Hemoglobin and hematocrit readings

495. A glaucoma patient indicates an understanding of discharge instructions by making which of the following statements?
① "I will avoid antihistamines for the treatment of a cold."
② "I will keep the affected eye patched at night."
③ "I will keep the lights dim so that I won't hurt my eyes."
④ "I will discontinue my medication if I feel well."

496. The nurse will expect the patient with a detached retina to report:
① Periorbital pain
② Flashes of light
③ Blurred vision
④ Rainbows around lights

497. The preoperative nursing care plan for a patient with a detached retina includes:
① Maintaining the patient on bed rest
② Having the patient cough every 2 hours
③ Irrigating the affected eye
④ Keeping one eye patched

498. The patient is immediately postoperative from a corneal transplant. The nurse will instruct the patient that the following activity may be done postoperatively:
① Sneeze
② Cough
③ Lift
④ Laugh

499. A patient is admitted with a diagnosis of Ménière's disease, which is:
① Characterized by recurrent episodes of vertigo, progressive unilateral nerve deafness, and tinnitus
② Acute disease of the inner ear
③ Most common in men who are 30 to 40 years of age
④ Diagnosed through specific blood tests

500. Which of the following factors is most related to the incidence of heat exhaustion?
① Gender
② Age
③ Activity
④ Weather

501. The physician suspects the patient's problem is heat exhaustion. Which of the following treatments should be completed by the nurse immediately?
① Administering oxygen
② Giving the patient a drink of an electrolyte solution
③ Loosening the patient's clothes
④ Elevating the patient's feet

502. Symptoms of heatstroke that the nurse will expect are:
① Double vision, nausea and vomiting, muscle incoordination, and dyspnea
② Muscle cramps; cool, pale, damp skin; tachycardia; and marked diaphoresis
③ Edema; discoloration of skin; blister formation; complaints of numbness, tingling, and burning of the skin
④ Hot, flushed, dry skin; hypotension; tachycardia; and hyperpyrexia

503. The nurse's aide reports a patient's blood pressure is 80/50. The nurse rechecks the blood pressure and obtains the same reading. The patient states that he feels fine; however, the nurse would:
① Call the physician immediately
② Check the blood pressure in the other arm
③ Ask another nurse to check the blood pressure
④ Document the blood pressure and retake it in 10 min

504. The patient was found comatose near his truck. His temperature is 106° F, and he has been diagnosed as having heat stroke. The nurse knows which of the following is the *most effective* method of heat reduction in the patient?
① Apply cool moist cloths to the forehead
② Apply ice to the groin, neck, and axillary areas
③ Put a fan near the patient's chest
④ Loosen the patient's clothing

505. Nursing interventions for a heatstroke should include:
① Removing constrictive clothing; providing warm soaks; and if conscious, giving warm liquids
② Ensuring adequate airway and ventilation, administering quick-acting carbohydrates, and recording vital signs
③ Maintaining adequate airway, breathing, and circulation; providing rapid cooling; and administering oxygen, if prescribed by a physician
④ Making sure the patient is in a cool area, giving salt water if the patient is conscious and not vomiting, and relieving muscle cramps

506. The patient's blood pressure is 80/50, pulse is 140/min, and respirations are 24/min. Her skin is cool and clammy, and she is bleeding from a large laceration across the top of her head. Which of the following types of shock would the patient most likely be experiencing?
① Hypovolemic
② Cardiogenic
③ Neurogenic
④ Septic

507. The patient is in critical condition as a result of blood loss due to an accident. Which of the following is *not* recommended in the initial treatment of the patient's hypovolemia?
① Control of bleeding at the source
② Administration of oxygen
③ Fluid replacement
④ Cleansing of the wound

508. The patient's hypovolemic condition has been improving. The nurse recognizes which of the following as objective criteria for clinical improvement?
① Continued mental disorientation
② Urine output of 25 ml/hr
③ Blood pressure of 88/46 mm Hg
④ Radial pulse of 74 beats/min

509. The physician has ordered an antihistamine to be given immediately to treat a patient's allergic reaction to an insect bite. In this situation, the emergency room nurse will expect which of the following drugs to be administered?
① Ephedrine
② Epinephrine
③ Neosynephrine
④ Hydroxyzine (Vistaril)

510. Emergency room nurses are always vigilant for a severe, allergic, systemic reaction to a foreign substance, which could cause a condition known as:
① Psychogenic shock
② Neurogenic shock
③ Cardiogenic shock
④ Anaphylactic shock

511. Which of the following symptoms will indicate to the nurse that the patient is in danger of anaphylactic shock?
① Increased pulse rate and drop in blood pressure
② Decreased pulse rate and increase in blood pressure
③ Sensation of being hot and feverish
④ Increased respiratory rate

512. When a patient who has been in good health suddenly experiences a sharp pain in the midsternal area, radiating down the left arm, and nausea, what is the most common patient response to chest pain?
① Dialing 9-1-1 immediately
② Lying down and delaying calling for help
③ Calling the physician
④ Ignoring the pain and continuing to work

513. The nurse knows that the immediate rescuer response to a patient experiencing chest pain should be which of the following?
① Walk with the patient to help him or her remain conscious
② Start CPR before the patient's heart stops beating completely
③ Put the patient in the car and drive to the hospital immediately
④ Keep the patient at rest and call 9-1-1

514. The nurse's first consideration when a patient has a cardiac arrest is:
① Airway
② Breathing
③ Circulation
④ Definitive therapy

515. A patient's heart rate is 100 to 160 beats/min, rhythm is regular, the P waves are normal, the P-R interval is normal, the QRS is normal. The nurse in the emergency room should interpret this rhythm as:
① Complete heart block
② Atrial fibrillation
③ Sinus tachycardia
④ Sinus bradycardia

516. Concerning emergency procedures, the nurse must know that elective cardioversion is a procedure performed by the physician to:
① Restore ventricular function
② Decrease the work of the right ventricle
③ Terminate heart block
④ Terminate rapid dysrhythmias

517. The first choice of treatment for ventricular fibrillation is:
① Emergency administration of IV atropine
② Immediate defibrillation
③ Endotracheal intubation
④ Cardioversion

518. When an electrocardiogram is done on a patient with severe chest pain, the nurse knows that this test:
① Records the flow of blood through the heart
② Measures the strength of the heartbeats
③ Records the activity of the heart muscle
④ Measures the rate at which oxygen is used

519. The patient with a diagnosis of coronary occlusion is very apprehensive and expresses fear of dying. Her husband asks the nurse why the patient is feeling this way. The nurse's *best* response should be:
① "Your wife realizes she had a heart attack and that it is probably serious."
② "This reaction is not unusual for patients with a heart attack, and she needs reassurance."
③ "So many people die when they have this condition. It's typical."
④ "Your wife's heart attack probably affected her mind, so don't worry."

520. In providing appropriate nursing care to patients with cardiac disease, it is helpful for the nurse to understand that arteries supplying heart muscle tissue receive their oxygenated blood from the:
① Ascending aorta
② Left subclavian artery
③ Carotid arteries
④ Intercostal arteries

521. During a team conference, patient data are reviewed as a means of planning care. Of the following, which indicates myocardial damage?
① Decrease in heart rate
② Elevated cardiac enzyme levels
③ Severe cyanosis
④ Decreased cardiac enzyme levels

522. To protect a rape victim, what is the most important measure the nursing staff should follow?
① Personally take evidence to the laboratory
② Obtain an account of what happened in the patient's own words
③ Do not allow people around the patient
④ Arrange for the patient to be escorted home by someone she trusts

523. In the emergency room, a physical examination of the rape victim is recommended for early detection of:
① Dysuria
② Dysmenorrhea
③ Pregnancy
④ Venereal disease

524. A 70-year-old man is admitted to the hospital with a diagnosis of drug toxicity. His nurse remembers that medication effects are significantly different in the elderly. The rationale(s) for medication reaction differences in the elderly are based on:
    ① The effects of aging such as alteration of absorption/metabolism, structural and physiologic changes, diminished immune system, and polypharmacy
    ② The effects of aging such as forgetfulness, expense of medications, greater reliance on faith healing, and decreased libido
    ③ Decreased renal and central nervous system function
    ④ Decreased renal and musculoskeletal system function

525. When providing nursing care for elderly people in institutions, which of the following is a major consideration?
    ① Providing personal hygiene
    ② Eliminating all patient responsibilities
    ③ Fostering social privacy
    ④ Making decisions for the patient

526. The nurse knows the importance of assessing hydration status in an elderly person because dehydration can occur when:
    ① The body is unable to excrete sufficient amounts of sodium
    ② There is inadequate food or fluid intake
    ③ The kidneys are unable to excrete wastes normally
    ④ The bladder is unable to hold urine

527. The nurse knows changes in the elderly that translate into a greater risk of adverse drug reactions are:
    ① An increase in total body water, decreased muscle mass, and a decrease in body fat
    ② A decrease in total body water, increased muscle mass, and an increase in body fat
    ③ An increase in total body water, increased muscle mass, and increased body fat
    ④ A decrease in total body water, a decrease in muscle mass, and an increase in body fat

528. A patient is admitted to the nursing home with Alzheimer's disease. Which one of the following will be most important for immediate nursing care?
    ① Offer balanced meals and feed the patient
    ② Be sure the patient cannot leave the building
    ③ Keep a recent picture of the patient on the patient's door
    ④ Keep restraints on the patient at all times

529. The nurse is caring for a newly admitted geriatric patient. The patient tells the nurse that she has had nothing to eat this entire day. The nurse saw her eating lunch earlier. Which of the following explain the client's neurologic deficit?
    ① Recent memory loss is common
    ② Memory loss for past events is common
    ③ Medication has dulled her memory
    ④ She is hungry

530. The nurse knows that the greater the number of medications taken, the greater the risk of drug interactions and adverse drug reactions in the elderly. Identify those factors that contribute to polypharmacy in the elderly:
    ① Inexpensive cost of medications, use of primary care physicians, and decreased use of over-the-counter products
    ② Availability of medications, changes in patient expectation, use of multiple physicians, and changes within the health care system
    ③ Co-morbidities, decreased availability of medications, lack of education regarding medications, and increased use of over-the-counter products
    ④ The elderly are more likely to seek second opinions and seek medical assistance as soon as symptoms appear

531. The nurse is caring for an elderly, bedridden client who receives continuous full-strength tube feeding. What complication is most common?
    ① Nausea
    ② Diarrhea
    ③ Constipation
    ④ Abdominal pain

532. The cardinal rule the nurse will follow when administering medications in the elderly is:
    ① To achieve the maximum therapeutic benefits while giving the smallest necessary amount of medication
    ② To achieve the minimum therapeutic benefits while giving the largest amount of medication
    ③ To achieve minimum therapeutic effects while maximizing dosage strength
    ④ To follow the physician's orders

533. One of the most common myths associated with aging is that:
    ① The majority of elderly people reside in their own home
    ② Most elderly people have at least one chronic condition
    ③ All people become senile when they become old
    ④ Most elderly people are isolated and alone, averaging one weekly contact with family

534. Which of the following is *not* a common myth associated with aging?
    ① All people become senile when they become old
    ② Most older people are not isolated and alone
    ③ Most elderly are in nursing homes or care facilities
    ④ Old people are ill and disabled

535. To meet the Health Care Financing Administration (HCFA) mandates, nursing homes throughout the country have developed the Minimum Data Set (MDS) for Nursing Home Resident Assessment and Care Screening, and 18 Resident Assessment Protocols (RAPs) for problem identification. The MDS is a tool regarding resident care that:
    ① Has added a great deal of paperwork to caring for the elderly
    ② Provides a simple list of problems that a nurse uses to assess each resident
    ③ Is a functionally based assessment tool identifying pertinent information needed to develop a comprehensive care plan
    ④ Is the same for all states

536. Nursing home administrations developed 18 Resident Assessment Protocols (RAPs) for problem identification. The RAPs specify "trigger" definitions that:
① Have added a great deal of paperwork to caring for the elderly
② Provide a simple listing of problems that a nurse uses to assess each resident
③ Are the same as the MDS
④ Explicitly suggest specific care that requires implementation

537. HCFA received a federal mandate through the Omnibus Budget Reconciliation Act (OBRA) to ensure that the MDS and RAPs systems are implemented. These requirements are for:
① All long-term care facilities participating in Medicare or Medicaid programs
② All long-term care facilities participating in Medicare programs
③ All long-term care facilities participating in Medicaid programs
④ For everyone covered by Medicare, Medicaid, and private insurance plans

538. OBRA requires that each assessment be conducted or coordinated by:
① Any staff members directly caring for the resident
② Any licensed persons
③ Only registered nurses
④ Any staff members caring indirectly for the resident

539. The nurse documents the following on the chart of a 56-year-old patient: "Speaks frequently of his children being 'all grown up' and being at home all alone with his wife. States he has always cared for his wife, has never been sick for any length of time, and is concerned about loss of his job because of illness." From this statement the nurse should conclude that the patient is:
① Having trouble adjusting to the hospital and will need help from a social worker
② Too concerned about his wife and should be more concerned about himself
③ Demonstrating the normal characteristics of middle adulthood and the demands of illness
④ Demonstrating pity for himself and does not want to admit that he is getting older

540. Of the following methods of charting, which one *best* describes the recording of events as they occur throughout the day?
① Narrative charting
② SOAP charting
③ Focus charting
④ PIE charting

541. In SOAP charting, the S is best represented by which of the following entries?
① WBC count is elevated
② Patient says, "I feel better today."
③ Temperature is 102.8° F (39.3° C)
④ Incisional line is well approximated

542. In most agencies, the use of a pencil to record patient information is acceptable on which of the following documents?
① Flow sheet
② Discharge summary
③ Medication record
④ Kardex

543. Which of the following documentation provides the *most* objective information about the patient's neuromuscular status?
① Limited response to painful stimuli
② Decreased strength of the lower extremities
③ Confused at intervals; lethargic most of the time
④ Not able to grip nurse's hand with right hand, but strong grip with left hand

544. Which of the following barriers to communication is being demonstrated by a nurse who says to a patient, "There, there . . . don't worry. Everything will turn out for the best."
① Disagreeing with the patient
② Offering a cliché as an expression of reassurance
③ Belittling the patient's feelings
④ Giving approval

545. When the nurse tried to assist the patient with his bath, the patient became adamant and stated that he was not used to bathing every day and did not want a bath this morning. Which of the following would be the *best* response by the nurse?
① "All of our patients are bathed every day. I'll help you so it won't take long."
② "I'll have the supervisor come and explain why you must bathe every day."
③ "I'll give you a moist cloth to wash your hands and face."
④ "I'll call the doctor and tell him you won't bathe."

546. As the nurse prepares the patient for surgery, the patient makes the comment "I don't want to have surgery now. I've changed my mind." Which of the following would be the *best* action by the nurse?
① Realize that the patient has been premedicated and probably doesn't know what she is saying
② Explain to the patient that the surgery must be done and send her to the operating room
③ Cancel the surgery and reschedule for the following week
④ Discuss with the patient the reason for the statement; then call the surgeon if the patient still doesn't want the surgery

547. The patient has come to the hospital for chemotherapy treatments to begin in the morning. As the nurse is assisting him with evening care, the patient states, "I don't think my doctor knows what he is doing." Which of the following would be the *best* response by the nurse?
① "Your doctor is very knowledgable."
② "Why do you think the doctor doesn't know what he is doing?"
③ "If I were you I would switch doctors if I felt like that."
④ "You don't believe your doctor is capable?"

548. While being prepared for a sigmoidoscopy because of suspected cancer of the colon, a patient asks, "Am I going to die?" The nurse's response should be:
① "It is too early to tell."
② "Do *you feel* you're going to die . . .?"
③ "Oh, don't say things like that."
④ "Have you discussed this with your family?"

549. Which of the following is an example of a communication technique that *best* expresses the nurse's interest in what the patient has to say?
① Maintaining direct eye contact with the patient during the interaction
② Sharing several personal experiences with the patient
③ Smiling throughout the interaction
④ Providing privacy so that the patient's concerns will not be overheard

550. A patient about to be admitted to the coronary care unit after experiencing chest pain says to the nurse, "I don't know what all the fuss is about. I'm sure this is just a bad case of indigestion." Which coping mechanism is this patient demonstrating?
① Rationalization
② Regression
③ Denial
④ Compensation

551. The nurse notes that a male patient who has had a stroke has expressive aphasia. A plan is developed to help him communicate his needs more effectively. Which nursing intervention is *most* appropriate?
① Associate words with physical objects
② Inform the family that he cannot communicate
③ Immediately correct any of his mispronounced words
④ Anticipate his needs to minimize efforts at talking

552. Which of the following diagnostic tests would be *excluded* in establishing a diagnosis for a patient who exhibits symptoms of stomach cancer?
① Cholecystogram
② Gastroscopy
③ Fluoroscopy
④ Gastric analysis

553. The nurse knows that when a serum blood urea nitrogen (BUN) test is done, BUN is:
① Elevated in renal failure
② Lowered in renal failure
③ Not related to kidney disease
④ Not a very significant test to measure kidney function

554. Which of the following enzyme studies are *most* specific for measuring cardiac damage?
① SGOT, SGPT
② CPK, SGPT
③ CK-MB, isoenzymes LDH_1 and LDH_2
④ CH, CPT

555. The nurse will tell the patient that early renal damage is detected by the presence of which of the following lab abnormalities?
① An elevated BUN
② An elevated hemoglobin
③ Proteinuria
④ Ketonuria

556. The nurse collects a clean-catch urine specimen on the patient. She then checks the pH and specific gravity on the urine before sending it to the lab. As the nurse is documenting the procedure, which of the following descriptions of the urine displays a potential abnormal urine specimen?
① Clear, straw-colored urine
② pH of 6.0
③ Specific gravity of 1.015
④ Ammonia smell to the urine

557. The nurse recognizes that which of the following lab tests is specific for pancreatitis?
① Serum glucose
② Glycosylated hemoglobin
③ Blood urea nitrogen
④ Serum amylase

558. The patient is SOB, has tachypnea of 40/minute, and reports respiratory difficulty for the past 4 hours. Blood gases are drawn. Which of the following will be the most likely result of the ABGs?
① Respiratory alkalosis
② Normal pH
③ Respiratory acidosis
④ Metabolic alkalosis

559. When administering a cleansing enema, the nurse will place the patient in which of the following positions?
① Prone
② Supine
③ Left Sims'
④ Right Sims'

560. The nurse's aid reports to the nurse that the patient's bedpan was accidentally emptied and the urine was not saved in the 24-hour collection container. Since the 24-hour collection was started 6 hours earlier, the nurse should:
① Continue with the specimen collection, making a note in the chart
② Start the collection over, obtaining a new container and making a note in the chart
③ Start the collection over, using the same container and adding to the urine already collected
④ Stop the collection and wait to start a new specimen the next morning

561. The nurse knows that the burning and gnawing sensation in the stomach associated with duodenal ulcers is known to:
① Be constant
② Be more severe when eating
③ Occur 2 hours before meals
④ Occur 2 hours after meals

562. The patient needs to be catheterized for residual urine. During the procedure, the nurse notes resistance to the catheter at the external urinary meatus. Which of the following actions is the *most appropriate* for the nurse to implement?
① Ask the patient to cough several times
② Remove the catheter, then try again
③ Have the patient take several deep breaths
④ Pull back the catheter, then push forward again

563. Urine that remains in the bladder after a person voids is called:
① Reflex incontinence
② Residual urine
③ Urge incontinence
④ Retention urine

564. Which of the following procedures would be appropriate for the nurse in obtaining and measuring a patient's residual urine?
① Empty the collection receptacle and record the amount q8h
② Remove the retention catheter and measure the amount the patient voids
③ Have the patient void and then catheterize her immediately, measuring the amount obtained from the catheterization
④ Instruct the patient to void, and then wait 2 hours and have her void again

565. When collecting a routine urine sample, the nurse should instruct the patient to:
① Completely fill the container
② Void 50 to 100 ml of urine
③ Add a few drops of water to the empty container
④ Use a sterile container

566. Two days after an appendectomy, the patient complains of nausea, shortness of breath, and light-headedness. The nurse's *first* action should be to:
① Notify the nurse in charge
② Take his vital signs and report them along with his symptoms
③ Wait a short time to see if he is feeling better
④ Inspect the abdominal dressing

567. A patient with a myocardial infarction complains of constipation. The nurse knows that the physician will most likely order:
① Fleet enema
② Saline solution
③ Oil-retention enema
④ 1500 ml soap solution

568. The patient recovering from general anesthesia after surgery is given oxygen to promote tissue perfusion. What is the best method of oxygen administration for the patient?
① Nasal cannula with the O_2 flow rate set at 1 to 4 L/min
② Face mask with the O_2 flow rate set at 6 to 12 L/min
③ Oxygen tubing held by his face with the O_2 flow rate set at 6 to 12 L/min
④ Deep breathing exercises with a paper bag

569. To help the patient correctly use the incentive spirometer, the nurse should:
① Encourage the patient to cough to remove as much mucus as possible before the treatment
② Have the patient breathe as rapidly as possible during the treatment
③ Have the patient lie flat in the side-lying position to use the spirometer
④ Ask the patient to use the spirometer only when he thinks he is able

570. When a dressing on a Penrose drain near the incision site becomes wet during the patient's bath, what is the *best* method for the nurse to use during the dressing change?
① With sterile gloves, remove the dressing layers all at once to avoid contaminating the wound
② With clean, nonsterile gloves, remove the dressing one layer at a time
③ With sterile gloves, remove only the outer dressing and apply additional gauze pads
④ Gloves are not needed as long as the gauze for the dressing change is not touched

571. The patient has been admitted for surgery for an aortic aneurysm. The surgery is to occur in 48 hours. The patient and her husband speak only Spanish. Which of the following would be the most immediate nursing intervention?
① Give preoperative medication
② Find an interpreter
③ Give an enema
④ Get a medical history

572. During a dressing change, the nurse observes the patient and the incision site for any signs of infection. Which of the following signs should the nurse report to the surgeon?
① An oral temperature of 99.2° F on the first postoperative day
② A small amount of clear, yellow exudate at the edges of the incision
③ Redness and swelling around the incision
④ A sudden drop in blood pressure on the day of surgery

573. Which of the following postoperative nursing measures will best help the nurse assess a patient for postoperative complications?
① Allowing bed rest for as long as the patient feels the need
② Removing the elastic stockings during the morning bath and reapplying them at bedtime
③ Dorsiflexing the patient's foot and evaluating the patient for lower leg pain
④ Rubbing the patient's lower leg as a response to any complaints of leg cramps

574. The nurse is providing a sitz bath for the patient. The nurse knows to establish the temperature of the water at:
① 75° to 80° F (23.8° to 26.6° C)
② 85° to 90° F (29.4° to 32.2° C)
③ 100° to 105° F (37.7° to 40.5° C)
④ 120° to 125° F (48.8° to 51.6° C)

575. Peer assistance programs are present in most states to assist nurses who are impaired by either alcohol or drugs. The goals of the peer assistance program include all the following *except:*
① To assist the nurse who is impaired to receive treatment
② To protect the public from the untreated nurse
③ To assist the nurse in pursuing other vocational options
④ To assist the nurse in monitoring continued recovery for a period of time

576. While transferring a patient with an indwelling catheter from the bed to the chair, the nurse should:
① Place the Foley bag on the overbed table
② Place the Foley bag in the patient's lap
③ Disconnect the Foley bag and clamp the tubing
④ Hang the bag on the side of the chair, below the bladder

577. While suctioning secretions from a tracheostomy, the nurse will follow which of the following procedures?
① Oxygenate, suction for 30 seconds, oxygenate
② Oxygenate, suction for 15 seconds, cough and deep breathe
③ Oxygenate, suction for 10 seconds, oxygenate
④ Oxygenate, suction for 25 seconds, allow to rest

578. The patient underwent surgery this morning for a tracheostomy. While caring for the tracheostomy, the nurse notes that the tracheostomy tube has an inflatable cuff. The nurse knows the purpose of this cuff is to:
① Prevent aspiration
② Prevent bleeding
③ Improve oxygen exchange
④ Prevent accidental removal

579. The nurse knows that food selection for dysphagia patients will be based on:
① Food consistency
② Patient preference
③ Hospital availability
④ Physician's order

580. The patient is admitted with confusion and headaches. As the nurse begins to formulate a plan of care, which of the following would be a priority in the patient's care over the next several days?
① Teach the patient the importance of daily foot care
② Teach the patient how to take all medications as ordered
③ Keep the side rails up and monitor the patient closely
④ Post a sign on the door indicating no visitors

581. An elderly patient fell while trying to get out of bed. The nurse is preparing to fill out an incident report. Which one of the following is the best reason for filling out the incident report?
① To document the occurrence for the patient chart
② To prevent lawsuits
③ To prevent a recurrence
④ To refresh the nurse's memory should legal action occur

582. As the nurse prepares the patient for surgery, he notices that the patient has not signed the operative consent form. After discussing the problem with the surgeon, the nurse sends the patient to surgery anyway. What could be the result of this action?
① An invasion of privacy charge
② A *res ipsa loquitor* charge
③ A corporate negligence charge
④ An assault and battery charge

583. The patient has received all her preoperative preparation, including a preop medication of Versed 2 mg. While checking her chart before sending her to surgery, the nurse notes that the operative consent has not been signed. What would be the best action by the nurse?
① Notify the surgeon so the case can be canceled
② Have the patient's husband sign the consent
③ Have the patient's children sign the consent
④ Have the patient sign her own consent

584. The nurse working in public health is responsible for teaching and evaluating health promotion techniques. Which of the following would best show that the patient has learned?
① The patient repeats after the nurse the directions given
② The patient watches a video on the topic
③ The patient makes lifestyle changes
④ The patient asks meaningful questions

585. The 45-year-old patient has come to the physician's office complaining of excessive weight loss in a very short time. She has also been experiencing fatigue and lack of appetite. As the nurse completes the assessment process, she suspects the patient may be suffering from:
① Anorexia nervosa
② Tuberculosis
③ Gastric ulcer
④ Cancer

586. Which of the following actions indicates the nurse is practicing nursing according to the Controlled Substance Act?
① The nurse checks the nameband of the patient before administering the narcotic
② The nurse examines the label of the medication twice before administering the narcotic
③ The nurse documents the administration of the narcotic on the medication administration record
④ The nurse documents the removal of the narcotic from the locked cupboard

587. The nurse is caring for a 75-year-old woman who is suffering from sensory deprivation. Which of the following nursing actions will be *most* appropriate?
① Place a clock in the room
② Limit visitors
③ Do morning care quickly
④ Remove hearing aids

588. The patient has become hostile and aggressive and has attacked a nurse. He has just been placed in restraints. The nurse knows it is important to:
① Check the restraints once during each shift
② Check that the restraints are secured tightly
③ Have all available staff in the patient's room
④ Remove the restraints as soon as the patient regains control

589. The patient returned from surgery 6 hours ago. She has not voided since her return to the room. The nurse knows the first thing she should do is:
① Administer a narcotic for pain
② Insert a Foley catheter
③ Institute simple measures to help the patient void
④ Reposition the patient

590. Simple measures to stimulate urination have failed, and the patient is now 8 hours postop and has not voided. The nurse will next:
① Administer a narcotic for pain control
② Get the patient up to ambulate
③ Wait to do something until at least 12 hours postop
④ Call the physician for an order to catheterize the patient

591. "Adults over the age of 30 frequently gain weight." Which of the following is the *best* explanation for this statement?
① Basal metabolic rate declines each decade
② Physical activity declines
③ Food intake increases
④ Carbohydrate and fat content increases

592. Which of the following would best indicate the patient has hypernatremia?
① Thirst, increase in body temperature
② Muscular twitching, cramping
③ Cardiac arrhythmia, palpitations
④ Numbness, tingling of the fingers

593. Which of the following patients would be most at risk for hypothermia during and following surgery?
① A 10-year-old child
② A 40-year-old man
③ A 20-year-old woman
④ An 80-year-old woman

594. The nurse will encourage the patient with COPD (chronic obstructive pulmonary disease) to lean forward over the tray table with a pillow placed on it to facilitate his breathing. This position is known as:
① Sims'
② Lithotomy
③ Orthopneic
④ Supine

595. The obese patient is predisposed to a multitude of physiologic dysfunctions. Obesity predisposes the patient to which of the following?
① Hypertension, hypoxia, and osteoarthritis
② Hypotension, asthma, and decreased heart rate
③ Hypovolemia, hypertension, and hypoglycemia
④ Hypervolemia, hypertension, and hypothermia

596. A patient recently suffered a CVA and has right-sided hemiplegia. He is noncompliant with his physical therapy. Which of the following nursing interventions would the nurse initiate to prevent immobility?
① Insist that the patient participate with the therapist twice daily
② Ambulate the patient to the bathroom before meals and at bedtime
③ Refer the patient to the social worker for follow-up
④ Allow the patient to participate in activities from his wheelchair

597. The nurse explains to the patient that the primary purpose of being NPO after midnight the night before surgery is:
① To prevent vomiting or aspiration
② To enhance the effects of anesthesia
③ To prevent postoperative constipation
④ To prevent postoperative nausea

598. A caller is requesting specific information about a patient. To release this information would be a breach of:
① Privacy
② Anonymity
③ Confidentiality
④ Telephone rules

599. A patient with asthma is being instructed before discharge about the use of a metered-dose inhaler. Which of the following should the nurse include in her instructions?
① Keep the inhaler in the refrigerator between uses
② Shake the canister before use
③ Rinse the mouth before use
④ Hold the breath for 30 seconds after use

600. The patient has been hospitalized for dehydration. He had not voided for 12 hours and had significant postural hypotension on admission. His blood pressure was 110/58 mm Hg lying, 100/46 sitting, and 92/42 standing. His pulse at rest was 88 beats per minute. The patient has been hydrated with IV fluids for 6 hours now. The nurse checks his blood pressure again. Lying it is 140/72, sitting 132/72, and standing 130/68. His pulse is 80 beats per minute, and urine output 30 cc per hour. Which of the following findings indicates his postural hypotension is under control?
① The diastolic blood pressure decreases 10 mm Hg when he lies down
② The systolic blood pressure drops 10 mm Hg when he stands up
③ The pulse rate decreases six beats per minute when he stands up
④ The urine output decreases when he stands up

601. The patient is admitted to the unit with dyspnea and orthopnea. He is coughing up thick, yellow secretions and smokes two packs of cigarettes per day. Which of the following is the first action the nurse needs to perform?
① Prepare the patient for a chest x-ray
② Position the patient in high Fowler's position
③ Give a sedative as ordered
④ Question the patient about his health history

602. Which of the following is the most important nursing function for a patient who is in protective isolation while undergoing chemotherapy?
① Post a "no visitors" sign on the door
② Remove all clocks from the room to decrease boredom
③ Limit carbohydrate intake
④ Use supportive measures to decrease feelings of isolation

603. A new nurse is given the daily assignment and realizes she is assigned a new patient who is HIV positive. She does not want to care for the patient. The nurse will:
① Tell the charge nurse she refuses to care for the patient
② Care for the patient as she would any other patient and use standard precautions
③ Call the supervisor at home to report the problem
④ Talk to the patient and ask the patient to request another nurse

604. The nurse is caring for a patient whose femoral artery has been severed. She puts on gloves to protect herself from the spraying arterial blood. What other protective gear will the nurse wear?
  ① A lab coat
  ② Paper shoe protectors
  ③ A face shield
  ④ A second pair of gloves

605. The nurse knows that chronic protein calorie malnutrition is defined as:
  ① Osteomalacia
  ② Obesity
  ③ Gastritis
  ④ Cachexia

606. The nurse knows that which of the following is the most common type of nosocomial infection?
  ① Respiratory tract infection
  ② Urinary tract infection
  ③ Surgical wound infection
  ④ Gastrointestinal infection

607. The nurse is preparing to move a patient from the bed to a stretcher. Which of the following is the first action the nurse will take to ensure the safety of the patient?
  ① Explain the procedure to the patient
  ② Raise the bed to the same height as the stretcher
  ③ Close the door or curtain
  ④ Raise the side rails

608. The patient talks to the nurse a lot and at times appears to forget the way her story was to go. To compensate it seems she makes up information to fill in the gap. The nurse knows the patient is:
  ① Lying
  ② Reminiscing
  ③ Confabulating
  ④ Seeking attention

609. General subjective signs and symptoms of infection are:
  ① Fatigue, loss of appetite, headache, nausea, or complaint of pain
  ② Fever, tachycardia, tachypnea, vomiting, and decreased breath sounds
  ③ Redness, swelling, and pain or tenderness on palpation
  ④ Loss of function of the affected body part, elevated white blood cell count, and elevated erythrocyte sedimentation rate

610. When teaching the patient and family how to prevent infection transmission, the nurse will provide the following information:
  ① Importance of maintaining a strenuous activity level, decreasing kilocalories, decreasing fluid intake, and returning to work as soon as possible
  ② Importance of monitoring white blood cell count, urinary output, and skin color, as well as taking antibiotics until symptoms are gone
  ③ Importance of recognizing the five symptoms of local inflammation
  ④ Ways in which the infection is transmitted, proper handwashing techniques, approved disinfectants, and methods for proper handling and disposal of contaminated articles, as well as importance of completion of all antimicrobial agents prescribed by the physician

611. The nurse knows that to work effectively with a recovering alcoholic, she must:
  ① Assess her own feelings
  ② Discuss the problem with the patient
  ③ Discuss the patient with co-workers
  ④ Talk to family members

612. The patient has fractured his left humerus and has significant pain from the injury. His left arm is in an immobilizer, and he takes a narcotic analgesic pill every 4 hours. His bowels have not moved in 4 days. Which of the following should the nurse include in the patient's care?
  ① Range-of-motion exercises for the left shoulder
  ② A diet low in fiber and sodium and high in protein
  ③ Increase in the analgesics to two tablets every 4 hours
  ④ Increase in the fluid intake to 2000 cc per day

613. The patient has been hospitalized with left-sided facial droop and loss of fine motor coordination. He is alert and oriented. He has been having difficulty feeding himself and frequently spills food before he can get it to his mouth. Which of the following interventions should the nurse perform to aid the patient with his dietary problems?
  ① Recommend changing his diet to include more finger foods
  ② Recommend a liquid diet so the patient may use a straw
  ③ Arrange for someone to feed the patient at mealtimes
  ④ Place a large bib on the patient's chest and lap before meals

614. When suctioning the nasopharyngeal area, the nurse knows which of the following is the most important nursing action?
  ① Lubricate the catheter with mineral oil
  ② Suction 30 seconds each time
  ③ Apply suction only after the catheter is introduced
  ④ Force the catheter through the nares

615. The nurse is planning care for the patient who has been admitted to the hospital with pitting edema in both feet and SOB. Which of the following would be the most effective way to monitor the patient's fluid balance status?
  ① Obtain daily I & O
  ② Measure abdominal girth daily
  ③ Weigh the patient daily
  ④ Monitor mental status

616. The nurse knows that the appropriate term for the condition of a patient with an invasion of microorganisms is:
  ① Inflammation
  ② Allergy
  ③ Infection
  ④ Immunity

617. Which of the following is the most important safety action when using oxygen on a patient?
  ① Be sure the oxygen goes through a water reservoir
  ② Use a face mask to administer the oxygen
  ③ Apply powder around the edges of the mask
  ④ Keep flow on 8 to 10 L/min

618. Which of the following would be contraindicated as an instruction for the patient regarding metered-dose inhalation?
    ① Open the mouth with the inhaler 1 to 2 inches from the mouth before inhaling
    ② Attach a spacer to the mouthpiece before inhaling
    ③ Attach oxygen to the mouthpiece before inhaling
    ④ Place the mouthpiece inside of the mouth before inhaling

619. At 11:00 AM the nurse notices that her patient's catheter bag is empty and has had no drainage since 7 AM. After checking to see that no one emptied the bag, the nurse should:
    ① Check for kinks in the tubing
    ② Notify the physician immediately
    ③ Question the patient about how he feels
    ④ Increase the patient's IV from keep vein open (KVO) rate to 50 ml/h

620. The amount of fluid used in the irrigation of a ureteral catheter is:
    ① 1 to 2 ml
    ② 5 ml
    ③ 15 to 30 ml
    ④ 20 to 50 ml

621. Perineal exercises are most often used to help:
    ① Reduce residual urine
    ② Relieve urinary retention
    ③ Overcome painful urination
    ④ Control urinary incontinence

622. When the nurse discovers a reddened area on the coccyx, an appropriate nursing intervention is to:
    ① Rub the area with alcohol
    ② Keep the patient in semi-Fowler's position
    ③ Massage the surrounding area gently with lotion
    ④ Apply warm compresses four times a day

623. The newly admitted patient has complaints of abdominal pain, nausea, and vomiting, temperature of 100.4° F (38° C), blood pressure 140/76 mm Hg, pulse rate 80, and respirations 24 and slightly shallow. When planning care, which of the following actions should the nurse implement *first*?
    ① Nursing actions necessary for achieving a goal
    ② Revising the plan of care
    ③ Collecting data
    ④ Formulating a nursing diagnosis

624. While collecting data for further assessment of a patient, the nurse notes a decrease in the number of red blood cells and in the hemoglobin level. This information is vital in planning nursing care because it could indicate that the patient has:
    ① Leukemia
    ② Anemia
    ③ Hemolysis
    ④ Leukocytosis

625. If a patient has the following symptoms, the one *most* indicative of a fluid imbalance is:
    ① Heartburn
    ② A skin rash
    ③ Swollen fingers
    ④ Excessive tearing

626. Nephrosis is characterized by a group of symptoms: proteinuria, hypoalbuminemia, and edema. The nurse knows that a patient who has a disorder characterized by a group of symptoms is said to have a(n):
    ① Subjective symptom
    ② Objective symptom
    ③ Sign
    ④ Syndrome

627. In using a sphygmomanometer to check the patient's blood pressure, the nurse helps to determine any significant changes. A symptom that is detected through special examination and is observed is termed a(n):
    ① Subjective symptom
    ② Objective symptom
    ③ Sign
    ④ Syndrome

628. The patient has complaints of abdominal pain, nausea, and vomiting, temperature of 100.4° F (38° C), blood pressure 140/76 mm Hg, pulse rate 80, and respirations 24 and slightly shallow. What information about the patient is an example of subjective data?
    ① Temperature elevation
    ② Complaints of nausea
    ③ Blood pressure measurement
    ④ Rapid, shallow respirations

629. The patient has complaints of abdominal pain, nausea, and vomiting; temperature of 100.4° F (38° C); blood pressure 140/76 mm Hg; pulse rate 80; and respirations 24 and slightly shallow. Which of the following best describes objective data?
    ① Anorexia
    ② Pain
    ③ Nausea
    ④ Temperature

630. The patient is a moderately obese woman who is recovering from midline abdominal surgery done 3 days ago. A priority nursing diagnosis for the patient is:
    ① Fluid volume deficit related to surgery
    ② Activity intolerance related to surgery
    ③ High risk for alteration in tissue integrity related to surgery and excess adipose tissue
    ④ Impaired gas exchange related to surgery

631. Which one of the following is the most important nursing diagnosis for the perioperative patient?
    ① Bathing/hygiene self-care deficit
    ② Hopelessness
    ③ Potential fluid volume deficit
    ④ Social isolation

632. An important component of evaluating a plan of care is to:
    ① Regularly review the plan of care to determine whether any changes are necessary in synergy with the individual's right to change the plan of care
    ② Review the plan of care when a major health status change has occurred
    ③ Maintain the plan of care until all goals have been met
    ④ Remember that once a plan of care is established it is not necessary to change it

633. The patient has just returned to his room after undergoing a colectomy. He will be NPO for 3 days, with a nasogastric tube in place and IV therapy. Select the most appropriate goal for the patient.
① Pain will be controlled with analgesia
② Patient will not experience wound infection
③ Patient will maintain adequate tissue perfusion
④ Patient will not develop fluid or electrolyte imbalance

634. The most appropriate nursing interventions for the patient with a nursing diagnosis of impaired skin integrity related to immobility and pressure over the left trochanter are:
① Keep side rails up at all times, place call bell and personal items within reach, and answer call light promptly
② Turn every 1 to 2 hours using a turning sheet, inspect pressure areas every 4 hours, and keep the reddened area clean
③ Perform ROM on all joints tid, assist to turn and reposition every 3 hours, and assist to high Fowler's position
④ Frequently reinforce instructions not to get up without assistance, assist to bedside commode, and keep low light on in the room at night

635. The nursing assessment is important to the complete care of the patient. Which of the following are the two components of the nursing assessment?
① Health history and physical assessment
② Cultural history and care plan
③ Physical assessment and blood work
④ Physical assessment and emotional state

636. The patient is an emergency medical technician (EMT) who has been careful to wear gloves, goggles, or masks whenever there was a lot of blood present at the scene of an accident. She recently had a cold with a runny nose and itchy eyes. She was constantly blowing her nose and rubbing her eyes. Today, she is admitted to the unit with fatigue, swollen joints, dark urine, and yellow skin and has been diagnosed as having hepatitis B. The nurse knows that a major reason for contamination was:
① Being on an ambulance run with a patient infected with the hepatitis B virus
② Being exposed to a person with hepatitis in the hospital
③ Rubbing her eyes after touching sheets contaminated with blood, vomitus, and urine
④ Being in contact with other EMTs who have been exposed to patients with hepatitis

637. In maintaining safe practice procedures, which of the following is the *best* nursing method for preventing an accidental puncture from a contaminated needle?
① Remove the needle from the syringe and discard in a special container
② Recover the needle with its cap and discard in regular containers
③ Leave the needle uncapped after use and discard the entire syringe in a special container
④ Bend or break the needle from the syringe and discard in a regular container

638. The Occupational Safety and Health Administration (OSHA) recommends that high-risk public safety workers be given hepatitis B vaccine. The nurse in a public health clinic knows this vaccine is:
① A cure for the disease once a person is infected
② Made from human blood plasma and can spread the disease
③ A method of controlling the virus
④ Good for both HBV and HAV

639. The patient has a physician's order that reads, "Restrict fluids." The nurse would understand that the patient's general fluid intake should probably be limited to:
① 200 to 400 ml/24 hr
② 800 to 1000 ml/24 hr
③ 2000 ml/24 hr
④ 3000 ml/24 hr

640. A patient is NPO and has a nasogastric tube in place with low intermittent suction. He complains that he is thirsty. An appropriate nursing intervention is to:
① Offer sips of water by mouth
② Increase the flow of IV fluids
③ Offer him mouth care
④ Decrease the force of the suction

641. Following surgery, the patient is to be given a clear-liquid diet. Which of the following *would not* be included in this diet?
① Tea and coffee
② Popsicles and gelatin
③ Ice cream
④ Chicken or beef broth

642. The nurse is teaching the patient about food selection related to complex carbohydrates. The nurse will know that her teaching was effective when the patient selects:
① Cabbage, spinach, zucchini, and okra
② Pasta, mashed potatoes, lima beans, and bagel
③ Sweet roll, chocolate cake, potato chips, and crackers
④ Oatmeal, alfalfa sprouts, applesauce, and yogurt

643. The nurse instructs the patient on the importance of including which of the following vitamins in her diet to help counterbalance the effects of osteoporosis?
① Vitamin A
② Vitamin C
③ Vitamin D
④ Vitamin K

644. The nurse knows that the food group that has the highest calcium content is:
① Canned salmon, ribeye steak, peanuts, and eggs
② Beef liver, chicken liver, yeast rolls, and green beans
③ Whole milk, green leafy vegetables, and cottage cheese
④ Waffle, croissant, English muffin, and corn chips

645. To supply food of equal nutrient value for a patient who does not like milk, the nurse will encourage the eating of:
① Fresh pineapple
② Fish
③ Potatoes
④ Pudding

646. Which of the following foods may be included in a clear-liquid diet?
① Lime sherbet
② Cream of celery soup
③ Oatmeal
④ Weak tea with skim milk

647. The patient has been instructed to lower her fat intake. The nurse is helping the patient prepare her menu. Which selection will the nurse question?
① A baked sweet potato
② Lima beans
③ Avocado
④ Blueberries

648. The diet most appropriate for a patient with congestive heart failure is:
① Regular, 2200 calories, and no fluid restriction
② No added salt, 1800 calories, and fluid restriction of 1000 ml/day
③ Low cholesterol, added salt, 2500 calories, and no fluid restriction
④ 1800-calorie ADA diet

649. Nutrition is one of the basic human needs that supplies energy and sustains life. Sound nutrition is considered to be a primary basis for:
① Promoting health and preventing disease throughout life
② Maintaining physical endurance, lifestyle, and activity
③ Maintaining adequate fluid intake and urinary output
④ Maintaining appetite and the sleep/wake cycle

650. Physical and psychologic causes related to diminished interest in eating include:
① Well-fitting dentures, excellent dentition, good health, and a positive mental attitude
② Poorly fitting dentures, poor dentition, stomatitis, halitosis, and a negative attitude
③ Eating too slow, eating too much red meat, eating alone, and excessive fluid intake with meals
④ Consistent diet of fast foods, poorly prepared meals, poor variety, and not enough money to buy foods

651. The physician has ordered a no-added-salt, low-cholesterol, 1800-calorie diet. Select the most appropriate meal selection from the following:
① Fried chicken breast, mashed potatoes, green beans, roll, chocolate cake, and whole milk
② Hamburger, French fries, chocolate milkshake, and apple turnover
③ Broiled chicken (4 ounces), white rice, broccoli, wheat roll, angel food cake, and unsweetened iced tea
④ Fried filet of flounder, cole slaw, applesauce, hushpuppies, and cola

652. The protein requirement for adults, both young and old, is 0.8 gm/kg body weight. Select the best food option that represents the daily protein requirement for women.
① 4 ounces of fish, meat, or poultry and 2 ounces of milk or 3 ounces of cheese
② 8 ounces of lean red meat, 4 ounces of dairy products, and 4 ounces of carbohydrates
③ 6 ounces of fish, meat, or poultry and 3 ounces of milk or 2 ounces of cheese
④ 16 ounces of meat, fish, or poultry and 2 ounces of milk or 3 ounces of cheese

653. The patient has a stage II sacral decubitus. Select the most appropriate meal for the patient:
① Hamburger, fries, apple turnover, and coffee
② Broiled chicken, baked potato, green beans, roll, egg custard pudding, and an Ensure Plus milkshake
③ Fried pork chops, scalloped potatoes, macaroni and cheese, roll, and cheesecake
④ Ground beef, pureed carrots, applesauce, corn muffin, and hot tea

654. The patient, an elderly Jewish woman, has recently been admitted to a nursing home. She is refusing to eat her meals and complains that the food is not properly prepared. The nurse recognizes that the patient may be refusing meals based on:
① The principles of feeling insecure in unfamiliar surroundings
② A self-reported history of poor eating habits
③ The fact that the nursing home has a bad reputation regarding meal preparation
④ Religious practice and personal preferences

655. When preparing for a nutrition class, the nurse remembers that she must address traditional principles of nutrition for the elderly, which are based on:
① Dietary patterns similar to those of the younger adult
② Dietary patterns that decrease calories, and nutrient-dense foods
③ Dietary patterns exactly the opposite of those of the younger adult
④ Dietary patterns that increase calories, fat, protein, vitamins, and minerals

656. The major nutrients essential for sustaining physiologic functioning in the elderly include:
① Protein, carbohydrates, iron, and iodine
② Protein, carbohydrates, fat, amino acids, and lipoproteins
③ Protein, carbohydrates, fat, minerals, vitamins, and water
④ Protein, sugar, milk, carrots, and plenty of bread

657. The following items will be found in the bread category:
① Non-fat, low-fat, and whole milk
② All non-starchy vegetables
③ Lean, medium-fat, and high-fat meat
④ Cereal, pasta, starchy vegetables, and prepared foods

658. Dietary guidelines to follow in the prevention of hypoglycemia include:
    ① Eat meals 4 to 5 hours apart, plus prescribed snack, and eat extra food if performing extra exercise
    ② See physician for illness
    ③ Follow diet, don't overeat, and don't eat concentrated sweets
    ④ Eat meals 8 to 10 hours apart, eat a nighttime snack, and drink a vanilla milkshake before bedtime

659. A patient is to have dressings changed on burned areas of his body. The procedure is extremely painful. To promote the patient's comfort, which of the following actions should the nurse take?
    ① Have the patient take a nap immediately before and after the procedure
    ② Assist the patient to use relaxation exercises immediately before the procedure
    ③ Arrange to have the patient's favorite television or radio program on during the procedure
    ④ Administer to the patient a prescribed pain medication 15 to 30 minutes before the procedure

660. Which of the following nursing techniques has been found *most* helpful when caring for the patient in pain?
    ① Leaving the patient to rest in a quiet, darkened room
    ② Asking the patient why he or she thinks there is pain
    ③ Asking family members to remain with the patient
    ④ Allowing the patient to describe the nature of the pain

661. When developing a teaching plan for a patient who is 40 pounds overweight, smokes two packs of cigarettes a day, and drinks 8 to 10 cups of coffee a day, the nurse should take which of these actions first?
    ① Explain the effects of smoking on the cardiovascular system
    ② Give him a pamphlet that explains the benefits of exercise in reducing stress
    ③ Talk with his wife regarding his intake of calories and cholesterol
    ④ Determine his understanding of the relationship between his behavior and his condition

662. Which of the following nursing behaviors *best indicates* that the nurse is meeting a patient's need for emotional support?
    ① The nurse spends time listening to the concerns of a patient scheduled for surgery
    ② The nurse assists an elderly patient in eating a meal
    ③ The nurse accompanies a patient to have an x-ray examination
    ④ The nurse avoids disturbing a patient who is praying

663. Hospice nurses often provide narcotic analgesics for patients in pain. One of the most common side effects of narcotic analgesics is:
    ① Constipation
    ② Anorexia
    ③ Nausea
    ④ Muscle weakness

664. The licensed practical nurse/vocational nurse (LPN/VN) is a secondary nurse in a primary hospice team. The LPN/VN's functions and responsibilities include:
    ① Providing physical assistance for the patient and emotional and spiritual support for the patient and family
    ② Providing instruction to the patient and family about health care management and the effects of medication and illness
    ③ Providing companionship, respite care for family relief, and emotional support
    ④ Providing opportunities for spiritual reconciliation and healing and prayer

665. A hospice nurse provides palliative care, which is defined as:
    ① Support care
    ② Curative care
    ③ Holistic care
    ④ Symptom-control care

666. The patient has been admitted to the hospital for incontinence and burning on urination. He is alert and oriented but occasionally has difficulty communicating his needs because of his heavy German accent. Who should make the decisions regarding his care?
    ① The patient
    ② The physician
    ③ The primary care giver
    ④ The patient's son

667. On admission to nursing homes, residents designate a person as having durable power of attorney. This means that the resident legally appoints a person on his behalf to:
    ① Make decisions regarding his finances
    ② Make health care decisions for him even when he is able
    ③ Make decisions as to how he will spend his money for health care
    ④ Make health care decisions for him when he is unable to do so

668. The status of durable power of attorney that a nursing home resident gives to a person shall include but is not limited to:
    ① Selling his home, property, and other possessions that he has while he is alive, whether he is mentally competent or not
    ② Obtaining, inspecting, receiving, and disclosing medical records and information related to his physical/mental health history and medications
    ③ Giving the nursing home all his finances once he has passed away
    ④ Taking care of all his property, finances, and other responsibilities upon his death

669. In planning for the pain management of a 1-day postoperative patient, the nurse should instruct the patient to inform her of the need for medication:
    ① Every time she is able to have a dose of medication, even if it is before she is aware of much pain
    ② As she begins to have the sensation of pain
    ③ When the pain has risen to 7 or 8 on a 10-point scale
    ④ When she has pain, but only if the 4-hour period is up

670. Before intramuscular injection of medication, the nurse should aspirate for blood. If blood returns in the syringe, the nurse should:
① Proceed with the injection of medication
② Withdraw the needle and prepare a new syringe
③ Slowly inject the medication and massage the site
④ Withdraw the needle and give the injection in another site

671. When preparing to administer medications to geriatric patients, the nurse knows that as a general rule, medications for elderly patients should be given in:
① Smaller doses, closer together
② Larger doses, closer together
③ Smaller doses, farther apart
④ Larger doses, farther apart

672. Which of the following actions that the nurse performs is most likely to decrease discomfort from an intramuscular gluteal injection?
① Rub the skin firmly with an antiseptic swab
② Pull the skin tissue taut
③ Aspirate for blood
④ Inject the medication rapidly but consistently

673. The nurse is preparing furosemide (Lasix) 40 mg PO for administration. The most important time the label should be checked is:
① When checking the medication record with the physician's orders
② Immediately before pouring the medication
③ After pouring the medication
④ After administering the medication

674. While on duty, the nurse notices that the medication refrigerator is very warm, registering 80° F (26.6° C), and that the vaccines stored inside are all warm. The nurse should:
① Notify the pharmacy and adjust the thermometer
② Close the door and report it later to the supervisor
③ Adjust the temperature and recheck in an hour to be sure the temperature has dropped
④ Remove all of the medication and return it to the pharmacy

675. The nurse obtains a scheduled drug from the narcotics cabinet and prepares to administer it as ordered. No one has seen her prepare the drug. She asks a co-worker to sign the record that the excess was wasted. The co-worker's correct response would be to:
① Sign the record because she trusts her co-worker
② Refuse to sign the record and inform the co-worker of this decision
③ Refuse to sign the record and hope the co-worker will forget about it
④ Sign the co-worker's name with her own initials next to the signature, indicating that the excess was wasted

676. An air lock should be used with a subcutaneous injection of insulin for a hospitalized patient if:
① The nurse prefers to use an air lock with insulin
② The patient is obese and needs a longer needle for administration
③ A pediatric patient is receiving insulin twice a day
④ The patient has been using an air lock during self-administration of insulin at home

677. The nurse recognizes that a maximum safe volume to be injected in the deltoid muscle is:
① 1 cc
② 2 cc
③ 4 cc
④ 5 cc

678. The patient had a total left hip arthroplasty after falling on an icy sidewalk. She returned from the operating room 3 hours ago after having spinal anesthetic. She has an IV running in her right hand and a hemovac drain from her left hip. She is complaining of pain in her operative site. The physician has left an order for meperidine (Demerol) 75-100 mg IM every 4 hours as needed for pain. The nurse prepares to administer the medication to the patient. Which of the following would be an appropriate site for the injection?
① Left gluteus medius
② Left ventral gluteal
③ Right deltoid
④ Right vastus lateralis

679. Which of these sites is preferred for the subcutaneous administration of heparin?
① In the deltoid muscle
② On the top of the thigh
③ In the buttocks at a 45-degree angle
④ Below the ribs to the iliac crest

680. To ensure that the correct patient is receiving a prescribed medication, it is *essential* that the nurse take which of these actions?
① Check the name on the patient's wristband
② Call the patient by name
③ Read the name of the patient on the bed card
④ Check the medication record for the patient's room number

681. The physician orders penicillin 250,000 U IM. The label on the vial reads 100,000 U/ml. How much medication should the nurse prepare to administer to the patient?
① 1 ml
② 1.5 ml
③ 2 ml
④ 2.5 ml

682. The physician orders penicillin liquid 500 mg PO tid. The bottle of penicillin that comes from the pharmacy is labeled 125 mg/tsp. Which of the following would be the appropriate dose for the nurse to administer to the patient?
① 15 ml
② 16 ml
③ 20 ml
④ 25 ml

683. Heparin 5000 U is to be given subcutaneously. In stock is heparin 10,000 U/ml. The nurse should administer:
① 0.5 ml
② 1 ml
③ 1.25 ml
④ 1.5 ml

684. The patient has codeine, 1.5 gr, ordered. On hand are scored tablets labeled 60 mg. The nurse should give:
    ① ½ tablet
    ② 1 tablet
    ③ 1½ tablets
    ④ 2 tablets

685. The order for penicillin 150,000 U IM is written on the medication record sheet. The drug label reads penicillin 1,000,000 U/6 ml. How many ml should the nurse give?
    ① 0.01 ml
    ② 0.5 ml
    ③ 0.9 ml
    ④ 1.5 ml

686. The nurse is to administer pain medication. The physician ordered Demerol 75 mg. The ampule reads Demerol 100 mg/2 ml. What quantity does the nurse administer?
    ① 0.6 ml
    ② 1 ml
    ③ 1.2 ml
    ④ 1.5 ml

687. The patient has an order for her IV to infuse at 1000 ml q8h. The drop factor is 10 gtt/ml. How many gtt/min will be needed for the IV to infuse?
    ① 12 gtt
    ② 13 gtt
    ③ 20 gtt
    ④ 21 gtt

688. The patient refuses to take the ordered medication. The nurse will tell the patient:
    ① "The physician has ordered this medication; you really need it."
    ② "You have the right to refuse this. I will respect your right."
    ③ "Let me give you this medicine now and in a while I will call your physician to see if we can hold it in the future."
    ④ "You do not have to take this medicine, but let me explain what this medication is for."

689. Besides an adequate diet with sufficient fluid intake, which of the following nursing interventions should be ordered to relieve a patient's constipation?
    ① Oil-retention enema every other day
    ② Strong laxative every third day
    ③ Stool softeners once a day
    ④ Saline enema as needed

690. The nurse instructs the patient that nitroglycerin:
    ① Is given only three to four times a day
    ② Cannot be used more frequently than every half hour
    ③ Takes approximately a half hour to relieve anginal pain
    ④ Should be taken at 5-minute intervals (up to three doses) to relieve anginal pain

691. The physician's written order is for the patient to have Maalox 1 hour before meals and at bedtime, and the patient is taking digitalis every morning. If breakfast comes at 8 AM, which schedule would be *most* effective for the patient?
    ① Maalox and digitalis at 9 AM
    ② Maalox at 8 AM and digitalis at 9 AM
    ③ Maalox at 9 AM and digitalis at 10 AM
    ④ Maalox at 8:30 AM and digitalis at 9 AM

692. On reviewing a patient's medication record, the nurse notices that there is an order for warfarin (Coumadin) 5 mg PO qd and an order for Fiorinal tablets PO q4h prn. The nurse's concern should result in which action?
    ① Leave the prn order on the medication administration record but note that the patient is on warfarin
    ② Inform the patient that he will not be able to receive any pain medication for a while
    ③ Call the physician and request an order for a different pain medication
    ④ Call the physician and request an order for heparin instead of warfarin

693. A patient is receiving warfarin (Coumadin) every day at 9 AM. Her laboratory work comes back with her prothrombin time four times the control. The nurse discovers that the patient's laboratory work was within normal limits the day before. The nurse's *first* action would be to:
    ① Call the physician immediately and then report to the charge nurse
    ② Check the time the laboratory work was drawn and report to the charge nurse
    ③ Prepare an injection of vitamin K while the charge nurse calls the physician
    ④ Prepare to administer protamine sulfate while the charge nurse calls the physician

694. The patient who had been drinking heavily all day is voiding large amounts in the evening. The nurse knows that this is because alcohol causes diuresis by:
    ① Increasing cardiac output
    ② Increasing renal blood flow
    ③ Inhibiting secretion of the pituitary antidiuretic hormone
    ④ Stimulating the posterior pituitary gland

695. Before administering digoxin (Lanoxin) to a patient with congestive heart failure, the nurse will hold giving the medication and report to the charge nurse if the patient:
    ① Complains of nausea and vomiting and has a pulse rate of 52
    ② Complains of nausea and vomiting and has a pulse rate of 80
    ③ Has a regular, strong pulse
    ④ Complains of nausea and vomiting

696. The following order is transcribed on a patient's medication record sheet: "Acetaminophen (Tylenol) tablets prn for pain or temperature of 102° F (38.7° C)." The nurse would:
    ① Assume that two tablets are to be given every 4 hours
    ② Give the acetaminophen if pain or fever occurs and note the reason in the nurses' notes
    ③ Call the physician to clarify the dosage and frequency of the medication before giving it
    ④ Call the physician to clarify the dosage and frequency of the medication after giving a dose for pain

697. Which of the following symptoms should concern the nurse if observed in a patient who received a bronchodilator?
    ① Fremitus
    ② Wheezing
    ③ Rales (crackles)
    ④ Yellow, thick sputum

698. The patient who has been placed on birth control pills should notify her physician before beginning which of the following medications?
    ① Propylthiouracil (Propyl-Thyracil)
    ② Ranitidine hydrochloride (Zantac)
    ③ Tetracycline hydrochloride (Achromycin V)
    ④ Gelusil (aluminum hydroxide, magnesium hydroxide, simethicone)

699. The nurse will teach the patient that the most effective way to use the rhythm method of birth control is to keep careful records of her:
    ① Weight
    ② Pulse rate
    ③ Body temperature
    ④ Blood pressure

700. The patient had enteric-coated salicylates ordered before having a nasogastric (NG) tube inserted. When preparing to administer the medication, the nurse should:
    ① Check with the physician regarding the status of this drug
    ② Hold the medication because it cannot be administered at this time
    ③ Crush the medicine and mix it in water; administer it down the NG tube and clamp the tube
    ④ Have the patient swallow the tablet with sips of water

701. Before administering penicillin VK, which question should the nurse ask the patient?
    ① "Do you understand how often you will be taking this medicine?"
    ② "Do you have any medication allergies?"
    ③ "Have you eaten recently?"
    ④ "Do you know what this medication is for?"

702. The patient has been using tetrahydrocannabinol for the past several years. When the patient asks, "What will happen to me if I suddenly quit?", the nurse will respond that all of the following symptoms may be experienced except:
    ① Tremors
    ② Increased perspiration
    ③ Increased appetite
    ④ Nausea

703. Which of the following is an accurate statement about diuretics?
    ① Diuretics act by increasing sodium reabsorption
    ② Osmotics are often used before eye surgery to increase intraocular pressure
    ③ Diuretics should be scheduled early in the morning or no later than 5 PM if possible
    ④ Carbonic anhydrase inhibitors are strong and frequently used to lower blood pressure

704. Which of the following statements indicates an understanding about the effects of oral anticoagulants?
    ① "I will brush my teeth with a soft toothbrush."
    ② "I will eat plenty of green, leafy vegetables each day."
    ③ "I will use aspirin if I get a headache."
    ④ "I will stop driving now that I'm on Coumadin."

705. In planning nursing care for a patient receiving warfarin (Coumadin), the nurse must be aware that the antidote for warfarin is:
    ① Protamine sulfate
    ② Vitamin K
    ③ Folic acid
    ④ Calcium gluconate

706. The drug trimethobenzamide hydrochloride (Tigan) is used to control nausea and vomiting and is classified as a(n):
    ① Antispasmodic
    ② Anticholinergic
    ③ Antiemetic
    ④ Cathartic

707. Drugs that lower body temperature when the patient has a fever are classified as:
    ① Antibiotics
    ② Antipyretics
    ③ Antiemetics
    ④ Antihistamines

708. The nurse knows that it is best to administer a diuretic at:
    ① 6 PM
    ② 1 PM
    ③ 9 AM
    ④ 4 PM

709. A potassium-sparing (retaining) diuretic used to reduce hypertension and/or edema is:
    ① Furosemide (Lasix)
    ② Spironolactone (Aldactone)
    ③ Sulfisoxazole (Gantrisin)
    ④ Methenamine (Mandelamine)

710. A patient receiving heparin must be observed for:
    ① Bleeding
    ② Numbness
    ③ Convulsions
    ④ Muscle twitching

711. The primary action of cimetidine (Tagamet) is to:
    ① Directly promote healing of an ulcer
    ② Neutralize gastric acidity
    ③ Inhibit the secretion of hydrochloric acid
    ④ Decrease gastric motility

712. What signs and symptoms should a nurse be alert for in detecting a patient's recent use of cocaine?
  ① Clear, constricted pupils
  ② White, patchy areas of the tongue
  ③ Red, excoriated nostrils
  ④ Seizure activity

713. After taking amitriptyline hydrochloride (Elavil), the patient tells the nurse that his mouth feels dry. An appropriate nursing intervention is to:
  ① Tell him that this is just his imagination and to ignore it
  ② Tell him to suck on hard candies
  ③ Recommend chewing sugarless gum or drinking plenty of fluids
  ④ Instruct the patient to rinse his mouth with salt water

714. Frequently used medications for myocardial infarctions are:
  ① Salicylates, antiinflammatory agents, and gold salts
  ② Antidysrhythmics, analgesics, and anticoagulants
  ③ Cardial glycosides, diuretics, and nitrates
  ④ Anticoagulants, vasodilators, and fibrinolytics

715. The physician orders promethazine (Phenergan) for a patient with nausea. The charting method for an injection of promethazine intramuscularly, Z-track would be which of the following?
  ① "Phenergan 50 mg IM given Z-track for complaint of nausea"
  ② "Phenergan 50 mg IM in the right dorsogluteal for complaint of nausea"
  ③ "Phenergan 50 mg IM given in the dorsogluteal Z-track for complaint of nausea"
  ④ "Phenergan 50 mg IM, Z-track in the right dorsogluteal for complaint of nausea"

716. The following medications are all ordered prn by the physician. Which should be administered when the patient complains of anxiety and inability to sleep?
  ① Nalbuphine hydrochloride (Nubain)
  ② Magaldrate hydroxymagnesium aluminate
  ③ Indomethacin (Indameth)
  ④ Flurazepam hydrochloride (Dalmane)

717. In planning care for a patient on acetazolamide (Diamox), the nurse will include instructions on:
  ① Photosensitivity effect of this drug
  ② Hypoglycemic effects of this drug
  ③ Diuretic effect of this drug
  ④ Cardiac effects of this drug

718. The patient has had a Hickman catheter inserted and is scheduled to begin antineoplastic chemotherapy. The nurse would plan to:
  ① Place the patient in strict isolation
  ② Offer frequent skin care of the site to promote comfort
  ③ Use strict infection-control procedures
  ④ Serve only bland foods

719. Which information would be appropriate for the nurse to assess as baseline data on a patient who is ordered to receive corticosteroids?
  ① Bone length and calcium levels
  ② Sleep patterns and understanding of disease
  ③ Abdominal girth and leg circumference
  ④ Weight and blood pressure

720. Before the nurse administers a preoperative injection that includes atropine, she nurse will explain that the medication will:
  ① Help to decrease secretions in the digestive tract, thus lessening the chance of complications with surgery
  ② Promote the cardiac response to stress
  ③ Help control anxiety and pain
  ④ Help him sleep and potentiate the anesthesia

721. The physician orders lanoxin (Digoxin) 5 mg for the patient. Recognizing this to be a high dose, the nurse's *most* appropriate action would be to:
  ① Transcribe the order as Digoxin 0.5 mg, because this is a normal dose for the patient
  ② Transcribe the order as written
  ③ Seek clarification now from the physician regarding the required dose
  ④ Hold the medication until the physician next makes rounds

722. Three patients need medication at the same time. They are: (a) the patient who receives Demerol 100 mg intramuscularly, which he has just requested for pain he describes as "pretty strong," (b) the patient who receives nitroglycerin sublingual stat, and (c) the patient who receives ampicillin IVPB q6h, and it was time for her dose 10 minutes ago. In which order should the medications be administered?
  ① Ampicillin IVPB, nitroglycerin SC, Demerol IM
  ② Nitroglycerin, Demerol, ampicillin
  ③ Demerol, nitroglycerin, ampicillin
  ④ Demerol, ampicillin, nitroglycerin

723. The patient is experiencing sudden, severe, sharp chest pain; shortness of breath; profuse perspiration; and nausea. The nurse administered morphine sulfate ¼ gr (15 mg) intravenously. The morphine was given primarily to:
  ① Relieve the severe chest pain
  ② Relieve the nausea
  ③ Relieve the vomiting
  ④ Relieve shortness of breath

724. A patient has a daily prothrombin time level ordered. The nurse gives the anticoagulant, warfarin (Coumadin). The main action of this drug is to:
  ① Prevent hemorrhage
  ② Prevent infection in the blood
  ③ Interfere with clotting mechanisms
  ④ Stimulate the heart action

725. When administering chloral hydrate, the nurse knows that the medication is a(n):
  ① Sedative
  ② Antiepileptic
  ③ Antidepressant
  ④ Tranquilizer

726. Minor tranquilizers are used mainly for the symptomatic treatment of:
  ① Common psychoneuroses
  ② Acute psychoses
  ③ Chronic psychoses
  ④ Epilepsy

727. The nurse's initial intervention when a patient has a seizure in her presence is to:
① Control the seizure
② Restrain the patient
③ Protect the patient
④ Increase circulation to the brain

728. After administering pentobarbital (Nembutal), the nurse expects the patient to fall asleep because the action of this drug is to:
① Depress the cough center of the brain
② Relieve moderate-to-severe pain
③ Allay apprehension
④ Increase blood pressure

729. The nurse knows that the brand name for meperidine hydrochloride is:
① Dilaudid
② Demerol
③ Dilantin
④ Dicumarol

730. The nurse is teaching the patient to administer her own insulin. She has been instructed to rotate the sites of injections. The purpose of site rotation is to:
① Reduce pain at the injection site
② Allow for absorption of the medication
③ Let nerve endings regenerate
④ Reduce the risk of injecting into superficial vessels

731. The patient has recently started treatment with an MAO inhibitor. As the nurse prepares him for discharge, it is important that emphasis is placed on:
① Avoiding caffeinated beverages
② Taking the medicine on an empty stomach
③ Avoiding aged cheeses
④ The fact that these drugs may be habit forming

732. The doctor has ordered cephalexin (Keftab) 250 mg IM q6h. The medication label reads "Cephalexin 2 gm/5 ml after reconstituted." How much should the nurse give?
① 25 ml
② 6 ml
③ 0.6 ml
④ 2 ml

733. A 70-year-old patient comes to the health clinic with chronic constipation. She has tried diet changes with no results. Which of the following will the nurse suggest for the resolution of the constipation?
① Metamucil
② Magnesium citrate
③ Daily enemas
④ Mineral oil

734. A patient has come to the clinic with digestion problems. The patient suffers from frequent bouts of constipation, bloating, and gas. Which of the following would be best to include in the nursing plan for teaching?
① Limit fluid intake to 600 ml per day
② Limit fat intake to 20% of calories per day
③ Increase carbohydrate intake
④ Set up a regular exercise schedule

735. The patient is being discharged from the hospital after treatment of angina and a cholesterol level of 350. Which of the following drugs will most likely be ordered as home medications and need to be included in the nurse's discharge planning?
① Lasix (furosemide)
② Zocor (simvastatin)
③ Atarax (vistaril)
④ Tagamet (cimetidine)

736. The patient had a total knee replacement yesterday. He is to be up in a chair twice per day and is taking morphine for pain. He begins to complain of nausea and vomiting. Which of the following would be the best nursing action?
① Give medication as ordered for vomiting
② Call the doctor to change the pain medication
③ Keep the patient NPO until the nausea passes
④ Keep the patient on bed rest until the nausea passes

737. The order reads digoxin (Lanoxin) 0.375 mg po qod. The pill comes supplied as 0.125 mg per tablet. The nurse interprets the new order to be:
① Take one pill every day
② Take three pills every day
③ Take one pill every other day
④ Take three pills every other day

738. The patient has an IV running at 125 cc/hr because of dehydration. The nurse walking by the patient's room notes the drip chamber is full to capacity. What can the nurse do to visualize the drops coming into the chamber?
① Change to a new tubing and drip chamber
② Invert the chamber and squeeze the fluid into the IV bag
③ Squeeze the drip chamber to get air from the IV bag
④ Insert a needle into the chamber and withdraw the fluid

739. The physician has ordered meperidine hydrochloride (Demerol) 75 mg IM every 4 hours. The nurse recognizes the intramuscular route is preferred because:
① This drug is less irritating to the subcutaneous tissue
② This route provides a slower rate of absorption
③ This route provides a more rapid rate of absorption
④ This route prohibits giving large volume of drug

740. The patient is 6 feet tall and weighs 178 pounds. The nurse is preparing to give him an injection in the vastus lateralis. Which size needle is appropriate for this site?
① ⅜ inch
② ⅝ inch
③ 1½ inch
④ 2½ inch

741. Which of the following drugs is a corticosteroid?
① Albuterol (Proventil)
② Methylprednisolone (Solu-Medrol)
③ Terbutaline (Brethine)
④ Theophylline ethylenediamine (Aquaphyllin)

742. The nurse prepares to administer a drug intramuscularly by identifying the anatomic landmarks of the deltoid muscle. The landmarks include:
① Anterior superior iliac crest
② Posterior superior iliac crest
③ The acromion process
④ The greater trochanter

743. When administering a drug into the subcutaneous space, the nurse knows that the space is located:
① Under the epidermis
② Into the dermis
③ Into the fibrous tissue above the muscle
④ Into the body of a striated muscle

744. The physician has ordered magnesium hydroxide (Milk of Magnesia) 1 ounce at HS daily. The nurse calculates the conversion of ounces to cubic centimeters and arrives at a dose of:
① 15 cc
② 30 cc
③ 45 cc
④ 60 cc

745. Which of the following medications would put a patient at a higher risk for a heat stroke?
① Digoxin (Lanoxin)
② Furosemide (Lasix)
③ Diazepam (Valium)
④ Amoxicillin/clavulanate potassium (Augmentin)

746. The physician has ordered aspirin (Ecotrin), 325 mg daily, for the patient who is in skeletal traction for the next 6 weeks; the nurse recognizes that the primary purpose of this order is to:
① Relieve pain
② Prevent headache
③ Prevent thrombus formation
④ Potentiate narcotic action

747. The nurse has an order to give crushed enteric-coated aspirin 650 mg down a nasogastric tube. A priority nursing action should be to:
① Give the medication as ordered
② Not give the medication
③ Hold administration of the medication until she has contacted the physician regarding how the medication is to be given
④ Give the medication only in whole tablet form

748. The nurse will recognize the following as adverse reactions associated with digoxin (Lanoxin) toxicity:
① Ravenous appetite, weight gain, tachycardia, and drowsiness
② Anorexia, nausea and vomiting, bradycardia, and headache
③ Tachycardia, weight loss, insomnia, and hyperkalemia
④ Complete third-degree heart block, hypertension, tachycardia, and hypokalemia

749. The patient admits to taking aluminum hydroxide (Amphojel) daily for 2 to 3 weeks. The nurse will be alert for what side effect?
① Anorexia
② Diarrhea
③ Nausea
④ Constipation

750. The patient has been given an overdose of heparin IV. The nurse will have which of the following medications on hand as an antidote?
① Vitamin K
② Protamine sulfate
③ Aspirin
④ Coumadin

CHAPTER 3

Maternal-Child Health Nursing Review Questions

1. As the nurse explains fetal circulation to the expectant parents, she notes their fascination with the fact that, during fetal circulation, blood flowing through the heart actually bypasses the:
   ① Liver
   ② Lungs
   ③ Brain
   ④ Kidneys

2. A patient who is pregnant for the first time asks the nurse questions on basic anatomy and physiology of pregnancy, such as "How much amniotic fluid will be in the bag of waters when I reach term?" The nurse responds:
   ① "300 ml, which is replaced on a continual basis"
   ② "500 ml, which is replaced at the rate of 250 ml/hr"
   ③ "1000 ml, which is replaced every 3 hours"
   ④ "2000 ml, which is replaced every 3 hours"

3. When working in a prenatal clinic, the nurse must be aware that during pregnancy there are definite changes that occur in all major body systems. Which of the following is a major change within the hematologic system?
   ① Decreased red blood cell count
   ② Increased hemoglobin level
   ③ Decreased white blood cell count
   ④ Increased coagulation factors

4. During a training session for childbirth educators, the following question was asked: "Which type of pelvis can be classified as the 'true' female pelvis?" Participants, demonstrating their readiness for their new role, would answer:
   ① Android
   ② Anthropoid
   ③ Gynecoid
   ④ Platypelloid

5. During childbirth classes, the nurse teaches the patients and their significant others that the fetus is fully developed in the:
   ① Third month
   ② Fourth month
   ③ Fifth month
   ④ Sixth month

6. When teaching patients about the processes of fertilization and implantation, the nurse must know that fertilization normally occurs in the:
   ① Ovary
   ② Fundus of the uterus
   ③ Upper third of the cervix
   ④ Distal end of the fallopian tube

7. A patient asks how oxygen gets to her baby in utero. The nurse's most appropriate response would be to:
   ① Show the patient a picture of the umbilical cord
   ② Show the patient a picture of the fetal circulation
   ③ Use a chart, explaining that the umbilical vein carries oxygen
   ④ Use a chart, explaining that the umbilical artery carries oxygen

8. During prenatal class, a patient asks the nurse just how the fetus receives nutrients from the mother. The nurse explains that the link between mother and fetus is the umbilical cord, which contains:
   ① One artery and one vein
   ② One artery and two veins
   ③ Two arteries and one vein
   ④ Two arteries and two veins

9. Which of the following available snack foods should the nurse suggest to a pregnant patient as the best source of complete protein?
   ① Cereal
   ② Peanuts
   ③ Cheese on crackers
   ④ Peanut butter on apple wedges

10. A 16-year-old pregnant high school student attends a prenatal clinic on a regular basis. During each visit the nurse emphasizes the patient's need for extra calcium because of her age. Which of the following statements correctly explains this need?
    ① During pregnancy, the calcium need is higher for this age-group than it is for an expectant mother who is age 21 or older
    ② During pregnancy, the calcium need is lower for this age-group than it is for an expectant mother who is age 21 or older
    ③ During pregnancy, the calcium need is the same as it is for an expectant mother who is age 21 or older
    ④ During pregnancy, the calcium need is always met naturally in persons of this age-group

11. During a routine prenatal examination, a patient complains of being constipated. Which of the following could the nurse suggest to minimize this discomfort?
    ① Increase her intake of milk and dairy products
    ② Increase her intake of refined cereals
    ③ Increase her intake of raw fruits and vegetables
    ④ Increase her intake of ground meats

12. A patient complains that she hates milk, but because she is pregnant she will drink a lot of it anyway. Which of the following could the nurse recommend as a milk substitute that supplies adequate amounts of calcium for the expectant mother?
    ① Liver and organ meats
    ② Cheddar-type cheeses
    ③ Dark yellow vegetables
    ④ Enriched macaroni products

13. A divorced, working mother with two small children at home is 8 months' pregnant with her third child and is having trouble making ends meet. She asks the nurse at the prenatal clinic if she knows of any organization that might provide food after the baby arrives. Which of the following responses by the nurse is the most appropriate?
    ① "The food stamp program will provide adequate food for your family; the social worker will help you to apply."
    ② "If you are eligible, there is a federal supplementary program that provides nutritional food for you and your children."
    ③ "The Women, Infants, and Children (WIC) program will provide plenty of food for you, your infant, and children under 5 years of age."
    ④ "You should apply for welfare immediately."

14. A 23-year-old patient is 2 months' pregnant with her first child and is visiting her physician for the first time. It is important that the nurse counsel the patient about the need for sufficient iron in her diet because in the last trimester the fetus stores iron that will be needed for the first:
    ① 3 Months of life
    ② 6 Months of life
    ③ 9 Months of life
    ④ Year of life

15. A patient who is 4 months' pregnant asks the nurse to recommend *economical* sources of protein. Which of the following foods would be most appropriate for the nurse to recommend?
    ① Red meats and fish
    ② In-season fruits and vegetables
    ③ Breads and macaroni
    ④ Dried beans and lentils

16. The patient has just received the test results that determined that she is HIV positive. She is 8 months' pregnant. Which of the following statements made by the patient during the counseling session would show she has a clear understanding of the diagnosis?
    ① "I will probably have to have a C-section to prevent the baby from getting the disease."
    ② "I must have gotten the disease from using public rest rooms."
    ③ "My baby will have a 50% chance of contracting the disease."
    ④ "I should not receive blood transfusions during the labor and delivery period."

17. A 30-year-old gravida 1 para 0 attends the prenatal clinic on a regular basis. The physician has ordered an ultrasound to confirm a multiple pregnancy. The patient appears anxious about this procedure and asks the nurse what she might expect. The best explanation the nurse can give is that:
    ① Radiopaque dye will be injected into her uterus and an x-ray will be taken
    ② A jelly-like substance will be applied to her abdomen, then a small device will be moved back and forth over the abdominal area
    ③ During the test she will be placed in several different positions so that the uterus can be viewed from different angles
    ④ A small area on her abdomen will be numbed; then a needle will be inserted and a small amount of fluid will be removed

18. The nurse would plan for all of the following tests to be routinely done on all expectant mothers during their initial prenatal visit *except:*
    ① Hemoglobin and hematocrit levels
    ② Abdominal ultrasound
    ③ Maternal blood type and Rh factor
    ④ Urinalysis

19. A patient who is 6 months' pregnant with her second child was exposed to rubella during her fourth month. The physician orders a rubella titer drawn. The patient exhibits anxiety over the prospect of this new test. In preparing to counsel the patient, the nurse must know that the test actually:
    ① Indicates active disease during this pregnancy
    ② Measures the level of maternal antibodies
    ③ Indicates teratogenic effects on the fetus
    ④ Protects the patient from getting active disease

20. Nursing assessment during routine prenatal visits includes a urinalysis, blood pressure check, and a weight check to:
    ① Prevent pregnancy-induced hypertension
    ② Ensure good prenatal care
    ③ Detect diabetes
    ④ Detect anomalies

21. A patient comes to the clinic for a pregnancy test, which is positive. Her last menstrual period began on July 8 and lasted 5 days. The nurse calculates her due date as:
    ① April 15
    ② March 20
    ③ April 20
    ④ May 15

22. A patient attends the prenatal clinic exhibiting presumptive signs of pregnancy. The nurse knows that these signs would most likely include:
    ① Urinary frequency, Chadwick's sign, and quickening
    ② Fatigue, positive gravindex, nausea, and vomiting
    ③ Amenorrhea, fatigue, and urinary frequency
    ④ Chadwick's sign, breast enlargement, and fetal movement felt by examiner

23. The clinic nurse can inform patients that a pregnancy can be positively confirmed by:
    ① A palpable enlargement in uterine size, and a change in shape
    ② A positive gravindex test
    ③ Fetal heart tones heard by the examiner
    ④ Amenorrhea for past 2 months

24. During the first trimester of pregnancy, the nurse can expect that a patient's complaints of nausea and vomiting can be controlled by:
    ① Antiemetics and rest
    ② Plenty of fluids and a well-fitting girdle
    ③ Increasing bulk in her diet and restricting salt
    ④ Rest periods and a high-carbohydrate diet

25. A patient is 6 months' pregnant with her second child. During her prenatal visit, she tells the nurse that her 5-year-old son is asking a lot of questions about the baby, particularly its sex. Which of the following suggestions by the nurse is the most appropriate approach to this situation?
    ① Divert his attention to his toys, telling him that there is time after the baby is born to answer his questions
    ② Tell him that the stork will decide whether the baby will be a boy or a girl
    ③ Tell him that she honestly doesn't know at this time and will not know until the baby is born
    ④ Refer him to his father for answers on a "man-to-man" level

26. When caring for the prenatal patient, the nurse should stress which of the following in her teaching plan?
    ① No sexual intercourse during the first trimester
    ② Weight gain of over 25 pounds by the due date
    ③ Need to report epigastric/abdominal pain
    ④ Need to participate in childbirth classes

27. A patient who is pregnant for the second time asks the nurse if it is really beneficial to attend natural childbirth education classes. The nurse explains that the primary benefit of such classes is that:
    ① Labor and delivery will be more rapid and less painful
    ② Most likely no pain medication will have to be administered
    ③ She will deliver the baby in a natural and quiet environment
    ④ Preparation will allow her to more fully assist in the birth

28. A patient is now in her seventh month of pregnancy, and the nurse notes that she is wearing high-heel shoes. The nurse should advise her to:
    ① Continue wearing the shoes she is now wearing
    ② Wear heels of a moderate height to prevent varicose veins
    ③ Wear low-heel shoes to avoid additional strain on her back
    ④ Wear athletic shoes for walking

29. During a routine prenatal visit to her physician's office, a patient asks if a thin, watery secretion that she has noted from her breasts is normal in the third trimester of pregnancy. The nurse reassures her that this is common at this time and that the proper term for this secretion is:
    ① Lochia
    ② Colostrum
    ③ Chloasma
    ④ Chorion

30. A patient has come to the obstetrician's office for her eighth-month prenatal examination. She learns that she has gained 32 pounds. How will the nurse use this information in developing a plan of care?
    ① Discuss diet with the patient to determine ways to increase her weight gain
    ② Discuss diet with the patient to determine ways to decrease her weight gain
    ③ Encourage the patient to continue eating as she has been since her weight gain is within normal limits
    ④ Explain to the patient that she will probably lose weight during the last 4 weeks

31. The patient tells the nurse that her EDC is January 5. When planning the essentials of prenatal care for this patient, the nurse knows that this means:
    ① Her expected delivery date
    ② The day her labor will begin
    ③ The first day of her last menstrual period
    ④ The date her pregnancy was confirmed

32. A woman who thinks that she is pregnant asks when she should consult the physician. The nurse's best reply would be:
    ① "As soon as lightening occurs"
    ② "As soon as you miss one or two menstrual periods"
    ③ "As soon as morning sickness stops"
    ④ "As soon as you feel movement"

33. A nonstress test has been ordered for a patient in the OB clinic. The most likely reason for this test is to determine:
    ① The presenting part
    ② Gestational age
    ③ Fetal well-being before labor begins
    ④ When labor is likely to begin

34. A patient who is 2 months' pregnant has just informed the nurse during the health history that her 2-year-old niece has German measles. The blood test results for the rubella titer show that the patient is not immune to the disease. Which of the following would be the best response by the nurse?
    ① "Do not be concerned; it is unlikely to damage the baby."
    ② "You should avoid being around the child until after the first trimester of your pregnancy."
    ③ "We will give you an immunization against measles."
    ④ "We will treat you with antibiotics to prevent infection."

35. A patient pregnant for the second time is concerned because she lost her first pregnancy during the fourth month. She is afraid that this will happen again and asks the nurse why this may have occurred. Although unable to give her a definite answer, the nurse can tell the patient that the major hormone necessary for maintaining a pregnancy is:
    ① Estrogen
    ② Progesterone
    ③ Luteinizing hormone
    ④ Follicle-stimulating hormone

36. A patient who is 6 months' pregnant has been experiencing back and leg pains. During a routine check-up she makes the statement, "I am afraid to take aspirin for the discomfort." What would be the most appropriate evaluation by the nurse of this statement?
    ① The patient has a good concept of prenatal care
    ② The patient is displaying early signs of paranoia
    ③ The patient does not understand prenatal drug use
    ④ The patient is confusing aspirin with Tylenol

37. A patient who is pregnant for the first time is approaching her estimated date of confinement (EDC). She is quite anxious and reports that although she has been able to breathe more easily for the past 2 days, she now has to void more frequently. The office nurse would:
    ① Explain that this is normal since lightening has occurred
    ② Obtain a urine sample for culture and sensitivity
    ③ Recommend that she restrict fluid intake
    ④ Report this to the physician immediately

38. A patient asks the nurse when she will most likely feel the baby move for the first time. The nurse responds that the fetus is most likely to move during which of the following months of pregnancy?
    ① Fifth
    ② Sixth
    ③ Third
    ④ Fourth

39. During the initial visit of a patient in a prenatal clinic, for which of the following assessments would the nurse be responsible?
    ① Enlargement of the uterus
    ② Examining for Goodell's sign
    ③ Enlargement of the breasts
    ④ Fetal heart tones

40. A patient is 35 weeks' pregnant and has ankle edema in the afternoon and evening but *not* when she arises in the morning. The nurse should inform the patient that:
    ① Edema with this pattern requires complete bed rest
    ② She is in the beginning stages of pregnancy-induced hypertension
    ③ She must restrict her sodium intake
    ④ This dependent edema that disappears after a night of sleep is not unusual during pregnancy

41. A patient is 8 months' pregnant with her second child. She tells the nurse that her 6-year-old son has been asking her why she is getting so fat. Which of the following responses should the nurse suggest?
    ① "I've been eating for two people, for me and the baby, so I'm gaining a lot of weight."
    ② "The baby is growing inside mommy's uterus, which is a special place where babies grow."
    ③ "The baby is growing inside mommy's stomach, so I am getting fat."
    ④ "The baby is getting so big that he is using up all my energy and I have to eat a lot more, which is making me fat."

42. A patient who is 6 months' pregnant tells the nurse that her 5-year-old son has been toilet trained for a while but is now wetting and soiling his pants like a new baby. The best guidance the nurse can give her is:
    ① That this will pass; it is just a phase he is going through
    ② To sit down and have a heart-to-heart talk with him, explaining that big boys don't do this
    ③ To scold him so he knows this is wrong
    ④ To include him when going to prenatal visits and in getting the baby's room ready

43. While giving her obstetrical health history, a patient who is new to the clinic states that she has a history of genital herpes simplex virus. Tests confirm that she is in the infectious stage. The patient is due to deliver her baby within the next 2 weeks. How will this diagnosis affect her care?
    ① She will be treated with antibiotics
    ② She will be treated immediately after delivery
    ③ She will need to have a C-section
    ④ She will need to be immunized

44. A patient who is a gravida 1 para 0 is a class B insulin-treated diabetic. She wants to know why she has to take more insulin during the second half of her pregnancy. The nurse tells her that:
    ① Hormonal activity tends to counteract the effects of insulin in the second half of pregnancy
    ② Because her activity level will increase, her insulin needs will also increase
    ③ Taking more insulin tends to prevent urinary tract infections
    ④ The baby is growing and needs extra insulin

45. A patient is 20 weeks' pregnant and has had persistent nausea and vomiting for the past 2 days. Her physician decides to admit her to the obstetric unit. In planning care for this patient, the nurse should know that the diagnosis is most likely to be:
    ① Pregnancy-induced hypertension
    ② Morning sickness
    ③ Hyperemesis gravidarum
    ④ Preeclampsia

46. The nurse caring for a patient with a diagnosis of hyperemesis gravidarum knows that, if left untreated, this condition could result in:
    ① A low-birth-weight infant
    ② Anorexia nervosa
    ③ Premature delivery
    ④ Maternal and/or fetal death

47. A patient calls the doctor's office complaining of nausea, vomiting, and a stabbing, tearing pain on her left side. She also indicates she has missed one menstrual period. The nurse's most appropriate action would be to:
    1. Recommend complete bed rest for 3 days
    2. Call an antibiotic order in to the pharmacy for the patient
    3. Have the patient come to the office immediately
    4. Send the patient to the hospital immediately

48. A patient is being evaluated for preeclampsia. Which of the following assessments would the nurse make first?
    1. Fundal height
    2. Blood pressure
    3. Urine for sugar/acetone
    4. Fetal heart tone

49. During her pregnancy a patient has developed a urinary tract infection. The nurse teaches the patient that it is important to:
    1. Drink four to six 8-oz glasses of fluid per day
    2. Eat extra carbohydrates and sugar
    3. Void before and after sexual intercourse
    4. Wear only nylon underwear

50. A patient who is a gravida 3 para 0 miscarried as a result of two preterm labors. To reduce the risk of preterm labor, the nurse teaches this patient to:
    1. Avoid salt in her diet
    2. Comply with the prescribed amount of bed rest
    3. Reduce calorie intake
    4. Reduce fluid intake

51. Patients in labor will need support and encouragement, especially during the:
    1. Second stage
    2. Third stage
    3. Early part of the first stage
    4. Transition phase of the first stage

52. When timing a patient's contractions, the nurse should place her hand:
    1. Just above the patient's pubis
    2. Just above the patient's umbilicus
    3. On either side of the patient's abdomen
    4. Between the pubis and the perineum

53. A patient is admitted to the labor room in what appears to be very early labor. She is anxious but excited because this is her first pregnancy. When planning care for this patient, the nurse knows that, once active labor begins, the patient can expect to give birth to her infant in approximately:
    1. 14 to 16 hours
    2. 18 to 20 hours
    3. 22 to 24 hours
    4. 26 to 28 hours

54. Accompanied to the delivery room by her husband, a patient gives birth to a female infant with an Apgar rating of 9 at 1 minute after birth. According to most states, the nurse legally identifies the infant by:
    1. Placing identification bracelets on mother and infant
    2. Attaching laboratory slips of the mother to the infant's chart to verify blood type
    3. Obtaining the signature of the physician on the identification sheet
    4. Obtaining the infant's footprints and the mother's fingerprint on the delivery record

55. After 16 hours of labor, a patient's first child has been delivered. The nurse knows that before a newborn takes the first breath, the physician will most likely:
    1. Clamp and cut the cord
    2. Evaluate the Apgar score
    3. Clear the infant's airway of mucus
    4. Repair the episiotomy

56. A newly admitted labor patient appears anxious and states, "I wish that my husband could be here. He's at work, and if he leaves, he'll lose his job." Which of the following interventions indicate caring and understanding on the part of the nurse?
    1. Ask the patient if there is another person she would like to have with her at this time
    2. Follow through with routine procedures according to hospital policy and procedure
    3. Explain that many women go through labor and delivery without their husbands
    4. Listen empathically, but say nothing in anticipation of being with her most of the time

57. A patient is to have a vaginal examination to determine how much the cervix has dilated. To prepare for the procedure, the nurse should include:
    1. Having a sterile speculum
    2. Cleaning the patient's vulva
    3. Placing the patient in lithotomy position
    4. Telling the patient to bear down

58. The physician has just completed his examination of a newly admitted patient in labor and requests that the nurse recheck the fetal heart tones. The nurse knows that the best location on the abdomen to hear the fetal heart tones is:
    1. Above the umbilicus
    2. Below the umbilicus
    3. The upper right quadrant
    4. The upper left quadrant

59. The nurse is administering an enema to a woman in early labor. An important reason for giving an enema at this time is to:
    1. Prevent constipation during labor
    2. Relieve pressure in case of an episiotomy
    3. Ease the contractions
    4. Provide for a clean delivery

60. A patient is admitted to the hospital in the first stage of labor. True labor is best described as having started when a patient's:
    ① Mucus plug is expelled from the cervical canal
    ② Membranes rupture spontaneously
    ③ Uterine contractions are regular and effective
    ④ Fetus drops into the brim of the pelvis

61. The nurse is caring for a patient in the latent phase of the first stage of labor. Which of the following situations would necessitate immediate notification of the physician?
    ① Meconium in the amniotic fluid
    ② No palpable movement of the fetus
    ③ Spontaneous rupture of the membranes
    ④ Fetal heart rate of 90 beats/min

62. A husband has been coaching his wife during labor. The patient now informs her husband and her nurse that she feels like pushing. The physician examines the patient and informs the nurse that the patient is completely dilated and ready to begin pushing. Which of the following instructions would the nurse be correct in giving the patient?
    ① Head back, arms forward, hips back, lips closed, and push down
    ② Inhale, head on chest, elbows out, push down toward anus and count to 10; pelvic tilt helps
    ③ Spread legs apart, take deep breath, and bear down while exhaling
    ④ Pant and blow until the fetus is completely delivered

63. A physician informs the nurse that the patient is 3 cm dilated and that the fetus is in cephalic presentation. In planning care for the patient, the nurse knows that this means the:
    ① Cervix is 3 cm thick, and the head of the fetus is high in the pelvis
    ② Fetal head is against the cervix, and the cervix is thinning
    ③ Cervix has opened 3 cm, and the fetal head is presenting
    ④ Fetal head is 3 cm above the ischial spines of the pelvis

64. A father-to-be tells the nurse that he has learned how to count fetal heart tones in childbirth classes and that he will record them for her on the labor record because she is so busy. The most appropriate action/response by the nurse would be to:
    ① Provide him with paper to record fetal heart tones and check his accuracy at intervals
    ② Tell him that this is the nurse's job and doing this would only increase his anxiety about the infant's condition
    ③ Explain that the nurse must monitor the fetal heart tones and ask him to assist in timing contractions
    ④ Explain that childbirth classes don't teach students everything they need to know about monitoring fetal heart tones

65. A patient has been in labor for 6 hours. Her membranes have just ruptured. The nurse's priority now is to assess:
    ① Amniotic fluid with nitrazine
    ② Duration of contractions
    ③ Fetal heart rate
    ④ Maternal vital signs

66. A 25-year-old gravida 2 para 1 is admitted to the labor room having contractions every 5 to 7 minutes, each lasting 30 to 35 seconds. She states that her contractions started about 2 hours ago and that her bag of waters (BOW) is intact. Vaginal examination reveals a cervix that is 2 cm dilated and 25% effaced. When planning care for this patient, the nurse knows that this patient is in:
    ① False labor; Braxton-Hicks contractions
    ② Early labor; latent phase
    ③ True labor; transitional phase
    ④ Active labor; third stage

67. A patient, gravida 12 para 10, is admitted to the labor and delivery suite in active labor. Contractions are approximately every 2 to 3 minutes, strong, lasting 45 to 50 seconds. She states that her membranes are still intact and that she has very fast labors. During her admission, which one of the following nursing actions would be contraindicated for this patient?
    ① Application of an external fetal monitor
    ② Requesting a urine specimen from the patient
    ③ Administering a small-volume enema
    ④ Requesting stat blood work

68. The nurse is timing a patient's contractions. To document correctly the nurse must know that the term used to describe the length of the contraction from beginning to end is called the:
    ① Duration
    ② Intensity
    ③ Frequency
    ④ Interval

69. Which one of the following choices would be the most important nursing function during the fourth stage of labor?
    ① Documenting the amount of time between contractions
    ② Assisting the doctor with the episiotomy repair
    ③ Sending umbilical blood samples to the lab
    ④ Checking the fundus for firmness

70. The delivery room nurse knows that a patient's labor is truly complete when the:
    ① Infant is delivered
    ② Cord is cut
    ③ Placenta is delivered
    ④ Uterus becomes inverted

71. Following the delivery of a healthy, 7 lb 7 oz (3375 g) baby girl, a patient begins to shiver and her teeth start chattering. Which of the following nursing interventions is appropriate?
    ① Check her temperature immediately
    ② Cover her with several warmed blankets
    ③ Administer oxygen via nasal canula
    ④ Administer acetaminophen

72. The physician delivers the baby, and the nurse gives an oxytocic drug to the new mother soon after the delivery of the placenta. This is done primarily to help:
① Decrease the likelihood of uterine spasms
② Strengthen contractions of the uterus
③ Hasten the process of involution
④ Prevent uterine inversion

73. A patient who is a 14-year-old primigravida has ruptured membranes, a slight, bloody show, and contractions that are 10 to 12 minutes apart, lasting about 20 seconds. She states that she was seen by a physician for the first time 3 weeks ago. The nurse notes that the patient's blood pressure is 150/98, her face is edematous, and her urine shows 2+ protein. The nurse would know that these are symptoms of:
① Normal delivery progress
② Impending delivery
③ Preeclampsia
④ Gestational diabetes

74. When planning care for cocaine-addicted mothers in labor, the nurse must know that they will experience:
① Fewer labor contractions than do nonaddicted mothers
② Stronger labor contractions than do nonaddicted mothers
③ No more or less discomfort than that experienced by nonaddicted mothers
④ Less need for sedation than do nonaddicted mothers, because of their cocaine addiction

75. A 15-year-old pregnant patient has just been admitted to the labor and delivery suite. She has had no prenatal care and on examination by the physician is noted to have an advanced case of herpes genitalis. In developing a plan of care for this patient, the nurse must:
① Suggest that the patient be placed in complete isolation
② Use extreme caution when preparing the patient for delivery
③ Implement universal precautions for blood and body fluids
④ Use strict handwashing procedures

76. A patient who is a gravida 2 para 1 has been in labor for the past 8 hours. During the last 2 hours, contractions have become progressively weaker, with no noticeable effect on cervical dilation or effacement. The physician orders an IV drip with oxytocin (Pitocin). Which of the following nursing interventions is of prime importance when observing a patient with an oxytocin drip?
① Time contractions; report to physician at frequent intervals
② Monitor the intervals during and after contractions; report if longer than 5 minutes apart
③ Monitor the blood pressure and patient reactions to IV drip
④ Monitor intervals carefully; if less than 1 minute or absent, stop IV and notify physician immediately

77. A patient who is 38 weeks' pregnant is admitted to the labor room following a seizure at home. The patient is extremely anxious and is complaining of epigastric pain. Her blood pressure is 190/112. The physician orders 4 g magnesium sulfate to be given intravenously in 250 ml D_5W. When planning care for this patient, the nurse knows that this medication will:
① Reduce the pulse rate
② Stimulate labor
③ Reduce edema
④ Increase peristalsis

78. A patient is admitted to the hospital with third-trimester bleeding. She is crying and very nervous. The appropriate nursing action is to:
① Ask the chaplain to talk to the patient
② Explain possible causes for the bleeding
③ Leave the patient and her husband alone after the initial assessment
④ Reassure the couple that everything will probably be all right

79. While working in the labor and delivery area, the nurse must be aware of the signs and symptoms of premature separation of the placenta from the uterine wall. This is known as a (an):
① Ectopic pregnancy
② Placenta previa
③ Abruptio placentae
④ Complete abortion

80. The patient asks if she will be able to breast-feed her baby after a cesarean delivery. The nurse's best reply would be:
① "You'd better bottle-feed, because you will probably be in a lot of pain."
② "You can still breast-feed, and we will help you."
③ "It's best that you ask your doctor."
④ "You don't have to decide now."

81. A patient is going to surgery for an emergency cesarean section. Which of the following anesthetics would the nurse recognize as being the best choice for both mother and infant?
① An epidural block
② A general anesthetic
③ A pudendal block
④ A Bier's block

82. A patient has just been admitted to the recovery room following a cesarean section for which she received spinal anesthesia. Which of the following actions by the recovery room nurse is appropriate in caring for this patient?
① Avoid palpating the uterine fundus
② Restrict oral fluids until the gag reflex returns
③ Catheterize the patient every 4 hours following surgery
④ Keep the patient lying flat for 8 to 12 hours following surgery

83. Nursing assessment of a patient with placenta previa often reveals:
① Pain with no bleeding
② Pain with passage of clots
③ Painless bleeding with a hard uterus
④ Painless bleeding with a soft uterus

84. A patient who is in her thirty-sixth week of pregnancy has had no contractions, but amniotic fluid has been slowly leaking from her vagina. Priority nursing assessment includes:
   ① Nutritional history
   ② Onset of contractions
   ③ Urinalysis
   ④ Vital signs

85. Labor progresses without incident, and a patient delivers a healthy baby boy and is taken to the recovery room. Because the patient was diagnosed as having preeclampsia, the nurse knows that she must still be observed for impending eclampsia for at least:
   ① 3 hours
   ② 24 hours
   ③ 36 hours
   ④ 72 hours

86. A gravida 1 para 0 patient has a diagnosis of preeclampsia and is receiving magnesium sulfate during early labor. The nurse observes that the patient's respirations are 9 and that her patellar reflexes (DTRs) have decreased. This information should be:
   ① Recorded and monitored
   ② Immediately brought to the physician's attention
   ③ Considered an indication for increasing the dose
   ④ Considered to be a normal result

87. A patient is admitted to the obstetric unit with a diagnosis of preeclampsia, and the physician orders IV magnesium sulfate. In planning care for this patient, the nurse knows that this drug is administered to:
   ① Prevent convulsions
   ② Relieve pain
   ③ Increase blood pressure
   ④ Induce labor

88. A patient is concerned that her other children have not shown any interest in the new baby when they have come to visit her in the hospital. The nurse responds to this concern with:
   ① "It's just as well, because babies need their rest. They can stay away until he's older."
   ② "It's just as well, because they may hurt him if they get too close to him."
   ③ "Time will take care of things; just wait, they will come around."
   ④ "Include them in the care and attention you give the baby."

89. An expectant couple are concerned that their 5-year-old daughter will have difficulty adjusting to the new baby. When counseling the couple, the nurse knows that it is important for them to:
   ① Buy presents for their daughter, equal to the number they feel the new baby will receive
   ② Allow their daughter to kiss and hold the new baby so she will begin to love the new baby
   ③ Tell their daughter that she is a big girl and can help mommy with some chores around the house
   ④ Plan to spend time alone with their daughter, doing the things that she wants to do

90. The nurse is giving postpartum instructions to her patient. She explains that for the first 2 to 3 days her lochia will be:
   ① Pale pink or brownish
   ② Yellowish, creamy discharge
   ③ Excessive and bright red
   ④ Dark red to bright red

91. A new postpartum patient's lochia has several clots and has saturated the perineal pad. When documenting, the nurse would describe this amount of lochia as:
   ① Moderate
   ② Gross
   ③ Scant
   ④ Heavy

92. A new mother has decided not to breast-feed her newborn son because of recurrent mastitis. She asks the nurse how much formula she should give the infant, and how often. Which of the following suggestions offered by the nurse is in line with the general guidelines for formula feedings?
   ① Allow the infant as much as he likes as often as he likes
   ② 30 ml every 1 to 2 hours for the first 2 months
   ③ 60 to 120 ml every 3 to 4 hours for the first 2 months
   ④ 180 to 280 ml every 3 hours for the first 2 months

93. In addition to using an anesthetic ointment, another common measure the nurse could suggest to relieve discomfort from an episiotomy is to have the patient:
   ① Ambulate frequently
   ② Take sitz baths
   ③ Elevate her hips while in bed
   ④ Apply cortisone ointment to the perineal area

94. A patient has decided to try "rooming in" with her first baby. In helping the patient prepare, the nursery nurse should inform her that rooming in means that:
   ① The baby's father will be allowed to stay in the room and assist in caring for his new baby
   ② A private duty nurse will care for her for the first few days
   ③ The patient will be sharing her room with another mother who is more experienced in infant care
   ④ The patient's infant will be at her bedside so that she may care for her as long as she feels up to it

95. A patient is breast-feeding her infant daughter and using the demand feeding method. In planning care for the baby, the nursery nurse understands that this method allows the baby to be fed:
   ① Whenever she cries
   ② Approximately every 4 hours
   ③ At the time and in the amount the newborn wishes
   ④ Whenever her mother feels her breasts to be full

96. The nurse knows that breast-feeding increases nutritional requirements. In planning care for a patient who plans to breast-feed, the nurse knows that this increase includes:
    ① An additional 1000 ml of fluids daily and increased protein
    ② An additional 3000 ml of fluids and an additional 640 calories daily
    ③ Additional vitamin supplements and protein every other day
    ④ An additional half-quart of milk and vitamin supplements daily

97. A new mother asks the nurse how soon it will be before she can start to breast-feed and is anxious to know when her milk will begin to flow. Which of the following statements by the nurse is the most appropriate in answering this patient's questions?
    ① "I really can't answer that; perhaps you should ask your physician."
    ② "Your baby will be brought to you for the next feeding; your milk will probably start right after that."
    ③ "We encourage you to nurse as soon as you can; your milk will probably start in about 3 days."
    ④ "The baby can nurse anytime after birth."

98. On the second day after delivery, a patient who is breast-feeding complains that her breasts feel tight and are tender. The correct nursing action in response to the patient's complaint is to:
    ① Offer to bottle-feed her baby in the nursery for the next several feedings
    ② Notify the physician, because this may be a sign of mastitis
    ③ Apply a breast binder and ice packs to the breasts
    ④ Tell her that nursing her baby will offer relief

99. A patient delivered her baby 1 hour ago. The anesthesia used was a spinal block. She calls the nurse to request help to the bathroom. Which of the following would be the best action for the nurse to take?
    ① Get someone to assist her in walking the patient to the bathroom
    ② Use a wheelchair to assist the patient to the bathroom
    ③ Take a bedside commode into the room for the patient to use
    ④ Assist the patient in using the bedpan

100. When caring for a postpartum patient, the nurse may best facilitate the return of normal bowel and bladder function by which of the following nursing interventions?
    ① Providing perineal care and administering sitz baths as ordered
    ② Encouraging ambulation and eating of a well-balanced diet
    ③ Obtaining orders for simple catheterization and a cathartic
    ④ Recording intake and output, and instructing the patient in perineal care

101. A patient who is 2 days postpartum tells the nurse she has not had a bowel movement since delivery. The most appropriate nursing intervention would be to:
    ① Obtain an order for a Fleet enema; encourage ambulation
    ② Check for fecal impaction; suggest additional fluids
    ③ Encourage fluids and bulk-forming foods
    ④ Check for fecal impaction; administer a laxative

102. Several hours after delivery, a patient's uterus lies to the right side of her abdomen. The nurse knows that the most likely reason for this position is that the:
    ① Stomach is distended
    ② Urinary bladder is full
    ③ Uterus has returned to normal position
    ④ Uterus is filling with blood

103. A variety of nursing interventions are implemented to help the patient void after delivery. An overdistended bladder is likely to predispose the patient to development of:
    ① A hematoma
    ② Phlebitis
    ③ Cystitis
    ④ A tumor

104. A patient is unsure as to whether she should have her newborn baby boy circumcised. Which of the following comments by the nurse is most appropriate in responding to the patient's uncertainty?
    ① "Circumcision is necessary for good hygiene."
    ② "Circumcision reduces the incidence of disease."
    ③ "Circumcision decreases the risk of sexually transmitted diseases (STDs)."
    ④ "Circumcision is a matter of the parents' personal choice."

105. A baby was circumcised the morning of discharge. The nurse's discharge teaching to the new mother should include the fact that:
    ① Frequent checking for bleeding and keeping the incision well-lubricated are important
    ② Complications frequently occur after the procedure
    ③ Voiding is frequently affected, causing the baby's abdomen to become distended
    ④ Healing takes a long time because circulation to the site is poor

106. A patient who is a gravida 5 para 3 ab 2 is being discharged after delivering a 9 lb 2 oz (4139 g) baby boy 2 days earlier. How many live births did this mother have?
    ① Three
    ② Five
    ③ Eight
    ④ Ten

107. A 36-year-old postpartum patient has come to the health department seeking contraceptives. She has no health problems and is seeking a method that does not have to be remembered each day or before intercourse. The best choice for this patient would be:
    ① Condoms
    ② Oral contraceptives
    ③ Diaphragm
    ④ Norplant system

108. A young patient's family is very supportive, but she expresses concern about how to financially support herself and the baby. She is only 14 years old. The best response by the nurse should be:
    ① "Why didn't you think about that before you got pregnant?"
    ② "Ask the baby's father to help; it's his responsibility too."
    ③ "Tell me some things you have considered so we can research some possibilities."
    ④ "Welfare seems to be the only answer."

109. On the second postpartum day, the nurse finds a new mother crying and complaining of feeling "down in the dumps." When caring for this patient, the nurse should:
    ① Leave her alone to work through her feelings
    ② Tell her to cheer up because she has a fine healthy baby
    ③ Explain that this is a normal response that many women experience
    ④ Consult the psychiatric clinical nurse specialist for guidance

110. A patient has just delivered twin sons via a normal vaginal delivery. The nurse is aware that she is now at increased risk for:
    ① Early postpartum hemorrhage
    ② Mastitis
    ③ Postpartum infection
    ④ Thrombophlebitis

111. Routine newborn care following delivery includes administration of an antibiotic ointment for the eyes. It is important that this be included in the nursing care plan for all infants, because these medications prevent blindness as a result of:
    ① Herpes
    ② Syphilis
    ③ Gonorrhea
    ④ Retrolental fibroplasia

112. Newborns have many needs. When planning for immediate care of a newborn, the nurse knows that the highest priority for the newborn following delivery is the need to be:
    ① Weighed
    ② Kept warm
    ③ Bathed
    ④ Circumcised

113. The nurse is to give the infant an injection of vitamin K. The best site to use for an intramuscular injection on an infant is:
    ① Biceps femoris
    ② Gluteus maximus
    ③ Vastus lateralis
    ④ Biceps brachii

114. The nurse is admitting a newborn to the well-baby nursery. The baby has an order for vitamin K intramuscularly. The nurse understands that this medication is given to newborns to prevent:
    ① Blood clots
    ② Bleeding
    ③ Gonorrhea
    ④ Anemia

115. When evaluating a newborn's heart rate, respiratory rate, muscle activity, reflex irritability, and color, the best possible score the team can obtain when using the Apgar scoring system is:
    ① 4
    ② 10
    ③ 14
    ④ 18

116. Capillary blood is often used to determine blood glucose levels and test for specific conditions such as phenylketonuria in the newborn. The site used to obtain the specimen is the heel. To increase blood flow to the area, the nurse should:
    ① Do nothing specific
    ② Elevate the foot of the crib
    ③ Wrap the foot in a warm wet cloth
    ④ Soak both feet in a saline solution

117. In observing a newborn the first 12 hours after delivery, the nurse notes that the infant's eyelids are puffy and red. The most appropriate nursing action is to:
    ① Notify the pediatrician immediately
    ② Culture any exudate noted at the inner canthus
    ③ Gently clean any exudate with warm sterile water
    ④ Review the labor record to see if any trauma to the head or eyes was noted

118. The nurse has just admitted a newborn baby girl from the delivery room. While reviewing the chart, the nurse notes the weight to be 8 lb (3632 g). In planning care for this infant, the nurse can expect that she will lose up to 10% of her birth weight. The nurse would be correct in estimating the newborn's weight to drop to:
    ① 7 lb 8 oz (3405 g)
    ② 7 lb 3 oz (3260 g)
    ③ 7 lb (3178 g)
    ④ 7 lb 5 oz (3317 g)

119. The nurse is preparing to give a baby his first bath following delivery. It would be appropriate for the nurse to:
    ① Hold the bath until he has begun taking PO fluids
    ② Initially clean only his face and torso
    ③ Provide cord care first
    ④ Use gloves throughout the entire procedure

120. The nursery nurse notes that a newborn baby girl has a small amount of pink vaginal discharge. The nurse knows that this is:
    ① Normal because of maternal hormones
    ② Normal because of birth trauma
    ③ Abnormal because of excessive hormones
    ④ The baby's first menses

121. The newest addition to the nursery, a baby girl, is noted to have an enlarged breast. Which of the following instructions would the nurse give the parents on how to care for this condition?
    ① Squeeze it daily
    ② Bind the breasts
    ③ Apply hot packs
    ④ Do nothing

122. When planning care, the nurse should be aware that all newborns should be burped (bubbled) during and after each feeding to prevent:
    ① Regurgitation of the feeding
    ② Gas pains/colic
    ③ Pneumonia
    ④ Pneumaturia

123. The nurse notices a 4-day-old infant tensing, throwing his arms out, and crying loudly. What should the nurse do?
    ① Nothing; this is a normal response of newborns
    ② Call the doctor; this may be an early sign of seizures
    ③ Restrain the baby so he will not hurt himself
    ④ Turn the baby to the left side to limit the reaction

124. When a baby's cheek is stroked, she turns her head in the direction of the stroked cheek. The nurse caring for the baby knows that this reflex, present at birth, is known as the:
    ① Rooting reflex
    ② Moro reflex
    ③ Tonic neck reflex
    ④ Sucking reflex

125. The nursery nurse meets all new mothers on a daily basis. During a recent encounter, a patient asked, "Why does she have such black, sticky stuff in her diaper? It looks awful and it's so hard to clean. Is she bleeding internally? I know something is wrong with her!" The nurse's response should be:
    ① "You should know that it is meconium. Didn't they cover that in your prenatal classes?"
    ② "That is meconium. It's baby's first bowel movement until the normal yellow stool comes through."
    ③ "Oh, that's nothing to worry about. It's normal."
    ④ "She's not bleeding. You're worrying needlessly."

126. A baby boy is admitted to the newborn nursery in good condition. On assessment, the nurse knows that the respirations of the normal neonate will be:
    ① Regular, 24 to 36 per minute
    ② Irregular, 40 to 58 per minute
    ③ Regular, 30 to 44 per minute
    ④ Irregular, 32 to 48 per minute

127. The physician orders phototherapy for a newborn who is 2 days old and has a bilirubin level of 13 mg/dl. Which of the following nursing interventions is of prime importance in caring for an infant undergoing phototherapy?
    ① Cover the eyes loosely with cotton balls
    ② Restrict fluids to enhance effects of therapy
    ③ Remove all clothing, including the diaper
    ④ Monitor skin temperature

128. Three days after birth a newborn appears to be slightly jaundiced. In caring for this baby, the nursery nurse is aware that this condition is most likely the result of:
    ① Rh incompatibility
    ② ABO incompatibility
    ③ Normal destruction of red blood cells
    ④ A liver malfunction

129. A new mother examines her baby and says, "Look, my baby's hands and feet are purple! She must have a heart condition. I know there is something wrong with her!" The nurse's response to this should be:
    ① "Bluish discoloration of the hands and feet occurs with newborns and usually lasts for a few days."
    ② "Your baby is cold because you've kept her undressed for so long."
    ③ "Your baby worked hard during delivery by kicking and pushing. She has bruised herself."
    ④ "Your baby probably does have problems. We will have to call the doctor."

130. A new mother puts her baby on the bed and begins to walk away, stating that she has to go to the bathroom down the hall. The appropriate nursing action would be to:
    ① Watch and say nothing
    ② Pick up the baby and put her in the crib
    ③ Sit on the edge of the bed next to the baby
    ④ Caution the new mother never to leave the baby unattended

131. One minute a new mother shows concern for her new baby by asking a lot of questions. The next minute she appears not to care as she leaves the baby unattended. Observation of this patient leads the nurse to assume which of the following?
    ① She has answered all of the patient's questions satisfactorily and doesn't need to do anything else
    ② She has taken care of all of the patient's concerns; she is all right
    ③ The patient's questions are the kind usually asked by new mothers, and there is no need for concern
    ④ The changes in the patient's behavior are of concern and should be reported to the charge nurse immediately

132. A patient who is a primipara and has just delivered a baby girl asks if something is wrong with her baby because she is breathing so fast. The nurse's most appropriate response would be:
    ① "A newborn's respirations vary, going up to 60 at times and as low as 30."
    ② "We should watch her closely. That seems high to me, too!"
    ③ "Why don't you let us check her vital signs for accurate information?"
    ④ "You don't need to worry; her color is okay."

133. Which of the following would the nurse recognize as the *normal* heart rate of a newborn at rest?
    ① 100 to 110 beats/min
    ② 110 to 120 beats/min
    ③ 120 to 140 beats/min
    ④ 160 to 180 beats/min

134. A newborn is being given a PO elixir. The best technique for the nurse to use would be to:
    ① Mix the medication with 1 mg of formula
    ② Place a small amount in a spoon and give slowly
    ③ Mix with a small amount of rice cereal and give slowly
    ④ Give through a 1-ml syringe placed against the buccal wall

135. An infant born with a cleft lip and palate has a multitude of problems to be considered when formulating a nursing care plan. Which one of the following would be the most pressing patient problem?
    ① Risk for infection
    ② Threat to body image
    ③ Potential for injury
    ④ Inability to feed

136. The nurse is assisting with the development of a preoperative care plan for an infant with a cleft lip. The plan should include which of the following interventions?
    ① Discouraging discussions of feelings about the defect by the parents
    ② Feeding the infant upright with the nipple well back into mouth
    ③ Describing surgical repair with the parents, emphasizing the poor appearance that could result
    ④ Feeding the infant by nasogastric tube until NPO for surgery

137. A newborn is admitted to the nursery with a confirmed diagnosis of Down syndrome. In preparing to care for the infant and to respond to questions the mother may have, it is important for the nursery nurse to know that this condition is:
    ① A congenital abnormality
    ② Caused by a bacterial infection
    ③ Caused by a viral infection
    ④ A result of oxygen deprivation

138. A couple anxiously awaited the birth of their first child. The infant was born with a myelomeningocele. As the delivery room nurse cares for the infant, the new father suddenly leaves the delivery room. The best way for the nurse to approach the father is to:
    ① Offer him a cup of coffee and leave him alone
    ② Sit down beside him and ask if he needs help
    ③ Tell him that, although deformed, the baby can live a normal life
    ④ Ask him several questions about the delivery to start conversation

139. Seeing his new son, who was born with a myelomeningocele, for the first time, the father asks, "What is that horrible thing on my baby's back?" An appropriate first response from the nurse would include:
    ① The term "myelomeningocele" and a simple description of the anomaly
    ② A description of the long-term care the infant will need
    ③ A full description of the condition, including complications
    ④ Conversation that would direct his attention away from the situation

140. In caring for a newborn with a myelomeningocele, it is important that the nurse observe closely for:
    ① Bowel elimination
    ② Moro's reflex
    ③ Relationship with the mother
    ④ Hemoglobin levels

141. The nurse can assist the physician in determining the extent of neuromuscular damage in an infant with spina bifida by:
    ① Observing movement of extremities
    ② Testing response to deep pain
    ③ Checking tendon reflexes
    ④ Recording the type of cry heard

142. In caring for a newborn addicted to cocaine, the nurse must know that the infant reacts to the drug because:
    ① Of the inability of the infant's immature liver to excrete the drug rapidly
    ② Of use of the drug by the mother just before conception
    ③ When taken by the mother in combination with other drugs, cocaine is doubly addictive
    ④ It impairs uterine growth and fosters respiratory distress syndrome problems following birth

143. A newborn has been diagnosed with ophthalmia neonatorum. It is important for the nurse to know that ophthalmia neonatorum refers to:
    ① Congenital cataracts
    ② Congenital syphilis
    ③ Gonorrheal infection of the conjunctiva
    ④ Congenital deformities

144. In caring for the newborn with hyperbilirubinemia, it is important for the nurse to know that this is a hemolytic disease caused by an:
    ① Rh-negative father and Rh-negative mother giving birth to an Rh-positive baby
    ② Rh-negative mother giving birth to an Rh-positive baby fathered by Rh-positive father
    ③ Rh-positive mother giving birth to an Rh-positive baby fathered by Rh-positive father
    ④ Rh-positive mother giving birth to an Rh-negative baby fathered by Rh-positive father

145. A newborn has been undergoing phototherapy for high bilirubin levels because of ABO incompatibility. In caring for this infant, the nurse might expect the baby's stools to be:
    ① Watery and green
    ② Golden yellow and loose
    ③ Greenish black and sticky
    ④ Pale yellow and soft

146. A new mother, a gravida 2 para 1, has a blood type of O positive, and her husband's is A negative. During the first day after delivery, the nurse observes slight yellowing of the sclera in the newborn. By the second day, the jaundice is more obvious and is noted over the infant's entire body. Laboratory studies indicate the unconjugated bilirubin level to be 9 mg/dl. When planning further care for this infant, the nurse must consider that the jaundice is most likely related to:
    ① Normal physiology of the newborn
    ② Rh incompatibility
    ③ Hepatitis B
    ④ ABO incompatibility

147. A baby was admitted to the newborn nursery at 5:01 AM. The infant's mother had an active case of syphilis diagnosed during her pregnancy but did not comply with the treatment protocol for the disease. In caring for a newborn possibly infected with syphilis, the nurse must observe for which of the following signs and symptoms?
    ① Rash and nasal discharge
    ② Vomiting and diarrhea
    ③ Central nervous system instability and seizures
    ④ Conjunctivitis and septicemia

148. In planning care for a newborn who has tested HIV positive, it is most important for the nurse to:
    ① Wash hands frequently
    ② Notify the Centers for Disease Control and Prevention
    ③ Implement universal precaution protocol
    ④ Wear mask, gown, and gloves at all times

149. The nurse is assisting the pediatrician in examining a 6 month old. The baby weighed 7 pounds 6 ounces at birth. The nurse would expect the child's weight to be approximately what now?
    ① 21 pounds
    ② 15 pounds
    ③ 10 pounds
    ④ 25 pounds

150. A 2-year-old's mother states that her son's favorite word lately has been "no!" The nurse can explain that according to Erickson's developmental stage, he is in a stage of:
    ① Industry vs. inferiority
    ② Autonomy vs. doubt
    ③ Trust vs. mistrust
    ④ Initiative vs. guilt

151. Knowledge of child growth and development principles is essential when planning care for a pediatric patient. Therefore the nurse knows that punishment is most effective when:
    ① The child knows that his mother loves him
    ② It is a logical consequence of wrongdoing
    ③ It enables the parent to constructively channel his or her anger
    ④ The child has been disobedient

152. In caring for pediatric patients, it is important that the nurse understand normal growth and development periods. A sense of trust is developed at a definite period in the life of the child. This period is primarily during:
    ① Adolescence
    ② Preschool
    ③ School age
    ④ Infancy

153. A new mother brings her 1-month-old son to the pediatric clinic. The nurse recognizes which of the following developmental achievements as normal for the infant?
    ① He rolls from his back to his right side
    ② He smiles and laughs aloud when talked to
    ③ He holds a rattle for a brief period
    ④ He turns his head from side to side while on his abdomen

154. The nurse observes an infant in the pediatric clinic to be competent in various developmental skills, including holding her head erect when in a sitting position, staring at an object when it is placed in her hand and putting it in her mouth, cooing and gurgling when talked to, and sustaining part of her own weight when held in a standing position. The nurse is correct when she assesses the infant's age to be approximately:
    ① 2 months
    ② 4 months
    ③ 6 months
    ④ 8 months

155. A mother states, "The soft spot near the front of my child's head is still big. When will it close?" The nurse's response should be guided by knowledge that most often the anterior fontanel closes when the infant is between the ages of:
    ① 2 and 4 months
    ② 4 and 8 months
    ③ 8 and 12 months
    ④ 15 and 18 months

156. Knowledge of the principles of child growth and development is essential in planning care for a pediatric patient. The nurse knows that language and speech development is promoted by speaking to the 18 month old:
    ① Clearly and simply
    ② With a rich vocabulary
    ③ In "baby talk"
    ④ As if he or she were an adult

157. In caring for a toddler, the nurse must know that a physiologic task that would be unrealistic for most toddlers between 12 and 14 months of age to achieve is:
    ① Helping to feed self
    ② Walking with assistance
    ③ Manipulating building blocks
    ④ Controlling the anal sphincter

158. When planning the care of a pediatric patient, the nurse knows that to facilitate readiness for toilet training, the child should wear:
    ① Diapers
    ② Rubber pants
    ③ Training pants
    ④ Overalls

159. When planning care for the pediatric patient, the nurse knows that toddlers often ingest or aspirate foreign bodies because they:
    ① Want to frighten their mothers
    ② Want to get attention
    ③ Have easy access to them
    ④ Learn through exploring

160. A toddler's mother expressed concern that her son, age 2, does not play with other children or share his toys. The nurse's appropriate response to the mother would be:
    ① "You'd better take him to counseling sessions."
    ② "He has probably inherited his father's behavior."
    ③ "You should strongly encourage him to share toys."
    ④ "He is demonstrating normal behavior for his age."

161. A mother brings her 14-month-old toddler to the health clinic for a checkup. During the assessment, she states that she is having difficulty toilet training her child. Which nursing action would be the most appropriate?
    ① Review various toilet training techniques with the mother
    ② Stress the importance of not punishing the child during toilet training
    ③ Encourage the mother to wait several months and try again
    ④ Suggest treats to be given after the child uses the toilet

162. When observing a pediatric patient, the nurse knows that gross motor coordination is demonstrated by:
    ① Running
    ② Tying shoelaces
    ③ Writing
    ④ Sewing

163. When caring for a 5 year old, the nurse knows that the normal pulse rate for a child of this age is:
    ① 76 to 90 beats/min
    ② 90 to 110 beats/min
    ③ 110 to 140 beats/min
    ④ 120 to 150 beats/min

164. When caring for a pediatric patient, the nurse knows that a major benefit a preschool child receives from attending nursery school is:
    ① Lessening of sibling rivalry
    ② Improvement in eating and sleeping habits
    ③ An opportunity to learn to play with peers
    ④ Decreased tension and anxiety for his age

165. The nurse knows that according to Erikson, when a child starts engaging in tasks in the real world (learning to win recognition by producing things), this change is a sign of the emergence of the child's sense of:
    ① Autonomy
    ② Industry
    ③ Initiative
    ④ Intimacy

166. The nurse knows that an important aspect of development of the child during the middle childhood years is his or her ability to engage in:
    ① Abstract thinking
    ② Logical thinking
    ③ Perceptual thinking
    ④ Preconceptual thinking

167. A nurse providing care for an infant realizes the baby's mother does not respond when the baby cries. As a result, the baby's basic needs are not being met, which the nurse knows may contribute to:
    ① Ability to trust others
    ② Poor interpersonal relationships
    ③ Self-confidence
    ④ No sense of purpose

168. It is important for the nurse working in the local well-baby clinic to know that the total number of deciduous teeth is:
    ① 18
    ② 20
    ③ 22
    ④ 24

169. While doing a history on a 3 year old the nurse notes that the toddler is drinking 24 ounces of milk per day. What would be the nurse's best response?
    ① "This is an appropriate amount for a 3 year old."
    ② "This is too much for a 3 year old to be drinking."
    ③ "You need to increase it to 38 ounces per day."
    ④ "You need to replace the milk with juices."

170. According to Piaget's stages of cognitive development, which of the following would be the best technique for preparing a child of 8 years for surgery?
    ① Have the mother stay with the child until anesthesia has begun.
    ② Explain in abstract terms what will happen in surgery and allow the child to reason out the outcomes.
    ③ Take the child to the operating room before the day of surgery so the child can touch and feel the equipment that will be used.
    ④ The child is too young to understand surgery, so explanations should be directed to the parents.

171. In caring for the adolescent, the nurse must understand adolescent characteristics. Which statement regarding adolescence is *least true*?
    ① Sexual experiences have repercussions on budding identity
    ② Adolescent rebellion is inevitable in our society
    ③ A major problem for adolescents today is pregnancy
    ④ Current sexual attitudes and behaviors are more liberal than in the past

172. Which of the following behaviors would the nurse expect to be characteristic of a 13 year old?
    ① Predictability
    ② Seclusive and moody
    ③ Accepting of parents' ideals
    ④ Moving from autonomy to dependency

173. In caring for the adolescent patient, the nurse must know that Erikson's theory of development states that adolescents are in the stage of:
    ① Industry vs. inferiority
    ② Trust vs. mistrust
    ③ Initiative vs. guilt
    ④ Identity vs. role confusion

174. The nurse working on an adolescent unit knows that, in planning care for patients, consideration should be given to the developmental tasks of the adolescent. These include all of the following *except:*
    ① Development of body image
    ② Being dependent on parents
    ③ Achieving proper social roles
    ④ Establishment of career goals

175. An 18 month old has seen the physician for a well-baby examination. The doctor has recommended that he receive his MMR (measles, mumps, rubella) vaccine. This vaccine provides:
    ① Passive immunity
    ② Active immunity
    ③ Artificial immunity
    ④ Temporary immunity

176. A preschool child's mother asks the nurse about immunizations and communicable diseases. Which of the following statements best describes the incidence of communicable diseases in children?
    ① Communicable diseases have been eradicated by immunizations
    ② Immunizations have reduced the incidence of communicable disease; however, communicable diseases are still a major cause of illness in children
    ③ Communicable diseases are absolutely necessary in a child's life
    ④ Communicable diseases are never severe

177. A 16 year old has been exposed to a friend with tuberculosis. His physician has ordered a Mantoux test for him. The nurse prepares the intradermal injection. In order for the bleb to form during the injection, the bevel of the needle should be facing:
    ① Up
    ② Down
    ③ Distally
    ④ Proximally

178. The U.S. Department of Health and Human Services publishes an immunization schedule for children. Which of the following schedules do they recommend?
    ① 1 month: DPT, OPV
       3 months: DPT, OPV
       5 months: DPT
       10 months: DPT, OPV, MMR
    ② 2 months: DPT, OPV
       4 months: DPT, OPV
       6 months: DPT
       15 months: DPT, OPV, MMR
    ③ 4 months: DPT, OPV
       8 months: DPT, OPV
       12 months: DPT
       16 months: DPT, OPV, MMR
    ④ 3 months: DPT, OPV
       6 months: DPT, OPV
       9 months: DPT
       12 months: DPT, OPV, MMR

179. In planning discharge instructions for a 2-day postpartum patient, the nurse needs to include instructions for the infant's immunizations. The best planning would include directions to begin the infant's immunizations at what age?
    ① 1 month
    ② 2 months
    ③ 4 months
    ④ 6 months

180. A 15 month old received a measles vaccine when she was 11 months old. The nurse informs the mother that the toddler will need to be revaccinated for measles because:
    ① There are fewer side effects at this age
    ② Children less than 1 year old do not get measles
    ③ Circulating maternal antibodies interfere with immunity
    ④ A new strain of measles has been identified

181. A mother brings her 10-month-old infant to the clinic for a check-up. During the history the mother mentions that the baby's food intake consists of breast milk only. What would be the best response by the nurse?
    ① "Breast milk is all the baby needs at this point."
    ② "You need to supplement with vitamins."
    ③ "Be sure you are eating enough iron in your food."
    ④ "The baby needs to be eating solid food."

182. The schedule for introduction of semisolid foods depends on the infant and the physician's recommendation. The nurse would instruct the mother to introduce cereal at:
    ① 1 to 2 months
    ② 2 to 3 months
    ③ 5 to 6 months
    ④ 7 to 8 months

183. When explaining an infant's diet and feeding schedule to a new mother, the nurse must include the following principles. Which is the *most* important for the nurse to emphasize?
    ① New foods are introduced one at a time to observe for allergies
    ② Pureed fruits and cereals are added when formula no longer satisfies the infant
    ③ Solid foods are added when the infant begins to chew
    ④ Formula feedings are supplemental, along with plenty of water

184. A high school student asks the school nurse what he can eat to increase the vitamin C content of his diet. His basketball coach suggested this because he seems to bruise easily. The nurse can suggest which of the following in response to his question?
    ① Milk, cheese, eggs
    ② Fats, oils, sugar
    ③ Breads, cereals, rice
    ④ Oranges, lemons, strawberries

185. A school-age child is receiving a low-sodium diet. She has requested an evening snack. In planning her diet, which of the following foods would the nurse consider?
    ① Banana
    ② Candy bar
    ③ Ham sandwich
    ④ Tuna salad

186. A 5 year old, ill with chicken pox, is running a temperature that fluctuates between 101° to 103° F and refuses to eat but will drink liquids. The mother asks the nurse what the best liquids are, stating the child prefers chicken broth, tea, 7-Up, and orange soda. The nurse suggests 7-Up and orange soda because the nutrients in these liquids will function to:
    ① Rebuild and repair cells
    ② Supply fuel for cell metabolism
    ③ Provide padding for vital organs
    ④ Insulate the body and help control temperature

187. The nurse is evaluating the diet of a 13 year old during a health promotion discussion. Which of the following are fat-soluble vitamins?
    ① Vitamin C, vitamin D, vitamin B_{12}
    ② Vitamin B_{12}, vitamin E, biotin
    ③ Vitamin B_6, folic acid, vitamin D
    ④ Vitamin A, vitamin K, vitamin E

188. A 5-year-old child does not like to drink milk. Which of the following foods would the nurse suggest to the child's mother to meet the need for essential amino acids provided by milk??
    ① Cereals
    ② Eggs
    ③ Lentils
    ④ Legumes

189. A urinalysis performed on a 5 year old shows a high bacteria count. Which of the following instructions should be included when teaching the child's mother?
    ① Bathe her daily in a tub, using soap and water
    ② Discontinue antibiotics as soon as symptoms disappear
    ③ Have her drink only cranberry juice
    ④ Wipe her perineum from front to back after she voids

190. While doing a physical examination on a 15-month-old child, which of the following should be included?
    ① Head circumference, blood pressure, and temperature
    ② Blood pressure, pulse, and temperature
    ③ Head circumference, temperature, and pulse
    ④ Oral temperature, pulse, and respirations

191. In caring for a child with rheumatic fever, the nurse must know that the most potentially serious complication from it is:
    ① Disintegration of the joints
    ② Cardiac involvement
    ③ Cerebral involvement
    ④ Paralysis of limbs

192. A 9-year-old boy is admitted to the hospital for further testing. He has been experiencing low-grade fevers, weight loss, and pain in his arms and legs. He recently had a sore throat and was diagnosed as having rheumatic fever. In planning care for this patient, the nurse knows that the organism most likely responsible for the sore throat is:
    ① A virus
    ② *Pneumococcus*
    ③ *Staphylococcus*
    ④ *Streptococcus*

193. The physician orders aspirin for a 9 year old with rheumatic fever. The nurse knows that the most probable reason for this medication is to relieve:
    ① Carditis
    ② Cardiac enlargement
    ③ Joint pain
    ④ Nausea

194. A 10 year old is in the acute stage of rheumatic fever. During this stage the nursing care should include:
    ① Assisting him to the shower
    ② Walking him to the bathroom
    ③ Protecting him from sunlight
    ④ Turning him in bed

195. Documentation that the nurse would make immediately after a child returns from a cardiac catheterization includes:
    ① Assessing insertion site
    ② Monitoring vital signs q2h
    ③ Frequent turning of patient
    ④ Recording preoperative medications

196. Following a cardiac catheterization, a child has an intravenous infusion running at 20 ml/hr. The infusion set delivers 60 drops (gtt)/ml. The nurse regulates the drops per minute at:
    ① 2 gtt/min
    ② 5 gtt/min
    ③ 10 gtt/min
    ④ 20 gtt/min

197. A 2-month-old infant has been in the neonatal ICU since birth. The nursing staff observes the infant closely because he exhibits symptoms such as a large pulse pressure, dyspnea on exertion, and growth retardation. These symptoms could be indicative of:
    ① Aortic stenosis
    ② Pulmonary stenosis
    ③ Coarctation of the aorta
    ④ Patent ductus arteriosus

198. A 6-week-old infant has been diagnosed with patent ductus arteriosus. In caring for this infant, the nurse knows that cyanosis is *not* present because of the connection between the:
    ① Right and left atria
    ② Right and left ventricles
    ③ Pulmonary artery and aorta
    ④ Pulmonary vein and right atrium

199. In planning care for a patient with leukemia, the nurse must understand that the disease is characterized by:
    ① An increase in the number of red blood cells (RBCs)
    ② Severe weight gain from edema
    ③ Increase in the number of white blood cells
    ④ Immature RBCs in circulating blood

200. A 6 year old has been diagnosed with acute leukemia. In planning care for this patient, it is important for the nurse to be aware of the signs and symptoms of this disease, which include:
    ① Decreased white blood cell (WBC) count, decreased hemoglobin, petechiae, and anorexia
    ② Decreased WBC count, pallor, lethargy, and fever
    ③ Increased WBC count, increased hemoglobin, petechiae, and pallor
    ④ Increased WBC count, pallor, anemia, and petechiae

201. A 6-year-old leukemia patient asks the nurse, "Am I going to die?" The nurse wants to help relieve the child's anxieties. Her best response would be:
    ① "Do you really feel that bad today?"
    ② "Tell me more about how you feel."
    ③ "Let's talk about something else."
    ④ "Don't worry about that; let's watch television."

202. A 4 year old admitted to the hospital for diagnostic tests is suspected of having leukemia. The nurse anticipates that the test most likely to be ordered to determine whether the child has leukemia is:
① Bone marrow aspiration
② Gastric analysis
③ Arterial blood gases
④ Cardiac echogram

203. Bed rest is ordered for a 4 year old with leukemia. The reason bed rest is ordered is to relieve:
① Cyanosis
② Palpitations
③ Painful joints
④ Blurred vision

204. A 9-year-old leukemia patient is not responding to treatment. Which of the following signs would indicate to the nurse that the disease is progressing?
① Edema
② Cyanosis
③ Rectal bleeding
④ Clubbed fingers

205. Prednisone (Meticorten) and vincristine sulfate (Oncovin) are prescribed for a 10-year-old leukemia patient. The nurse knows that this combination of drugs in the body acts to:
① Reduce symptoms of pain
② Induce prolonged remissions
③ Prevent infections
④ Promote white cell production

206. A 16-year-old high school student has not been feeling well. On the basis of her presenting symptoms, she is being given a diagnostic workup for leukemia. During the admission procedure, the nurse would closely observe the patient for symptoms of leukemia that include:
① Epistaxis, easy bruising, and malaise
② Gastrointestinal bleeding, nausea, and vomiting
③ Pruitis, rash, and fever
④ Petechiae, gastrointestinal bleeding, and rash

207. A major nursing goal in caring for a teenager diagnosed with leukemia includes assisting her to:
① Cope with the diagnosis/prognosis
② Deal with her body image
③ Continue with school
④ Go home as soon as possible

208. Discharge planning for a patient with leukemia will most likely include a treatment plan for:
① A diet high in vitamins
② Loss of weight by controlling edema
③ Home care as soon as possible
④ Antibiotics and blood transfusions

209. In planning postoperative care for a young patient following surgical intervention for removal of the structure that produces the growth hormone, the nurse plans care for which of the following?
① Hypophysectomy
② Thyroidectomy
③ Parathyroidectomy
④ Adrenalectomy

210. A 15-year-old patient tells the nurse he wants to be on the basketball team next year, but he has been told he is too short. He asks what can be done to make him grow taller. The nurse explains that growth occurs as a result of the growth hormone produced by the:
① Thyroid gland
② Anterior pituitary gland
③ Posterior pituitary gland
④ Adrenal medulla

211. The nurse should observe for potential complications following surgical intervention in the structure that produces the growth hormone. This will include assessing for:
① Adrenal insufficiency, diabetes insipidus, and hypothyroidism
② Thyroid storm, tetany, and respiratory obstruction
③ Ketoacidosis, hypoglycemia, and coma
④ Adrenal crisis, hypotension, tachycardia, convulsions, and coma

212. Which of the following would be an acceptable nutritional practice for a boy, newly diagnosed with diabetes, who wants to eat at a fast-food restaurant with his friends?
① Order only lettuce and tomato salads without dressing
② Order foods as desired, later adjusting the insulin dose based on the blood glucose check
③ When ordering, use a dietary exchange list specific to fast-food restaurants
④ Order whatever is desired; all adolescents need time away from restrictions

213. A 16-year-old high school student has been diagnosed with type I diabetes. The nurse knows learning has taken place when the patient states:
① "I will keep my insulin at my bedside."
② "I will shake the vial vigorously."
③ "I will draw up the regular insulin first, then the NPH."
④ "I use the top part of my leg because it's easy to reach."

214. A 17 year old diagnosed as a diabetic 3 years ago has been admitted with abdominal pain associated with her spleen. She has been very short of breath when performing any activity lately. On analysis of her blood, it is discovered that her erythrocytes are abnormally shaped. The nurse explains to the patient that abnormal erythrocyte function is expected because her serum has been:
① Hypoglycemic
② Hyperglycemic
③ Hyperkalemic
④ Hyponatremic

215. The nurse teaches a newly diagnosed diabetic teenage patient hypoglycemic prevention strategies. The patient verbalizes that the most important strategy to prevent episodes of hypoglycemia is to:
① Keep a glucose source available at all times
② Increase carbohydrate and protein intake thirty minutes before beginning an exercise program
③ Know that the peak insulin time is midafternoon
④ Eat meals including snacks at the same time every day

216. A 16-year-old diabetic patient would like to take driver's education and obtain his driver's license. What advice should the nurse give this patient about driving a car?
    ① He should not drive until he is older and is sure that he will not have problems with his diabetes
    ② He should carry a snack with him in the car in case he begins to feel hypoglycemic
    ③ He will need to have another driver with him at all times
    ④ A driver's license will not be issued

217. In counseling the parents of a child with celiac syndrome, the nurse would strongly recommend which of the following foods to be eliminated from the child's diet?
    ① Rye bread
    ② Lean meats
    ③ Green beans
    ④ Strawberries

218. Nursing management of the patient with Crohn's disease includes monitoring the patient's diet. Which of the following diets would the physician most likely order for this patient?
    ① Full liquid diet
    ② Clear liquid with potassium
    ③ Soft diet, no foods high in fiber
    ④ Soft diet with bulk-containing foods

219. A nurse in the emergency department is caring for a 5-year-old child with a urinary tract infection (UTI). What signs and symptom would the nurse expect the child to exhibit?
    ① Dizziness and drowsiness
    ② Frequency and dysuria
    ③ Polyuria and dysphasia
    ④ Nausea and anorexia

220. In planning care for a patient with nephrosis, the nurse knows that the proper diet for the condition would most likely contain:
    ① Decreased sodium and increased fluids
    ② Decreased protein and sodium
    ③ Increased fiber and vitamins
    ④ Increased protein and decreased sodium

221. In caring for a 4-year-old with nephrosis, the nurse would expect that the urinalysis would reveal:
    ① Gross hematuria
    ② Gross albuminuria
    ③ Glycosuria
    ④ No abnormalities

222. A 4 year old is admitted to the hospital with the diagnosis of nephrosis. During the admission process, the nurse knows that the prime presenting symptom of the child would be:
    ① Edema
    ② Hematuria
    ③ Petechial rash
    ④ Dehydration

223. A child's burned areas have healed enough so that he can receive skin grafts. After skin grafting, the most important nursing action to promote acceptance of the graft is to:
    ① Debride the outer edge of the recipient site to facilitate healing
    ② Restrict movement of the graft site to prevent dislodging of graft
    ③ Apply a heat light to decrease drainage
    ④ Change the petroleum gauze dressings daily

224. In caring for a burn victim who has just received skin grafts, the nurse must encourage the patient to drink fluids to prevent:
    ① Renal calculi
    ② Dehydration
    ③ Electrolyte imbalance
    ④ Weight loss

225. A 2 year old enters the emergency room with a burn to the left hand. The skin appears blistered and red, and the child is experiencing severe pain. To what degree is the skin most likely burned?
    ① First degree
    ② Second degree
    ③ Third degree
    ④ Fourth degree

226. A 10 year old has sustained second- and third-degree burns over 43% of his body. Before the burn dressing is changed, he is to receive 20 mg of Demerol elixir. The elixir has 50 mg of Demerol per teaspoon. How many milliliters of the elixir would the nurse administer to the child?
    ① 1 ml
    ② 2 ml
    ③ 4 ml
    ④ 6 ml

227. A 7-year-old child comes to the clinic with pediculosis capitis. This is the second infestation in the past month. Which of the following would be the best evaluation of the previous treatment?
    ① Everyone in the family was not treated
    ② The treatment was not effective on the child
    ③ The child is not kept clean
    ④ The child is allergic to the medication

228. A recent graduate has taken a summer job as a nurse for the local childrens' camp. As the camp nurse, she must know that a common fungal infection of the skin on the scalp, body, and feet is:
    ① Ringworm
    ② Pediculosis
    ③ Herpes
    ④ Urticaria

229. In caring for a child with tinea capitis, it is important for the nurse to know that the organism responsible for causing the condition is a:
    ① Virus
    ② Bacillus
    ③ Bacterium
    ④ Fungus

230. A 5 year old has been admitted to the pediatric unit with a diagnosis of eczema. Nursing care for the child should include which of the following nursing interventions?
    ① Maintaining the child in one position
    ② Keeping the child fully clothed
    ③ Maintaining skin integrity
    ④ Applying moist dressing

231. A new mother brings her 6-week-old newborn to the clinic because of an apparent red rash on the infant's arms. The earliest indication of an allergic response in an infant is:
    ① Impetigo
    ② Acne vulgaris
    ③ Eczema
    ④ Dysplasia

232. A 2 year old is in the hospital with a fractured right femur. The physician has ordered Bryant's traction. In planning care for a child in Bryant's traction, the nurse must know:
    ① The type/purpose of traction
    ② The function of the traction only
    ③ The method used to order the traction
    ④ That she need not be concerned with the age of the child

233. In caring for a child in traction, it is important to maintain proper use of the traction. Therefore, the nurse should check:
    ① That the weights rest on the floor
    ② The pulleys and correct weights
    ③ The splints, and reposition them as necessary
    ④ The position of the bed

234. While bathing a 2 year old in traction with a fractured right femur, the nurse carefully assesses the child's.
    ① Skin condition
    ② Circulation to the left lower extremity
    ③ Immobility in bed only
    ④ Mother's reaction to the situation

235. The nurse develops a plan of care for a 2 year old in Bryant's traction. Because bed rest is ordered, the plan should include which of the following?
    ① Promote as little activity in bed as possible
    ② Change the weights on the traction daily
    ③ Administer pain medication q2h
    ④ Change position, still maintaining proper traction

236. In planning care for a child in traction as a result of a fracture, the nurse must understand that the purpose of the traction is to:
    ① Cure the fracture immediately
    ② Keep the patient in bed
    ③ Promote comfort in bed
    ④ Align/immobilize the limb

237. An 18-year-old male injured his right arm while wrestling. The nurse suspects the arm is fractured. In addition to immobilizing the arm and applying ice, the nurse should assess:
    ① Warmth, sensation, movement, and color
    ② Capillary refill, wetness, and touch
    ③ Sensation, motion, and touch
    ④ Color, stiffness, and wetness

238. A 10 year old was admitted to the emergency room with a suspected fracture of the right wrist. Following confirmation of the diagnosis by x-ray examination, the physician applied a cast. The nurse in the emergency room shows his mother the correct way to check for tightness of the cast. Which of the following statements made by the nurse is an appropriate teaching statement?
    ① "After the cast has dried, insert your fingers between the skin and the cast."
    ② "Pull the cast up and down to determine movement."
    ③ "Insert a gauze dressing as far down in the cast as possible."
    ④ "Insert a rigid object as far down inside the cast as possible."

239. A 17-year-old patient who had been wrestling with a friend when he felt his arm snap was brought to the emergency room by his parents complaining of severe pain in his right forearm. The nurse is concerned that he has broken his arm. Which of the following pieces of information should be reported to the physician about this patient?
    ① Patient's age
    ② Patient was wrestling with a friend
    ③ Patient heard a snapping sound
    ④ Patient has broken his arm

240. A 3 year old has been admitted to the pediatric unit with a fractured left femur. He was placed in Russell traction and is having a difficult time adjusting to being immobilized. His grandmother is concerned about his wetting the bed at night. The most appropriate response by the nurse in answer to the woman's concern would be:
    ① "He may need to be toilet trained again after his discharge from the hospital."
    ② "Don't worry about his wetting the bed at night. We change his sheets frequently."
    ③ "He has had a traumatic experience. When he gets used to being in the hospital he will stop wetting the bed."
    ④ "Wetting the bed is not unusual for a child his age. Children often regress in some behaviors in the hospital."

241. A 12 year old is brought to the pediatric clinic by her mother, who states the child appears to be "walking funny." On further examination, the physician discovers that the child has a lateral S-shaped curvature of the spine. In planning home care for this patient, it is important for the nurse to know that this condition is called:
    ① Scoliosis
    ② Nephrosis
    ③ Lordosis
    ④ Kyphosis

242. In caring for a child with scoliosis over a period of time, the nurse knows that which of the following statements regarding the condition is true?
    ① Pain is a common presenting symptom
    ② Disability is confined only to the spine
    ③ Detection is difficult and requires radiography
    ④ A compensatory curve usually results in an effort to maintain an erect posture

243. Of the following symptoms, which should the nurse watch for in cases of possible spinal cord compression?
    ① Severe headaches
    ② Changes in sensation
    ③ Unconsciousness
    ④ Convulsions

244. A 14 year old suffered a spinal cord injury following a dive into a shallow pond while on a family outing. In planning care for a patient with a spinal cord injury, the nurse would consider which of the following interventions to lower the blood pressure quickly in the event the child experiences autonomic dysreflexia?
    ① Get the patient to a sitting position
    ② Call the physician immediately
    ③ Administer oxygen immediately
    ④ Put the patient in Trendelenburg's position

245. In caring for a patient with head or neck injuries, the nurse is aware that a drug frequently used in the management of such injuries is:
    ① Methylprednisolone (Solu-Medrol)
    ② Dexamethazone (Decadron)
    ③ Acetazolamide (Diamox)
    ④ Chlorothiazide (Diuril)

246. When planning to teach patients with spinal cord injuries about the action of certain foods in their bodies, the nurse would make a point to include that the liquid least likely to cause formation of urinary calculi is:
    ① Cranberry juice
    ② Tomato juice
    ③ Coffee
    ④ Milk

247. With some spinal cord injuries, patients often have a great deal of pain. When caring for these patients, the nurse is aware that narcotics are contraindicated for long-term use because of the possibility of:
    ① Respiratory complications
    ② Addiction to narcotic drugs
    ③ Abscesses from frequent infections
    ④ Circulatory complications

248. With the increasing occurrence of head injuries, it is important for the nurse to know that:
    ① Head injuries are a common cause of mental illness
    ② Concussion is a bruising of cerebral tissue
    ③ Negative symptomatology is unrelated to the extent of organic damage
    ④ Psychic effects of brain injury are a reaction to the trauma

249. The nursery nurse has just admitted a newborn with a congenital disorder in which the abdominal organs have protruded through the abdominal wall and have formed a sac on the abdomen. In developing a plan of care for this infant, it is important for the nurse to know that this is a(n):
    ① Diaphragmatic hernia
    ② Umbilical hernia
    ③ Omphalocele
    ④ Esophageal atresia

250. A baby born with a myelomeningocele usually requires a lengthy hospital stay. Because of the length of hospitalization and separation of the parents from their infant, the nursing staff would foster the child-parent relationship by:
    ① Encouraging both parents to see the infant during the specified visiting hours
    ② Explaining the process of parent bonding and how the parents should treat the child at home
    ③ Encouraging the parents to touch and hold the newborn as much as possible
    ④ Ignoring the parents' statements indicating their grief at not having a normal baby

251. A mother tells the nurse that her infant daughter vomits frequently. Knowing this can happen with a child who has a myelomeningocele, the nurse would advise the mother to promote adequate nutrition by:
    ① Holding the infant while supporting the head; offering small frequent feedings
    ② Witholding feedings until the baby stops vomiting, then giving thickened feedings
    ③ Increasing the carbohydrates in each feeding by adding sugar to the formula
    ④ Inserting a nasogastric (NG) tube to give the formula; instructing the mother in the proper care of the NG tube

252. An infant with a myelomeningocele is scheduled for insertion of a ventriculoperitoneal shunt to decrease accumulation of cerebrospinal fluid causing hydrocephalus. In planning postoperative care, the nurse knows that the infant would be positioned:
    ① On the operative side
    ② In Trendelenburg's position
    ③ On the nonoperative side
    ④ In high-Fowler's position

253. A mother asks the nurse, "Why do you keep measuring my baby's head every day? I thought after the shunt was put in, everything would be all right." The most appropriate response by the nurse would be:
    ① "The baby's head size should have decreased immediately after surgery. I am checking to see if the shunt helped your baby."
    ② "By measuring the baby's head, I will know if there is an increase in intracranial pressure."
    ③ "As cerebrospinal fluid drains from the ventricles of the brain, the head circumference will gradually decrease."
    ④ "You need not be concerned with what we are doing. Your baby is all right and will be going home soon."

254. While assessing a child having a petit mal seizure, the nurse is most likely to observe:
① Body stiffening
② Jerking movements
③ Lip smacking
④ Urinary incontinence

255. In caring for a child admitted with recurrent seizures that are a result of uncontrolled epilepsy, the nurse is aware that an anticonvulsant drug commonly used to control such seizures is:
① Cimetidine (Tagamet)
② Hydroxyzine pamoate (Vistaril)
③ Prochlorperazine (Compazine)
④ Phenytoin (Dilantin)

256. A 10-year-old patient, diagnosed with epilepsy, is discharged on 100 mg. of phenytoin (Dilantin) tid. Which remark by his mother would indicate she understands the potential side effects of the drug?
① "My son will be sensitive to sunlight."
② "The medicine will discolor my son's teeth."
③ "My son may have an overgrowth of gum tissue."
④ "The medication may make my son hyper."

257. A 14 year old is admitted to the pediatric unit after experiencing a grand mal seizure at school and is scheduled to have an electroencephalogram. The patient's mother states "I am afraid for my son to have this test." Which of the following responses by the nurse would be most appropriate at this time?
① "Has someone given you false information?"
② "Can you tell me more about your fears?"
③ "Have you told the doctor this?"
④ "Your son really needs to have this test."

258. The nurse is caring for an 11 year old who was admitted for evaluation of seizures. The nurse enters her room and finds the patient on the floor having a grand mal seizure. What should the nurse do *first?*
① Put her back to bed
② Place a padded tongue blade in her mouth
③ Place pillows around her
④ Hyperextend her head to open her airway

259. Developing family relationships is important for a child with cerebral palsy. The nurse knows this goal has been achieved when:
① Ritualization management is accepted
② There is acceptance of his growing independence
③ A study is completed to determine how much help the parents need in caring for him
④ There is acceptance of him as he is now

260. A 10 year old has cerebral palsy and is cared for at home by his parents with the assistance of home-care nurses. Nursing management of his care should include:
① Educational and social programs
② Long-term planning and care
③ Patience and tolerance
④ Knowledge of the general disease processes

261. A major nursing consideration that the nurse must deal with during the early years of a cerebral palsy patient's life is:
① Seizure activity
② Increased muscle tone
③ Decreased muscle tone
④ Sensory impairment

262. A 7-year-old boy has cerebral palsy. He is cared for at home by his parents with the assistance of home-care nurses. He has a gastrostomy tube in place for his feedings. In planning care for this patient, it is important for the nurse to know that cerebral palsy may be caused by:
① Premature birth
② Injury to the brain
③ A genetic disorder
④ Erythroblastosis fetalis

263. A 5 year old is a cerebral palsy patient who has a gastrostomy tube in place for his feedings. When giving him his gastrostomy feeding, the nurse would:
① Push the formula in with a 50 ml syringe to ensure that the feeding gets into the stomach
② Aspirate formula in the stomach and discard it
③ Allow the formula to flow in by gravity and flush with 10 ml of water
④ Reinsert the gastrostomy tube each feeding

264. An infant is admitted with a suspected diagnosis of meningitis. Several diagnostic laboratory tests are ordered, and preparation is made for a lumbar puncture. To prepare the infant for a lumbar puncture, the nurse would:
① Restrain the infant in a side-lying position with the head hyperextended during the procedure
② Administer 10 mg of Demerol intramuscularly to sedate the infant before the procedure
③ Hold the infant in a sitting position with head flexed during the procedure
④ Place the infant in a mummy restraint and hold the neck flexed during the procedure

265. A 17 month old is admitted to the hospital with a diagnosis of meningitis. In planning care for this child, the nurse knows that his symptoms will most likely include:
① Fever, stiff neck, and elevated white blood cell (WBC) count in blood and spinal fluid
② Dyspnea, lethargy, and elevated pulse and blood pressure
③ Vomiting, diarrhea, dehydration, and red raised rash
④ Red raised rash, fever, diarrhea, and elevated WBCs in spinal fluid

266. The physician orders blood cultures to be drawn on an infant with suspected meningitis. Following the puncture for collection of the blood specimens, the nurse would immediately:
① Take the specimens to the laboratory
② Obtain an arterial blood specimen for comparison
③ Apply a warm compress to decrease pain and ecchymosis
④ Apply direct pressure to the area until bleeding has stopped

267. An infant diagnosed with meningitis is placed in isolation. The baby's mother asks the nurse how long her baby will stay in isolation. The nurse's response is based on the knowledge that:
    ① Isolation will be maintained until a negative cerebrospinal fluid bacterial growth culture is returned
    ② Isolation is not necessary 24 hours after antibacterial therapy
    ③ Preventing the spread of infection is the primary objective in the care of the infant
    ④ Isolation is maintained until completion of 7 days of IV antibiotics

268. While providing daily care for an infant with meningitis, the nurse would observe for:
    ① Skin integrity, inflammation of IV site, and infiltration of IV
    ② Increase in temperature and urine specific gravity and decrease in urinary output
    ③ Change in vital and neurologic signs and increased urinary output
    ④ Frequent bowel movements, signs of nuchal rigidity, and hypothermia

269. The physician has ordered 125,000 U of aqueous penicillin q6h intravenously for an infant who has been diagnosed as having meningitis. Before each administration of the medication, the nurse would:
    ① Check the IV tube site for signs of phlebitis and infiltration
    ② Flush the IV line with 30 ml of IV fluid to test patency of line
    ③ Verify the amount of reconstituted solution to be administered
    ④ Ask the mother to leave the room during the procedure

270. A 2 year old has been admitted to the pediatric unit with a diagnosis of meningitis. Of prime importance is nursing observation for seizures. In the event that the child has a seizure, it is important that the nurse remember to:
    ① Document and notify the charge nurse immediately
    ② Restrain the child to prevent injury
    ③ Insert a padded tongue blade to prevent possible respiratory complications
    ④ Observe movements and document the time and length of the seizure

271. A 5 year old has been admitted to the pediatric unit with a diagnosis of croup. When planning care for this child, the nurse would most likely expect the treatment of choice to include:
    ① Warm, humidified air and antibiotics
    ② Humidified oxygen and sedatives
    ③ Humidified oxygen and antiemetics
    ④ Cool, humidified air and syrup of ipecac

272. On the basis of results of a sweat test, chest x-ray examinations, and the decreased amount of duodenal pancreatic enzymes, a child is diagnosed with cystic fibrosis. Which of the following does the nurse correctly recall as the primary factor responsible for the symptoms of cystic fibrosis?
    ① Increased viscosity of mucous gland (exocrine) secretions leads to the mechanical obstruction of the glands
    ② The fetal lungs do not develop properly
    ③ There are multiple untreated episodes of upper respiratory infections
    ④ There are multiple treatments of upper respiratory infections with antibiotics and suppression of the immune system

273. What is the primary reason that cystic fibrosis patients do not gain weight even though they may eat voraciously?
    ① They eat the wrong foods for their health problem
    ② They have constant diarrhea because of the use of multiple antibiotics
    ③ They have continual vomiting due to strictures of the upper gastrointestinal tract
    ④ Their intestines are unable to digest fats and proteins

274. In caring for a child with cystic fibrosis, the nurse knows that the foul-smelling, frothy stools often associated with this condition result from large amounts of undigested:
    ① Minerals
    ② Carbohydrates
    ③ Fats
    ④ Vitamins

275. The nurse prepares a 4 year old with cystic fibrosis for her bath. The nurse notes several bruises on both of the child's lower legs. The child's mother states that every time she is bumped or falls down she seems to get another bruise. What is the most likely cause of the bruises on the child's legs?
    ① The child is developing a neurologic deficit
    ② There is deficient absorption of vitamin K
    ③ The child does not have sufficient supervision during play
    ④ At age 4, most children fall and bruise easily

276. In caring for a child with asthma, the nurse must know that asthma can be caused by extrinsic or intrinsic factors. Intrinsic factors include:
    ① Injury to the nose
    ② Pollen from flowers
    ③ Respiratory infections
    ④ Allergens in the environment

277. In planning care for a young asthmatic patient, the nurse would include all of the following nursing care measures *except:*
    ① Monitoring intravenous fluids
    ② Administering aminophylline
    ③ Bed rest in supine position
    ④ Assisting with intermittent positive-pressure breathing treatments

278. A 10 year old has been complaining of breathlessness. He is alert, oriented, and pale, with a respiratory rate of 44/minute. Use of accessory muscles is noted. His lungs have tight wheezy sounds noted in all fields. He has used a metered dose inhaler 4 puffs every 20 minutes for the last hour. The nurse notes improvement in his condition based on which of the following:
    ① Continued complaints of breathlessness
    ② Absence of intercostal retractions
    ③ Respiratory rate of 50 breaths per minute
    ④ Presence of nasal flaring

279. A 3 year old is admitted to the emergency room in obvious respiratory distress. The admitting physician is talking to the medical student, telling him the child has a respiratory disease that is characterized by spasms of the bronchial tubes caused by hypersensitivity of the airways. In planning care for this child, the nurse prepares for nursing interventions specific to the diagnosis of:
    ① Pneumonia
    ② Asthma
    ③ Cystic fibrosis
    ④ Allergic rhinitis

280. The pediatrician orders acetaminophen 40 mg PO. On hand is acetaminophen 160 mg/tsp (5 ml). The nurse would administer:
    ① 0.5 ml
    ② 2 ml
    ③ ¼ tsp
    ④ ½ tsp

281. A 2 year old was admitted to the pediatric hospital with respiratory difficulty. After the child's respiratory problems worsened, the physician performed a tracheostomy. When aspirating the child's tracheostomy, the nurse should:
    ① Apply suction to the catheter only while withdrawing it
    ② Remove both the inner and outer cannulas before inserting the catheter
    ③ Twirl the catheter rapidly while withdrawing it slowly during removal
    ④ Untie the twill neck tapes while cleansing the skin edges of the wound

282. A 7-year-old child with asthma was brought to the emergency room while having an acute attack. During the attack the nurse is aware that the child's breathing is most likely characterized by:
    ① Noisy inspirations
    ② Wheezing on expiration
    ③ Frequent periods of apnea
    ④ Labored abdominal breathing

283. The physician ordered epinephrine (Adrenalin) stat for a child in severe respiratory distress. The epinephrine was ordered to:
    ① Relax the smooth muscles of the bronchi
    ② Produce vasodilation of the blood vessels of the skin
    ③ Decrease cardiac output as a result of its vasopressor action
    ④ Stimulate constriction of the smooth muscles of the respiratory tract

284. The physician ordered epinephrine (Adrenalin) to be administered subcutaneously. The injection is administered using a:
    ① 19-gauge, 1-inch needle
    ② 22-gauge, 1-inch needle
    ③ 25-gauge, ⅝-inch needle
    ④ 27-gauge, ½-inch needle

285. A mother brought her 5-year-old son to the clinic to have his eyes checked. On examination, the nurse finds them to be red and inflamed, with a green crusty discharge. The physician has diagnosed him as having "pinkeye." In planning care for this child, it is important for the nurse to know that "Pinkeye" is:
    ① Degeneration of the conjunctiva
    ② Inflammation of the lacrimal sac
    ③ Inflammation of the conjunctiva
    ④ Opacity of the lens

286. In caring for a 5 year old with pinkeye, the nurse is aware that the medication of choice is usually:
    ① Pilocarpine eye drops
    ② Photocoagulation
    ③ Normal saline eye drops
    ④ Neosporin ophthalmic drops

287. An 8 year old has been diagnosed with pinkeye. The nurse is teaching the child's mother the proper procedure for administering eye drops. Before the child's mother puts the medication in his eyes, the nurse should instruct her to:
    ① Wash the eyes from the inner canthus outward with a cotton ball and warm water
    ② Wash the eyes back and forth several times with a cotton ball and warm water to get all the crusted material off
    ③ Just put in the medication, which will take care of the crusting
    ④ Wash the eyes with hydrogen peroxide to clear away the crusting

288. A child has been diagnosed with pinkeye. The mother asks how long she should put the antibiotic into her son's eyes. The nurse's response should be:
    ① "Continue until the medication is finished."
    ② "For 10 days only."
    ③ "Use your own judgment."
    ④ "Continue until 5 days after the eyes appear clear."

289. A 2 year old has otitis media, which the nurse knows is often a common complication of a(n):
    ① Ear injury
    ② External ear infection
    ③ Myringotomy
    ④ Upper respiratory infection

290. A 2 year old has been admitted to the pediatric unit with a history of recurring episodes of otitis media. In planning care for this child, the nurse is aware that repeated episodes of otitis media in infants and toddlers can result in:
    ① Chronic strep throats
    ② Delayed speech development
    ③ Mastitis
    ④ Sleep walking

291. Instructions to the parent of a child with otitis media following a myringotomy should include having the child lie on his or her:
① Abdomen
② Affected side
③ Back
④ Unaffected side

292. A new mother asks the nurse if her 2-week-old baby can die from impetigo. The nurse knows that impetigo can become a life-threatening systemic infection, although this is a rare happening. The nurse should answer:
① "I'm sure your baby will respond to medication."
② "You really don't have anything to worry about now."
③ "Medication usually works; however, I would be happy to call your minister."
④ "The nursing staff will keep a close eye on your baby and check his response to the medicine."

293. A young mother is concerned with possible adverse effects her child may experience as a result of chicken pox. The nurse knows that chicken pox is associated with:
① No serious complications
② Loss of hearing
③ Loss of visual acuity
④ Muscular system involvement

294. When caring for a child with mumps, it is important for the nurse to know that the child must be considered contagious until:
① All swelling has disappeared
② The rash has completely disappeared
③ Fever subsides
④ Two months after the onset of symptoms

295. A 13 year old is taken to his pediatrician with a suspected case of mumps. His mother appears quite concerned about the child's condition. To respond appropriately to the mother's concerns, the nurse must know that the child may be in danger of which of the following complications?
① Orchitis
② Meningitis
③ Myositis
④ Pyelonephritis

296. In planning care for a child with acquired immune deficiency syndrome (AIDS), the nurse must know that the causative organism of AIDS is:
① Cytomegalovirus
② Human immunodeficiency virus
③ Human papilloma virus
④ Herpes virus

297. A nurse is teaching a health education class in one of the local high schools, and a student asks the nurse, "What is the name of skin cancer that AIDS victims usually get?" The nurse answers:
① Kaposi's sarcoma
② Malignant melanoma
③ Basal cell carcinoma
④ Squamous cell carcinoma

298. The nurse is caring for a 9-year-old child recently diagnosed with attention deficit disorder (ADD). The child is taking Ritalin and attends family counseling. Which statement by his parents indicates additional teaching is needed?
① "We must set limits and be firm with him."
② "We need to simplify his home environment."
③ "We administer his medication at bedtime so he won't get drowsy."
④ "The medication allows him to pay closer attention to his school work."

299. A 5 year old is choking and cannot expel the foreign object. The child is unconscious and turning blue. The nurse performs the Heimlich maneuver five times. What should she do next?
① Continue to perform the Heimlich maneuver until the object is expelled from the mouth
② Look in the mouth and do a finger sweep if she sees the object
③ Continue to perform the Heimlich maneuver while sweeping the mouth with her finger
④ Give five deep breaths into the child's mouth

300. When explaining ways to prevent a recurrence of Lyme disease to the mother of an active 10 year old, which of the following would be the most appropriate directions for the nurse to offer the mother?
① Repeat the vaccine every 5 years
② Avoid swimming in contaminated water
③ Wear long pants while in the woods
④ Take corticosteroids

301. A 6-month-old infant is admitted to the emergency room in what appears to be a severe state of dehydration. Nursing assessment of severe dehydration would likely reveal:
① An elevated blood pressure; sunken fontanel
② A rapid pulse and marked oliguria
③ A slow pulse and parched mucous membranes
④ Slow respirations and loss of skin elasticity

302. A 17-year-old patient is recovering from heat stroke and is anticipating discharge tomorrow. The nurse should include which of the following in his discharge instructions?
① Wear a hat when outdoors.
② Drink at least one gallon of water daily.
③ Avoid re-exposure to heat.
④ Resume any type of activities.

303. A mother brings her baby to the well-baby clinic for the first time. The mother gives a history of a difficult pregnancy and relates that the baby seemed to move around a lot before she was born and now doesn't seem to be growing. The nurse notes that the baby is small for her age and has altered facial features. In planning care for this mother and baby, the nurse knows these signs and symptoms to be typical of:
① Failure to thrive
② Hereditary defect
③ Cocaine addiction
④ Alcohol addiction

304. As a nurse in a pediatric clinic, it is important to be knowledgable about child abuse. Which of the following statements is true relative to battered child syndrome?
    ① Child abuse is physical, not emotional abuse
    ② Parents who abuse their children were usually abused as children
    ③ Statistics indicate that child abuse is not evident in middle-class families
    ④ Abused children always have congenital defects or other abnormalities

305. A nurse in the emergency department assesses a 3 year old with multiple bruises on her back. The patient's mother tells the nurse she doesn't know how the child was injured. Child abuse is suspected. What should the nurse do first?
    ① Report her suspicions to the proper authority
    ② Explain her concerns to the parents
    ③ Refer the family to the social worker on call
    ④ Document findings relative to the bruises in detail

306. While waiting for surgery, a 10 year old was left alone on the stretcher in the hallway. When the nurse returned to take the child to the operating room, the child was gone. What are the legal ramifications of this action?
    ① A charge of abandonment
    ② A charge of malpractice
    ③ A breech of the borrowed servant rule
    ④ A breech of the Respondeat Superior

307. A 3-month-old infant is being discharged on continuous home oxygen therapy. The nurse is reinforcing home care teaching. Which of the following statements by the infant's mother indicates she *does not* understand home oxygen therapy?
    ① "I won't be able to smoke in the room with the baby."
    ② "If my baby turns blue, I'll just turn up the oxygen."
    ③ "I need to have extra full oxygen tanks in case my weekly delivery is late."
    ④ "The oxygen won't work as well if my baby's nose is stuffy."

308. After a 6-year-old patient's surgery for a ruptured appendix, her physician has written an order to maintain the patient in a semi-Fowler's position. The nurse knows the importance for maintaining this position is to:
    ① Promote drainage and prevent abscess formation
    ② Decrease stress on the suture line
    ③ Decrease the likelihood of aspiration if vomiting occurs
    ④ Encourage deep breathing and prevent respiratory complications

309. A mother brings her 7-year-old child to the emergency room with a fever and a sore throat. The child's temperature is 38.5° C (101.5° F). The physician orders cooling measures to be taken while waiting for the acetaminophen (Tylenol), which was given at home, to begin working. Which of the following cooling measures would the nurse most likely implement?
    ① Offer the patient sips of ice water
    ② Apply cold compresses
    ③ Bathe the patient with refrigerated alcohol
    ④ Bathe the patient with tepid water

310. When preparing to administer medications, the nurse is aware that the preferred site for administering an intramuscular injection to a toddler is the:
    ① Deltoid
    ② Dorsogluteal
    ③ Vastus lateralis
    ④ Ventrogluteal

311. A 5-year-old child is taught coughing and deep-breathing exercises before surgery. Which of the following methods used by the nurse would indicate the best teaching approach?
    ① Placing information in a logical sequence
    ② Presenting material from simple to complex
    ③ Building on the child's level of knowledge
    ④ Using actual equipment for the demonstration

312. In observing skin conditions, it is important for the nurse to be able to describe the various lesions for documentation. Lesions that are circumscribed elevations of the epidermis, less than 1 cm in diameter, and contain a clear liquid are described as:
    ① Mascules
    ② Vesicles
    ③ Maculopapules
    ④ Papules

313. To obtain a urine specimen from an infant, the nurse would:
    ① Clean and dry the genitalia, perineum, and skin; and apply a self-adhesive plastic bag
    ② Clean and dry the perineum and catheterize infant
    ③ Apply a disposable diaper and aspirate urine from the diaper with a needle and syringe
    ④ Place the infant on a small container to void and pour the urine into a specimen tube

314. Of the following data, which is most important for the nurse to know in monitoring the respiratory rate of children?
    ① Average respiratory rate for age
    ② The child's developmental level
    ③ Side effects of bronchodilators
    ④ The child's theophylline level

315. A 2 year old has an order for temperature readings q4h. Because of this patient's age, the nurse would take his temperature by which of the following methods?
    ① Axillary/rectal
    ② Oral/rectal
    ③ Rectal only
    ④ Axillary only

316. A 5 year old is admitted to the hospital with vomiting and diarrhea lasting 24 hours. As the nurse begins to plan care, which of the following would be the most important nursing diagnosis?
① Nutrition, altered
② Health maintenance, altered
③ Fluid volume deficit
④ Incontinence, functional

317. The nurse is caring for a 9 month old and receives orders to give a preoperative intramuscular injection of a medication. The best site for this injection would be:
① Deltoid
② Ventrogluteal
③ Dorsogluteal
④ Vastus lateralis

318. While administering an intramuscular injection to a 9 month old, the nurse would most likely need:
① A second individual to secure the child
② Antibiotic ointment for the site
③ A toy to distract the infant during the procedure
④ The patient's hospital number to ensure identification

319. The pediatrician orders aspirin 5 gr PO. On hand the nurse has aspirin 300 mg in tablet form. Which of the following would the nurse be correct in giving her young patient?
① ½ tablet
② 1 tablet
③ 1½ tablets
④ 2 tablets

320. An 8 year old weighs 75 pounds. The nurse is to administer a medication for which the average adult dose is 300 mg. Using Clark's rule, which of the following doses would the nurse be correct in administering to this child?
① 75 mg
② 125 mg
③ 150 mg
④ 200 mg

321. An 8 year old is to receive a medication for which the average adult dose is 500 mg. By implementing Young's rule, the nurse would select which one of the following as the correct dose for this child?
① 200 mg
② 250 mg
③ 325 mg
④ 375 mg

322. The nurse is caring for a 17-year-old surgical patient who needs to have a postoperative chest x-ray. Which of the following would be an important safety measure for the nurse or x-ray technician to carry out?
① Place a radiation warning on the door before the x-ray is taken
② Cover the patient from the waist down with a lead apron
③ Place amber-colored eye shields over the patient's eyes
④ Clear the hall outside the room before the x-ray is taken

323. The nurse working on the pediatric floor needs to follow standard precautions on which of the following patients?
① Children who are diagnosed HIV positive
② Children who are over the age of 2 years
③ All surgical patients
④ All patients when exposed to body fluids

324. It is important for the nurse to know that for toddlers, temper tantrums can be avoided or decreased in number and severity by:
① Letting the toddler have his own way
② Providing regular periods of active physical exercise
③ Giving him what he wants to quiet him down
④ Making him understand that this is unacceptable behavior

325. Following discharge from the hospital, a child's mother calls the nurse at the clinic and tells her that the child is having frequent temper tantrums. Which of the following statements by the nurse best describes the way to handle the situation?
① "Offer her a cookie if she will stop."
② "Ignore her until the tantrum is over."
③ "Spank her and send her to her room."
④ "Try to find what the problem is during the tantrum."

CHAPTER 4

Mental Health Nursing Review Questions

1. The determination that an individual's pattern of behavior is evidence of either mental health wellness or illness is made on the basis of which of the following considerations?
   ① Observations of the persons who know the individual best or those who live with him or her
   ② The degree of intelligence and the amount of education the individual has acquired
   ③ The specific behavior, as well as the context in which it takes place
   ④ The degree to which the behavior is pleasing to others

2. Behavior of a psychiatric patient is assessed on the basis of the nurse's understanding that:
   ① Adults must conform to certain societal norms and beliefs
   ② Behaviors of mentally ill individuals are exaggerations of normal human behavior
   ③ Behaviors of mentally ill individuals are sufficiently bizarre that they cannot be understood by a rational person
   ④ Behaviors of a mentally ill individual are the result of failure in his or her moral training

3. Which of the following statements *best* describes mental health?
   ① The absence of worry and pain and the ability to get along with others
   ② A cheerful, positive outlook on life and its problems; the capacity for happiness
   ③ An individual's ability to manage life's problems and to derive satisfaction from living throughout various life stages
   ④ The ability to win power over others; to control the lives of other people

4. The nurse-patient relationship is marked by which of the following characteristics?
   ① It is a warm, close friendship in which the patient has his or her needs met
   ② It is a reciprocal relationship in which both the nurse and the patient have needs met
   ③ It is a purposeful relationship that has a therapeutic goal for the patient
   ④ It exists solely to permit the patient to depend on the nurse

5. The nursing process with the mentally ill patient begins with which of the following?
   ① Establishing firm limits to control the patient's behavior
   ② A thorough assessment, including physical, psychologic, and emotional state
   ③ Communicating with the patient so that the patient knows he or she is in good hands
   ④ Finding out the patient's preferences for room assignment

6. To be an effective practitioner in the mental health field, the nurse should possess the ability to:
   ① Point out the patient's moral shortcomings and effect a change in his or her personal value system
   ② Solve one's own personal and family problems without the assistance of others
   ③ Understand oneself, be aware of how one affects others, and have the capacity to treat other people with respect
   ④ Bring others into compliance with society's rules and expectations

7. In caring for patients in a mental health setting, the nurse is aware that communication:
   ① Is talking and listening in an attentive way that is satisfying to the parties involved
   ② Is a complex activity resulting in a negotiated understanding between two or more people
   ③ Is an exchange of information
   ④ Consists of verbal and nonverbal messages

8. A new patient on the unit is depressed and not eating or sleeping well. As the nurse approaches one morning, the patient, sitting on the side of the bed in her night clothes, states, "I can't go on. I just can't go on." The *best* response by the nurse should be:
   ① "I understand how you feel. We all feel that way from time to time."
   ② "Let me help you shower and dress. It will make you feel better."
   ③ "You'll feel better once you are up and active."
   ④ "You're feeling hopeless and very sad."

9. The patient is able to state that she is at the mental health clinic and knows the date and time. She can tell the nurse her own name and recognizes the nurse as a nurse. This patient's ability to do this tells the nurse about her:
   ① Mental function
   ② Emotional function
   ③ Communication style
   ④ Coping style

10. A patient being interviewed is becoming agitated but is still able to write her name and draw a circle, square, and triangle on a piece of paper. On the basis of this observation, the nurse can conclude that the patient's:
    ① Mood and affect are stable
    ② Ability to communicate is intact
    ③ Coordination is unaffected
    ④ Agitation is not drug-induced

11. One morning, as the nurse walks into a patient's room, the patient says, "I didn't get any sleep last night. I finally dozed off around 5 AM." The *best* response by the nurse is:
    ① "Don't worry. You'll sleep better at home in your own bed."
    ② "Can you tell me more about what kept you awake?"
    ③ "Why didn't you ask for a sleeping pill?"
    ④ "It's not that bad. You'll be able to take a nap this afternoon."

12. A patient is scheduled for gastrointestinal surgery. Which of the following statements by the nurse should encourage the patient to verbalize her feelings about her impending surgery?
    ① "Everything will be okay; keep your chin up."
    ② "Things have a way of working out."
    ③ "This must be a difficult time for you."
    ④ "You have a very competent physician."

13. A patient has an episode of nausea before entering his first group therapy session. He states to the nurse, "I feel worse today than ever before. I wonder why this is happening to me." The nurse's *most appropriate* reply would be:
    ① "I'll ask the doctor for some medication."
    ② "I see your symptoms worry you."
    ③ "It will be okay. You'll feel better in a few minutes."
    ④ "Think about something pleasant."

14. A patient has been pacing up and down the corridor for several hours. The nurse observes him yell at another patient, "Get out of my way, moron." The *most appropriate* nursing response would be to tell him:
    ① That his behavior is unacceptable and won't be tolerated
    ② That if he doesn't cool it, he'll be put in seclusion
    ③ That if he doesn't stop bothering the other patients, his afternoon privileges will be taken away
    ④ To come to the medication room for his Ativan

15. A patient has lung cancer, and a pneumonectomy is performed. Later in the day, a nursing assistant reports that she observed the patient's wife crying. When the nurse approaches, the patient's wife states, "What made my husband so sick? I think God is punishing me for something I did." An appropriate response by the nurse would be:
    ① "Don't worry about what caused this. Pull yourself together and give him support."
    ② "I see no need to blame yourself."
    ③ "You appear to be very distraught."
    ④ "Why do you feel guilty about your husband's illness?"

16. A patient asks the nurse to keep a secret and not tell the other staff members what she's about to reveal. The nurse's *most* appropriate response would be:
    ① "Let's move to a more private area."
    ② "Be careful that no one overhears you."
    ③ "I'll have to hear what you have to say before I can promise that."
    ④ "I cannot make that promise. It might be information important for other staff to know."

17. The nurse is meeting with her assigned patient. Another patient approaches and interrupts the meeting, stating she must speak with the nurse. The nurse's most appropriate response to the second patient should be:
    ① "Why don't you sit with us until we're finished talking?"
    ② "I'm with this patient for the next 15 minutes. When our time is up, I'll talk with you."
    ③ "I'm sorry; I'm sure you can see that I'm busy right now."
    ④ "You'll have to ask my patient if it is alright for you to join us."

18. Just as the nurse's contracted time with her patient is up, he says, "I have to tell you something horrible that happened to me yesterday." Which of the following statements is an appropriate response by the nurse?
    ① "You'll have to tell me quickly because our time is up."
    ② "Our time is up; I'm leaving now."
    ③ "I'll give you no more than 5 more minutes to tell me what happened."
    ④ "Our time is up now. This would be a good place to start at our next session."

19. During contracted time with the nurse, a patient who was admitted to the unit 10 days ago reveals an elaborate elopement plan. The nurse's *priority* action is to:
    ① Try to talk the patient out of eloping
    ② Let the patient know she understands his feelings
    ③ Tell the patient that this is serious and the information needs to be reported to other staff
    ④ Tell the patient that it's important that he discuss his feelings with his psychiatrist at their next session

20. To facilitate a patient's ability to form more healthy relationships, the nurse should:
    ① Encourage the patient to talk with him or her only about the patient's problems
    ② Discourage the patient from forming any close attachments to others to avoid getting hurt
    ③ Let the patient know that the nurse accepts the patient but does not endorse all of his or her behaviors
    ④ Allow the patient to spend time only with other patients with similar problems

21. When caring for a patient who appears to have poor self-esteem, it is important for the nurse to know that poor self-esteem may be described as being the difference between:
    ① Identity and body image
    ② Role and body image
    ③ Ego ideal and perceived self
    ④ Body image and ego ideal

22. A patient who is being evaluated for a tumor in the frontal region of his brain complains of the odor of cigar smoke in his room. After examining the room and finding no odor, the nurse's *most* important nursing action would be to:
    ① Inform him that she does not smell cigar smoke in the room
    ② Observe, report, and record the clinical symptom
    ③ Ask if he has had an important relationship with a cigar smoker
    ④ Provide a room deodorizer that is more pleasing to the patient

23. A patient on the unit believes that another patient has stolen her watch, and she wants to talk about this with the nurse. The nurse's *best* response is:
    ① "You really can't prove anything."
    ② "Tell me what you believe happened."
    ③ "I'm sure no one here would do a thing like that."
    ④ "No one likes to feel accused."

24. The nurse finds a patient in her room crying. Which of the following responses by the nurse is *most* appropriate?
    ① "Why are you crying?"
    ② "You appear to be feeling sad."
    ③ "What's the matter with you?"
    ④ "Dry up those tears. It's time for group therapy!"

25. With a smile on her face, a young patient tells the nurse that she has just failed her final history exam. This is an example of:
    ① An attempt to be cheerful in the face of adversity
    ② A discrepancy between verbal communication and facial expression
    ③ A lack of seriousness on the patient's part
    ④ An indication that the patient had a desire to fail

26. A patient whose history reflects a reluctance to be hospitalized for a work-up verbalizes anger over a delay in his testing. The nurse's *most* appropriate response would be:
    ① "Believe me, I know just how you feel."
    ② "I'm sorry for the delay, but there are other patients ahead of you."
    ③ "Why don't you read one of these magazines while you're waiting."
    ④ "You seem upset about being here."

27. For the past hour a new patient on the unit has been observed sitting in the corner of her room, staring out the window. A supportive nursing measure should include:
    ① Asking her if there is something the nurse can do for her
    ② Encouraging her to go to the dayroom and interact with the other patients
    ③ Leaving her alone with her thoughts, but checking on her periodically
    ④ Taking a few minutes to sit with her in case she wishes to talk

28. A patient tells the nurse she has received a letter from her boyfriend in which he says he wants to break up with her. The *most* appropriate response by the nurse would be:
    ① "Tell me how you feel about this."
    ② "He must not have loved you enough."
    ③ "You're better off without him."
    ④ "A good-looking girl like you can find a new man in no time!"

29. A very distraught patient tells the nurse a rather confusing story of a recent event. The nurse's *best* response is:
    ① "Settle down and tell me this straight."
    ② "You must be very angry."
    ③ "Let me see if I understand what you're telling me."
    ④ "You always overreact."

30. A patient has been on the mental health unit for 3 weeks. In working with this patient, the nurse-patient relationship is enhanced when the nurse uses both verbal and nonverbal methods of communication to provide:
    ① Understanding, attention, and recognition
    ② Self-esteem, love, and security
    ③ Persuasive techniques for reducing resistance to therapeutic intervention
    ④ Knowledge of the patient's difficulties

31. During an assessment interview, the patient becomes increasingly confused and seems to have a difficult time paying attention and concentrating. The patient becomes easily distracted when being questioned. The nurse realizes that the patient:
    ① Is probably hallucinating
    ② Is becoming fearful of the nurse
    ③ Does not understand the questions
    ④ Is becoming disoriented

32. In talking with a 15-year-old patient, the nurse notes that the patient states that she and her friends occasionally use dexies, bennies, uppers, and speed for fun and excitement. The nurse recognizes these drugs as:
    ① Stimulants
    ② Hallucinogens
    ③ Amphetamines
    ④ Types of street cocaine

33. A patient comes to the local mental health clinic with multiple complaints. The nurse assigned to assess the patient notes the patient's dress, grooming, posture, and facial expressions. These observations help the nurse to assess which of the following?
    ① The patient's emotional state
    ② The patient's thought content
    ③ The patient's general affect
    ④ The patient's level of consciousness

34. Which of the following should a community mental health nurse assess that a nurse practicing on an inpatient mental health unit should not?
    ① Sociocultural influences
    ② Client support systems
    ③ Individual psychosocial stressors
    ④ Economic and political factors

35. The role of the nurse in community mental health is *best* described as:
    ① Functioning mostly as a primary therapist
    ② Controlled by physicians and social workers
    ③ Varied according to location and customs
    ④ Stressful and not well-defined by law

36. A consistent set of behaviors unique to an individual (i.e., the sum total of the individual's thoughts, feelings, physical characteristics, and sociocultural biases) *best* defines which of the following:
    ① Mental status
    ② Psychologic state
    ③ Educational level
    ④ Personality

37. According to Sigmund Freud, the three elements of personality structure are:
    ① Id, ego, and superego
    ② Preconscious, conscious, and unconscious
    ③ Child, adult, and parent
    ④ Oral, anal, and phallic

38. According to Eric Berne, the three elements of personality structure are:
    ① Id, ego, and superego
    ② Preconscious, conscious, and unconscious
    ③ Child, adult, and parent
    ④ Oral, anal, and phallic

39. Personality functions performed by the id/child should include which of the following?
    ① Societal values; may be judgmental and critical
    ② Objective reality with the needs of the individual; objective and rational
    ③ The perception of the individual's role in his world
    ④ The basic innate psychic energy and drive; the emotional responses of love, anger, and passion

40. A 16 year old has a chemistry test in the morning. His friends want to go to the lake for a party. The teen's decision to study or go to the party is a function of which of the following personality functions?
    ① Id/child
    ② Ego/adult
    ③ Superego/parent
    ④ Unconscious

41. There are negative functions of the superego/parent that include the judgmental, punitive aspects of the personality. The positive aspects are known as:
    ① Maintenance of a positive attitude and a sense of humor
    ② The incorporation of societal values and norms; the inclusion of religious values
    ③ The ability to maintain rational objectivity
    ④ The playful, spirited aspect of the personality

42. A child is brought to the mental health center because, according to his mother, "He is slow for his age." While observing him during the first interview, the nurse notes that the child is able to tie his own shoelaces. The nurse knows that this is an example of:
    ① Mental illness
    ② Coping behavior
    ③ Cognitive dysfunction
    ④ Autism

43. The psychoanalytic theorist who founded the client-centered therapeutic school that uses the nondirective interview as a technique is:
    ① Carl Rogers
    ② Harry Stack Sullivan
    ③ Eric Berne
    ④ Erik Erikson

44. Two women have been in a committed relationship for 20 years. They are happy together and have many friends as a couple. One recently experienced a tragedy in which two close members of her family died in a motor vehicle accident. One month after the tragedy, she requests psychiatric care for depression and panic-like symptoms as a result of her grief. In performing a comprehensive nursing assessment, the nurse might view this patient's homosexual lifestyle in what way?
    ① It is a psychiatric disorder that may require therapy
    ② It is an alternative lifestyle that may be a healthy choice for some individuals
    ③ It is a form of character defect that is an indication of moral inferiority
    ④ It is a lifestyle that undermines the well-being of the traditional family

45. Adjustment mechanisms or ego defense mechanisms serve the individual by managing anxiety. These mechanisms become a problem when they:
    ① Cause the individual to draw attention to himself
    ② Interfere with the individual's day-to-day functioning
    ③ Create social embarrassment
    ④ Advance the individual's interest above the interests of others

46. An adolescent patient on the pediatric unit reports that she has recently failed a math test. She tells the nurse, "Next time I will cheat like everyone else does." The nurse recognizes she is using which defense mechanism?
    ① Compensation
    ② Minimization
    ③ Projection
    ④ Rationalization

47. The nurse is in a group therapy session with a young adult who was raped as a young child. She is unable to recall the event. The nurse recognizes this as which defense mechanism?
    ① Reaction formation
    ② Projection
    ③ Repression
    ④ Regression

48. An 8 year old got into trouble at school for wearing an Elvis Presley outfit almost daily. He also hummed some of Elvis Presley's hits during class. The nurse, in talking with the child's newly divorced mother, explains that the child is using a mechanism known as:
    ① Displacement
    ② Dissociation
    ③ Identification
    ④ Compensation

49. A nurse is making home visits to new mothers who were discharged early. The young mother the nurse just visited expressed concern because her 2 year old has started wetting her pants since the new baby arrived. The nurse explains to the mother that the child is using which defense mechanism?
    ① Repression
    ② Regression
    ③ Reaction formation
    ④ Projection

50. A patient had an unpleasant interchange with her mother-in-law. She decides to set the matter aside and go on as if the event had never occurred. The nurse recognizes that this patient is using which of the following defense mechanisms?
    ① Denial
    ② Suppression
    ③ Repression
    ④ Rationalization

51. A couple has been married for 10 years. The husband is very attractive and has had a number of affairs with other women. He is very jealous of his wife and frequently accuses her of seeing other men. Which of the following defense mechanisms is he using?
    ① Denial
    ② Repression
    ③ Rationalization
    ④ Projection

52. A young woman is scheduled for a mastectomy. A well-trained nurse, she studies her anatomy books and knows the procedure in detail. She denies having any feelings about the loss of her breast. The ego defense mechanism the patient is using is:
    ① Rationalization
    ② Denial
    ③ Intellectualization
    ④ Fantasy

53. A man presents himself to his co-workers as morally self-righteous. He is rather judgmental and critical of others and continually portrays himself as superior. His co-workers are surprised when he is arrested at work for having robbed a drug store. This individual's ego defense mechanism is:
    ① Denial
    ② Repression
    ③ Reaction formation
    ④ Regression

54. A 3 year old and her family moved to another state. Though she had been fully toilet trained, the child began to have frequent episodes of wetting herself. The child's ego defense mechanism is:
    ① Regression
    ② Denial
    ③ Repression
    ④ Reaction formation

55. A woman has had a bad day at work but finds it unacceptable to tell her boss how angry she is. She comes home and throws her cat out the door. The defense mechanism she used is:
    ① Identification
    ② Displacement
    ③ Introjection
    ④ Reaction formation

56. A middle-aged woman went through a painful divorce in which she lost her home and most of her possessions. She spends much of her day imagining herself decorating her lovely home using her unlimited wealth. Which of the following cognitive dimensions is the woman implementing?
    ① Fantasy
    ② Denial
    ③ Repression
    ④ Reaction formation

57. An 80-year-old woman has been a resident in Westhaven Nursing Home for the past year, after having lived with her daughter for 5 years. She tells the nurse caring for her, "All the people around here mumble when they talk; no one speaks clearly; they ought to take a course in speaking correctly!" The nurse knows that the resident could be using which of the following defense mechanisms?
    ① Projection
    ② Denial
    ③ Withdrawal
    ④ Compensation

58. According to Kübler-Ross, the dying child who turns her face toward the wall when the nurse enters the room would be in which stage of the grieving process?
    ① Denial
    ② Depression
    ③ Anger
    ④ Acceptance

59. A patient is admitted to the hospital for an open biopsy of the left lung and possible pneumonectomy. During the admission process, the nurse asks him if he has any questions concerning the surgery. The patient says "no" and then starts to talk about his daughter's upcoming wedding. The nurse understands that he is using which of the following defense mechanisms?
    ① Denial
    ② Compensation
    ③ Repression
    ④ Suppression

60. Freud described the psychosexual development of humans and categorized these into five stages. The patient who smokes two packs of cigarettes per day could best be categorized as having difficulty with which one of these stages?
    ① Oral stage
    ② Anal stage
    ③ Phallic stage
    ④ Latency stage

84. A 42-year-old man was involved in a plane crash 5 years ago. In addition to surviving the crash, he was able to help save the lives of two other people. After the events of the crash, he returned to his family and his job. On the outside, he had appeared to be doing well. But he has just been admitted to the mental health unit with a diagnosis of posttraumatic stress disorder. The nurse should assess for which of the following symptoms?
    ① Lethargy and disorientation
    ② Paranoia and suspiciousness
    ③ Mutism and immobility
    ④ Nightmares and anxiety

85. Hallucinations are perceptual experiences and are distressing symptoms that may be present in several types of mental illness. The perceptual experience of hallucinations occurs:
    ① As a result of ingestion of street drugs
    ② In the absence of external stimulus
    ③ As a result of conflict
    ④ As a result of frustration

86. The nurse is caring for a patient on the psychiatric unit. In group this morning the patient reports that she is a millionaire and her family owns the Xerox corporation. The nurse recognizes this as an example of:
    ① Confabulation
    ② Delusions of grandeur
    ③ Delusions of persecution
    ④ Flight of ideas

87. A patient tells the nurse that FBI agents are after him and plan to kill him. The *best* nursing action would be to:
    ① Point out the irrationality of his belief and assure him that there are no enemy agents trying to get his secret
    ② Focus on his feelings and encourage ways to verbalize them
    ③ Recognize that there is no verbal response that will make this belief go away, and therefore say nothing
    ④ Tell him that his belief is amusing

88. A 32-year-old patient has trouble getting to work on time due to obsessive-compulsive behavior. How should the nurse interpret his behavior?
    ① He is lazy and doesn't want to work
    ② He is trying to decrease his anxiety by trying to control his environment
    ③ He is responding to voices that tell him what to do
    ④ He needs behavior modification training

89. A 75-year-old man arrives in the emergency room seeking help. When asked the date, he says it is April 1886. The nurse can *best* describe this patient as:
    ① Oriented × 3
    ② Not oriented in time
    ③ Confused
    ④ Dishonest

90. The nurse begins to plan care for a patient who is said to have scattered thought processes. To substantiate this, the nurse should base the observation on:
    ① Frequent changes of topic
    ② Rapidity of speech
    ③ Physical appearance
    ④ Recent history

91. A woman has been hospitalized on a psychiatric unit for 6 years as a committed patient with a diagnosis of schizophrenia. The nurse should expect the patient to be receiving which of the following medications?
    ① Buspirone (Buspar)
    ② Chlorpromazine (Thorazine)
    ③ Lithium carbonate
    ④ Fluoxetine (Prozac)

92. A 48-year-old man was admitted to the mental health unit because his family was concerned that he had been withdrawn, apathetic, and careless of his personal body needs. Since his admission, the nurse notes his behavior as isolated and that he talks aloud to no one in particular. This patient's symptoms are characteristic of behavior associated with:
    ① Dissociative reaction
    ② Manic depressive reaction
    ③ Schizophrenia
    ④ Paranoid reaction

93. A newly admitted patient is diagnosed as a paranoid schizophrenic. In planning his care, the nurse should:
    ① Offer him several choices for his morning activity
    ② Discuss his care with the charge nurse while standing outside the patient's room
    ③ Offer him few choices, as she is aware of ambivalence as a symptom of his disease
    ④ Have a male attendant accompany her when giving care to this patient.

94. A patient is suffering from schizophrenia. She has been hearing voices telling her she is "no good." The nurse notices that she is becoming more agitated. She tells the nurse that the voices are louder now and they are telling her to "jump off the bridge over the freeway." The nurse's *priority nursing intervention* should be to:
    ① Involve the patient in group activities so that her mind will be occupied and the hallucinations will be less troublesome for her
    ② Explain to the patient that she is a worthwhile human being and that the staff of the hospital is genuinely concerned about her as a person
    ③ Notify her attending psychiatrist and implement immediate suicide precautions
    ④ Spend time with the patient and teach her techniques for handling the hallucinations

95. The medication of choice in treating patients with schizophrenia comes primarily from a group of drugs classified as:
    ① Antipsychotic agents
    ② Antidepressant agents
    ③ Antianxiety agents
    ④ Mood-stabilizing agents

96. A patient has been receiving chlorpromazine (Thorazine) for treatment of auditory hallucinations associated with schizophrenia. Which of the following statements by this patient would indicate to the nurse that the chlorpromazine is effective?
    ① "I hear a different voice now."
    ② "I'm not hearing any voices right now."
    ③ "Sometimes I hear voices; sometimes I don't."
    ④ "The voices aren't as loud as they were."

97. A patient is diagnosed as paranoid schizophrenic. He refuses to eat, telling the nurse the food is poisoned. The *most appropriate* nursing intervention should be to:
    ① Allow food brought from home
    ② Ignore him; he'll eat when he's hungry
    ③ Provide foods in their own containers
    ④ Tell him that feeding tubes are used on patients who don't eat

98. A patient with a 3-month history of depression is admitted to a psychiatric unit. Physician's orders include a monoamine oxidase inhibitor and a tyramine-restricted diet. Of the following foods, the nurse knows that the patient is allowed to have:
    ① Chocolate cake
    ② Cottage cheese
    ③ Green beans
    ④ Summer sausage

99. When caring for a psychiatric patient on chlorpromazine (Thorazine), the nurse would recognize which of the following as a central nervous system side effect of chlorpromazine?
    ① Dry mouth
    ② Dyspnea
    ③ Hypotension
    ④ Syncope

100. A patient is diagnosed with schizophrenia. When the nurse is formulating a teaching plan for the patient and his family, what is the *best* thing to tell them about the action of his antipsychotic medication?
    ① The medication works on the nervous system
    ② The medication stabilizes the patient's mood and behavior
    ③ The medication increases the patient's sense of reality
    ④ The medication blocks adrenaline uptake

101. A 21-year-old male is admitted to the mental health unit with a diagnosis of schizophrenia. In the initial interview, his parents indicate he has isolated himself from the family, quit his job, and dropped out of college. The nurse knows which of the following data to be *most characteristic* of schizophrenia?
    ① Unstable mood and delusions of grandeur
    ② Auditory hallucinations and altered thought processes
    ③ Depressive thoughts and low self-esteem
    ④ Lack of judgment and involvement in complicated legal problems

102. A patient, diagnosed as schizophrenic, is withdrawn, negativistic, and hallucinating. In attempting to activate him, the *most appropriate* nursing intervention should be to:
    ① Invite him to play a simple card game
    ② Insist that he join a group activity
    ③ Explain the benefits of activity
    ④ Mention that his "voices" would want him to participate

103. A schizophrenic patient is experiencing racing thoughts, looseness of association, and the belief that he is being controlled by others. He is easily distracted, has trouble with abstract reasoning, and is hearing voices. To help the patient get through his day at his best level of functioning, the nurse plans to:
    ① Provide him with a simple structured schedule to follow
    ② Engage him in talking about the feelings he is experiencing
    ③ Allow him to remain in his room until he feels better
    ④ Offer him the use of mechanical restraints to help him control himself

104. Following a thorough medical and psychiatric evaluation, a patient diagnosed as schizophrenic receives a prescription for haloperidol (Haldol), a major tranquilizer. In planning care with this patient, the nurse cautions her to expect which of the following common side effects?
    ① Headache and nausea
    ② Skin rash and itching
    ③ Increased sex drive and breast size
    ④ Dry mouth and blurred vision

105. After the first two doses of haloperidol (Haldol), a patient begins to pace and states that she feels "antsy" and can't sit still. Her neck becomes stiff and twists to one side, then her eyes roll upward. These symptoms are consistent with:
    ① A severe allergic reaction
    ② An extrapyramidal reaction
    ③ A worsening of the patient's psychosis
    ④ A rare side effect

106. A patient's reaction to haloperidol (Haldol) is most likely to be controlled by which medication?
    ① Acetylsalicylic acid (Aspirin)
    ② Lorazepam (Ativan)
    ③ Benztropine (Cogentin)
    ④ Lithium carbonate

107. A 37 year old works as an air traffic controller at a local airport. He was recently suspended from his job when he told his supervisor that his co-workers had a plot to steal his wife and kill his dog. Delusions of persecution are associated with which type of schizophrenia?
    ① Catatonic
    ② Disorganized
    ③ Paranoid
    ④ Undifferentiated

108. On admission to the hospital, a patient is hearing command hallucinations directing him to kill the men whom he believes to be a threat to his family. The *priority* nursing intervention should be to:
    ① Attempt to engage him in therapeutic activities to distract him from these distressing thoughts
    ② Notify all staff immediately so that elopement precautions can be instituted
    ③ Attempt to establish a rapport with the patient, hoping to be able to influence him not to kill anyone
    ④ Contact a chaplain who can discuss with the patient the moral consequences of killing

109. A patient treated for paranoid schizophrenia was discharged from a psychiatric facility 2 months ago with the medication thiothixene (Navane) 30 mg PO hs. He calls the unit and complains that "Every time I turn around, I have to go to the pharmacy to have my prescription filled." He becomes verbally abusive and insists on a 6-month supply of thiothixene so he doesn't have to go to the pharmacy so often. The *best* nursing response to this patient should be:

① "Relax. We'll send you a prescription for a 6-month supply."

② "You sound upset. Why don't you come to the hospital and we'll discuss your problem?"

③ "You're on a highly potent medication, and the doctors here never prescribe more than a 30-day supply at one time."

④ "You're not working, so you have plenty of time to go to the pharmacy."

110. A patient diagnosed as paranoid schizophrenic is being treated with chlorpromazine (Thorazine). Which statement by the patient would indicate that she has an appropriate understanding of necessary precautions to take while receiving chlorpromazine?

① "How can I control this runny nose?"

② "I'll be sure to take my medication before each meal."

③ "I'll be sure to increase my food intake."

④ "Which sunscreen should I buy?"

111. A schizophrenic patient is experiencing delusions of persecution. The nurse recognizes that delusions are a source of protection for the patient and she can expect these delusions to be abandoned under which of the following circumstances?

① When the nurse can joke with the patient about his beliefs

② When the patient feels safe and secure

③ When the patient gains insight into his delusional state

④ When the patient is convinced that the nurse likes him

112. A 20 year old is having an acute psychotic episode. He is hearing voices that direct him to run from the hospital and jump off a freeway overpass. He is unable to control the impulses that result from the voices he hears. If the patient is placed in seclusion against his will, the nurse is aware that this intervention raises an ethical issue because it is:

① Considered to be a crime

② A decision based on moral belief

③ Viewed as control of personal freedom

④ An obligation of the nurse to protect him from manifestations of illness

113. A patient with bipolar disorder has been on lithium for approximately 10 days. He is brought to the emergency department by his family because he is still depressed. How would the nurse evaluate the patient's behavior?

① The patient needs to be changed to another medication

② The nurse needs to check the patient's lithium level

③ It is too soon to see the desired effect of the drug

④ The physician should consider increasing the lithium dose

114. The medication of choice in treating a patient with a diagnosis of schizophrenia comes from the group of antidepressants known as:

① Tricyclics

② Tetracyclics

③ Monoamine oxidase inhibitors

④ Trazodone hydrochlorides

115. Side effects of the antidepressant group monoamine oxidase inhibitors that the nurse must observe for are:

① Lowered blood pressure, increased ocular pressure, and tachycardia

② Flushing, diaphoresis, and dry mouth

③ Drowsiness

④ Confusion

116. In caring for a patient who is receiving monoamine oxidase inhibitors, the nurse is aware that the drug can be dangerous when combined with certain foods. The substance in these foods is called:

① Histamine

② Phenylalanine

③ Lysine

④ Tyramine

117. The *best* intervention for the nurse when a manic patient is acting out while playing cards with another patient is to:

① Ask both of them to leave the game area with her

② Ask the other patient to leave the game area

③ Scold the patient for her inappropriate behavior

④ Explain the rules of the game to the patient

118. A patient's mother asks what she should do if her son threatens to hit or hurt her after she takes him home from the hospital. The nurse's *best* response would be:

① "Yell for someone's help when he threatens you."

② "In a calm voice, direct him to leave the area."

③ "Ignore his threats. He wouldn't really hit you."

④ "Call the authorities to have him restrained."

119. A patient receiving lithium complains of blurred vision and frequent urination. The nurse also notices that the patient is having difficulty maintaining her balance. Which of the following nursing actions is appropriate?

① Administer an antiparkinsonian drug, such as benztropine (Cogentin)

② Take the patient's vital signs and administer high-potassium fluids

③ Hold the patient's next dose of medication and call the physician immediately

④ Sit with the patient to teach her about the side effects of lithium

120. A 45-year-old woman has been admitted for treatment of bipolar disorder, manic phase. She exhibits constant activity and pressured speech. She has been sleeping only 2 hours a night for weeks and is physically exhausted. The *priority* nursing intervention should be to:
   ① Show her to her room and insist that she remain there and take a nap
   ② Show her to her room and remain with her, talking calmly and showing her some relaxation exercises
   ③ Administer the prescribed medication and wait until its effects cause her to become drowsy
   ④ Show her to the dayroom where several patients are engaged in activity

121. The psychiatrist has prescribed haloperidol (Haldol) and lithium carbonate to treat a patient's bipolar disorder. The nurse knows the primary purpose of haloperidol is to:
   ① Provide sedation
   ② Provide a "chemical restraint"
   ③ Stimulate the patient's appetite
   ④ Alleviate anxiety

122. Lithium, commonly used to treat bipolar disorder, is effective as a mood stabilizer. In planning care for the patient receiving lithium carbonate, the nurse should monitor for which of the following side effects?
   ① Food cravings
   ② Fine tremors
   ③ Worsening of psychotic symptoms
   ④ Sensitivity to sunlight

123. A patient is admitted to the psychiatric unit with a diagnosis of bipolar disorder, manic phase. The physician orders lithium carbonate 500 mg PO tid. In planning care for this patient, when should the nurse schedule serum lithium levels to be drawn?
   ① Any time of day
   ② In the evening after the last dose of the day
   ③ In the morning before the first dose of the day
   ④ Only when the previous level exceeds 1.5 mEq/L

124. The *best* way for the nurse to see if the manic patient is beginning to attain normal nutritional status is to verify that:
   ① Her appetite is maintained
   ② She eats at scheduled times
   ③ Her weight is maintained
   ④ Her meals are finished

125. The nurse observes her patient playing cards with another patient, noting she is smiling and conversing quietly. The patient loses a game and begins to curse and scream at her partner. This demonstrates which of the following?
   ① Flight of ideas
   ② Ideas of reference
   ③ Mood instability
   ④ Loose associations

126. When monitoring a patient for side effects of lithium carbonate, which of the following manifestations should the nurse observe for?
   ① Dry mouth
   ② Blurred vision
   ③ Dysarthria
   ④ Muscular weakness

127. A patient is receiving lithium carbonate 500 mg PO tid for treatment of bipolar disorder, manic phase. After 3 days of lithium carbonate treatment, the patient's husband approaches the nurse and says, "I don't see any difference in my wife since she was started on lithium." The nurse's *best* response should be:
   ① "Let me call the physician to discuss this with you."
   ② "It can take up to several weeks for mood-stabilizing effects to occur."
   ③ "We can add a neuroleptic to achieve more rapid treatment."
   ④ "Some bipolar patients require long-term therapy with lithium."

128. A patient is on salt lithium carbonate 500 mg PO tid. Her last serum lithium level was 0.3 mEq/L 4 weeks ago. On routine rounds, the nurse observes that the patient is lethargic and unresponsive to verbal and tactile stimuli. The nurse's *priority action* should be to:
   ① Call a code
   ② Increase her fluid intake
   ③ Notify the physician
   ④ Take her vital signs

129. A patient is soon to be discharged with the medication lithium carbonate to be taken 500 mg PO tid. Which statement by the patient indicates that she understands the importance of compliance with her medication regime?
   ① "If I miss a dose, I'll have to take an extra dose before I go to bed."
   ② "If I miss a dose, I'll have to go to the lab and have a lithium level drawn."
   ③ "If I miss a dose, I'll have to increase the sodium in my diet."
   ④ "If I miss a dose, what should I do besides notify my physician?"

130. Approximately one third of patients with bipolar disorder do not respond to lithium carbonate therapy. Carbamazepine (Tegretol) is sometimes prescribed in such cases. When caring for a patient who is receiving carbamazepine, the nurse should plan to regularly check which of the following diagnostic data?
   ① Blood sugar level
   ② Complete blood cell count
   ③ Gastric analysis
   ④ Urine for culture and sensitivity

131. A patient is admitted to the psychiatric unit with a diagnosis of bipolar disorder, manic phase. She is hyperactive, restless, agitated, and hostile. The *priority* nursing diagnosis for this patient would be:
   ① Altered nutrition: less than body requirements, related to inattention to need for food
   ② Potential for injury: falls, related to hyperactivity
   ③ Potential for violence: self-directed related to hostility
   ④ Sleep pattern disturbance related to hyperactivity

132. During periods of extreme elation and overactivity, the manic patient needs a structured environment. In planning activities, the nurse considers which of the following?
    ① Asking the patient for suggestions in planning unit activities
    ② Keeping her from assuming more responsibility than she can handle
    ③ Putting her in charge of a unit project with a group of patients
    ④ Suggesting activities that require concentration; limiting physical activity

133. A patient on the mental health unit is disruptive. He overturns tables and throws anything he can get his hands on. When planning care for this patient, it is important for the team to set limits on behavior. Setting limits on the patient's behavior can be done when the team:
    ① Considers the morale and safety of other patients
    ② Considers the degree of the staff's responsibility from a legal point of view
    ③ Adheres strictly to all rules and regulations
    ④ Appreciates the value the patient attaches to each situation

134. A patient is admitted to the mental health unit. During the admission process, the nurse notes that he speaks quite rapidly while frequently changing topics. This patient's speech pattern is described as:
    ① Unintelligible
    ② Disorganized
    ③ Variable
    ④ Pressured

135. A manic patient has begun to call other patients derogatory names and uses profanity in her conversations. The most appropriate nursing intervention should be to:
    ① Ignore the comments
    ② Tell the patient that her behavior will be reported to the physician
    ③ Set limits to this behavior
    ④ Instruct the other patients to ignore her behavior

136. The nurse observes that a patient moves very quickly from one idea to another and that there is no connection between them. The nurse knows that the patient is demonstrating:
    ① Confabulation
    ② Primary process
    ③ Flight of ideas
    ④ Neologisms

137. When the nurse checks a manic patient's chart for his lithium level, she finds that it is 2 mEq/L. The interpretation/action by the nurse should be:
    ① This level is within therapeutic range; do nothing
    ② This level is below therapeutic range; call the physician
    ③ This level is slightly high but does not require action
    ④ This level is high; he should be assessed for signs/symptoms of toxicity

138. After leaving the unit during a visit, a manic patient's mother calls the nurse from home to report that her son threatened to hit her. Which of the following diagnoses would the nurse add to the patient's care plan?
    ① Ineffective family coping related to hospitalization
    ② Anxiety related to inability to cope with their son's illness
    ③ Potential for violence related to unstable mood and affect
    ④ Potential for self-injury related to loss of control

139. A patient is diagnosed with bipolar disorder, manic phase. Lithium carbonate is prescribed for her, along with a neuroleptic. The nurse understands the action of lithium carbonate to be that of:
    ① Decreasing her depression
    ② Increasing her libido
    ③ Increasing her affect
    ④ Stabilizing her affect

140. A patient has just been admitted to the psychiatric unit with a diagnosis of bipolar disorder, manic phase. In assessing the patient's emotional status, which of the following should the nurse expect her to say when asked if she is concerned about her family?
    ① "I'm worried about their welfare."
    ② "I'm a failure as a wife."
    ③ "Why should I be worried?"
    ④ "I just hope they're okay."

141. One of the primary diagnoses for the patient with mania is altered nutrition: less than body requirements related to hyperactivity. The nurse's *best* intervention should be to:
    ① Provide her with small, easily carried foods
    ② Provide large, high-protein meals
    ③ Provide a quiet mealtime environment
    ④ Provide her with extra vitamin supplements

142. An appropriate nursing intervention for a patient with a paranoid personality disorder would be to:
    ① Maintain honest, clear, open communication
    ② Reduce social contact because interactions precipitate further distortions
    ③ Make decisions for him to reduce added stress
    ④ Avoid discussing his treatment plan with him

143. The nurse is sitting with a patient one day when he turns and says, "Isn't that singing beautiful!" The nurse does not hear anything and concludes that the patient is probably experiencing a hallucination. The *best response* by the nurse would be:
    ① "I understand you think you hear singing; however, I don't hear anything."
    ② "Tell me the words to the song."
    ③ "What are you talking about? I don't hear any singing."
    ④ "Yes, I'm enjoying the song."

144. Which of the following is *most appropriate* when the nurse is aware that a patient is hallucinating?
    ① Tell him that there is no one there
    ② Ask him to describe his feelings at this time
    ③ Use simple statements in communicating with him
    ④ Encourage him to participate in self-care

145. The nurse is working the night shift on a general surgery floor. A patient who had surgery 2 days ago for an acute bowel obstruction calls the nurse to her room to report that she sees green snakes coming from the heater vents. There have been no previous reports of the patient experiencing visual hallucinations. The priority nursing intervention should be to:
    ① Turn on the light and reassure her that there are no snakes in the hospital
    ② Notify the charge nurse or her attending physician of her visual hallucinations
    ③ Observe and record the nature and quality of her hallucinations
    ④ Check her chart to see if there is any indication of a history of mental illness

146. A patient reports "seeing the face of Satan" on the wall of his room. This is an example of:
    ① Delusion
    ② Illusion
    ③ Hallucination
    ④ Regression

147. A patient believes that he holds the secret to solving the problem with the hole in the ozone layer. Unfortunately, he says, enemy agents are pursuing him in order to steal his secret. The nurse knows that this patient is experiencing which of the following?
    ① Panic
    ② Stress
    ③ A delusion
    ④ A hallucination

148. A patient is brought to the hospital by two friends. He is a 19-year-old college student who is known to have experimented with drugs. He is in a psychotic, violent, and agitated state. His pupils are dilated and he is having vivid visual hallucinations. His skin is flushed and is hot and dry to touch. On the basis of these assessment data, the nurse suspects intoxication with:
    ① Heroin
    ② PCP, or angel dust
    ③ Barbiturates
    ④ Marijuana, or grass

149. Two police officers escort a patient to the emergency room. He has some minor injuries from an automobile accident that he has caused. After the physician has examined him and his injuries are treated, the physician requests a blood alcohol level. The nurse knows the blood alcohol that legally indicates intoxication is usually:
    ① 0.25 mg/dl
    ② 0.5 mg/dl
    ③ 0.10 mg/dl
    ④ 0.05 mg/dl

150. The patient's withdrawal from diazepam (Valium) is complicated by her use of alcohol. The nurse understands that the reason for this is that:
    ① She is becoming an alcoholic and is therefore less motivated
    ② Alcohol and diazepam are cross-tolerant drugs
    ③ She began using the diazepam as a prescription drug and the alcohol is a nonprescription drug
    ④ Once she is no longer receiving diazepam, the alcohol will not be a problem for her

151. A patient, in the hospital for 3 days, is experiencing withdrawal symptoms from alcohol and diazepam (Valium). The nurse should expect to see which of the following symptoms?
    ① Confusion, disorientation, and stupor
    ② Irritability, restlessness, and insomnia
    ③ Gregariousness, euphoria, and irritability
    ④ Seizures, coma, and death

152. A patient is withdrawing from alcohol and diazepam (Valium). The *priority* nursing intervention for patients experiencing withdrawal would be:
    ① Monitoring the vital signs and providing emotional support and encouragement
    ② Insistence on attendance at all group therapy sessions
    ③ Strict enforcement of mental health unit rules
    ④ Exploration of feelings about the experience

153. A 27-year-old dancer in the city ballet feels her profession demands that she keep her weight down. After the birth of her last child, she had difficulty losing weight. She acquired some amphetamines from a friend to help her lose weight. After 6 months of steady use, she has become dependent on the drugs. On admission to the hospital, this patient is malnourished and exhausted. On assessment, which additional signs of amphetamine use should the nurse expect to find?
    ① Mild-mannered and compliant
    ② Disoriented and disheveled
    ③ Psychotic and delusional
    ④ Mildly paranoid and irritable

154. A patient is experiencing amphetamine withdrawal. The nurse knows which of the following to be classic signs of amphetamine withdrawal?
    ① Chest pain, diaphoresis, and palpitations
    ② Euphoria, hyperactivity, and alertness
    ③ Profuse sweating, gooseflesh, and diarrhea
    ④ Depression, fatigue, and lethargy

155. A 36-year-old woman who is a successful artist began to experiment with cocaine, believing that it improved her ability to be creative in her work. The recent death of a friend from cocaine abuse has convinced her to seek treatment to discontinue using the drug. In addition to cravings from the drug, what should the nurse expect this patient to experience during her withdrawal from cocaine?
    ① Palpitations
    ② Paranoia
    ③ Euphoria
    ④ Depression

156. A 36 year old has been using heroin for several years. He sells drugs and commits other antisocial acts to support his habit. Arrested for robbing a convenience store, he is still intoxicated with heroin when he is involuntarily admitted to the mental health unit. The nurse should expect to see which of the following symptoms of drug intoxication?
    ① Dilated pupils
    ② Hostility
    ③ Pinpoint pupils
    ④ Profound depression

157. A patient is recovering nicely from alcohol withdrawal. The nurse attempts a conversation with him. When the nurse begins to speak of alcoholism, the patient lapses into a period of silence. To be *most* helpful, the nurse should:
    ① Sit in silence with him
    ② Suggest they talk later
    ③ Change the topic of the conversation
    ④ Acknowledge his silence and encourage him to speak

158. A patient is experiencing delirium tremens. The nurse should implement which of the following *priority actions?*
    ① Discussing benefits of Alcoholics Anonymous (AA)
    ② Keeping him awake and oriented
    ③ Monitoring vital signs
    ④ Recording hourly outputs

159. To relieve some of the serious neurologic symptoms of delirium tremens, the nurse should anticipate the physician ordering which of the following medications while the patient is in withdrawal?
    ① Disulfiram (Antabuse)
    ② Calcium
    ③ Magnesium sulfate
    ④ Morphine sulfate

160. A patient is hospitalized for heroin intoxication. Four hours after admission, what change should the nurse expect to notice in this patient's condition as a result of the beginning of his withdrawal syndrome?
    ① Dilated pupils
    ② Hostility
    ③ Pinpoint pupils
    ④ Profound depression

161. The nurse working in an inner-city emergency room is called on to present a community education program on drug abuse. She presents the fact that drugs of the opiate class include medicinal drugs. She discusses heroin, which is also in this class but is not used medicinally in the United States. The nurse will discuss the clinical symptoms of the effect of the opiate class of drugs, including:
    ① Sweating, abdominal pain, and diarrhea
    ② Pinpoint pupils, euphoria, and respiratory depression
    ③ Dilated pupils, drowsiness, and visual hallucinations
    ④ Hypervigilance, hallucinations, and heightened capacity to concentrate

162. While the nurse is planning for a patient's discharge from alcohol treatment, the patient's mother asks if she will have to make her daughter attend Alcoholics Anonymous (AA) meetings. The nurse should:
    ① Tell the mother that attending AA meetings will help the patient stay sober
    ② Ask the mother how she feels about her daughter attending these meetings
    ③ Emphasize that it is the patient's responsibility to decide whether to attend AA meetings
    ④ Remind the mother that attending AA meetings is a condition of discharge

163. A 45-year-old man has been a severe alcoholic for years. Hospitalized for 3 days, he is in alcohol withdrawal. He complains of bugs and rats crawling on his skin. The nurse knows that he is experiencing which of the following types of hallucinations?
    ① Olfactory
    ② Visual
    ③ Auditory
    ④ Tactile

164. A patient was admitted to the mental health unit because he was withdrawn and apathetic. After 3 weeks of taking prescribed medication, he appears to be receptive to further therapy. The *best type* of therapy should include:
    ① Therapeutic group sessions
    ② Transactional analysis group sessions
    ③ Relaxation therapy group sessions
    ④ Reality orientation group sessions

165. A 19 year old is brought to the crisis center after being bailed out of jail for acts of vandalism. His father is requesting a mental health evaluation. The nurse should assess the patient for what additional characteristics of antisocial personality disorder?
    ① Difficulty maintaining employment
    ② Impulsive, unpredictable behavior
    ③ Dramatic, attention-seeking behavior
    ④ Intentional inefficiency

166. The antisocial personality presents numerous problematic behaviors. The nurse knows that to decrease manipulative behavior, an appropriate nursing intervention should be to:
    ① Immediately set limits on all behavior
    ② Set limits only in those areas necessary to protect the patient
    ③ Let the patient decide the limits to be set
    ④ Allow the community to set limits on the patient's behavior

167. On the basis of his knowledge of the causes of mental illness, the nurse knows that the development of a personality disorder is *most likely* caused by:
    ① A biochemical imbalance
    ② A genetic predisposition
    ③ A parental/family dysfunction
    ④ A birth complication

168. On the basis of her knowledge of personality disorders, the nurse should expect which of the following to be the *primary* problem for these patients during hospitalization?
    ① Participating in activities
    ② Withdrawal from substances
    ③ Observing unit rules
    ④ Relationships with others

169. "Addiction" to a substance means that a person has:
    ① Physiologic dependence
    ② Psychologic dependence
    ③ Both physiologic and psychologic dependence
    ④ Either physiologic or psychologic dependence

170. Of the following systems, which is the most seriously affected by long-term alcohol abuse?
     ① Endocrine
     ② Cardiovascular
     ③ Musculoskeletal
     ④ Reproductive

171. The son of a delirious patient states, "I feel so helpless. I just don't know what to do." Which of the following is the *best way* to help the patient's son deal with his mother's illness?
     ① Reassure him that his mother will be fine in a few days
     ② Suggest that he not visit her until she improves
     ③ Role model how best to interact with his mother
     ④ Refer him to the physician to answer his concerns

172. A 36 year old is diagnosed with multiple personality disorder. The nurse understands that the basic explanation of a personality disorder is:
     ① A maladaptation that is most apparent within an interpersonal or social context
     ② The capacity to induce others to feel extreme irritation and annoyance
     ③ A self-centered, inflexible approach to work and interpersonal relationships
     ④ The tendency to be overly concerned with having a good time and entertaining others

173. A 25 year old is an outpatient at the local mental health clinic. Although he appears witty and charming, he has had several "scrapes" with the law. He has been unable to hold down a job for any length of time and is a high school dropout. He is an habitual liar and has broken off many relationships with young women. The nurse recognizes these behaviors as consistent with which of the following personality disorders?
     ① Avoidant personality
     ② Schizotypal personality
     ③ Antisocial personality
     ④ Impulsive personality

174. A patient is identified as having a disruptive lifestyle. The nurse understands that this patient can be expected to manifest which of the following behaviors?
     ① An illness
     ② A perceptual or affective disorder
     ③ A maladaptive coping style
     ④ A genetically inherited dysfunction

175. A 24 year old is diagnosed as having an antisocial personality disorder. An expected treatment goal for this patient should be:
     ① Success with medication regime
     ② Highly successful group therapy
     ③ Long-term psychotherapy
     ④ Decrease in his anxiety

176. A 36 year old has been a patient on the mental health unit for 1 week and is diagnosed with a paranoid personality disorder. He exhibits mistrust, hypersensitivity, and restricted feelings. The nurse should expect the patient's restricted feelings to be evidenced by which of the following behaviors?
     ① Sentimentality
     ② Lack of a sense of humor
     ③ Self-indulgence
     ④ Attention-seeking behavior

177. A patient just admitted for detox has a hangover. The nurse would expect which of the following signs and symptoms as evidence of this condition?
     ① Prolonged, elevated blood levels of alcohol
     ② Hyperglycemia and decrease in lactic acid in the blood
     ③ Prolonged sense of euphoria
     ④ Headache and irritability

178. Several years ago a 42-year-old man began the use of alcohol. Recently he has been drinking on a daily basis. On the morning following a binge, he has no memory of events of the evening before. This patient is experiencing which of the following signs of alcoholism?
     ① Social impairment
     ② Wernicke's syndrome
     ③ Blackout
     ④ Selective memory

179. For nervousness, a patient has been given diazepam (Valium) for several years by her physician. Over the past year, she has begun to use the medication daily. In addition to daily use of Valium, the patient has begun to drink alcohol daily. The nurse knows diazepam (Valium) to be the second most commonly abused drug classified as:
     ① Amphetamines
     ② Cocaine
     ③ Narcotic
     ④ Sedative/barbiturate

180. When setting limits on a patient's behavior, the nurse must identify the consequences to the patient should he exceed the established limits. The nurse knows that the *most appropriate* time to establish consequences is:
     ① Just before the anticipated behavior
     ② After the patient has exceeded the set limits
     ③ At the time the limits are set
     ④ When the staff can no longer tolerate the patient's behavior

181. An appropriate goal toward which the patient with personality disorder can work during hospitalization is:
     ① Establishing a stable marital relationship
     ② Planning for productive employment
     ③ Understanding the consequences of substance use
     ④ Finding nondestructive ways to meet needs

182. The primary mechanism by which a patient with a personality disorder will attempt to have needs met by others is:
     ① Manipulation
     ② Projection
     ③ Repression
     ④ Sublimation

183. After her husband's death, a widow is experiencing physical symptoms of loss of appetite, nausea, and vomiting. The nurse should assess her stage of grieving as:
     ① Shock and denial
     ② Developing awareness
     ③ Restitution
     ④ Distorted

184. A patient has a leg paralysis for which no physiologic cause can be identified. Because of the patient's psychosocial history, the physician suspects a conversion reaction. The nurse understands that a conversion reaction enables an individual to:
    ① Dismiss uncomfortable thoughts or feelings
    ② Find an acceptable excuse for his behavior
    ③ Blame someone or something for his action
    ④ Express emotions through physical symptoms

185. While he is waiting to have a computed tomography (CT) scan performed, a patient with Alzheimer's disease becomes anxious and restless and cannot follow the instructions that the staff gives him to prepare for his examination. Which of the following is the *best* nursing intervention at this time?
    ① Allow him to respond to instructions when he feels ready
    ② Give him written rather than verbal instructions
    ③ Tell him he will have to leave if he cannot cooperate
    ④ Take him to a quiet place to wait for his scan

186. During his admission assessment, a patient with Alzheimer's disease tells the nurse, "You ask too many questions. Why can't you just leave me alone?" What is the *best* way for the nurse to respond?
    ① "These are important questions. We have to continue."
    ② "I know that you don't really feel that way."
    ③ "You sound upset. Would you like to rest for a while?"
    ④ "You know your family wants you to cooperate."

187. The family of an Alzheimer's disease patient asks the nurse how long it will take him to recover. What is the *best* answer?
    ① "With proper treatment and care, not that long."
    ② "There is no way to tell how long he will be ill."
    ③ "He will not be able to regain what was lost."
    ④ "He will continue to get progressively worse."

188. A 90-year-old widow is experiencing forgetfulness, confusion, and bouts of disorientation that are worse at night. A medical diagnosis of Alzheimer's disease has been made. The nurse serves the meal and later returns to find the tray untouched. On the basis of the nurse's understanding of this patient's condition, the nurse believes the most likely cause of refusal to eat is that the patient:
    ① Does not care for hospital food
    ② Is too forgetful to remember to feed herself
    ③ May believe the food is poisoned
    ④ Is too depressed to eat

189. A 52-year-old woman has Alzheimer's disease. To support her nutritional needs, the nurse's *priority* nursing intervention should be to:
    ① Have a staff member feed the patient
    ② Have the nutritionist come to talk with her about her food preferences
    ③ Have a staff member or a family member remain with the patient while she is eating
    ④ Talk with the patient about her nutritional needs

190. A newly admitted patient has just been diagnosed with Alzheimer's disease. With which of the following would he experience the most difficulty in stage one of Alzheimer's disease?
    ① Getting dressed
    ② Remembering telephone numbers
    ③ Walking up and down stairs
    ④ Brushing his teeth

191. Which of the following would be the most appropriate nursing intervention for a patient with a compulsive personality disorder?
    ① Teaching relaxation techniques
    ② Avoiding discussion of compulsive behavior
    ③ Contracting for an amount of time spent doing compulsive behavior
    ④ Joining an assertiveness training group

192. A patient is diagnosed with a compulsive personality disorder. The nurse understands that the patient's interpersonal relationships are most apt to be negatively affected by which of the following behaviors characteristic of compulsive personality disorders?
    ① Perfectionistic
    ② Decisive
    ③ Empathetic
    ④ Cooperative

193. A 32-year-old woman is a buyer for a local department store. She is good at her job, but she annoys her co-workers with her rigid, detail-oriented manner. She has definite characteristics of a compulsive personality disorder. Which of the following behaviors should the nurse expect the patient to also demonstrate as a result of this disorder?
    ① Attention seeking
    ② Impulsiveness
    ③ Magical thinking
    ④ Superior attitude

194. The nurse is caring for a patient who is diagnosed with agoraphobia. What symptoms would the nurse expect to see?
    ① Psychotic symptoms
    ② Fear of leaving home
    ③ Fear of physical symptoms
    ④ Bradycardia

195. A 34-year-old single parent is hospitalized for obsessive-compulsive disorder and depression. Her compulsion is washing. She repeatedly scrubs her hands, arrives late for meals, and neglects her nutritional intake. An appropriate nursing intervention to increase this patient's nutritional intake should be to:
    ① Interrupt the patient's ritual and tell her she must come to the dining room
    ② Tell the patient how silly she's being and that eating is the priority
    ③ Instruct her to hurry up; her meal is getting cold
    ④ Provide her with nutritious between-meal snacks

196. A short-term goal for an obsessive-compulsive disorder patient should be to decrease the incidence of compulsive behavior. The patient is considered to be responding positively to treatment if she:
    ① Outwardly attempts to ignore or suppress impulses
    ② Decreases repetitive performance of ritualistic acts
    ③ Verbalizes difficulty in being self-reflective
    ④ Expresses a need to control the immediate environment

197. A 20-year-old college student is physically attractive, although she worries excessively about her weight. She has learned that she can eat anything she wants as long as she can go to the bathroom and make herself vomit after eating. The nurse suspects that the patient is suffering from:
    ① Anorexia nervosa
    ② Bulimia
    ③ Agoraphobia
    ④ Narcissistic personality disorder

198. A 14 year old is diagnosed with anorexia nervosa and characteristically performs elaborate rituals with her food. She primarily performs these rituals to:
    ① Reinforce feelings of wellness
    ② Control feelings of anxiety
    ③ Increase calorie expenditure
    ④ Maintain personal boundaries

199. Anxiety related to fear of weight gain is the primary nursing diagnosis for a patient with anorexia nervosa. The best nursing intervention for this diagnosis should be to:
    ① Discuss how she uses weight to control anxiety
    ② Point out how unattractive her extreme thinness is
    ③ Explain that being slightly overweight is more healthy
    ④ Discuss the danger she is in from extreme dieting

200. The nurse is caring for a 16-year-old patient diagnosed with anorexia nervosa. What observation by the nurse would indicate that the patient is improving?
    ① She no longer weighs herself daily
    ② She requests favorite foods at meals
    ③ She has gained weight
    ④ She eats all the food on her tray

201. The nurse is caring for a 14 year old diagnosed with anorexia nervosa. The nurse is assigned to be with the patient at meal time to monitor what she eats. The patient accuses the nurse of not trusting her. What response from the nurse is best?
    ① "I will check back on you in 15 minutes."
    ② "This is good food; you need to eat."
    ③ "There are a lot of starving people in the world."
    ④ "I will sit quietly while you eat."

202. The self-concept of patients with restricting anorexia is based mainly on the idea that thinness will:
    ① Increase their acceptability to others
    ② Increase their mental abilities
    ③ Increase their feelings of power over others
    ④ Increase their feelings of safety

203. The nurse is caring for a shy 16 year old admitted to the psychiatric unit weighing less than 90 lbs. The patient nibbles at her meals, exercises extensively each day, and wears oversized clothes. What statement by this patient causes the nurse to suspect she is suffering from anorexia nervosa?
    ① "I'm really not very hungry today."
    ② "I feel okay, but I haven't had my period for 2 months."
    ③ "I feel fine and have no reason to complain."
    ④ "You know my parents don't even know how much I weigh."

204. A patient's parents have agreed to participate in a case conference. Knowing that family dynamics play a role in the illness of the patient with anorexia nervosa, the nurse would expect this patient's parents to display which of the following behaviors?
    ① Immature and eager to please
    ② Overprotective and rigid
    ③ Passive and nonassertive
    ④ Secretive and stubborn

205. Many psychiatric therapies involve a holistic emphasis. The nurse must understand that the concept of holism is *best* explained by which one of the following statements?
    ① The individual's role in his world determines his health
    ② Illness results from a complex interaction between the mind and body
    ③ The individual is both separate from and part of society
    ④ A community is whole

206. Multifaceted approaches to treatment are used in mental health nursing. In planning patient care, the nurse knows that these approaches comprise which of the following dimensions?
    ① Financial resources, cost effectiveness, efficiency, and efficacy
    ② Bed availability, potential for recovery, potential benefit to society, and therapies available
    ③ Medication, group therapy, milieu therapy, and rehabilitation
    ④ Physical, psychologic, cultural, and socioeconomic

207. An appropriate nursing goal for a patient who is in the terminal stages of an illness would be:
    ① Assisting the patient through each stage of the death and dying process
    ② Reassuring the patient that he has nothing to fear in death
    ③ Secluding the patient from others
    ④ Engaging the patient in future planning

208. A patient was admitted to the psychiatric unit involuntarily. The nurse understands this to mean:
    ① The patient has lost all his civil rights
    ② The patient cannot leave the hospital unless discharged
    ③ The patient is incompetent
    ④ The patient can no longer vote

209. In evaluating the outcome of care, the nurse reads the following in the care plan: "Patient will understand his medication regimen in 5 days." Although this is a desirable goal, the nurse auditing the care plan knows that:
    ① This goal is not an achievable outcome
    ② This goal is not directly observable
    ③ This goal is unrealistic
    ④ This is a behavioral goal

210. A patient has just been told that the illness he is experiencing is inoperable lung cancer. He is advised to get his affairs in order because he has no more than 3 months to live. The nurse should anticipate which of the following reactions from this patient?
    ① Shock and denial
    ② Anger and rage
    ③ Sadness and insomnia
    ④ Acceptance and compliance

211. A 43-year-old woman who is mentally retarded works in a sheltered workshop where she has friends and feels productive. Her mother has just died of cancer. What reaction should the nurse expect to see in the patient at this time?
    ① No reaction
    ② Tendency to abuse alcohol
    ③ Psychotic depression
    ④ A normal grief reaction

212. The nurse is caring for a 24-year-old psychotic patient. As part of the treatment plan, the patient is given tokens for appropriate behavior. The nurse realizes this is a form of:
    ① Bribery
    ② Role modeling
    ③ Positive reinforcement
    ④ Negative reinforcement

213. The nurse is admitting a 17 year old to the surgical unit. As she orients the patient to the unit she chats and tries to learn some things about her. The nurse's rationale for doing this is to:
    ① Establish a trusting relationship
    ② Foster nonverbal communication
    ③ Ease the tension in the room
    ④ Show compassion for the patient

214. A nurse receives her daily assignment and realizes that she has 10 of the 20 patients on the floor to care for that day. There are two other nurses and an aide scheduled to work that day on the floor. She goes to the charge nurse and states "I realize we're very busy today, but I feel like I cannot possibly give good nursing care to 10 patients. I would like to have a few patients reassigned." This statement is an example of which type of behavior?
    ① Aggressive
    ② Passive
    ③ Manipulative
    ④ Assertive

215. A patient is attending the group therapy sessions on the psychiatric unit. Following the meeting the patient states, "I don't think I'll ever get better." The nurse responds by saying "Don't be ridiculous. You shouldn't even think that way!" This is an example of which type of block to therapeutic communication?
    ① Changing the subject
    ② Belittling
    ③ Disagreeing
    ④ Reassuring clichés

216. A nurse working on a psychiatric unit knows which of the following statements to be true?
    ① Most mentally ill patients require extensive hospitalization
    ② Some mentally ill patients do not require hospitalization
    ③ Most mentally ill patients remain in long-term care
    ④ The majority of mentally ill clients reside in state institutions

217. The nurse is admitting a patient to the psychiatric unit. He is very agitated and anxious. What should the nurse do first?
    ① Involve the patient in group therapy
    ② Take the patient to the gym for exercise
    ③ Place the patient in a quiet area away from others
    ④ Introduce the patient to the others on the unit

218. Neuroleptic malignant syndrome is an unusual reaction to neuroleptic medications (antipsychotic drugs). The nurse should expect a person with this diagnosis to manifest which of the following classic symptoms of neuroleptic malignant syndrome?
    ① Convulsions, headache, and fever
    ② Hyperthermia, muscle rigidity, and stupor
    ③ Severe headache, fever, and neck stiffness
    ④ Shaking chills, temperature, and hypotension

219. A patient is ordered to receive phenelzine (Nardil), a monoamine oxidase inhibitor (MAOI). Which of the following statements by the patient should indicate to the nurse that he understands his tyramine-restricted diet?
    ① "It will take me a while to develop a taste for hot dogs with sauerkraut only."
    ② "I like my salads moist. I guess I can use any salad dressing as long as it isn't made with MSG or cheese."
    ③ "I love pizza, but I guess I can only have it on special occasions now."
    ④ "My wife and I always have a glass of sherry after dinner. I guess we'll be losing some weight now that we can only have a glass a week."

220. A patient admitted 3 days ago has been observed by the nursing team as not being interested in becoming involved in the treatment program or in following unit rules. She clearly prefers some staff members over others. In planning for her nursing care, which consideration is *most important?*
    ① If the patient prefers some staff members over others, those are the ones who should work with her
    ② Patience is required to work with this patient; when she is ready, she will begin to appreciate the value of the treatment program
    ③ The nursing team must confer and decide which rules are important to enforce in this patient's care; all staff must enforce the same rules equally and consistently
    ④ Because the patient is an adult, the staff has no responsibility in enforcing any of the rules; she will decide for herself when she desires treatment

221. Thirty minutes after a patient receives the antipsychotic drug fluphenazine (Prolixin), his tongue becomes thick, he drools, his jaw becomes rigid, and his speech is slurred. Which of the following prn orders should the nurse give immediately?
    ① Diazepam (Valium), 15 mg IV
    ② Benztropine (Cogentin), 2 mg IM
    ③ Chlorpromazine (Thorazine), 25 mg IM
    ④ Lorazepam (Ativan), 1 mg PO

222. A patient's family brings him to the emergency room after he stops taking his antipsychotic medications and starts to hallucinate and become agitated. The emergency room physician orders haloperidol (Haldol) 20 mg intramuscularly. Why does the nurse refuse to give the medication as ordered?
    ① The dose is too low to relieve his symptoms
    ② Haloperidol is only available in oral form
    ③ Haloperidol is an antidepressant and as such is not indicated
    ④ The dose is too high to be given intramuscularly

223. A patient receiving antipsychotic medication tells the nurse, "I feel so nervous, like I can't sit still." The nurse should suspect that this patient is describing the common side effect of:
    ① Dystonia
    ② Akathisia
    ③ Tardive dyskinesia
    ④ Pseudoparkinsonism

224. It is important to include the family when teaching a patient about medications, primarily to:
    ① Provide information and support for the patient
    ② Ensure that members of the family will not undermine treatment
    ③ Have the family take responsibility for the patient
    ④ Gain the family's approval for the treatment

225. For a hospitalized patient who has had dysfunctional grieving for 2 years, which of the following times/conditions would be *best* to encourage verbalization of feelings?
    ① At discharge
    ② Monthly, with her social worker
    ③ Daily, with her primary nurse
    ④ Weekly, with her psychiatrist

226. A 38 year old is a psychiatric patient with a history of medication noncompliance. The nurse knows the physician will order medications for this patient in which of the following dosage forms?
    ① Capsule
    ② Liquid
    ③ Tablet
    ④ Parenteral

227. Which of the following statements indicates the nurse's understanding of what it means to establish a contract with a psychiatric patient?
    ① It emphasizes what the nurse will do for the patient
    ② It emphasizes what the nurse will not do for the patient
    ③ It states the nurse's level of participation
    ④ It states the patient's responsibilities

228. A patient is being prepared for discharge and follow-up visits at the community mental health center. A goal of community mental health is to:
    ① Quickly return patients to their community
    ② Ensure that the whole community is mentally healthy
    ③ Hospitalize patients away from their communities
    ④ Restructure the community

229. The patient is responding well to drug therapy and is placed in group sessions. Group activities can be expected to be effective if they are:
    ① Democratic in principle, permitting change and providing spontaneity and variety
    ② Structured and purposeful
    ③ Practical and presented at the patient's level of function
    ④ Structured to repress aggressive behavior

230. A patient has an inoperable brain tumor and is in the terminal phase of his illness. While being helped with his morning bath, he begins to talk about dying. The best response by the nurse should be to:
    ① Ask if he would like to see a member of the clergy
    ② Say little and listen to what the patient has to say
    ③ Act as if she did not hear him and excuse herself from the room
    ④ Encourage the patient to keep his hope up and think positively

231. Crisis intervention therapy is short term. A crisis is usually resolved in which of the following time frames?
    ① 24 to 48 hours
    ② 2 to 4 days
    ③ 4 to 6 weeks
    ④ 6 to 12 months

232. The *first priority* for the nurse to address when a battered woman comes for treatment is the woman's need to:
    ① Feel physically and mentally safe
    ② Reestablish feelings of control
    ③ Obtain accurate legal advice
    ④ Discuss her living situation

233. A patient asks the nurse if her abusive husband can ever change, or should she just "give up hope?" The *best* nursing response is:
① "Leaving is your only real option for survival."
② "You are fooling herself to stay with him."
③ "I understand you are dependent on him."
④ "Batterers can learn more effective ways of relating."

234. A patient tells the nurse that her husband gets violent with her after he's been drinking with his friends. Which of the following is the appropriate information for the nurse to give the patient regarding the relationship between abuse and alcohol use?
① If he didn't drink, he wouldn't beat her
② Use of alcohol can increase the likelihood of abuse
③ There is no relationship between these two things
④ Alcohol use is the primary cause of battering

235. Women from lower socioeconomic status (SES) groups are more frequently identified as victims of battering than women from middle or upper SES groups. This is because:
① Women from lower SES groups are more frequently victimized
② Women from middle and upper SES groups conceal their battering
③ Women from middle and upper SES groups obtain better police protection and intervention
④ Men from lower SES groups are naturally more violent

236. The nurse should expect a 7-year-old's mother to reveal which of the following characteristics of abusive parents?
① Low socioeconomic level
② Realistic expectations of a child's behavior
③ History of abuse as a child
④ Socially interactive

237. Which of the following behaviors in individuals who were abused children should be indications that they suffered *physical* abuse as opposed to other types of child abuse?
① Apprehension when other children cry
② Habit disorder such as rocking
③ Poor peer relationships
④ Developmental lag

238. An appropriate therapy for a sexually abused child that is *least* threatening should be:
① Group therapy
② Hypnosis
③ Art therapy
④ Desensitization therapy

239. A patient comes to the clinic after being beaten by her husband. Battered women are most frequently encountered in which of the following settings?
① Emergency rooms
② Obstetric services
③ Mental health clinics
④ Legal aid services

240. After coming on duty, the nurse learns that one of her patients has lapsed into depression after seeming to progress well. The nurse finds the patient sitting in her room with her hands on her lap and her head bowed. The patient does not respond to the nurse's greeting. The *best response* by the nurse should be:
① "Chin up, it can't be all that bad."
② "I understand that you seem troubled."
③ "You must pull yourself together."
④ "You were doing so well; what happened to you?"

241. A 6 year old is hospitalized for treatment of depression. The nurse would expect which of the following treatment modalities to be used for the child?
① Cognitive therapy
② Insight-oriented psychotherapy
③ Play therapy
④ Work therapy

242. After 3 weeks of treatment in the hospital for major depression, a patient feels much better. She is very appreciative of the nurse's work with her and she wants to call the nurse to have lunch outside the hospital after she is discharged. The nurse's *best response* to the patient's request should be:
① "It would be a pleasure to have lunch with you. When would you like to go?"
② "It would not be appropriate for me to be seen having lunch with a former patient."
③ "Our relationship has been a professional one. It would not be appropriate for me to meet you for lunch."
④ "Perhaps after you have been out of the hospital for a longer period of time, we could consider having lunch together."

243. A patient's husband asks what he can do to reduce the likelihood of his wife being hospitalized for depression in the future. Which of the following will the nurse tell him is the *best* preventive measure?
① Learn the signs and symptoms of the onset of depression
② Keep her busy and distracted from her problems
③ Hire household help so she is not stressed
④ Give unconditional acceptance of her behavior

244. A patient is admitted to a psychiatric facility with a history of depression. He tells the nurse, "I can't eat; I have no appetite." Which of the following responses by the nurse should be *most appropriate?*
① "If you have no appetite, how come you're not underweight?"
② "You have difficulty eating?"
③ "Why do you feel this way?"
④ "Why don't you try eating just a little?"

245. A 34 year old is receiving antidepressant therapy. She tells the nurse that the medication she is receiving makes her mouth dry, and she asks the nurse to get her something to drink. The nurse's *best response* should be to:
    ① Tell her there's juice in the refrigerator and she may feel free to help herself
    ② Remind her that she just had a drink a short time ago
    ③ Get her a cup of water from the fountain
    ④ Tell her that it's important that she not concentrate on the side effects of her medication

246. A recently retired banker is brought to the emergency room by his wife, who reports that he constantly complains that he has nothing to do. He has recently lost weight and is sleeping only 3 or 4 hours each night. The patient is admitted for depression. What would the nurse assess *first?*
    ① Physical appearance
    ② Risk for suicide
    ③ Lack of motivation
    ④ Nutritional status

247. A 20-year-old woman is admitted to the hospital with a diagnosis of major depression. She has suffered multiple losses within a 2-year period and states there is nothing left to be taken from her. The *priority* nursing diagnosis for this patient should be:
    ① Altered nutrition: less than body requirements related to loss of appetite secondary to emotional stress
    ② Ineffective individual coping related to internal conflicts
    ③ Sleep pattern disturbance related to emotional stress
    ④ High risk for violence: self-directed related to feelings of loneliness

248. A young mother has been admitted for treatment of major depression. She believes that she was never a good mother or wife and that she has let her family down. She believes that she is responsible for any bad luck that has come their way. The nurse understands that this patient is experiencing:
    ① Delusions of grandeur
    ② Delusions of persecution
    ③ Delusions of guilt or sin
    ④ Flight of ideas

249. A 57-year-old man is admitted to the unit with a diagnosis of severe depression. His son states that his father always appeared to have poor self-esteem. In planning care for this patient, the nurse knows that poor self-esteem is described as the difference between:
    ① Identity and body image
    ② Role and body image
    ③ Ego ideal and perceived self
    ④ Body image and ego ideal

250. A patient voluntarily admitted himself to a private psychiatric facility for treatment of depression. Three weeks after admission, he decides he wants to leave. Which response by the nurse is *most accurate?*
    ① "You may sign yourself out against medical advice."
    ② "You may appeal for discharge through the court."
    ③ "You're free to leave at any time."
    ④ "You must give 72 hours' written notice."

251. A patient's diagnosis is major depression. Her psychiatrist prescribes the tricyclic antidepressant nortriptyline (Pamelor). In addition to administering the medication on time as ordered, the nurse is able to answer the patient's questions about the side effects she is experiencing. The nurse's teaching plan for this patient should emphasize the need for her to report the following common side effects:
    ① Rash across her face
    ② Constipation
    ③ Sudden, rapid change in mood
    ④ Jitteriness

252. A patient has been brought to the hospital following a suicide gesture in which he ingested a quantity of sleeping pills. After gastric lavage is performed and a complete physical examination is accomplished, the nurse makes an assessment of the patient's suicide gesture. The *most appropriate* question to ask him would be:
    ① "Don't you realize how you will hurt your family if you kill yourself?"
    ② "Do you still want to hurt yourself?"
    ③ "Are you trying to manipulate other people to get your way?"
    ④ "Why are you being such a big baby?"

253. The head nurse informs the nurse that her patient is having suicidal thoughts and instructs the nurse to initiate suicide precautions. The nurse's *first nursing action* should be to:
    ① Apply ambulatory restraints
    ② Begin one-to-one observation
    ③ Place the patient in seclusion
    ④ Remove dangerous possessions

254. When planning care for a suicidal patient, the nurse assists by:
    ① Being aware that most attempts are gestures
    ② Teaching problem-solving strategies to the patient
    ③ Reporting the patient to local authorities
    ④ Asking for the patient's reasons for suicidal thinking

255. A nurse is caring for a patient who was admitted for depression. The nurse should be aware that the patient is most likely to entertain suicidal thoughts when:
    ① In deepest depression
    ② The depression is lifting
    ③ No longer depressed at all
    ④ The depression is controlled by medication

256. A 42-year-old man who recently lost his job has been drinking more than usual. His father was a suicide victim. Now he reports thinking of suicide. The nurse knows that this patient is at which level of risk?
    ① Low
    ② Moderate
    ③ High
    ④ Very high

257. A 62-year-old woman is admitted to the hospital following an unsuccessful suicide attempt. She has been non-responsive to antidepressant medication and is scheduled for electroconvulsive therapy (ECT). Information in the nurse's pretreatment plan should emphasize which of the following?
    ① ECT cures depression
    ② Memory loss is permanent
    ③ On awakening, the patient will be confused
    ④ Depressive symptoms usually disappear after the first treatment

258. A patient is brought to the hospital after threatening to kill herself. She admits to several years of substance abuse and arrests for shoplifting and prostitution. She has healed scars on her wrists and states that she is angry because "my boyfriend dumped me." The nursing diagnosis with *highest priority* for this patient is:
    ① Ineffective individual coping related to poor impulse control
    ② Anxiety related to unstable relationships
    ③ Knowledge deficit related to effects of substance abuse
    ④ Potential for violence: self-directed related to impulsiveness

259. A nurse volunteers on a crisis hot line and receives a call from a man threatening suicide. What question would the nurse ask first?
    ① "How do you plan to kill yourself?"
    ② "When did you decide to commit suicide?"
    ③ "Do you want me to get help?"
    ④ "What has happened to make you want to end your life?"

260. Which one of the following is required at all community mental health centers?
    ① Family therapy programs
    ② Partial hospitalization
    ③ Suicide prevention programs
    ④ Alcohol detoxification

261. All of the statements below indicate that an individual is at some degree of risk for suicide. The nurse knows that the statement that indicates the *highest suicide risk* is:
    ① "I haven't been able to get the education I've wanted. I can't earn the money I need, and my family doesn't appreciate me. Now and then I feel so frustrated I think of suicide."
    ② "Since the death of my husband, life has lost its meaning. I've gotten a large supply of sleeping pills and I will take them tomorrow, which would have been his birthday."
    ③ "My girlfriend is threatening to leave me because I am so jealous. I told her that if she leaves me, I'll kill myself."
    ④ "It takes a real man to kill himself. I don't have that kind of courage right now. If things don't get better, I may just have to find it."

262. A newly admitted patient has been placed on one-to-one observation for suicidal intentions. Which of the following items should the nurse remove from the patient's possession?
    ① Daily newspaper
    ② Hairbrush
    ③ Metal nail file
    ④ Shoes

263. After initial assessment determines that a rape victim did not suffer any life-threatening injuries, which of the following should be the next intervention for the nurse to perform?
    ① Prepare her for a vaginal examination
    ② Give her towels to go and shower
    ③ Inform her of her rights and options
    ④ Photograph her cuts and bruises

264. An 18 year old is brought to the emergency room after having been raped by her date. Her mother asks the nurse for advice in helping her daughter cope with this experience. Which of the following responses by the nurse would be *most appropriate?*
    ① "It is important to help her move on to new and healthy experiences. She will eventually come to better understand her experience."
    ② "A period of counseling or therapy might help her and the family recover more fully."
    ③ "It is sometimes better to let a person work things out by herself."
    ④ "You might anticipate that she will be reluctant to trust males until she resolves her experience."

265. A nurse in the emergency room is assigned to work with a young girl the doctor believes may have been sexually abused. The girl is not communicating with the nurse or the social worker. The nurse suggests giving her some paper and drawing materials. The rationale for this is:
    ① The ER is busy, and the nurse needs to see to other patients at this time
    ② The nurse wants to distract the girl and hopes she will open up and talk
    ③ The nurse is using the drawing materials to bribe the patient to talk
    ④ Children frequently communicate their feelings through their play

266. A 9-year-old boy has entered the hospital following an episode of possible sexual abuse by a close family member. The child is withdrawn and depressed. No one is staying with him. While formulating a plan of care, which of the following would be best to include in the care plan?
    ① Covering the patient with a blanket and sitting quietly with him
    ② Holding the child and rocking in the rocking chair
    ③ Giving the child privacy by leaving him alone
    ④ Insisting on the child describing the incident

267. Special legal consideration is given to the relationship between psychiatric nurses and their patients. This is called:
    ① Privileged communication
    ② Habeas corpus
    ③ Malpractice
    ④ Locus tenens

268. The nurse is caring for a patient scheduled for electroconvulsive therapy (ECT). The patient has expressed concern about the procedure. The nurse knows some patients perceive ECT as:
    ① A form of punishment
    ② A painful experience
    ③ An escape from reality
    ④ Having a potential for electrocuting them to death

269. A severely depressed patient is scheduled for electroconvulsive therapy (ECT). While the nurse is preparing the patient for treatment, the patient asks "How long is this procedure going to take?" The *most appropriate* response by the nurse should be:
    ① "Just a few minutes. You'll be finished before you know it."
    ② "It can take anywhere from a few hours to all day, depending on how things go."
    ③ "Actually it only takes a few seconds."
    ④ "The average treatment time is 15 minutes."

270. A patient's physician is considering electroconvulsive therapy for her. The nurse should expect that the patient has which of the following disorders?
    ① Agonophobia
    ② Severe anxiety
    ③ Severe depression
    ④ Substance dependency

271. A 60-year-old man with a history of depression has just been admitted to the unit. His physician has ordered electroconvulsive therapy. When planning immediate posttreatment care for this patient, the *priority nursing action* would be to:
    ① Assist him to become oriented on awakening
    ② Assure him that memory loss is temporary
    ③ Implement seizure precautions
    ④ Monitor intake and output

272. A nurse is assigned to a patient who has haloperidol (Haldol) 1 mg ordered PO tid. The nurse understands the medication is ordered to:
    ① Reduce psychotic symptoms
    ② Induce sleep
    ③ Decrease hypertension
    ④ Increase alertness

273. Lorazepam (Ativan) is ordered for a patient by his physician. A common central nervous system side effect to Ativan is:
    ① Drowsiness
    ② Dry mouth
    ③ Dizziness
    ④ Urine retention

274. A patient who is a known alcoholic arrives at the local emergency room requesting admission for detoxification. He states he has been drinking daily for at least 2 weeks. The nurse should observe the patient for impending delirium tremens (DTs) and plan to monitor him for which of the following physiologic indications of DTs:
    ① Constricted pupils, subnormal temperature, and bradycardia
    ② Hallucinations, fear, and agitation
    ③ Hypertension, diaphoresis, and elevated temperature
    ④ Hypotension, tachycardia, and diaphoresis

275. The nurse is caring for a chronic alcoholic who is experiencing auditory hallucinations. He admits himself to the hospital for treatment. The nurse realizes that this type of admission is:
    ① Voluntary
    ② Involuntary
    ③ Commitment
    ④ Limited

CHAPTER 5

Comprehensive Examinations

COMPREHENSIVE EXAMINATION ONE: PART 1

1. The patient asks the nurse the purpose of the urine culture. The appropriate response would be:
   ① It is used to test kidney function
   ② The urine is checked for albumin
   ③ Residual urine is measured
   ④ Urine is checked for bacteria

2. In preparing to teach a class on nutrition in a prenatal clinic, the nurse knows it is suggested that the pregnant mother increase her caloric intake by:
   ① 300 calories per day
   ② 500 calories per day
   ③ 800 calories per day
   ④ 1200 calories per day

3. A patient is admitted to the hospital for treatment of cirrhosis of the liver. The nurse who admits the patient tells the nursing assistant that he must be an alcoholic. This is an example of:
   ① A mental set
   ② An ideology
   ③ A halo effect
   ④ A stereotype

4. Several hours after delivery a patient's uterus is firm and lies to the right side of her abdomen. The most likely reason for this uterine position is that the patient's:
   ① Stomach is overdistended
   ② Uterus is returning to a normal position
   ③ Urinary bladder is distended
   ④ Uterus is filling with blood

5. Which of the following techniques is *most* important in preventing infections in the newborn nursery?
   ① Sterilize all baby linen
   ② Use scrub attire for all nursing personnel
   ③ Wash hands before and after each infant contact
   ④ Have individualized newborn equipment

6. The nursing diagnosis that should receive priority for a thought-disordered patient in the emergency room is:
   ① Ineffective individual coping related to disordered thought processes
   ② Anxiety related to perceived environmental threat
   ③ Violence, potential for, related to confusion
   ④ Knowledge deficit related to new onset of illness

7. A 40-year-old female patient is ordered to have a retention catheter inserted before surgery. Which catheter should the nurse select for this procedure?
   ① Straight catheter, 16 to 18 gauge
   ② Foley catheter, 14 to 16 gauge, with a 5 ml balloon
   ③ Foley catheter, 8 to 12 gauge, with a 10 ml balloon
   ④ Coude catheter, 14 to 18 gauge, with a 10 ml balloon

8. Central to the principle of restorative/rehabilitative care in the elderly is:
   ① Establishing priorities based not on the nurses' values but on the older adult's values, which ensures that all nursing care is patient/resident focused
   ② Following organizational policies and procedures and meeting patient/resident expectations strictly according to agency policy
   ③ Requiring that patients/residents perform those tasks directed by nursing
   ④ The health care team having total authority and direction regarding a patient's/resident's care

9. An 87-year-old has recently moved into a nursing home and is feeling depressed. His physician has prescribed amitriptyline hydrochloride (Elavil). An adverse effect of this antidepressant may be:
   ① Diarrhea
   ② Insomnia
   ③ Hypertension
   ④ Urinary retention

10. An infection occurring after the patient enters the hospital is called:
    ① Communicable
    ② Inflammation
    ③ Carrier
    ④ Nosocomial

11. Although lactation will cease within a few days to a week without stimulation of the breast, some physicians still may order which of the following to aid in suppressing lactation?
    ① Ibuprofen (Motrin)
    ② Docusate sodium (Colace)
    ③ Oxytocin (Pitocin)
    ④ Bromocriptine mesylate (Parlodel)

12. The nurse is starting an IV on the patient and needs to calculate the flow rate. The order reads "Give 1000 ml lactated Ringer's over 10 hours." The nurse has on hand an Abbott Macrodrip that delivers 15 gtt/ml. Calculate the flow rate.
    ① 25 gtt/min
    ② 15 gtt/hour
    ③ 15 gtt/min
    ④ 10 gtt/min

13. A patient admitted to the hospital for treatment of cirrhosis of the liver is prescribed large doses of niacin. This patient should be observed for side effects of niacin that include:
   1. Retention of body fluids
   2. Eyelid irritation
   3. Swelling of the tongue
   4. Flushing of the skin

14. During one of her prenatal visits, a patient complains of "heartburn." She claims that it happens every day and she really does not want to eat because of it. The nurse's *best* response should be to advise the patient to:
   1. Eat one large meal in mid-day
   2. Eat frequent, small amounts of foods that are not greasy or fried
   3. Take ½ tsp of sodium bicarbonate in water to relieve the heartburn
   4. Buy an antacid in the drugstore and follow the directions on the label

15. On the morning of a patient's scheduled surgery, the nurse is to administer preoperative medication. Which of the following nursing actions is appropriate after the medication is given?
   1. Change the patient's gown
   2. Give the last preoperative instructions
   3. Have the patient sign the consent form for surgery
   4. Pull up the bed side rails

16. The patient in the long-term care facility is able to ambulate with walker assistance, and her cognitive abilities are intact. Every time the nurse enters the room the patient talks about her flower garden. The patient has refused to participate in individual or group activities since admission. A possible solution may be to:
   1. Force the patient to participate in group activities
   2. Tell the patient that if she doesn't participate in activities, she will not be allowed to have visitors
   3. Suggest that she grow her own flower garden in a designated area of the long-term care facility's outdoor area
   4. Tell the patient that she will have to be content with activities provided by the facility

17. A patient with a depressive disorder is sitting in the dayroom knitting when the nurse approaches her to ask if she would like to talk. When she doesn't respond, the nurse replies, "I'll just sit down with you for a while in case you feel like talking." The nurse is using which of the following techniques when dealing with the patient?
   1. Open-ended questions
   2. Empathetic understanding
   3. Therapeutic use of self
   4. Reflection

18. While checking a patient's fundus, the nurse notes that it is soft (boggy); the nurse's *first* clinical priority is to:
   1. Immediately notify the charge nurse
   2. Check the perineum for vaginal bleeding
   3. Check the patient's blood pressure and pulse rate
   4. Massage the fundus immediately

19. A 32-year-old patient has delusions of persecution involving the CIA and the KGB. Following occupational therapy one day, the patient asks if he can work on his woodburning activities on the unit. The nurse's *primary* consideration in response is:
   1. Encouraging participation in activities
   2. Concern for patient safety
   3. Unit rules on activities
   4. Other patients' response to his privileges

20. The hypertensive patient has diuretics ordered daily and is on a low-sodium diet. The nurse is helping the patient fill out her breakfast menu. Which of the following selections would indicate additional teaching is needed?
   1. Orange juice
   2. Cranberry juice
   3. Grape juice
   4. Tomato juice

21. A 26-year-old schizophrenic is discussing her relations with her estranged husband. She discusses making a complete break and then discusses their future while she laughs and cries throughout the conversation. The nurse recognizes this as:
   1. Apathy
   2. Ambivalence
   3. Paranoia
   4. A simple defense mechanism

22. The nurse knows that an important part of nursing care for a patient with a spinal cord injury is:
   1. The administration of analgesics and antiinflammatories as ordered, application of heat and cold, and the provision of range-of-motion exercises
   2. The maintenance of spinal cord alignment, log rolling, and frequent observations of respiratory and neurologic functioning
   3. Application of heat, administration of analgesics as ordered, use of a back brace, and bed rest
   4. The administration of antiinflammatory and uricosuric agents as prescribed, weight loss if indicated, and provision of patient education

23. A 54-year-old disorganized schizophrenic is walking around complaining of hornets stinging her all over her body. The nurse should note which of the following actions on the plan of care?
   1. Keep the patient away from areas where insects may be present
   2. Discuss with the patient the sensation of stinging hornets
   3. Place medication on sting areas
   4. Frequently assess the skin for integrity

24. Discharge teaching to a patient 6 days after an arterial myocardial infarction will include:
   1. "You may return to your normal level of activities in 1 week."
   2. "Feeling guilt over disease is a normal process."
   3. "You may resume sexual relations in 1 week."
   4. "Having a heart attack will not significantly alter your lifestyle."

25. A skin infection that is characterized by red vesicular lesions often found in children and caused by *Streptococcus* or *Staphyloccus* bacteria is known as:
    1. Infantile eczema
    2. Pediculosis
    3. Urticaria
    4. Impetigo

26. A patient is ordered to take metronidazole (Flagyl) 250 mg tid for 7 days. Which of the following statements made by the patient indicates her understanding about this medication?
    1. "I can discontinue the medication if the symptoms disappear."
    2. "I should not drink alcohol while I'm using this medication."
    3. "It is probably not necessary to treat my sexual partner with this medication."
    4. "I should avoid dairy products, which could cause nausea while using this medication."

27. A patient in early labor is very anxious about the outcome of this pregnancy. She asks the nurse, "Do you think that the baby will be okay?" The nurse should respond appropriately by saying:
    1. "Oh, I wouldn't be too concerned. Your other children are fine."
    2. "I really don't know. I hope so."
    3. "Yes, but I'm sure you're worried. Would you like to talk about what concerns you have?"
    4. "Why would you be concerned? You have a very good physician."

28. A 5-year-old has been exposed to chicken pox while in school today. His mother inquires how long the time frame is from exposure to onset of symptoms. The correct response would be:
    1. 2 to 5 days, sometimes longer
    2. 2 to 3 weeks
    3. 4 to 15 days
    4. 12 to 26 days

29. A 33-year-old is admitted to the hospital with a diagnosis of thrombophlebitis. While assessing the patient, the nurse is aware that the problem of thrombophlebitis most commonly occurs:
    1. In superficial peripheral veins
    2. In deep leg veins
    3. As a result of exercising while pregnant
    4. Only in large arteries

30. The nurse knows that a patient who has an obsessive compulsive disorder has begun to identify her feelings when she states:
    1. "I don't use compulsive activities as often in the hospital."
    2. "I try to involve myself in other activities when obsessive thoughts enter my consciousness."
    3. "I will never have compulsive behavior again."
    4. "Anxiety is so unpredictable that I stay prepared all the time."

31. A 49-year-old is admitted to the hospital for treatment of cirrhosis of the liver. After several days in the hospital, the patient complains of "bugs all over my bed." When completing her charting, how should the nurse best express the patient's behavior?
    1. Seeing "bugs" on her bed
    2. Out of contact with reality
    3. Restless and disoriented; hallucinating
    4. Agitated; auditory hallucination

32. The nurse is gathering information on a patient who has fallen on the sidewalk and injured her left arm. She notes that the patient's left forearm is deformed. There is also a hematoma forming on the medial side of the patient's left jaw. Which of the following pieces of additional data should the nurse immediately notify the physician about?
    1. The absence of a radial pulse on the left
    2. The presence of an abrasion on the left palm
    3. The presence of pain in the patient's knee
    4. The patient has a pulse of 100 beats per minute

33. A patient is admitted to the emergency department with a history of increased seizure activity during the last 48 hours. Nursing diagnoses for a patient with seizures may include, but *need not be* limited to:
    1. Ineffective airway clearance, anxiety, and potential for injury
    2. Altered nutrition, potential for powerlessness, and loss of body control
    3. Constipation related to intestinal mobility, and potential for aspiration
    4. Anxiety as a result of cognitive impairment, functional incontinence, and potential for injury related to cognitive problems

34. If the nurse observes an infant gagging on mucus and becoming cyanotic, she should *first:*
    1. Call the charge nurse
    2. Aspirate the pharynx with a bulb syringe
    3. Raise the baby's head and pat the infant on the back
    4. Give oxygen by positive pressure

35. The nurse prepares to give a drug in the gluteus medius muscle. The nurse uses the landmarks of the greater trochanter, posterior superior iliac spine, and the iliac crest to identify the proper location of the muscle. Which of the following nerves is the nurse trying to avoid injury to by using these landmarks?
    1. Sciatic
    2. Vagal
    3. Trigeminal
    4. Radial

36. A patient has been diagnosed as having congestive heart failure. He can best avoid weight from fluid retention by:
    1. Taking his prescribed diuretic before bedtime
    2. Limiting his salt intake
    3. Reducing all food intake
    4. Following a high-calorie diet and forcing fluids

37. Before administering acyclovir (Zovirax) and metronidazole (Flagyl), the nurse should confirm that:
① The patient's hemoglobin level is above 15 gm/dl
② The patient is not pregnant
③ The patient is not allergic to eggs
④ The patient is able to tolerate a normal diet

38. A major nursing goal for a patient with osteoporosis would be:
① Increasing calcium in her diet
② Prevention of injury
③ Prevention of further bone demineralization
④ Restricting activities

39. When documenting the type of pain in a patient with Buerger's disease, the term that most accurately describes such pain is:
① Claudication
② Intermittent claudication
③ Homans' sign
④ Hyperemia

40. To appropriately teach prenatal patients good health behaviors, it is important for the nurse to know that the fetus is most susceptible to malformation from teratogens during the:
① First trimester
② Second trimester
③ Third trimester
④ Last half of pregnancy

41. The drug that the nurse would most likely administer in the emergency room to a patient with a thought disorder is a(n):
① MAO inhibitor
② Tricyclic antidepressant
③ Hypnotic
④ Antipsychotic

42. The nurse decides to instruct a patient, diagnosed with active genital herpes, on safe sex practices. Which of the following instructions indicate that the patient understands the nurse's teaching?
① "Condoms need only be worn when the lesions are present."
② "I should not have sex at all if the lesions are present."
③ "The use of a diaphragm will help prevent the transmission of herpes."
④ "There is no relationship between genital herpes and an increased risk of cervical cancer."

43. Patient education is an important aspect of patient care, and the nurse must remember to:
① Have answers to anticipated questions written out so she can read them to the patient
② Involve the patient in decision making concerning her care
③ Identify community resources available to the patient
④ Encourage involvement of family and significant others

44. A patient has a large abdominal dressing and a closed-suction drain following an anterior repair of the bladder. During the first evening after surgery, the nurse notes a 2-cm spot of blood on the abdominal dressing. What should her next action be?
① Notify the team leader or physician immediately
② Remove the dressing and inspect the wound
③ Reinforce the dressing with a sterile ABD pad
④ Mark the spot and assess the dressing for further bleeding

45. A newly admitted patient has a history of multiple sclerosis. Signs and symptoms of multiple sclerosis are:
① Impaired chewing and eating, excessive sweating, and tremors
② Aphasia, syncope, and seizures
③ Blurred vision, dysphasia, and ataxia
④ Splenomegaly, hepatomegaly, and elevated white blood cell count

46. A 20-year-old enters an outpatient clinic in an agitated state. He reports that his best friend has been diagnosed as HIV positive. The nurse knows that AIDS is best described as:
① A disease of the immune system
② A chronic and incurable disease that is multicausal in origin
③ A neoplastic immunodeficiency disease
④ An inflammatory skin response to certain allergenic offenders

47. The psychiatrist in the emergency room decides that a patient needs to be admitted to the hospital. She refuses to sign herself in, saying "it is a plot by the aliens." Her parents ask what the possible options are in this situation. Which is the *best* answer for the nurse to give?
① She can be sent home with her roommate because she does not want to stay in the hospital
② Her parents can sign her out of the hospital if they are willing to take responsibility for her safety
③ She will be kept in the emergency room under nursing supervision until she feels better
④ She can be involuntarily committed to the hospital if the physician judges that she is a danger to herself or others

48. A long-time alcoholic is going home on a weekend pass. His physician has ordered disulfiram (Antabuse A). Which statement made by the patient shows understanding regarding his medication?
① "I can drink, but if my blood alcohol level gets above 0.1, then I will be ill."
② "The Antabuse will keep me from wanting a drink and I can more effectively participate in AA and other therapy."
③ "I should not take any over-the-counter cough syrups."
④ "The Antabuse will alter my metabolism so the alcohol will have no effect on my system."

49. A patient is being discharged from the hospital with three new medications. A teaching plan for administering medications will include the following priority information:
    1. Take the medications whenever she thinks about it, call the doctor only if she experiences an allergic reaction, and double up on medications if she forgets to take the medications
    2. Take the medications as prescribed, do not take with food, and take with the smallest amount of water necessary to swallow the medications
    3. She may share her medications in order to help other people, and it's not important to know the names of the medications; just take the medications at the right time of day
    4. The trade/generic drug name, time of drug administration, how much drug to take, and what actions to take if side effects occur

50. When educating a patient with a pneumothorax, the nurse explains that the purpose of the chest tube is to:
    1. Instill antibiotics
    2. Drain secretions
    3. Remove blood
    4. Remove air

51. A mother brings her 1-month-old son to a well-baby clinic. Which of the following developmental achievements is normal for this infant?
    1. Smiling and laughing out loud
    2. Rolling from his back to his side
    3. Holding a rattle for a short period of time
    4. Turning his head from side to side

52. The nurse knows that physiologic jaundice, which is often seen on or about the infant's third day of life, indicates:
    1. An incompatibility of the mother's and infant's blood
    2. Damage to the infant's liver
    3. Destruction of the excessive number of red blood cells present at birth
    4. Improper care of the infant at birth

53. As the nurse is preparing to give the preoperative medication, her patient states, "I'm afraid of the anesthesia, going to sleep and maybe having trouble waking up, or getting sick." What is the *best* response by the nurse?
    1. "Tell me more about this worry."
    2. "There is nothing to be afraid of, this is done every day."
    3. "You have an excellent anesthesiologist. He'll take good care of you."
    4. "I'll call your physician."

54. A patient who is 5 months' pregnant has some problems with constipation. The nurse would teach her that she could decrease constipation by:
    1. Eating an adequate diet that includes fluids, fresh fruits and vegetables, and fiber
    2. Administering a Fleet enema when necessary
    3. Maintaining good posture while standing and working
    4. Using a glycerine suppository as necessary

55. While making rounds, the nurse notices that the Salem Sump is not draining into the suction apparatus properly for a new postoperative patient. The nurse should perform which of the following measures?
    1. Irrigate the blue pigtail with air
    2. Irrigate the blue pigtail with water
    3. Disconnect the suction and irrigate with air through the tube
    4. Disconnect the suction and irrigate with water through the tube

56. A 72 year old has been admitted to the hospital with symptoms that include rapid, shallow, dyspneic respirations. He has been diagnosed as having congestive heart failure. What cardiac drug would the nurse expect to be ordered for this patient?
    1. Inderal
    2. Aspirin
    3. Lanoxin
    4. Atropine

57. A mother brings her 4-month-old healthy infant to a well-baby clinic. What would the nurse *not* expect the infant to be demonstrating at 4 months of age?
    1. Responding to pleasure with smiles
    2. Grasping a rattle
    3. Sitting up without support
    4. Turning himself from his side to his back

58. A patient in a psychiatric unit is a substance abuser and has been avoiding talking about his abuse of chemicals. He says, "I am just bored," or "I can get along fine," or he makes similar statements when asked about his use of chemicals. The nurse recognizes that:
    1. He is attempting to manipulate her into not confronting him
    2. Denial is a common defense mechanism for substance abusers
    3. Strict limits on activities may be needed so he will communicate more effectively
    4. Alteration of this patient's reward system may be needed to get him to verbalize his feelings

59. A patient tells the nurse that he will be the most popular patient in the unit once everyone gets to know him. The nurse responds, "It sounds like you are concerned with how others feel about you." The technique the nurse used is:
    1. Seeking clarification
    2. Encouraging comparisons
    3. Summarizing
    4. Focusing

60. A patient is exhibiting signs of anxiety and apprehension because of the diagnosis of essential hypertension. The best nursing intervention is to:
    1. Teach the patient about hypertension
    2. Let the patient express her feelings
    3. Explain that everybody has the same feelings
    4. Avoid the subject of her disease

61. An 18-year-old comes to the health clinic complaining of "blisters" on her perineal area and difficulty voiding. The physician diagnoses active genital herpes and *Trichomonas vaginalis*. The patient is ordered to take acyclovir (Zovirax) 200 mg, five times per day. What instructions should the nurse give the patient about this medication?
    ① This medication is the only cure for genital herpes
    ② The patient should decrease her fluid intake because voiding will irritate her lesions
    ③ The lesions should resolve in 2 to 6 weeks
    ④ No showers or tub baths should be taken while the lesions are present

62. A patient returns from bladder surgery with a Foley catheter. What is the *best* procedure in caring for his catheter?
    ① Extra tubing should be coiled to prevent urinary stasis
    ② For sanitary reasons, the drainage bag should be disconnected and the urine drained in the bathroom
    ③ The drainage bag should be attached to the bed at a level lower than the bladder
    ④ The catheter should be taped to the patient's thigh for comfort

63. A patient was receiving an antibiotic supplied in 50-mg capsules. How many capsules should be given per dose if 0.2 g PO is ordered daily in four divided doses?
    ① ½
    ② 1
    ③ 2½
    ④ 4

64. A 4-month-old is seen at a local clinic because of severe diarrhea. Because of the diarrhea, she presents signs and symptoms of dehydration that include:
    ① Slow, labored breathing; bulging anterior fontanel; glassy eyes; and low-grade fever
    ② Rapid, shallow breathing; depressed anterior fontanel; hollow eyes; and high fever
    ③ Failure to gain weight, delayed motor activities, and inadequate growth weight
    ④ Anemia, listlessness, and an appearance of malnourishment

65. A patient who is recovering from bladder surgery is ordered promethazine (Phenergan) 50 mg intramuscularly for nausea. What is the best method for administering this medication?
    ① The ventrogluteal site should be chosen for the injection
    ② Hold the syringe at a 45-degree angle
    ③ Mark the site for the injection with an index finger
    ④ Use a ⅝ inch needle for greater patient comfort

66. To promote measures directed at reversing inappropriate health behaviors in the patient, the nurse should:
    ① Inform the patient that unhealthy behaviors can harm other people
    ② Ask the patient to explain why she still engages in this unhealthy practice
    ③ Supply the patient with educational materials aimed at reducing the unhealthy practice
    ④ Realize that the patient may resist changing a behavior that has become a habit

67. An 8-month-old is brought to the clinic because he has had diarrhea for the past 24 hours. Potential causes for his *acute* diarrhea could include:
    ① Cystic fibrosis, celiac disease, or carcinoid tumors
    ② Parasites, protein-calorie malnutrition, or chronic pancreatitis
    ③ Irritable colon syndrome, hyperthyroidism, or immune deficiencies
    ④ Changes in formula, milk protein intolerance, or URI (upper respiratory tract infection–otitis media)

68. A 13-year-old comes to the school health office to see the nurse and tells her that she has some questions about "being a woman." She also states that she cannot talk about this with her mother because her mother doesn't understand her. Which of the following statements about early adolescent development helps the nurse understand the child's statement?
    ① The child is developing a disrespectful attitude toward her mother
    ② Young adolescents sometimes normally reject parental efforts at guidance
    ③ Seeking independence from the family is normally a task of late adolescence
    ④ Professional therapy is often needed at this age to control the adolescent child

69. A 2-year-old is brought into the clinic for a well-baby check-up. The child's physical growth would be expected to show:
    ① A decrease in rate of growth, but an increase in rate of development
    ② A gain of less than 5 lb and less than an inch in height each year
    ③ An increase in rate of growth and a decrease in rate of development
    ④ A rapid language development, and talking to himself and other people

70. A patient weighs 260 lbs and is 6 ft tall. On the third postoperative day, which of the following signs would indicate a postoperative complication?
    ① The catheter is draining very light yellow urine
    ② The patient requests medication for incisional pain
    ③ The dressing becomes damp with serosanguineous drainage
    ④ The patient complains about his full-liquid diet

71. The physician orders a patient to have an IV of 5% dextrose in lactated Ringer's solution. The IV is to run at 125 ml/hr. The IV tubing has a ratio of 15 gtt/ml. An infusion pump is not currently available, so the IV will run by gravity. The IV should be running at how many gtt per minute?
    ① 15 gtt/min
    ② 25 gtt/min
    ③ 31 gtt/min
    ④ 46 gtt/min

72. Two days postoperatively a patient begins to cough and tells the nurse, "I just felt something 'give way' under this bandage." What *appropriate* action should the nurse take next?
    ① Ask the patient why he coughed so hard
    ② Check the incision
    ③ Reassure the patient that he is okay
    ④ Obtain the ordered pain medication for the patient

73. The newborn's movements are jerky and uncoordinated. The nurse understands that this is a result of:
① A warm, comfortable environment
② An immature nervous system
③ No muscle tone
④ Injuries received during birth

74. A 14 year old is wearing clothes in the newest fashion, with her hair stylishly combed. She states that looking attractive at school is very important to her. What understanding of adolescent development should the nurse have before responding to the 14-year-old?
① She is unduly influenced by peer pressure at this age
② She is behaving in a narcissistic manner
③ Peer responses are normally important to early adolescents
④ Promiscuous tendencies are evident in the child's attitude

75. A 13 month old is admitted to the hospital with a fracture of the right femur. She is accompanied by both parents, each of whom provides a different story. Child abuse is suspected. The nurse should be alert to which of the following that may indicate abuse?
① Thumb-sucking
② Underdevelopment for her age
③ Interacting well with others
④ Eating well without urging

76. Before bathing a 5-year-old child, the nurse suggests to his mother that she step out to have coffee and stretch during the boy's morning care. On seeing his mother leave the room, the child begins to cry and ask for her repeatedly. The nurse should offer assurance to him, knowing that he is likely experiencing:
① Temper tantrum
② Loss of self-image
③ Separation anxiety
④ Dependent coping mode

77. A new mother brings her 5-month-old infant into the well-baby clinic. The infant appears healthy, and the mother asks when she should wean him from breast feeding. The nurse should inform her that he will show readiness to be weaned when he is:
① Sleeping through the night
② Taking solid foods well
③ Eating on a regular schedule
④ Around 6 months of age

78. A 13 year old tells the school nurse that her menses began 6 months ago but that her periods are irregular. What advice can the nurse *appropriately* give the adolescent?
① For the first year or so after menses begins, periods are commonly irregular
② Something may be wrong; it is best to schedule an appointment with a physician
③ She should not worry so much about menses; nature and time take care of minor problems
④ She should ask her mother for advice

79. Three characteristic behaviors an active 2 year old may exhibit are:
① Display of negativism, ritualism, and temper tantrums
② Display of stranger anxiety, cries easily, laughs easily
③ Reaction to adult anger, has definite social attachments, and presents imitative and repetitive speech
④ Development of imagination, acute awareness of sexuality, and learning through play

80. A postpartum patient complains to the nurse, "My stitches really hurt." Which action would be most appropriate for the nurse to take *first?*
① Medicate for pain
② Examine the perineum
③ Apply a heat lamp
④ Notify the nurse in charge

81. An 85-year-old patient with a stroke has an order for turning q2h. When the nurse goes into the room to turn her, the family refuses and states that she has "had enough" and that she needs to rest. The nurse should:
① Call for assistance and turn the patient; instruct the family that physician orders must be followed
② Wait an hour or so and hope the family members will change their mind; if not, insist that the patient be turned
③ Explain that it is the physician's order and it must be continued; family members will need to speak to the physician on his next rounds
④ Explain the importance of turning to the family and arrange for the patient to rest uninterrupted for the next 2 hours

82. The nurse observes a patient's IV for signs of possible infiltration. Which of the following descriptions most likely indicates that the IV is infiltrated?
① Blood backflows into the tubing when the IV bag is lowered
② The IV appears to be dripping too slowly
③ The skin around the infusion site is cool to touch and slightly swollen
④ The connection between the IV catheter and the tubing is leaking

83. The nurse is preparing to administer the varicella vaccine subcutaneously. She cleans the site with alcohol and inserts the needle at a 45-degree angle. The rationale for inserting the needle at this angle is:
① The medication is beneath the epidermis
② To prevent injection into the muscle
③ To prevent blood from tracking back
④ To prevent the vaccine from tracking back

84. An 18-year-old male patient has second-degree burns over 85% on the entire posterior aspects of his body to the mid-axilla on each side. He was admitted to the step-down unit from ICU and is complaining of severe pain and requests medication. The physician has ordered meperidine (Demerol) and hydroxyzine (Vistaril) intramuscularly for his pain. The nurse should use which site for the injection?
① Deltoid
② Dorsogluteal
③ Ventrogluteal
④ Vastus lateralis

85. A 4 year old has been exposed to chicken pox while in daycare. The nurse knows that clinical signs and symptoms should include:
   ① Severe cold with high temperature, nasal congestion, cough, and conjunctivitis
   ② Headache, stiff neck, malaise, sore throat, and coryza
   ③ Slight fever, anorexia, and malaise
   ④ Low-grade fever, malaise, edema, and pain in salivary glands

86. In preparing a patient for testing related to Buerger's disease, the nurse explains that the three diagnostic tests are Doppler ultrasonography, arteriography, and:
   ① Echocardiography
   ② Stress test
   ③ Electrocardiography
   ④ Oscillometry

87. A 32 year old is admitted to the hospital with a fractured hip. Appropriate nursing diagnoses would include:
   ① Anxiety, knowledge deficit, and potential for injury
   ② Sleep pattern disturbance, activity intolerance, and altered thought processes
   ③ Pain, impaired physical mobility, and altered peripheral tissue perfusion
   ④ Knowledge deficit, alteration in self-concept, and impaired physical mobility

88. A 55-year-old patient who is a heavy smoker and is obese is admitted with the diagnosis of Buerger's disease. When assessing the patient for symptoms typical of Buerger's disease, the nurse should observe for:
   ① Leg pain at rest (not associated with activity)
   ② Redness and pain along a vein pathway
   ③ Dilated veins and ankle edema
   ④ A positive Homans' sign

89. A 2 year old has been exposed to chicken pox while in daycare today. If she develops varicella, which of the following patient teachings should the nurse offer the child's mother?
   ① Keep her in bed; photophobia is common, so keep window shades down and lights dim
   ② Keep her isolated; relieve her discomfort with Tylenol; avoid giving her spicy or sour foods
   ③ Keep her hospitalized and isolated; avoid sudden noises
   ④ Keep her in strict isolation at home until crusts form

90. A 71-year-old woman uses timolol (Timoptic) for glaucoma at home. While visiting her on a home visit, the nurse observes that the patient's apical pulse rate is 50 beats/min. What action should be taken?
   ① Contact the patient's physician and discuss her heart rate and parameters for continuation of the medicine
   ② Instruct the patient to continue the drug as prescribed and continue to monitor the heart rate
   ③ Tell the patient to stop taking the drug and to discuss it with her physician during her next weekly appointment
   ④ Tell the patient to stop taking the drug, then reassess her pulse rate the next day

91. A postpartum patient asks the nurse when she may resume sexual intercourse. The nurse responds that it is a common practice to recommend that sexual intercourse be avoided after delivery for a period of approximately:
   ① 2 weeks
   ② 4 weeks
   ③ 6 weeks
   ④ 12 weeks

92. When caring for a 2 year old, the nurse should be aware that the most common accidents for a child this age involve:
   ① Falls, drownings, and suffocations
   ② Suffocations, burns, and falls
   ③ Foreign body aspiration, injury from toys, and burns
   ④ Falls, lacerations, and abrasions

93. Quality indicators have become very important in nursing care. What is the main purpose for quality indicators?
   ① Provide for good patient care
   ② Set standards for reimbursement
   ③ Address financial loss
   ④ Focus on infections and causes

94. Triazolam (Halcion) 0.25 mg is ordered qhs for rest. Available are 0.125 mg tablets. How many scored tablets should be given?
   ① ½ tablet
   ② 2 tablets
   ③ 2½ tablets
   ④ 4 tablets

95. The newborn's skin is bright red following delivery because of:
   ① Irritation during delivery
   ② Large amounts of pigment that are characteristic of all newborns
   ③ Anemia, which is common in newborns
   ④ The large number of red blood cells present in the infant's blood

96. A culture reveals the presence of *Escherichia coli* (*E. coli*) and *Candida* in a patient's urine. What is the most likely cause of the presence of the *Candida* organism?
   ① Increased intake of yogurt with an active culture
   ② Multiple uses of antibiotics
   ③ Use of deodorant soaps
   ④ Use of scented toilet paper

97. A new mother tells the nurse that she is really disappointed now that she can't breast-feed her daughter because of a cesarean delivery. The nurse's *best* response should be:
   ① "You can still breast-feed your baby. We will help you do this."
   ② "Yes, it is more difficult to breast-feed if you have had a cesarean section."
   ③ "Some mothers do and some don't. It depends on how you feel about it."
   ④ "You are going to need time to recover. It might be best if you thought of yourself first."

98. A patient says that she is frightened of aliens. The *best* response by the nurse should be:
① "I don't see anything like that."
② "Where do you see them, exactly?"
③ "I understand that you are feeling afraid."
④ "Don't worry, you'll feel better soon."

99. The nurse has an order for acetaminophin (Tylenol) chewable tablets, two PO q4h for T >101° F (38.3° C) for a pediatric patient. The nurse assistant reports a rectal temperature of 39.2° C. The nurse would proceed with which of the following?
① Give two Tylenol tablets
② Give one Tylenol tablet
③ Do not give any Tylenol tablets
④ Check the temperature orally first

100. In prenatal clinics, the nurse is responsible for teaching patients the danger signals of pregnancy. Which of the following symptoms is *not* considered a danger signal of pregnancy?
① Excessive swelling of the feet
② Persistent vomiting
③ Increased vaginal discharge
④ Persistent headaches

101. Methenamine (Urex) 1 g qid is prescribed for a patient with a urinary tract infection. Which of the following statements by the patient indicates an understanding of the instructions given by the nurse about this medication?
① "I will expect my urine to be a red-orange color from the medication."
② "I should reduce the amount of fluids I take so that the medication will remain in my bladder longer."
③ "My urine may appear pink or slightly bloody as a result of the cleansing action of this medication."
④ "My urine will have a blue or blue-green coloration."

102. During preparations for discharge a patient's daughter voices concern over use of the wrist restraints and posey vest. The nurse should instruct the daughter to:
① Use the restraints only at night
② Loosen the posey vest and turn the patient every 6 to 8 hours
③ Release the restraints every few hours, checking circulation to the hands
④ Release the restraints q2h or more often and check circulation to the hands

103. A 44 year old is admitted to the gynecology unit for an exploratory laparotomy and possible abdominal hysterectomy. The patient brings her laboratory workup with her. The nurse notes that her potassium level is 3.0 mEq/L. What action should the nurse take?
① Notify the team leader or physician
② Tape the laboratory results on the patient chart
③ There is no needed action
④ Give the patient a drink of orange juice

104. A patient has a physician's order to increase fluids to 2880 ml q24h. How many 8-oz glasses of liquid can she have over a period of 24 hours?
① 10
② 12
③ 16
④ 21

105. A 20 year old, who is completely incoherent, is admitted to the emergency room. Her roommate asks the nurse whether she should contact the patient's parents to come to the hospital. The nurse's best response would be:
① "It's better for them not to see her when she is so confused."
② "Please call them; perhaps they can give us some helpful information."
③ "No; she is an adult and is responsible for her own care."
④ "No; that would violate her confidentiality."

106. Which of the following should the nurse be sure is done before a scheduled gallbladder series?
① An IV should be started the evening before the test
② The upper abdominal area should be prepped and shaved
③ The patient should be NPO after the evening meal
④ A low-fat, high-carbohydrate breakfast should be given before the test

107. A 13 year old asks the nurse if soaking in a tub bath is "okay" during menses because she heard that water could be harmful at that time. What would be the *best* response by the nurse?
① "It is always better to take a shower during menses rather than a tub bath."
② "Tub bathing, as well as showering, is a good hygiene practice during menses."
③ "Immersion in water is not safe during menses."
④ "It's best to take a sponge bath during menses to avoid contamination of the perineal area."

108. During the evening shift a patient asks the nurse for assistance with writing a living will. The nurse recognizes which of the following as the primary purpose of a living will?
① It provides that the family may make all decisions regarding the patient's health care when the patient is no longer able to decide for himself or herself
② It provides for the distribution of all the patient's material possessions
③ It states exactly what measures are to be taken to save the patient's life
④ It provides that extraordinary measures not be taken to save a patient's life if he or she becomes terminally ill

109. A 50 year old was involved in a motor vehicle accident. During the accident, the buckle on the seatbelt caused a blunt injury to his bladder. Following an anterior repair of his bladder, the patient is admitted to the surgical unit. During the transfer of the patient from the operating room to his bed, he complains of nausea and begins vomiting. Which of the following should be the *first* nursing action?
① Obtain the antiemetic medication as ordered
② Turn his head to the side
③ Quickly place him on the bed
④ Notify the team leader or physician

110. The physician orders nitroglycerin ointment for his patient to prevent any further chest pain. Soon after applying the ointment to the patient, the nurse begins to have heart palpitations and feels faint. After noticing the ointment on her hands, the nurse realizes that she is probably experiencing:
① A local effect
② A systemic effect
③ An additive effect
④ A teratogenic effect

111. Approximately 1 year ago a 50 year old was diagnosed as having ovarian cancer with distant metastases (stage IV). Since her initial diagnosis, she has undergone chemotherapy and radiation therapy. She is now admitted to the hospital with respiratory distress. What should the *priority* nursing action be upon admission of this patient to the hospital?
① Resumption of her physician-ordered chemotherapy
② Pain relief
③ Assistance with breathing
④ Orienting her to the unit and her room

112. Factors the nurse should consider when assessing an older adult's restorative/rehabilitative abilities are:
① Appropriate available resources, time constraints of the nurse, preferences of significant others, and ability to understand the importance of rehabilitation
② Level of consciousness, cognitive and emotional status, developmental stage, functional status, knowledge, physiologic status, health status, nutritional status, and attitude
③ Available space, adequate ventilation, adequate lighting, appropriate room temperature, and the presence of pets
④ Presence of an illness, level of energy, ability to perform manual tasks, and type of dwelling the individual lives in

113. During the evening visiting hours, the family remains out in the hall across from a patient's room. The nurse hears the family arguing, "This is your fault; you didn't take care of her well enough," "No, this is your fault, you are only concerned with yourself." The family continues bickering for 10 minutes before entering the patient's room. What would be an appropriate nursing diagnosis for this family?
① Anxiety related to the patient's medical diagnosis
② Hopelessness related to patient illness
③ Altered family processes related to inadequate coping behaviors
④ Social isolation as a result of many hospital visits and length of the patient's illness

114. In planning care for a patient with a diagnosis of thrombophlebitis, the nurse should include which of the following measures?
① Notify physical therapy that the patient will need exercises several times a day
② Observe for the symptoms of pulmonary embolism
③ Reduce fluid intake in order to reduce the circulatory volume
④ Keep the affected leg completely flat in bed

115. After a patient is admitted to the inpatient psychiatric unit, she asks if she can keep her personal belongings. What is the *best* response for the nurse to make?
① "Of course you can. This is not a prison."
② "Of course not; this is a psychiatric unit."
③ "You will be allowed to keep anything that is not harmful to you or anyone else."
④ "Everything will be sent home with your family to keep until your thinking is clearer."

116. A patient is admitted following an attempted suicide. In planning suicide precautions for this patient, the nurse should include:
① Providing occupational therapy to keep her active and to keep her thoughts away from suicide
② Sedation when the patient shows agitation and anxiety
③ Limiting her activities to her room or to strictly supervised activities
④ Walks and outdoor activities to promote physical fitness

117. A 28 year old reports to the urology clinic with a history of repeated urinary tract infections (UTIs). She states that she has had these many times before and has taken "lots of antibiotics." She believes she currently has another infection. While assessing the patient, which of the following symptoms would the nurse expect her to report?
① Feeling faint or dizzy while in the bathroom
② Inability to void when away from home
③ A "burning" sensation when voiding
④ Unusual thirst

118. The nurse is to administer morphine sulfate to the patient. What should the nurse assess first before administering the medication?
① The pain level
② The blood pressure
③ The pulse
④ The respiratory rate

119. A 2-day postpartum patient has been crying most of the evening. The nurse notes a decrease in her verbalizations and less eye contact than before. The *most appropriate* nursing action should be to:
① Avoid any discussion of what is bothering her
② Question her concerning mental illness history
③ Tell her to discuss this with her physician, enabling him to order tranquilizers
④ Offer support and try to discover her concern through therapeutic communication

120. A 26 year old was brought to the emergency room by her roommate after she stayed up all night telephoning the police to report that she was being spied on by aliens who had taken over their town. The idea that aliens are spying on her is an example of:
① Loose association
② Autistic thinking
③ Persecutory delusion
④ Conversion reaction

121. Several evenings before a patient's death, she confides to the nurse, "I just keep on hoping that someone will find a cure for this so I can continue to raise my family." What should be an appropriate response by the nurse?
    ① "I'll keep praying for you. There must be a cure somewhere."
    ② "I'll try to do everything I can to help you and keep you comfortable."
    ③ "I just read an article in a nursing journal about all the work being done at another hospital. I'll see what I can find out."
    ④ "Try to have more peace of mind with what you have accomplished."

122. To provide effective intervention for the most serious side effects of antipsychotic medications, the nurse should:
    ① Recommend high-calorie snacks between activities
    ② Administer antiparkinsonian drugs as ordered
    ③ Restrict potassium intake at meals and snacks
    ④ Provide extra exercise periods as requested by the patient

123. A patient has a diagnosis of ovarian cancer and has undergone chemotherapy and radiation therapy. Two days after her admission with respiratory distress, the patient is able to breathe without a great deal of difficulty. While assisting her with morning care, the nurse notes that she is very quiet, difficult to engage in any conversation, and seems "lost in her thoughts." The nurse recognizes this as part of the grief process. The patient seems to be in which stage of the grief process?
    ① Denial
    ② Anger
    ③ Bargaining
    ④ Depression

124. In providing nursing care for a patient with Buerger's disease, the nurse should stress:
    ① Restricting salt and eggs in the diet
    ② Substituting margarine for butter
    ③ Wearing cotton socks and gloves
    ④ Avoiding smoking and cold temperatures

125. A patient has been diagnosed with placenta previa. Considering the diagnosis, the nurse expects to find the patient complaining of which of the following?
    ① Abdominal pain
    ② Painless vaginal bleeding
    ③ Uterine tenderness
    ④ Tetanic contractions

COMPREHENSIVE EXAMINATION ONE: PART 2

126. An important part of the care of the family of an infant who has died of SIDS includes which of the following?
    ① Preparing the family for an autopsy of the infant
    ② Preparing the family for genetic testing
    ③ Refering the family to hospice care
    ④ Preparing the family to undergo blood tests

127. Nursing interventions following the application of a cast include:
    ① Helping the drying process by using a heat lamp positioned 24 inches away
    ② Handling cast with the fingertips rather than the flat part of the hand
    ③ Making a "window" to ensure the relief of pressure
    ④ Keeping the cast exposed to air

128. Which of the following precautions reflects an understanding of the methods of transmission of the AIDS virus?
    ① Precautions are limited to individuals with respiratory problems
    ② Necessary precautions should be taken with any patient known to be HIV positive
    ③ Precautions should be used with all patients, assuming that they could be HIV positive
    ④ Only needle and blood precautions are necessary

129. An HIV-positive patient shows the nurse two reddish-purple bumps on the top of his mouth. This finding is most probably which opportunistic infection associated with immunosuppression?
    ① Tuberculosis
    ② Herpes simplex
    ③ Kaposi's sarcoma
    ④ *Pneumocystis carinii*

130. A 36-year-old man has a history of difficulty with personal relationships; he does not grow or learn from experience or punishment; he has no real loyalties to any person, group, or code; and he has a tendency to rationalize behavior. In planning care for this patient, the nurse recognizes that these actions are characteristic of which type of personality disorder?
    ① Abusive personality
    ② Paranoid personality
    ③ Borderline personality
    ④ Antisocial personality

131. Recent modern developments in the treatment of mental illness include:
    ① Gradual re-entry of patients back into their homes, enabling certain change in society's attitudes, discovery of tranquilizing drugs, and development of support systems
    ② Mistreatment and banishment from the community as a result of the individual being possessed by supernatural spirits and forces
    ③ Deinstitutionalization, concept of humors, isolation from society, mistreatment, and major change in attitude of society
    ④ Returning patients to their homes as quickly as possible, development of support systems, and discovery of tranquilizing drugs

132. Which of the following would be the best nursing intervention for a patient having difficulty sleeping?
    ① Encourage the patient to take sleeping medication as needed
    ② Instruct the patient on relaxation techniques
    ③ Encourage the patient to do strenuous exercise every evening
    ④ Encourage the patient to drink warm milk before bedtime

133. Appropriate nursing interventions for the patient in skeletal traction include:
① Restricting movement and turning until the pin is removed
② Releasing traction weights q8h
③ Manipulating slipped pins back into place
④ Ensuring that the weights hang freely

134. A 16-year-old male has just been diagnosed as having insulin-dependent diabetes mellitus. If the patient receives NPH insulin at 7 AM, when would he be most likely to have a hypoglycemic reaction?
① 8 AM to 11 AM
② 12 noon to 3 PM
③ 11 AM to 7 PM
④ 12 midnight to 4 AM

135. Which of the following actions should the nurse initiate if she suspects that a child's condition may be the result of an abusive situation?
① Ask the mother to go to the waiting room
② Undress the child and help her into a hospital gown
③ Send for any of the child's old medical records and x-ray studies
④ Call the hospital business office for a bill estimate to give to the mother

136. When performing range of motion on the patient, the nurse bends the patient's wrist so the fingers are pointing toward the antecubital area. The bending motion is known as:
① Hyperextension
② Extension
③ Flexion
④ Supination

137. An antibiotic, ordered for a pediatric patient, is dispensed in liquid form. The label reads 125 mg/5 ml. The physician orders 150 mg q6h. How many ml would the nurse give for each dose?
① 0.5 ml
② 5 ml
③ 6 ml
④ 10 ml

138. A mother calls about her child's appointment to receive her 15-month measles, mumps, and rubella immunization (MMR). The child is coughing, running a fever of 102° F (38.8° C), and vomiting. The nurse should instruct the mother to:
① Keep the appointment and let the physician decide about administering the injection
② Give the child two baby aspirins and report for the injection at the appropriate time
③ Skip the injection; because of the illness, she will not be able to receive the vaccine at 15 months
④ See the physician for the increased temperature and reschedule the MMR

139. Teaching the mother of a child being discharged on antibiotic therapy should include giving the antibiotic:
① Until the child feels better
② Only while the child is awake
③ Until all the medication has been taken
④ Until the fever remains below 99° F (37.2° C) for 2 days

140. Following application of a plaster cast for a fractured radius and ulna, the nurse evaluates which of the following?
① Patient's respiratory rate
② Color, movement, and sensation of the fingers
③ Range of motion of the fingers
④ Patient's ability to sign her discharge instruction form

141. While a patient is in surgery for an appendectomy, the nurse plans for her postoperative recovery and gets her room ready. Because the patient has active tuberculosis and she will need to do deep breathing and coughing exercises following surgery, what type of precautions should the nurse be prepared to take?
① Isolation; the nurse need only wear a mask, carefully washing her hands after providing care
② Isolation; the nurse must wear a mask, gown, and gloves while providing care
③ Isolation is not necessary; the patient must wear a mask while in the hospital
④ No specific precautions are needed, only good hygiene by both the patient and nurse

142. A patient with a colostomy is afraid to have the nurse clean around his stoma during routine change of his dressing and appliance. He states that, if the stoma is touched, it will hurt too much. Which of the following statements by the nurse is most appropriate?
① "The stoma and the area around it must be cleaned. I'll be as gentle as possible to avoid causing you pain when I touch the stoma."
② "This is something that you'll have to get used to for the next several months. I'll be careful."
③ "I'll be as gentle as possible. You should also know that the stoma has no pain receptors."
④ "I'm trying very hard to do this correctly. Please tell me if I hurt you."

143. A call is placed to a clinic by a mother who says her 16-year-old daughter has a boyfriend who has mononucleosis. When asked the symptoms of this condition, the nurse should indicate which of the following?
① Chronic infections, urinary tract infections, pneumonia, weight loss, and hepatosplenomegaly
② Fatigue, enlarged lymph nodes, fever and sore throat, and stiff neck
③ Polyphagia, polyuria, fatigability, and polydipsia
④ Changes in behavior patterns, poor academic performance, and wearing long-sleeved shirts

144. When the nurse takes the initiative for making an independent decision about her patient's care, it is known in nursing practice as:
① Independence
② Accountability
③ Responsibility
④ Autonomy

145. A 22 year old undergoes a variety of tests for evaluation of a persistent dry cough, night sweats, and weight loss. Testing reveals that he is HIV positive. The positive HIV result indicates:
① An infection of unknown etiology
② The presence of AIDS wasting syndrome
③ That he has a definitive diagnosis of AIDS
④ Exposure to the virus known to cause AIDS and antibody development

146. When planning restorative care for the elderly, a *priority* consideration for the nurse is:
① The nurse's attitude concerning how much the elderly are capable of contributing to their own care
② The nurse's attitude is not important when planning care of the elderly
③ That the patient is old and should not have any input into the plan of care
④ To follow the physician's orders

147. The nurse is aware that her 22-year-old patient with a diagnosis of active tuberculosis will need specific instruction about good nutrition, including the food guide pyramid. Why is this instruction particularly important for the patient?
① The patient will be unable to cook at home for the next few weeks and will need to rely on others to bring meals
② Patients with tuberculosis usually have anorexia, nausea, and weight loss; they need proper nutrition to heal
③ Because of her age, the patient often relies on "fast foods" for nutrition
④ The medication needed to treat the patient's tuberculosis often causes patients to experience a rapid weight gain

148. A 5 month old is admitted to the hospital because of severe diarrhea. The nurse would describe the infant as having diarrhea on the basis of:
① Color and consistency of stools
② Consistency and frequency of stools
③ Amount and color of stools
④ Frequency and amount of stools

149. Which of the following will the nurse be aware of concerning women and heart disease?
① The typical onset of heart disease is 10 years later than it is in men
② About one fourth of those dying of heart disease are women
③ Women's mortality after age 65 is 50% higher than men's
④ Six times as many women die from breast cancer as they do from heart disease

150. Before discharge, a patient who has a colostomy asks the nurse to help him review the foods he should eat at home. Which statement by the patient indicates a good understanding of his nutritional needs now that he has a colostomy?
① "I should avoid citrus fruits because they contain acetic acid."
② "I should avoid foods like cabbage, cucumbers, and radishes because they will make me have more gas."
③ "I should avoid foods like spinach, oatmeal, and cream of wheat because food high in iron will make me constipated."
④ "I should avoid juices like apple and cranberry because they may cause diarrhea."

151. A patient is being discharged with her first child. She tells the nurse she is afraid she might not know how often to feed the baby. The nurse responds that it is generally agreed that an infant should be fed:
① On a demand schedule when he becomes hungry
② Every 4 hours even if he has to be forced to eat
③ At least every 2 hours for the first 2 months of life
④ At the convenience of the mother

152. A 35 year old is an outpatient in a mental health clinic. She exhibits a range of behaviors and presents characteristics of poor impulse control. She exhibits a total disregard for rules and regulations. When planning care for this patient, the nurse recognizes these symptoms as characteristic of which of the following mental disorders?
① Personality disorder
② Panic disorder
③ Thought process disorder
④ Bipolar affective disorder

153. A patient has just had her second child and has a 2-year-old daughter at home. She is afraid her 2-year-old will be jealous of the baby. Of the following suggestions, which one is *most appropriate* for the nurse to include in her conversation with this patient?
① "Divide your time equally between the two children."
② "Ignore any signs of jealousy to diminish the behavior."
③ "Give your daughter undivided attention, for a short period, several times a day."
④ "Keep the children apart to prevent your daughter from harming the baby."

154. Just before discharge, a patient tells the nurse that she is anxious to return to work because she needs the income to pay her hospital bills and living expenses. What can the nurse tell the patient about returning to work while being treated for tuberculosis?
① She should be able to return to work about 3 to 4 weeks after beginning therapy and will need follow-up treatment for 1 year
② She will be able to return to work after completing a year of therapy at home
③ She will be able to work after a year's therapy in a special tuberculosis hospital/sanitorium
④ She will be able to return to work as soon as she is started on therapy and feels well enough to work

155. Meperidine hydrochloride (Demerol) is ordered for the patient every 4 hours as needed. The nurse knows that the purpose of Demerol is:
    ① For pain relief
    ② For nausea and vomiting
    ③ To increase urine output
    ④ To dissolve a kidney stone

156. The process of constructing plausible reasons to explain and justify one's behavior is a commonly used defense mechanism of:
    ① Reaction formation
    ② Compensation
    ③ Conversion
    ④ Rationalization

157. A patient reports that she was tested for tuberculosis several years ago because her grandmother had it. She further stated that she thought the test was negative. What would indicate a positive response to the tuberculin skin test (Mantoux test)?
    ① An area of induration appearing at the site of the intradermal injection 48 to 72 hours after administration
    ② A maculopapular rash appearing on the inner aspect of the forearm 36 to 72 hours after the test
    ③ A reddened, raised area on the deltoid muscle where the injection was given
    ④ An increased cough and sputum production 24 to 72 hours after the test is administered

158. A patient asks the nurse when her baby's umbilical cord will drop off. The nurse answers that the cord will normally drop off when the infant's age is between:
    ① 3 and 4 days
    ② 7 and 10 days
    ③ 12 and 14 days
    ④ 15 and 20 days

159. Which of the following nursing diagnoses would be top priority for a patient receiving neuromuscular blocking agents?
    ① Alteration in thought processes
    ② Alteration in respiratory function
    ③ Alteration in tissue perfusion
    ④ Altered level of consciousness

160. A patient arrives in the emergency room with tachycardia, weak pulse, falling blood pressure, scant urinary output, and cool, clammy skin. The nurse knows these are most likely symptoms of:
    ① Cardiogenic shock
    ② Pulmonary edema
    ③ Pulmonary embolism
    ④ Right-sided heart failure

161. A patient is admitted to the gynecologic unit for a dilatation and curettage (D&C) following an incomplete abortion of a desired pregnancy. Following the D&C, the patient's hematocrit is 29%, and her hemoglobin level is 8.5 g/dl. How should the nurse interpret these laboratory findings?
    ① Higher than normal
    ② Average
    ③ Lower than normal
    ④ Life threatening

162. The Lamaze instructor teaches mothers about the various positions the fetus may assume while in utero. To fully explain a "breech position," she states that the presenting part is the:
    ① Back
    ② Shoulder
    ③ Buttocks
    ④ Head

163. A patient calls the nurse from home and states that he has gained 10 lb since his discharge 4 days ago from the hospital. He is taking his diuretic faithfully, but is concerned about what to do. The nurse's *first* action should be to:
    ① Tell him to report to the hospital immediately
    ② Assess for consistency in his routine to monitor his weight
    ③ Encourage him to make an appointment with his doctor as soon as he can
    ④ Tell him to decrease his fluids and weigh himself again in the morning

164. A 4 month old is admitted to the hospital because of severe diarrhea. When providing treatment, the nurse should initially plan to:
    ① Offer Pedialyte (electrolyte solution) and clear liquids progressing up to half-strength formula
    ② Observe closely, keep the baby NPO, and follow isolation procedures
    ③ Note time, type, and character of vomitus; weigh daily; and check patency of the IV
    ④ Provide large amounts of fluids, remove all blankets, and monitor temperature hourly

165. All of the following observations in a newborn infant are important. Which one should take *highest* priority in terms of planning his care?
    ① Skin eruptions
    ② Frequent crying
    ③ Cyanotic hands and feet
    ④ Respiratory difficulties

166. A nurse is about to administer Halcion, 0.125 milligrams, qhs PO to a patient in bed 2. She correctly verifies the physician's order, goes into the room, and instructs the patient to take his medicine. She then documents administration of the medication. Upon exiting the room, the nurse recognizes that she has made a major medication error as she notes the patient ambulating in the hall. Identify which medication principle was compromised.
    ① The right dosage
    ② The right route
    ③ The right patient
    ④ The right time and right medication

167. In caring for a patient who has had cataract surgery, the nurse should observe for what complication that might occur?
    ① Refractive errors
    ② Conjunctivitis
    ③ Retinal detachment
    ④ Optic atrophy

168. On the fourth day following a colon resection, a nurse changes a patient's dressing and pouch. The nurse notices that the patient turns his head and refuses to look at the incision or stoma. What would be the best action by the nurse?
    ① Get a mirror and show the patient the stoma so he can get used to its appearance
    ② Quickly finish the dressing change so he doesn't have to see the stoma
    ③ Ask the patient if he would like to see or touch the stoma
    ④ Start discussing the at-home care of the colostomy

169. The nurse knows that the following is a thrombolytic agent.
    ① Nitroglycerin (Nitroglyn)
    ② Propranolol (Inderal)
    ③ Streptokinase (Streptase)
    ④ Heparin (Heparin)

170. A 7 month old has severe diarrhea and is brought to the local neighborhood clinic. The nurse should expect that in addition to dehydration, the infant also has:
    ① An electrolyte imbalance
    ② Retention of urine
    ③ Hyperactive reflexes
    ④ Pulmonary congestion

171. A patient asks the nursery nurse what the "white spots" on her baby's nose are. The nurse tells her that plugged sebaceous glands on the nose and cheeks of the newborn are called:
    ① Vernix caseosa
    ② Milia
    ③ Lanugo
    ④ Mongolian spots

172. An 80-year-old man who has recently moved into a nursing home is depressed. The nursing assistants have expressed frustration in working with him because of his depression. The nurse should explain to the assistants that it could be difficult to maintain an effective relationship with this patient when he is depressed primarily because:
    ① People who are depressed are very lazy
    ② His poor personal grooming results in disgust from others
    ③ Independence and pride prevent him from asking for any kind of assistance
    ④ His pessimism arouses frustration and anger in others

173. A 3 month old is admitted to the hospital with a diagnosis of diarrhea. The infant is very irritable and is kept NPO. Which nursing intervention would be most beneficial for her irritability?
    ① Putting a mobile above the crib
    ② Talking quietly to the infant
    ③ Giving a pacifier
    ④ Placing the infant with other infants

174. A 19 year old was injured in a motor vehicle accident. X-ray examination reveals a comminuted fracture of the patient's left arm, and a long arm cast is applied. The most effective way to control swelling in the left arm is through:
    ① Cast application
    ② Medication therapy
    ③ Elevation of the extremity
    ④ Heated massage q4h

175. While visiting with a newly admitted nursing home resident, a nurse learns the patient is very depressed and feels worthless and unloved by his family. He is receiving amitriptyline (Elavil) prescribed by his physician. When would this drug be most likely to achieve the goal of lifting his depression?
    ① After a 6- to 7-week period
    ② In 2 to 4 weeks
    ③ Within a few days
    ④ Almost immediately

176. Nursing interventions for a child with upper respiratory tract infection may include:
    ① Antibiotics, ear drops, encouraging fluids, and eliminating environmental allergies
    ② Providing emotional support for the parents, decreasing fluids, positioning on the side, and decreasing stimuli
    ③ Antipyretics, bed rest, oral decongestants, cool air humidifier, proper nutrition, and encouraging fluids
    ④ Breathing exercises, liquid diet, steroid medications, bronchodilator medications, and intermittent positive-pressure breathing treatments

177. As the nurse is finishing her shift assessment, a patient who is HIV positive begins crying. He states he has lost most of his close friends and that his family doesn't want to see or talk to him anymore. What would be the nurse's *best* action?
    ① Tell him not to worry; there are many community agencies that can help
    ② Guide the conversation toward the acceptance phase of his illness
    ③ Encourage him to establish a relationship with another patient
    ④ Sit down and listen to his concerns and frustration

178. Considering a patient's hematocrit of 29% and hemoglobin of 8.5 g/dl, what postoperative nursing measures should most concern the nurse?
    ① Intake of oral fluids
    ② Adequate pain control
    ③ Ambulation
    ④ Assessment of voiding

179. A patient is admitted in active labor with a known breech presentation and is scheduled for a cesarean section (C-section). In planning care for this patient, the nurse knows that if her membranes rupture, she would be at risk for which of the following?
    ① A prolapsed cord
    ② Hemorrhage
    ③ A precipitate delivery
    ④ A nuchal cord

180. A patient, scheduled for an electroencephalogram in the morning, questions the nurse about what he might expect to occur. Which of the following statements by the nurse is *most accurate?*
① "You will be placed in a cylindrical apparatus, and brain wave activity will be evaluated."
② "You will be given a radiopaque mixture to drink, and brain wave activity will be evaluated."
③ "Electrodes will be placed on your head, and brain wave activity will be evaluated."
④ "An intravenous injection containing a radiopaque substance will be given, and evaluation of brain wave activity will be measured 2 hours after the injection."

181. A patient has been hospitalized for over a week for deep vein thrombosis. He is near discharge, and the physician is beginning warfarin (Coumadin) therapy for prophylaxis at home. Which of the following orders would require the nurse to report to the supervising nurse before implementation?
① Give all medication ac
② Collect daily prothrombin level
③ Ambulate in the hall bid
④ Demerol 50 mg IM for pain q4h prn

182. All states in this country require that 1% silver nitrate or erythromycin ophthalmic ointment be instilled into every newborn's eyes. The *primary* reason is to prevent:
① Gonorrheal infection of the eyes
② Syphilitic infection of the eyes
③ Development of retrolental fibroplasia
④ Development of cataracts

183. Discharge nutritional counseling for a patient with low postoperative hemoglobin and hematocrit levels should include an emphasis on which of the following types of foods?
① Citrus fruits
② Milk and other dairy products
③ Breads and pasta
④ Leafy green vegetables

184. A 30 year old is HIV positive. Significant others include his mother, father, two sisters, his lover, and a cat. He is now ready for discharge. He asks questions about living in a household with other individuals. Which of the following statements by the patient indicates his understanding of teachings relative to home care?
① "I'll have someone else clean the cat's litter pan."
② "I'll use gloves when preparing meals."
③ "My clothes and bed linens should be washed and dried separately."
④ "I'll avoid contact with others so the risk of AIDS transmission will be decreased."

185. A patient is ordered to take ferrous sulfate following surgery. Which of the following statements made by the patient indicates an understanding of the nurse's instructions about this medication?
① "I can only take the pill between meals to promote absorption."
② "I must take the pill with a laxative to prevent constipation."
③ "I must take the pill only with meals or a snack."
④ "I can only take the pill with liquids."

186. Which of the following conditions is an example of a patient response that a nurse can treat independent of physician or nursing orders/supervision?
① Sepsis
② Hypertension
③ Fatigue
④ Pneumonia

187. A patient has a cataract extraction with an intraocular lens implant. Immediate postoperative care includes having the patient:
① Turn, deep breathe, and cough
② Lie in high-Fowler's position with knees flexed
③ Lie on the unoperated side and in low-Fowler's position
④ Lie on the operated side and in high-Fowler's position

188. After checking for placement of an enteral feeding tube, the nurse prepares for the next enteral feeding of Ensure, 480 ml. The residual feeding is assessed, and 500 ml is aspirated from the stomach. The nurse should proceed as follows:
① Hold the feeding and notify the physician
② Give the 480 ml of feeding as scheduled
③ Hold this feeding and give extra the next feeding
④ Give half of the feeding and the other half in an hour

189. A patient is admitted with pancreatitis. His family tells the nurse he uses alcohol in unknown amounts daily. In addition to safety measures and prescribed care, the nurse should include which of the following in the plan of care?
① Report intake and output (I & O) to the supervising nurse q2h
② Perform neurologic checks qh
③ Observe for withdrawal symptoms from alcohol
④ Provide sedation prn

190. A nurse's aide on the unit mentions that a patient has a pulse rate of 42 beats/min. She checked the radial pulse for 15 seconds. She asks the nurse to check the pulse rate again to confirm her findings. The nurse should assess the:
① Radial pulse for 1 minute
② Apical pulse for 15 seconds
③ Apical pulse for 1 minute
④ Radial pulse in each arm for 15 seconds

191. A patient is being discharged after being diagnosed with diabetes mellitus type II. She has been stabilized on glipizide (Glucotrol). Which statement shows she has good understanding of this drug's effects and side effects?
① "This drug will keep my blood sugar stable all the time."
② "I must report the use of this drug to my doctor any time I am to receive another medication."
③ "I will need to take this drug after meals."
④ "I may frequently feel drowsy while I am taking this medication."

192. The nursing staff has reviewed a patient's progress to date and has written several short-term goals. Of the following outcome (goal) statements, which one is *most appropriately written?*
    ① The nurse will walk the patient whenever necessary
    ② The patient will take 15 steps, unassisted, by 5/19
    ③ The patient will be given a complete bath every day
    ④ The patient will want to be discharged by 5/16

193. A 20-year-old heroin addict is brought to the emergency room. When this patient leaves the hospital, she needs to learn new social and living skills. This is primarily because she previously has been living in a state of:
    ① Fear of authorities
    ② Minimal contact with friends and family
    ③ Preoccupation with obtaining and taking drugs
    ④ False sense of security

194. A patient is admitted to the unit with cholecystitis and a bipolar manic disorder. She arrives in a wheelchair, claiming she is a great actress like Betty Davis and will remember all of the little people in her future. She asks the nurse to draw her bath and have the kitchen send up pheasant for her supper. The nurse's *best* response is:
    ① "I'll check your diet orders."
    ② "I'll get you some more lithium."
    ③ "I'll be glad to draw your bath, but you must get into bed as soon as you are through. We have to prepare for your exam in the morning."
    ④ "You are in the hospital. I need to get some information from you, then I will help you bathe."

195. The nurse recognizes which of the following is the recommended angle of entry for an intradermal injection?
    ① 90 degrees
    ② 60 degrees
    ③ 45 degrees
    ④ 15 degrees

196. The external fetal-maternal monitor is applied to a patient's abdomen. The phonotransducer indicates a fetal heart rate (FHR) of 140 beats/min. The labor room nurse knows the normal range for the FHR is:
    ① 70 to 90 beats/min
    ② 80 to 120 beats/min
    ③ 120 to 160 beats/min
    ④ 170 to 190 beats/min

197. The nurse would caution a concerned parent not to be alarmed about which of these side effects of her child's recent immunization?
    ① Convulsions, fine tremors, and malaise
    ② Malaise, soreness, and a raised red area at the injection site
    ③ Urticaria, arthritic-type pain, and severe vomiting
    ④ Temperature of 104° F (40° C), welts over the entire body, and malaise

198. To prevent the spread of organisms and protect other patients, the nurse should always do which of the following?
    ① Use sterile gloves
    ② Use isolation gowns
    ③ Practice proper handwashing
    ④ Provide nonsterile gloves to the family

199. A 23-year-old patient with a toothache is given the antibiotic erythromycin to be taken tid for 10 days. Which set of instructions offered by the nurse would be correct to give her while taking this antibiotic?
    ① Take the antibiotic until the tooth stops hurting
    ② Take the antibiotic on an empty stomach, perhaps 1 hour before meals
    ③ Regardless of allergies, erythromycin is a relatively safe drug
    ④ Concurrent use of this drug with oral contraceptives may render the contraceptives ineffective

200. A 19-year-old patient is brought into the emergency room. She appears to be frightened of everyone and is hallucinating. The nurse discovers that she took LSD several hours ago. If the patient continues to use LSD for an extended period of time, she should be warned that she may:
    ① Become physically addicted
    ② Suffer symptoms of withdrawal
    ③ Have flashbacks
    ④ Suffer from acute organic brain syndrome

201. After a patient on IV therapy receives a calcium channel blocker, her blood pressure drops to 78/50. She says she feels all right but was dizzy when she stood. The nurse should take which nursing action while notifying the physician?
    ① Place her in a low-Fowler's position and increase her IV fluids
    ② Place her in a high-Fowler's position and increase her IV fluids
    ③ Place her in Trendelenburg's position and increase her IV fluids
    ④ Place her in reverse Trendelenburg's position and decrease her IV fluids

202. During the postoperative period following a lumbar laminectomy at the L4-L5 level, nursing care should include:
    ① Instructing the patient to turn as a unit
    ② Maintaining the patient's legs in an adducted position
    ③ Limiting range-of-motion exercises to the lower extremities
    ④ Turning the patient from side to side using the log-rolling technique

203. A patient is admitted to the hospital for acute appendicitis. Admission testing reveals that she also has active pulmonary tuberculosis. To plan the nursing care for this patient, the nurse must be aware of the route of tuberculosis transmission. Which of the following statements is *most accurate?*
    ① A single contact with an infected person will usually cause the disease
    ② Feces and stool can also contain the organism for pulmonary tuberculosis
    ③ A tine tuberculin test or tuberculin skin test (Mantoux test) can cause a person to develop active tuberculosis
    ④ Tuberculosis is spread via aerosolization such as coughing, sneezing, or singing

204. A 22 year old is brought into the emergency room by his wife. She reports that he had been with friends who were using LSD and he is having "a bad trip." Which of the following symptoms should the nurse expect to find in this patient?
    ① Slurred speech, blurred vision, light-headedness, ringing in the ears, loss of coordination, and excessive nasal secretions
    ② Drying of the mouth, increased appetite, reddening of the eyes, and short-term memory impairment
    ③ Tremendous confusion, unpleasant sensory images, and extreme panic
    ④ Stomach pains, chills, hallucinations, headache, and delirium tremens

205. A patient puts on his call light and complains of his arm burning severely at the IV site that is infusing 1000 cc D_5W with 20 mEq KCl at 150 cc/hour. He says he cannot tolerate the pain anymore. The nurse should *first:*
    ① Assess the site, discontinue the IV, and notify the team leader
    ② Assess the site, slow the IV until it is infused, and notify the team leader
    ③ Slow the IV, assess the site, and notify the team leader
    ④ Tell him the physician ordered the medication, assess the site, and keep the IV rate the same

206. In her eighth month of pregnancy a patient is admitted through the emergency room with a diagnosis of eclampsia. The nurse might expect the physician to order:
    ① A magnesium preparation
    ② A potassium preparation
    ③ A sodium preparation
    ④ A calcium preparation

207. A patient on the long-term floor has been unconscious for 2 months. The nurse knows the following action is the most important for this patient?
    ① Feed the patient three meals per day
    ② Give eye care at least every 4 hours
    ③ Allow the patient to sit up in a chair for at least 8 hours per day
    ④ Give frequent back rubs at least four times per shift

208. An 18 year old reports being raped at age 11 by a stranger. She speaks of this event with little affect. The characteristic of posttraumatic stress disorder being demonstrated is:
    ① Anxiety
    ② Rumination
    ③ Reliving the event
    ④ Numbness

209. A patient was admitted to the unit following an attempted suicide with sleeping pills. Her husband had arrived home early from a business trip and discovered her deeply sedated. In evaluating this patient's level of risk for future suicide attempts, the nurse is aware that this attempt:
    ① Was not planned out thoroughly
    ② Was intended to bring about emergency care and intervention
    ③ Was most serious, because a lethal method was used and there appeared little chance for discovery
    ④ Was less serious, because she used pills rather than a gun or more lethal method

210. A newly admitted depressed patient is found sitting alone in the dining room. He has eaten very little of his meal. What nursing measure should the nurse do first?
    ① Ask the family to bring favorite foods from home
    ② Offer diversional activities
    ③ Have the patient's meals served in his room
    ④ Order small frequent meals

211. When teaching health promotion activities, the nurse realizes that eating behavior is influenced by a variety of factors. These factors can be classified as biologic, psychologic, sociocultural, and environmental. Which of the following are examples of environmental factors?
    ① Accessibility, convenience, and cost
    ② Metabolic rate, hypoglycemia, and growth spurts
    ③ Ethnic foods, holiday get togethers, and birthday parties
    ④ Habits, self-esteem, and perceptions of control

212. On the basis of the admitting diagnosis, the psychosocial and physical assessment data, and the presence of an old, healing fracture found on x-ray examination, the physician and nurse suspect child abuse. In addition to the medical treatment of this 2-year-old child, which of the following nursing actions should also be initiated?
    ① An appointment should be made with the family pediatrician
    ② Child protection services should be notified
    ③ Family counseling services should be recommended to the mother
    ④ The mother should be counseled in the emergency department before the child's discharge

213. Nursing intervention for heat exhaustion includes:
    ① Removing constrictive clothing; providing warm soaks; and if conscious, giving warm liquids
    ② Ensuring adequate airway and ventilation, administering quick-acting carbohydrates, and recording vital signs
    ③ Maintaining adequate airway, breathing, and circulation; providing rapid cooling; and administering oxygen, if prescribed by physician
    ④ Making sure the patient is in a cool area, giving salt water if the patient is conscious and not vomiting, and relieving muscle cramps

214. A mother brings her sobbing 18 month old to the emergency room because she believes she has broken her arm while trying to get out of her crib. The nurse notices several bruises on both of her upper arms, in addition to what appears to be a broken forearm. Why does the nurse realize that it is important to obtain a well-documented history from the mother?
① Infants and toddlers do not normally sustain fractures while climbing into or out of a crib
② The child is crying and cannot talk to the nurse
③ The nurse needs to know what kind of first aid was given to her
④ The nurse needs to determine the child's health and need for a tetanus immunization

215. A nurse preparing to take a patient's fetal heart rate palpates the abdomen to determine fetal position. This procedure is called:
① Homans' sign
② Leopold's maneuver
③ Chadwick's sign
④ Ritgen's maneuver

216. A nursing mother often does not menstruate for several months after delivery or until she discontinues breast-feeding. Of the following information, which would be appropriate for the nurse to include in discharge planning for this nursing mother?
① Although she is breast-feeding, ovulation is not suppressed, and pregnancy is possible
② Ovulation is suppressed, and pregnancy is not possible while breast-feeding
③ Breast-feeding should be stopped if she does not menstruate in 3 months
④ The uterus will not return to normal size while she is breast-feeding

217. The nurse verifies rupture of the membranes (ROM) by testing the:
① Fluid in the vagina with Nitrazine paper and obtaining an alkaline reaction
② Fluid in the vagina with Nitrazine paper and obtaining an acid reaction
③ Condition of the vagina
④ Urine for protein

218. A nurse's personal friend says during coffee that she is very stressed with her job. The nurse knows that stress can be best defined as:
① Another way of coping with anxiety; used to block conscious awareness
② A specific response of the body to any demand made on it
③ A universal emotion; a general state of apprehension
④ Anything that interferes with goal achievement

219. A patient has a medical history of peptic ulcer disease. During a recent upper GI series, it was discovered that the patient has cancer of the stomach. She is admitted to the hospital for gastrectomy surgery. On the second postoperative day, the patient's nasogastric (NG) tube has drained only a small amount of clear greenish-tinged fluid. The *most appropriate* nursing action should be to:
① Do nothing; this amount of drainage is expected with this type of surgery
② Call the physician immediately to report an impending complication
③ Irrigate the tube with 100 ml of normal saline solution to ensure patency
④ Connect the tube to high suction on the Gomco machine for 15 minutes

220. A 25-year-old gravida 3 para 1 is admitted to labor and delivery with ruptured membranes. She is having contractions 6 to 7 minutes apart, lasting 30 seconds. The nurse obtains her temperature, pulse, blood pressure, respirations, and fetal heart rate on admission because:
① This information is part of the admission record
② Obtaining this information is a hospital policy
③ A baseline is necessary for further assessment
④ The nursing care plan depends on this information

221. A 23-year-old man is brought into the emergency department dead on arrival from drowning. The bereaved family arrives within minutes after the ambulance and requests to see the body immediately. The nurse's response should be to:
① Allow the family to see the body as requested
② Tell the family that viewing the body will make the grieving more painful
③ Suggest waiting until the mortician has cared for the body
④ Suggest that the family call other close relatives or friends to be with them when they see the body

222. Following a subtotal gastrectomy, a patient has physician's orders to receive vitamin B_{12} injections. The primary reason for this is to:
① Provide relief from gastric irritation and distention
② Assist in the repair and healing of the gastric mucosa
③ Stimulate appetite and decrease anorexia
④ Provide the body with the factor necessary to promote red blood cell production

223. A nurse's neighbor calls her about a headache and asks if she should take a pain reliever. She mentions that she is breast-feeding her baby. The nurse's advice should be to:
① Take the drug and watch the baby closely for side effects
② Take half the drug dose instead of the whole dose and watch for side effects
③ Check with the physician because some drugs are excreted in breast milk
④ Take the medication as needed; it shouldn't harm the child

224. While a nurse is working in the emergency room, a patient is brought in by friends. He is hallucinating, and the nurse discovers that he has been using LSD. What statement made by the nurse would be *most* beneficial to help the patient recover and regain control?
    ① "You're all right; don't worry."
    ② "You're having a bad trip, and the main reaction is about over."
    ③ "You were using acid and shouldn't have."
    ④ "You've taken a psychedelic and are suffering a mild psychosis that will last only a short time."

225. A patient is in the early stage of labor and is 2 cm dilated and 50% effaced. As the nurse times contractions, the patient asks her what effacement really means. The nurse explains that effacement is the:
    ① Position of fetus
    ② Size of the fetus
    ③ Irregular contractions of the uterus
    ④ Thinning and shortening of the cervix

226. An 18 year old is brought into a local clinic by friends. The nurse discovers she has taken LSD. On recovery, the patient says that she enjoys taking LSD because it helps in numerous ways. Which statement by the patient *would be most doubtful* as to why she enjoys taking the drug?
    ① It seems to increase creativity
    ② It seems to make time pass more slowly
    ③ It seems to make sounds be portrayed in color
    ④ It seems to create visual hallucinations

227. A patient with complaints of low back pain is admitted for evaluation. Which question by the nurse would obtain the *best* assessment data?
    ① "Do you feel like you need to urinate?"
    ② "Does the pain interfere with your daily activities?"
    ③ "Describe your pain and any associated feelings of discomfort."
    ④ "Is there any increase in pain when you have a bowel movement?"

228. An 82-year-old patient with a history of diabetes and hypertension comes into the clinic with a piece of steel embedded in his right foot. In setting up for the physician to anesthetize the foot, the nurse should offer which of the following?
    ① Betadine
    ② Benzoin spray
    ③ Lidocaine with epinephrine
    ④ Lidocaine without epinephrine

229. A 21 year old is brought into the emergency room by friends who state she is hallucinating and is frightened of everyone. The nurse discovers that the patient took LSD 3 hours ago. What terminology is also used for hallucinogens or psychedelics?
    ① Bennies, speed, hash
    ② Buttons, PCP, acid
    ③ H, smack, junk
    ④ Rainbows, downers, M

230. A 16-year-old patient who has been taking anticonvulsants for seizures reports to the office for a routine visit and lab work. She reports that because she has not had a seizure in a year and does not feel that she needs to take the medication every day, she skips a dose now and then. The nurse's reply should be:
    ① "You should be more careful in your drug treatment regimen."
    ② "I know that you are glad that the seizures are under control now."
    ③ "It is important that you follow your treatment plan on a strict basis and avoid skipping any doses."
    ④ "It may help you to buy a pill organizer that allows you to place the medicine necessary for each day of the week."

231. A colleague and confidant says her job is very stressful. The nurse is aware that:
    ① Health factors do not directly affect a person's response to stress
    ② The nurse should be a resource in helping her friend develop maladaptive patterns of behavior
    ③ Most changes in situations or events are not directly related to stress
    ④ The meaning an individual gives to stress determines whether the person feels distress

232. Which of the following represents an example of tertiary prevention in health promotion?
    ① Immunizations against hepatitis and polio
    ② Yearly flu vaccination
    ③ Breast self-examinations
    ④ Moving and positioning to prevent complications

233. In planning care for a patient diagnosed with ulcerative colitis, it is important that the nurse knows that the term "ulcerative colitis" is defined as:
    ① An inflammatory process in the sigmoid colon
    ② An ulcerative disorder of the terminal ileum
    ③ Inflammation and ulceration of the colon and rectum
    ④ A condition with alternating bouts of diarrhea and constipation

234. A myelogram is ordered for a patient with low back pain that has not responded to bed rest. Which of the following *best* describes the procedure?
    ① A contrast medium is injected via a lumbar puncture
    ② Small needles are inserted into the back muscles being evaluated
    ③ An amplified recording of the electrical activity of the brain is obtained
    ④ A noninvasive, painless procedure provides cross-sectional views of the spine

235. Following an 18-hour induced labor, a 38-year-old woman delivers her fourth child. Soon after birth, the pediatrician informs the patient she suspects that the baby has Down syndrome. Which of the following factors most likely contributed to the development of Down syndrome?
    ① Pitocin induction
    ② Prolonged labor
    ③ Maternal age
    ④ Multiparity

236. The nurse knows that mental illness may be evidenced by:
    ① A pattern of behavior disturbing to the individual or the community in which one lives
    ② The development of mature patterns of problem solving
    ③ The ability to cope with crisis
    ④ Having satisfying work and work relationships

237. The nurse places the patient into which position in preparation for administration of an enema?
    ① Lithotomy
    ② Sims'
    ③ Dorsal recumbent
    ④ Right lateral

238. A patient with congestive heart failure has been taking digoxin 0.125 mg orally when at home. The nurse realizes that to administer this medication in the hospital she must complete which of the following actions?
    ① Place the patient on a cardiac monitor
    ② Obtain the radial pulse and notify the physician of the results
    ③ Obtain the apical pulse for 60 seconds and withhold the medication if the pulse is below 60
    ④ Check the patient's mouth after administration to be sure he has swallowed the medication

239. Pulmonary therapy is ordered for a patient with cystic fibrosis. Her mother was taught the techniques of postural drainage and breathing exercises. Which of the following responses by the mother indicates an understanding of these techniques?
    ① "Therapy should be done immediately before meals to open air passages and make eating easier."
    ② "Therapy should only be done if she has difficulty breathing."
    ③ "Therapy should not be done immediately before or after meals."
    ④ "Therapy should be done only if she feels like she wants to."

240. A patient was admitted with pitting edema of both ankles and dyspnea. Her orders include bed rest, oxygen at 4 L, morphine sulfate 10 mg q4h, Lasix 40 mg IV stat, and a chest x-ray examination stat. The diagnosis is pulmonary edema, and the patient is extremely restless. On the basis of written physician's orders, the nurse should:
    ① Administer morphine sulfate 10 mg subcutaneously
    ② Increase the amount of oxygen from 4 to 8 L
    ③ Talk with her to decrease her level of anxiety
    ④ Elevate both legs

241. Besides the appearance of a high sodium and chloride content in sweat, what additional information should the nurse be sure to obtain when cystic fibrosis is suspected?
    ① The type of diapers or underpants the child wears at night
    ② The time the child goes to bed and wakes up in the morning
    ③ The kind of bowel movements the child has
    ④ The kinds of food the child enjoys eating

242. A gravida 5 para 5 is having difficulty accepting her newborn who has Down syndrome. During the early neonatal period, which nursing action would be the *most helpful* to the patient and her baby?
    ① Keeping the baby in the nursery for care
    ② Assisting the patient to hold and cuddle the baby
    ③ Leaving the patient and the baby alone so the mother can begin grieving
    ④ Completing the infant care in an Isolette rather than letting the patient do it

243. A new patient arrives on the floor and the nurse helps the charge nurse admit him. After the health history is taken, the patient states that he cannot remember if he is allergic to any medications but thinks he might be. On the basis of this information, the nurse would want to have on hand which classification of drug in case of an allergic reaction?
    ① Ganglionic blocking agents
    ② Sympathomimetic drugs
    ③ Parasympathetic blocking agents
    ④ Neuromuscular blocking agents

244. A 74-year-old patient is diagnosed with bilateral senile cataracts and is scheduled for surgery. He is admitted to the surgical unit because he also has congestive heart failure and is receiving multiple cardiac medications. The patient is able to see only shadows, but he has delayed having this surgery because, he says, "I was afraid. Since I have this heart problem, I just figured I was going to die." Which of the following represents an *appropriate* response by the nurse?
    ① "This must be frightening for you."
    ② "People do not die from cataract surgery."
    ③ "I can understand how you feel. I'd be afraid of dying too."
    ④ "How did you live at home when you couldn't see?"

245. A 4 year old has had multiple episodes of upper respiratory infections (URIs) since birth. She is thin and in the 30th percentile on the pediatric growth charts for height and weight. Which comment made by her mother during the check-up indicates the need for immediate follow-up?
    ① "When I kiss her, she tastes salty."
    ② "She drinks plenty of fluids."
    ③ "She occasionally wets the bed at night."
    ④ "She really seems to dislike vegetables."

246. The afternoon following an incomplete abortion and a dilatation and curettage (D&C), a patient confides to the nurse, "This baby meant so much to my husband and me. We were so excited about having a baby and had already started thinking about decorating a nursery and everything. I feel so disappointed and hurt." What is the *best* response by the nurse to this patient?
    ① "I know you feel bad now, but as time goes by you will feel better."
    ② "Somehow nature takes care of problems. There had to be something wrong with how the baby was growing."
    ③ "I can see that you feel bad about this. Let's talk about it."
    ④ "If you give your body about 6 months to recuperate, you should be able to get pregnant again."

247. The nurse notices after report that one of the other nurses on the unit is talking excessively. She complains of not sleeping well last night, appears restless, and has slight hand tremors when pouring medications. The nurse knows that this co-worker has been going through some difficult times in her personal life lately. The nurse might suspect her co-worker of misuse of which of these agents?
    1. Alcohol
    2. Diphenhydramine (Benadryl)
    3. Amphetamines
    4. Sympathomimetic drugs

248. When assessing a patient's lochia 12 hours after delivery, the nurse notes a foul smell. Which of the following actions would be most appropriate for the nurse to take?
    1. Do nothing because this is normal
    2. Administer vaginal douches
    3. Report this immediately because the patient could have an infection
    4. Count the perineal pads used

249. To evaluate heparin therapy, the nurse will monitor which of the following laboratory values?
    1. Bleeding time
    2. Platelet count
    3. Prothrombin time
    4. Clotting time

250. A 3 year old is seen at a clinic and is diagnosed with an upper respiratory infection. Symptoms of an upper respiratory infection include which of the following?
    1. Dehydration, vomiting, and irritability
    2. Fever, sore throat, and sneezing
    3. Restlessness, fever, and pulling at the ears
    4. Vomiting, pale color, and sharp abdominal pains

COMPREHENSIVE EXAMINATION TWO: PART 1

1. A 5 year old is admitted for removal of her tonsils and adenoids. Before surgery, the nurse should keep an accurate record of the child's temperature and vital signs. This is done primarily because:
   ① The child needs intravenous fluids before surgery
   ② Hemorrhage is quite common in tonsillitis before surgery
   ③ An elevated temperature or changes in vital signs may mean an infection and a need to postpone surgery
   ④ Any change in vital signs or temperature may indicate need for immediate surgery

2. An abused child's mother cries and tells the nurse that she "feels upset and responsible" for what has happened. What is the *best response* for the nurse to make to this statement?
   ① "Don't blame yourself. It could happen to anyone."
   ② "She's young, so it won't affect her that much."
   ③ "If you don't act upset, she won't be upset."
   ④ "It sounds like you feel you weren't there for her."

3. The patient receives morphine sulfate IV for pain. Which medication will the nurse have on hand to counter possible complications?
   ① Epinephrine (Adrenalin)
   ② Naloxone (Narcan)
   ③ Diphenhydramine (Benadryl)
   ④ Meclizine (Antivert)

4. After performing range-of-motion exercises on a 19-year-old paraplegic, the nurse notices that his right foot is in plantar flexion most of the time. The nurse should initiate which of the following interventions?
   ① Position the patient in proper alignment while he is asleep; increase his exercise while he is awake
   ② Inform the charge nurse of the need for intervention; increase exercise
   ③ Offer range of motion more frequently; change the type of exercise
   ④ Apply podus boots; position the feet in a dorsal flexion position

5. A patient with a history of seizures takes phenytoin (Dilantin). Which statement made by the patient indicates that he understands self-care related to his anticonvulsant medication?
   ① "I will take an additional dose when I feel stressed."
   ② "I will consume only a moderate amount of alcohol."
   ③ "I will keep my medication with me at all times."
   ④ "I will need an ongoing plan of oral hygiene."

6. A patient's hyperthyroidism is not controlled with medications, and a subtotal thyroidectomy is performed. Postoperatively, the nurse assesses the patient's wound for bleeding. Which technique is *most* appropriate?
   ① Inspect the dressing for any dried blood
   ② Monitor the hemoglobin and hematocrit levels for changes
   ③ Loosen dressing on both ends and check the wound directly
   ④ Slip a hand behind the patient's neck and check for blood on the back of the neck and on the bed linens

7. A patient who is 2 days postpartum indicates she has not had a stool since delivery. She had a normal labor, delivered an 8 lb. 4 oz. baby, and had an episiotomy. In an effort to assist her with elimination needs, the nurse should provide which of the following?
   ① Adequate analgesia to allow comfortable bowel elimination while the episiotomy heals
   ② Adequate fluids and exercise to promote peristalsis and soft stools
   ③ Rest and calories to promote healing
   ④ Laxatives and sitz baths to promote elimination

8. A 38 year old is pregnant for the first time and schedules an appointment with her obstetrician. During the initial visit, she appears healthy and gives an unimpressive medical history. The nurse explains to the patient that because of her age, special tests will be done. Which of the following tests would be indicated because of the patient's age?
   ① Test for gestational diabetes
   ② Alpha-fetoprotein level
   ③ Heterozygote testing
   ④ Estriol levels

9. The nurse can initiate a Moro reflex by implementing which of the following actions?
   ① Grasping the newborn's hand
   ② Stimulating the newborn's feet
   ③ Causing a banging noise
   ④ Turning the newborn's head to the right side

10. Which of the following assessment findings would *most likely* be associated with a diagnosis of delirium?
    ① Patient has been taking antibiotics for a sinus infection
    ② Patient has been taking furosemide (Lasix) for congestive heart failure
    ③ Patient had a hip replacement 12 months ago
    ④ Patient has lost 10 pounds over the past year

11. A patient who had a subtotal thyroidectomy is brought back to the nursing unit from the postanesthesia care unit. The nurse asks the patient to state her name and repeats this request frequently. The *primary* reason the nurse includes this intervention in the postoperative plan of care is to monitor for signs of:
    ① Hemorrhage
    ② Laryngeal nerve damage
    ③ Lower airway obstruction
    ④ Level of consciousness change

12. The nurse is reviewing foot care with a patient with diabetes. Instruction should be given to:
    ① Keep the toenails short and rounded at the edges
    ② Apply alcohol after washing her feet every day
    ③ Keep her feet warm at night by using a heating pad set on low
    ④ Select absorbent socks/stockings that allow for toe motion

13. A patient comes to the physician's office complaining of recurring headaches and abdominal pains. She states that her youngest son just left for college, that her mother-in-law has moved into her home, and that she and her husband are fighting constantly. She says, "I just can't take it anymore!" The problem that this patient presents is an example of a(n):
    ① Depressive episode
    ② Anxiety disorder
    ③ Situational crisis
    ④ Schizophrenic relapse

14. A newborn admitted to the nursery had an initial Apgar score of 4. The nurse interprets the Apgar score to indicate:
    ① A vigorous newborn
    ② A depressed newborn
    ③ Respiration had to be initiated
    ④ A respiratory rate of 20

15. A 15 year old visits the clinic for a physical examination required to play sports. The physician orders a clean-catch specimen for a urinalysis. The nurse should instruct the teenager to:
    ① Void a small amount in the toilet, then a small amount in the cup; cleanse her hands with the wipe
    ② Cleanse with the wipes; void a small amount in the toilet and a small amount in the cup; urinate the remainder in the toilet
    ③ Urinate a small amount in the toilet, stopping in midstream; cleanse from front to back with each wipe, then urinate the remainder in the cup provided
    ④ Use each individual wipe only once, cleansing from front to back; urinate a small amount in the toilet, stopping in midstream; urinate the remainder in the cup provided

16. The nurse is preparing an obstetric patient for an initial physical examination. The patient states that she has been having nausea and vomiting for the past 2 months. The term the nurse would note on the patient's medical record to indicate this would be:
    ① Pernicious vomiting
    ② Vomitus marinus
    ③ Morning sickness
    ④ Hyperemesis gravidarium

17. The nurse and a diabetic patient are reviewing exchange lists for meal planning. The patient shows an understanding of instructions by which of the following statements?
    ① "I should cut out desserts other than fresh fruit."
    ② "I should decrease my food intake during periods of heavy exercise."
    ③ "I should use only designated dietetic foods."
    ④ "I should schedule regular meals."

18. A patient returns for a follow-up obstetric visit about 6 months into her pregnancy. The nurse checks her weight and blood pressure, noting that the patient has gained 10 lb since her last visit and that her blood pressure is 200/90. The patient also states that her fingers and feet have become swollen. The nurse knows that these symptoms may be an indication of:
    ① Preeclampsia
    ② Eclampsia
    ③ Hypertension
    ④ Hypersthenia

19. The physician orders a pregnancy test to be done to determine the presence of a hormone that is excreted in the urine only during early pregnancy. In filling out the requisition form for the laboratory, the nurse should mark which hormone?
    ① ACTH
    ② FSH
    ③ HCG
    ④ TSH

20. A young mother, who is very apprehensive with her first child, tells the nurse that her 3-week-old baby girl sleeps most of the day. The nurse should inform her that newborns:
    ① Should have only brief naps
    ② Sleep all day and stay awake most of the night
    ③ Need at least 12 hours of sleep in a 24-hour period
    ④ Usually sleep about 18 to 20 hours during the first month

21. Which of the following questions asked by the nurse is *most appropriate* to reassess the level of orientation of a patient hospitalized for delirium?
    ① "Tell me what time of day it is."
    ② "Tell me how you are feeling right now."
    ③ "What did you have for breakfast yesterday?"
    ④ "What would you do if there was a fire?"

22. A patient is started on thyroid replacement therapy. Which of the following would indicate an undesirable effect from taking levothyroxine (Synthroid)?
    ① Chest pain
    ② Constipation
    ③ Decreased activity
    ④ Sore throat and fever

23. Which of the following nursing diagnoses should receive priority for a patient who is delirious?
    ① Self-care deficit related to confusion
    ② Activity intolerance related to weakness
    ③ Alteration in comfort related to dry mucous membranes
    ④ Potential for injury related to impaired judgment

24. A spinal cord–injured patient is now ready for the application of a halo brace. Which of the following *best relates* to the use of the halo fixation device?
    ① Infection is less of a problem because skull pins are not required
    ② The patient will have normal head and neck range-of-motion capability
    ③ The patient must remain in bed so that the weights can hang freely
    ④ Stabilization of the spine is provided without the use of a frame or special bed

25. A 70-year-old patient is being treated for chronic glaucoma. Data from the history would *most likely* reveal that the patient had:
    1. Acute attacks of eye pain
    2. A loss of her peripheral vision
    3. Tearing and redness after reading
    4. A decreased ability to focus on near objects

26. The nurse is teaching the patient how to instill eye drops. The nurse should tell the patient to:
    1. Apply light pressure to the eye after instilling the drops
    2. Cover the eye for at least 10 minutes after the drops are instilled
    3. Place the eye drops in the conjunctival sac that is opened by gently pulling the lower eyelid outward
    4. First remove any excess fluid by wiping the eye from the outer to inner canthus

27. The 92-year-old patient is being discharged home on furosemide (Lasix) and digoxin (Lanoxin). When providing discharge instructions, the nurse will carefully consider the following principle(s):
    1. Side effects associated with the use of diuretics are common in the elderly due to decreased total body water content and reduced renal function
    2. Side effects associated with the use of diuretics are uncommon in the elderly
    3. The two drugs should not be given together
    4. Side effects associated with the use of diuretics are common in the elderly due to an increase in total body water and an increase in renal reserves

28. A mother calls the clinic and in a panic-stricken voice states that her 2-year-old daughter has just ingested "some" Clorox. The mother states that she has syrup of ipecac at home. The nurse should instruct her to:
    1. Administer 10 ml of syrup of ipecac with milk
    2. Administer 10 ml of syrup of ipecac with water
    3. Not give syrup of ipecac; bring her daughter to the emergency room
    4. Not give syrup of ipecac; observe her daughter at home for the next hour

29. Which of the following statements would be *best* for the nurse to use when describing findings in relation to the onset of puberty in males and females?
    1. "Males and females experience the onset of puberty at about the same age."
    2. "Males experience the onset of puberty about 1 to 2 years earlier than females."
    3. "Females experience the onset of puberty about 1 to 2 years earlier than males."
    4. "Males and females experience the onset of puberty at the same age, but females decline in development 1 year after males."

30. To promote comfort and optimal functioning to a 14 month old who is placed in a Croupette, which of these actions would be *most appropriate* for the nurse to take?
    1. Change the bed linens and the patient's gown as often as necessary to keep him dry and comfortable
    2. Establish continuous drainage from the ice chamber as the ice melts
    3. Restrain the child to prohibit changing position in bed
    4. Maintain the child in a prone position

31. Otitis media is a common complication of an upper respiratory infection in infants. It occurs primarily because:
    1. The sinuses of an infant are not fully developed
    2. The digestive system is not fully developed
    3. The infant's eustachian tube is shorter, wider, and straighter than that of an adult
    4. The infant's eustachian tube is longer and more narrow than that of an adult

32. Upper respiratory infections are potentially more serious in infants than in adults primarily because:
    1. Infants cannot be given a well-balanced diet
    2. Infants have no ability to build up an immunity to disease
    3. Most infants cannot be given antibiotics
    4. The air passages of an infant are very small and are easily obstructed with mucus

33. An insulin-dependent diabetic tells the nurse she is thinking about beginning an exercise program and asks about the role of exercise in relation to her diet and medication. The nurse's response is based on the knowledge that:
    1. Exercise prevents hypoglycemia attacks
    2. Fruit or juice should be limited before exercising
    3. The blood sugar should be monitored before and after exercise
    4. Physical exercise is discouraged for insulin-dependent individuals

34. The *most* accurate method of evaluating fluid status in the patient with chronic renal failure is:
    1. Intake and output
    2. Daily BUN levels
    3. Daily weight
    4. Skin turgor

35. A patient is admitted with a diagnosis of delirium secondary to dehydration. Which of the following nursing interventions would be the *most appropriate* for her in her present condition?
    1. Acquaint her with the unit and her room
    2. Have her son leave a list of family numbers
    3. Explain the use of the call light and side rails
    4. Reorient her frequently to person and place

36. A patient is recovering from a right total hip arthroplasty. She uses a walker to aid her mobility. She has never been incontinent before but now finds herself having trouble making it to the bathroom on the second floor in time. Which type of incontinency is the patient experiencing?
    1. Functional incontinence
    2. Overflow incontinence
    3. Stress incontinence
    4. Urge incontinence

37. The physician has prescribed pilocarpine eye drops for the patient with glaucoma. This medication is given to:
    1. Dilate the pupil
    2. Decrease inflammation
    3. Promote drainage of aqueous humor
    4. Increase the production of aqueous humor

38. A patient with a pneumothorax has had a chest tube in place for 32 hours. Which finding would indicate that his lung has re-expanded?
    1. Fluctuation in the water-seal chamber
    2. Drainage changes in color from red to yellow
    3. Absence of bubbling in the water-seal chamber
    4. Continuous bubbling in the water-seal chamber

39. A 52 year old comes to the physician's office for a routine health screening. During the initial assessment, the nurse takes the patient's blood pressure. Where should the nurse position the stethoscope to best hear the blood pressure sounds?
    1. Over the radial artery
    2. Over the brachial artery
    3. Over the outer aspect of the antecubital fossa
    4. One half inch below the edge of the cuff

40. A child is to receive D_5RL at 50 ml/hr. A 500-ml bag of solution is available for the charge nurse to start the IV. How many hours will it take to infuse the 500 ml?
    1. 4 hours
    2. 6 hours
    3. 10 hours
    4. 15 hours

41. The nurse is reviewing the results of the CK-MB enzymes 6 hours after the admission of a patient with an acute myocardial infarction (MI). The nurse notes that the enzymes are elevated. These findings are indicative of the:
    1. Presence of infection
    2. Location of the myocardial infarct
    3. Evolution of the myocardial infarct
    4. Effects of heart disease on the kidneys

42. The physician orders a 1-day postoperative patient to sit in a dangling position for breakfast and sit in a chair for lunch. The patient asks if he can shower after breakfast. The *most appropriate* nursing response should be:
    1. "A shower will be alright, but I would like to assist you in dressing."
    2. "As long as you feel up to it, you may shower. Warm water may make you feel better."
    3. "Surgery often makes patients feel dizzy the first few times they get up; let's wait until you've been up longer."
    4. "You cannot take a shower until your dressing and stitches are removed completely by the doctor, probably before you go home."

43. A 1-day postoperative cesarean patient is reluctant to cough and deep-breathe because her "stomach hurts." Which of the following should the nurse do to help the patient cooperate with this nursing measure?
    1. Place the patient in a dangling position before the procedure
    2. Check her last pain medication time to see if she could have something to relieve the pain
    3. Explain the reasons why coughing and deep-breathing are necessary; stay with her and encourage her while she is trying to deep-breathe
    4. Tell the patient she will come back later when the patient is feeling better

44. A patient's daughter reports that her father has not had a formed bowel movement in several days and that he passes small amounts of water only. The nurse should proceed with which of the following?
    1. An order for a laxative
    2. An order for an antidiarrheal
    3. Assessment for a fecal impaction
    4. Assessment of the daughter's concern

45. The physician orders carbamazepine (Tegretol) 1.2 g/day in three divided doses. The medication is supplied in 100-mg tablets. How many tablets should be given per dose?
    1. 2 tablets
    2. 3 tablets
    3. 4 tablets
    4. 6 tablets

46. A mother asks if her daughter will ever be "cured" of her alcohol addiction. The nurse's *most appropriate* answer would be:
    1. "Yes, after she is sober for a long period of time."
    2. "No, because alcohol addiction is a chronic illness."
    3. "Alcohol addiction is not a disease."
    4. "Yes, if she does not already have permanent damage."

47. The long-term goal of rehabilitative nursing care in the elderly is to:
    1. Keep the patient alive as long as possible
    2. Help the patient achieve and maintain maximal physical, psychosocial, and spiritual health
    3. Help the patient maintain function within the home for as long as possible
    4. Promote compliance with the health care plan

48. Patient teaching for a patient receiving an anticonvulsant should include which of the following?
① Refraining from driving if drowsiness and dizziness occur
② Taking the medicine between meals and with milk
③ Stopping the medication if drowsiness occurs, and calling the physician
④ Use of sunscreen for photosensitivity only if the sun is extremely hot

49. A new mother asks if she can use a bottle prop when she is too busy to feed the baby. The nurse should base her response on the knowledge that bottle propping is:
① All right if the mother stays with the baby
② Considered dangerous because the baby might aspirate some of the formula while sucking
③ A safe and time-saving practice for busy mothers
④ Better than holding the baby during feeding

50. A patient had an emergency cesarean section under general anesthesia for cephalopelvic disproportion (CPD) at 3 AM this morning. She was delivered of an 8 lb 12 oz female infant with an Apgar score of 6. When the nurse first enters the patient's room, the patient asks, "Is my baby all right?" The nurse's *best response* should be:
① "I really don't know. When you see the nurse from the nursery, why don't you ask her?"
② "I'm sure the pediatrician will be in soon to give you a progress report."
③ "The nursery report this morning said she was progressing well. I will ask the nurse from the nursery to come and speak with you soon."
④ "Oh, I would not be too concerned. We give such good care that all our babies do real well."

51. A 27 year old woman is having contractions at 36 weeks' gestation. She asks if this is premature labor or false labor. The nurse tells her false labor:
① Often begins in the back
② Has a regular pattern
③ Often eases with ambulation
④ Is easily controlled with breathing techniques

52. A 5-year-old child has been hospitalized for a hernia repair in the morning. After his parents have left to eat supper, the child urinates in the bed. Which of the following best explains this occurrence?
① The child is spoiled
② The child is acting out
③ The child is regressing
④ The child is manipulative

53. A 32-year-old female is a homemaker and the mother of two boys. She complains of fatigue, nervousness, and irritability. A tentative diagnosis of hyperthyroidism is made. A finding that the nursing assessment is *most likely* to reveal is:
① Anorexia
② Weight gain
③ Constipation
④ Heat intolerance

54. The nurse suspects that tetany may be occurring if, following a thyroidectomy, the patient complains of:
① Joint pains and backache
② Excessive perspiration
③ Her fingers tingling
④ Voice weakness

55. The nurse evaluates the success of the postoperative interventions to maintain oxygenation. She knows that which of the following is indicative of decreased oxygen level?
① Bradycardia
② Ruddy complexion
③ Decreased breath sounds
④ Mental confusion, drowsiness

56. A rape victim asks the nurse what her options are if she is pregnant as a result of her assault. Which of the following is the *most appropriate* answer?
① The physician can prescribe hormone therapy
② Pregnancy as a result of rape is unlikely
③ An early abortion is her only option
④ She will be given a spermicidal douche

57. During a physical examination, an 8-year-old girl describes several incidents of sexual abuse by one of her teachers. Which of the following is the *first priority* of the nurse in this situation?
① Explain the psychologic effects of sexual abuse to her parents
② Prepare her for a pelvic examination by a physician
③ Inform local child protection authorities
④ Suggest that her parents confront the teacher

58. A patient returns from surgery following a tonsillectomy and adenoidectomy. In planning nursing care, the nurse knows the *best position* for this patient immediately after surgery is the:
① Prone position
② Side-lying position
③ Lithotomy position
④ Fowler's position

59. A patient in a situational crisis asks why the physician can't give her something like Valium to make her feel better. The nurse knows that the most important reason antianxiety drugs such as this are not prescribed to patients in crisis is:
① They have a high potential for abuse
② They do not address the underlying problem
③ They cause personality changes
④ They do not effectively treat the symptoms

60. Which of the following statements is the *best indication* that a patient with bipolar disorder has improved enough to be safely discharged to outpatient treatment?
① "I'm going to take lithium until I feel better."
② "I'm going to keep my therapy appointments every week."
③ "I'm going to pursue my dream of taking over IBM."
④ "I'm going to begin a new diet and redecorate my house."

61. A patient who has had a stroke is attempting to feed himself. He becomes easily frustrated as he tries to explain what he wants to eat. He cries and throws down his fork. This behavior supports a nursing diagnosis of:
① Anxiety, severe
② Diversional activity deficit
③ Sensory-perceptual alteration
④ Coping, individual ineffective

62. A patient, diagnosed with a deep vein thrombosis, is placed on strict bed rest with close observation. As the nurse prepares the thrombolytic agent, the patient asks what the medicine does and how it will help her leg. The nurse explains by stating:
    ① "The medicine thins the blood so that it will not clot anymore."
    ② "The agent inhibits the aggregation of platelets in the bloodstream."
    ③ "The medicine will prevent the formation of fibrin, which forms clots."
    ④ "The agent helps to dissolve the clot and will provide relief of the discomfort in your leg."

63. A 43 year old has been brought into the hospital because of a severe motor vehicle accident in which he suffered minor trauma. He states he is comfortable, with only slight shortness of breath, but is very anxious. He knows that he could have died and talks about it constantly. *From highest to lowest priority,* how should this patient's problems be ranked?
    ① Fear, anxiety, gas exchange
    ② Anxiety, gas exchange, fear
    ③ Gas exchange, fear, anxiety
    ④ Fear, gas exchange, anxiety

64. A pregnancy test is done, and the results are positive. The physician tells the nurse to position the patient for a vaginal exam. The nurse should place her in what *preferred* position?
    ① Horizontal recumbent
    ② Supine position
    ③ Dorsal recumbent
    ④ Lithotomy

65. Nursing implications for a patient on heparin include:
    ① Rotating sites in the abdomen if ordered subcutaneous
    ② Rubbing the site after a subcutaneous injection
    ③ Administering the medicine intramuscularly in the arm
    ④ Administering a continuous infusion by gravity

66. For a patient who abuses substances, inflicts frequent self harm, has multiple abusive/unstable relationships, and frequently threatens suicide, the nurse should suspect which of the following disorders?
    ① Character disorder
    ② Anxiety disorder
    ③ Borderline personality disorder
    ④ Substance abuse disorder

67. The nurse is to give heparin 8000 U SQ. The label reads 10,000 U/ml. How many ml should the nurse administer?
    ① 0.08 ml
    ② 0.8 ml
    ③ 0.825 ml
    ④ 1.8 ml

68. While caring for a fresh postoperative tonsillectomy and adenoidectomy patient, the nurse knows that the most common postoperative complication of a tonsillectomy is:
    ① Hemorrhage
    ② Abdominal pain
    ③ Loss of hearing
    ④ Loss of speech

69. A patient has been receiving a CNS depressant every 8 hours for several days. Upon entering the room to give him the 9 AM dose, the nurse notices that his pulse and respirations are slow, and he is drowsy and difficult to awaken. Upon further examination, the nurse notices that his pupils react sluggishly to light. The nurse should:
    ① Withhold the medication, raise the side rails, and call the physician
    ② Withhold the medication and observe him carefully over the next few hours
    ③ Administer the medication and observe him carefully over the next few hours
    ④ Administer the medication, raise the side rails, and instruct him not to get out of bed

70. The nurse is caring for a patient following a myocardial infarction (MI). The patient is to receive morphine sulfate 1/6 gr every 3 hours as needed for pain. The vial reads 15 mg/ml. How many milliliters will the nurse give?
    ① 1.0
    ② 0.5
    ③ 0.7
    ④ 1.5

71. In the nursing care plan for a patient who is suffering from an infected decubitus ulcer, the nurse would list which of these interventions as an independent nursing action?
    ① Arrange for a whirlpool bath qd by physical therapy
    ② Turn q2h (8 AM, 10 AM, 12 noon, etc), rotating right, left, and back
    ③ Administer penicillin PO q6h at 6 AM, 12 noon, 6 PM, 12 AM
    ④ Cleanse with hydrogen peroxide and apply Betadine q4h and with each dressing change

72. The *most important* nursing intervention in a situation of suspected child abuse in a school is:
    ① Discourage the keeping of secrets in the family
    ② Ensure the safety of the patient and other students
    ③ Help the child express her feelings about the abuse
    ④ Have the teacher removed from his or her position

73. A patient who just had a cesarean section asks why she cannot have something to drink, stating, "I have not had any water since 6 hours before I had my C-section." She begs for some ice water. The nurse's *best response* would be:
    ① "I know you are very thirsty. I will give you mouth care, and I'm sure you'll feel better."
    ② "I know you are very thirsty, and I would like to give you some water, but it is important that you not have anything by mouth until you are fully recovered from the effects of the anesthesia."
    ③ "The physician's orders said you cannot have any water until at least tomorrow, and then we will start with ice chips first."
    ④ "The IV handles all of your fluid needs, so why don't you rinse your mouth with mouthwash?"

74. When assessing a child's emotional response to alleged abuse, the nurse would be most likely to find that the child:
    ① Expects her parents to support and not blame her
    ② Uses familiar rituals to decrease her anxiety
    ③ Uses rationalization to cope with the abuse
    ④ Feels responsible for not stopping the abuse

75. A 24-hour-urine collection for creatinine clearance is ordered. The test is scheduled to end at 9 AM. The nurse would:
    ① Discard the 9 AM voiding and send the entire specimen to the laboratory
    ② Collect a final voiding at 9 AM and send with all the other collected urine to the laboratory
    ③ Instruct the patient to collect a specimen at 8:30 AM before sending it to the laboratory at 9 AM
    ④ Instruct the patient to obtain a clean-catch, mid-stream urine for the final urine specimen

76. Which of the following is of *primary importance* during the detoxification phase of the substance-addicted patient's hospitalization?
    ① Increase interpersonal skills
    ② Encourage group participation
    ③ Increase the patient's sense of responsibility
    ④ Prevent or treat symptoms of acute withdrawal

77. A patient is to receive intermittent feedings q4h through the Levine tube. The physician orders a total of 2800 calories and no more than 3000 ml in 24 hours. The feeding is supplied in 240-ml cans, with 1 ml = 1 calorie. How many cans should be given q4h?
    ① 1.5 cans
    ② 2 cans
    ③ 2.5 cans
    ④ 6 cans

78. Which of the following signs would alert the nurse that a postoperative tonsillectomy and adenoidectomy patient is bleeding excessively?
    ① Flushed face; bright red bleeding; loss of consciousness
    ② Tarry stools; restlessness; loss of consciousness
    ③ Frequent swallowing; restlessness; spitting up bright-red blood
    ④ Elevated temperature; decreased respirations; decreased pulse

79. In caring for a child with croup, it is necessary for the nurse to know that croup is characterized by:
    ① An infection of the pharynx
    ② Spasms of the larynx with partial obstruction of the respiratory tract
    ③ Contractions of the trachea
    ④ Inflammation of the lung tissue

80. When a postoperative tonsillectomy and adenoidectomy patient is allowed liquids, it would be best to give her:
    ① Fresh orange juice
    ② A popsicle or Gatorade
    ③ Hot tea or coffee
    ④ Ice cream

81. A patient is started on iron therapy. A liquid preparation is prescribed. Which patient statement indicates the need for additional teaching?
    ① "I will take the medication with meals."
    ② "A straw is necessary to prevent teeth staining."
    ③ "I'll report diarrhea and light-colored stools."
    ④ "Taking orange juice will help with absorption of the medication."

82. An infant patient is scheduled to receive ampicillin 250 mg orally. The label on the bottle reads "125 mg/5 ml." How much does the nurse administer?
    ① 1.5 ml
    ② 4 ml
    ③ 2.5 ml
    ④ 10 ml

83. A patient is being discharged on a monoamine oxidase inhibitor. During the patient teaching session, the nurse should instruct the patient to:
    ① Avoid bananas and yogurt; take the medicine prn
    ② Avoid seasonings and milk; be compliant in taking the medication
    ③ Avoid aged cheese, red wines, and beer; be consistent in taking the medication
    ④ Avoid colas and fruit; be consistent in taking the medication

84. Which of the following problems commonly results from chronic renal failure?
    ① Anemia
    ② Hypotension
    ③ Hypokalemia
    ④ Weight loss

85. A 35-year-old insulin-dependent diabetic is admitted to the hospital because her blood sugar has been difficult to regulate. The nurse knows that significant hyperglycemia is often manifested by:
    ① Dehydration, nausea/vomiting; elevated serum glucose levels
    ② Pale, cool, clammy skin; restlessness and irritability
    ③ Lowered serum glucose levels; negative urine glucose
    ④ Drowsiness, moist skin, perspiration, and tremors

86. The patient is started on hemodialysis three times a week. An arteriovenous fistula is created in the right arm. Specific nursing interventions include:
    ① Palpating the access for a thrill
    ② Keeping the right arm in a dependent position
    ③ Taking the blood pressure in the affected arm
    ④ Teaching the patient to keep the arm protected and covered

87. Considering the age factor, which of the following blood pressure values should the nurse recognize as abnormal and report for a 52-year-old patient?
    ① 128/84
    ② 136/74
    ③ 118/64
    ④ 132/94

88. A postpartum patient with an episiotomy has a heat lamp ordered to the perineal area. To provide this treatment the nurse should:
    ① Warm up the heat lamp thoroughly before applying heat
    ② Use a 60-watt bulb
    ③ Place the light 18 to 24 inches from the site
    ④ Allow the patient to use the light for 30 min

89. The condition of a pediatric patient with croup has improved with treatment, and he is ready for discharge from the hospital. To promote rest, which of these instructions should the nurse give the mother?
    ① Sedate him every 4 hours
    ② Place him in a dark room
    ③ Allow him to stay with her at all times
    ④ Provide a quiet environment as much as possible

90. A 15-year-old girl is admitted to the hospital after losing 25% of her normal body weight in a 2-month period. The diagnosis is restricting anorexia. What is the nurse's *first priority* for this patient?
    ① Exploring her feelings about her body
    ② Assessing her physiologic status
    ③ Discussing her relationship with her family
    ④ Planning a meal and exercise schedule

91. In which situation would the nurse anticipate using NPH insulin?
    ① For "sliding scale" coverage
    ② For managing acute hypoglycemia
    ③ For daily injection to control disease
    ④ In the emergency of diabetic ketoacidosis

92. Dietary management for the patient with chronic renal failure usually includes:
    ① Providing high-carbohydrate liquid supplements
    ② Restricting protein, sodium, and potassium
    ③ Increasing protein and sodium intake
    ④ Decreasing fat intake

93. Which of the following is the *most appropriate* short-term goal for a person with restricting anorexia?
    ① To encourage expression of feelings
    ② To alter the patient's body image
    ③ To promote peer relationships
    ④ To restore safe nutritional status

94. Which of the following statements is *most* descriptive of hemodialysis?
    ① Blood is circulated through a filter by the patient's own arterial system
    ② Chemical substances are removed from the blood through a vascular access
    ③ Toxic substances are removed from the body through the peritoneal cavity
    ④ The process is continuous through a permanent peritoneal catheter

95. The respiratory therapist explains the use of the incentive spirometer to a surgery patient who is a smoker. When the therapist leaves, the patient states the device is not needed and is a waste of money. The nurse should explain that the spirometer:
    ① Is a standard procedure for patients his age
    ② Provides better aeration to the lungs after surgery
    ③ Is needed to expand the alveoli after surgery because of the anesthetics given and his smoking history
    ④ Loosens the secretions that could exist as a result of the anesthetics given in surgery and his smoking history

96. A patient is brought to the emergency department by her son for evaluation after she becomes suddenly ill. The examining physician makes a diagnosis of delirium. Which of the following statements made by the patient's son best supports this diagnosis?
    ① "Mom has become so forgetful over the past 6 months."
    ② "She was perfectly fine until late this afternoon."
    ③ "Maybe we should expect this; she's 75."
    ④ "My uncle's death has made her very depressed."

97. The nurse would explain to a surgery patient about to be discharged when to report to the physician concerning changes in the incision. The nurse's explanation should include reporting:
    ① Any coolness or swelling at the incision site
    ② Soreness and bruising at the incision site
    ③ Signs of inflammation or infection
    ④ Redness, warmth, or severe pain at the incision site

98. A 60-year-old man being treated through the outpatient clinic is receiving external radiation therapy to the chest area. The skin over the treatment area is dry and red. The nurse instructs him in skin care. Which of the following statements indicates that he understands the teaching?
    ① "I will apply lotion to the dry areas daily."
    ② "I will make an effort to wear loose-fitting clothing."
    ③ "An astringent will be used after washing the site thoroughly."
    ④ "To help strengthen the skin, I will use rubbing alcohol on the area."

99. On entering the patient's room, the nurse finds the 9 month old being rocked by his mother. The mother is crying softly. After the nurse checks the vital signs, she asks the mother, "How is the baby doing today?" The mother replies, "I thought he was going to die when his respirations were so fast this afternoon." What is the *best response* by the nurse?
    ① "Yes, we too thought he would die."
    ② "It must have been very frightening for you."
    ③ "Don't be silly, we don't let 9-month-old kids die."
    ④ The nurse should say nothing and just finish the assessment

100. The immediate short-term goal for a patient in situational crisis should be to:
    ① Explore family relationships
    ② Decrease any somatic symptoms
    ③ Get her started with insight-oriented therapy
    ④ Encourage her to verbalize concerns

101. A 2-day postoperative patient, who has a vascular access in her right arm for dialysis due to renal failure, is scheduled to begin dialysis when the incision heals. Which of the following should be reported *immediately?*
    ① Abnormal blood pressure in the right arm
    ② Absence of a thrill over the vascular access
    ③ Complaint of soreness in the right arm
    ④ Fear of catching AIDS from the dialysis procedure

102. The nurse begins teaching the patient with angina about the use of sublingual nitroglycerin (NTG). Which statement indicates that the patient understands how to use the medication?
    ① "I'll take it after doing any exercising."
    ② "I'll take it at bedtime to prevent nighttime attacks."
    ③ "I'll take it every 6 to 8 hours to prevent any chest pain."
    ④ "I'll take it as soon as I notice any sign of chest pain."

103. Discharge teaching has been completed for the patient who has had a total laryngectomy. Which written statement by the patient indicates the need for additional teaching about home care?
    ① "When coughing, I will cover my stoma instead of my mouth."
    ② "I will check my stoma for signs of redness or swelling."
    ③ "I will clean the stoma area daily with a deodorant-type soap."
    ④ "A protective cover will be needed when I shave or have my hair cut."

104. The plan of care for the patient with hyperthyroidism should include:
    ① Limiting caloric intake
    ② Providing a restful environment
    ③ Applying emollients for dry skin
    ④ Maintaining the room temperature at above normal levels

105. The way in which patients in a situational crisis handle their current problem is *most determined* by:
    ① The level of support from their family
    ② The way that they have coped in the past
    ③ Their ability to change their life-style
    ④ The amount of therapy they receive

106. A friend's daughter comes home with a note that she has head lice. The mother doesn't know what to do other than buy some lindane (Kwell) to shampoo her daughter's hair. The nurse should also advise the mother to:
    ① Shampoo the hair for 15 minutes before rinsing
    ② Shampoo the hair again the next day and repeat the same process
    ③ Use a comb dipped in vinegar to comb out the nits after the shampoo
    ④ Wash linen and clothing only if desired; the head lice was confined to the child's hair

107. Early signs of exophthalmos are observed in the patient with hyperthyroidism. Which symptom is typical of this condition?
    ① Blurring of vision
    ② Protrusion of the eyeballs
    ③ Watery discharge from the eyes
    ④ Inability to distinguish colors

108. In preparation for a patient's home care following a cervical spinal injury, the nurse is teaching the patient and his family how to recognize signs and symptoms of complications that can develop because of his spinal injuries. He is encouraged to increase his intake of fluids *mainly* because:
    ① The replacement is needed for fluids lost during perspiration
    ② Fluids decrease the incidence of pulmonary infection
    ③ Fluids decrease the formation of urinary calculi
    ④ Fluids reduce the possibility of spinal shock

109. A patient who is in isolation due to constant coughing and suspected tuberculosis is scheduled for a chest x-ray tomorrow morning. The nurse will initiate which of these plans?
    ① Place a mask and gown on the patient as he travels to the radiology department
    ② Notify the charge nurse about requesting an order for a portable chest x-ray
    ③ Contact the infection control nurse about the scheduled test
    ④ Contact the radiologists and suggest that the technicians wear masks during the procedure

110. A finding characteristic of spinal shock is:
    ① Hypertension
    ② Bradycardia
    ③ Spasticity
    ④ Seizures

111. A patient has a laceration to the lower part of her leg and an ulcer at her ankle that needs irrigating every day. The nurse should prepare her for the treatment by placing her in which position?
    ① Lying down flat on the stretcher
    ② Dangling her leg over the side of the stretcher
    ③ Lying down with the foot of the stretcher elevated
    ④ Sitting in a chair with the leg elevated on the stretcher

112. Which of the following nursing assessments is a *priority* following spontaneous rupture of membranes?
    ① Station
    ② Contractions
    ③ Fetal heart tones
    ④ Maternal vital signs

113. While assisting a diabetic patient with morning care, the nurse notices the patient's toenails are long and unkempt. After talking to her about her nails, the nurse realizes she does not understand correct foot care for a diabetic patient. The nurse should instruct the patient to:
    ① Assess her feet occasionally for cuts
    ② Wear clean socks and carefully trim her nails
    ③ Wear socks if preferred and trim her nails when desired
    ④ Assess her feet occasionally and wear clean white socks

114. A 35-year-old multipara at term is admitted to the emergency department having contractions every 4 to 6 minutes lasting for 30 to 40 seconds. She states that her physician told her she has a marginal placenta previa. Which of the following is *most important* for the nurse to note on her plan of care?
    ① Schedule for ultrasound immediately
    ② No vaginal examinations
    ③ Pad count
    ④ Type and cross match for 2 units of packed red blood cells

115. A patient is receiving a blood transfusion. Thirty minutes after the transfusion started, the patient complained of respiratory distress and dyspnea. His pulse rate increased from 80 to 110. These symptoms *most likely* indicate what type of problem?
    ① Febrile reaction
    ② Allergic reaction
    ③ Hemolytic reaction
    ④ Circulatory overload

116. Neurologic assessment of the lower extremities of a patient with an acute spinal fracture at the cervical level would reveal:
    ① Absent deep-tendon reflexes
    ② Hyperactive deep-tendon reflexes
    ③ Increasingly higher levels of sensory paralysis
    ④ Absent temperature sensation bilaterally above the injury

117. The physician orders a loading dose of aminophylline. The order reads "aminophylline 250 mg in 100 ml D₅W to infuse at 33 gtt/min, followed by an aminophylline drip." The drop factor is 10. The charge nurse hangs the loading dose. How long will this intravenous piggyback take to infuse?
    ① 20 min
    ② 30 min
    ③ 45 min
    ④ 60 min

118. A 20 year old is brought to the hospital following a diving accident. He states that he is unable to move or feel his legs. His neck has been immobilized. Initial diagnostic studies indicate a C5-C6 fracture. Crutchfield tongs are inserted, and 10 lb of traction applied. The parents ask the nurse about the seriousness of the injury. The nurse's *best* response is to:
    ① Inform them that their son will be confined to a wheelchair and will require mechanical ventilation
    ② Reassure the family that he will be back to his pre-injury status but it will take a couple of months
    ③ Inform the parents that it is too early to know the full extent of the injury
    ④ Reassure the parents that their son will regain function before long

119. The nurse is caring for a patient in the third stage of labor. Signs of placental separation include:
    ① Increase in vaginal bleeding
    ② Shortening of the umbilical cord
    ③ Softening of the uterus
    ④ Increase in pulsations of the umbilical cord

120. The incorporation of Crutchfield tongs and traction into the plan of care following an acute cervical injury/fracture is to:
    ① Allow the patient to maintain normal head and neck movement
    ② Align the injured vertebrae and reduce muscle spasm
    ③ Provide support for the lower extremities
    ④ Prevent the development of spinal shock

121. A patient in active labor is in a supine position and on a uterine and fetal monitor. Vital signs show a pulse of 88, blood pressure of 130/82, and respirations of 24. Her labor progresses, and 2 hours later the nurse notes a pulse of 98 and blood pressure of 102/70. The nurse's next action should be:
    ① Place the patient in modified Trendelenburg's position
    ② Turn the patient to the left side
    ③ Administer oxygen and notify the physician
    ④ Check for fetal heart rate changes

122. A newborn has tested positive for phenylketonuria (PKU). The nurse knows that a sample of the infant's blood will contain abnormal amounts of:
    ① Tyrosine
    ② Phenylalanine
    ③ Phenylpyruvic acid
    ④ Phenylalanine hydroxylase

123. Phenylketonuria (PKU) is caused by an inherited error of metabolism which, if untreated, will result in:
    ① Hepatic coma
    ② Renal shutdown
    ③ Mental retardation
    ④ Epileptic seizures

124. A patient with hyperthyroidism begins taking propylthiouracil (PTU). The nurse should instruct the patient to report a(n):
    ① Pulse rate above 100
    ② Increased body weight
    ③ Metallic taste in her mouth
    ④ Sore throat, rash, or fever

125. In planning a diet for a patient with phenylketonuria, the nurse knows that the diet therapy will be based on the knowledge that the nutrients to be controlled are:
    ① Fats
    ② Minerals
    ③ Proteins
    ④ Carbohydrates

COMPREHENSIVE EXAMINATION TWO: PART 2

126. Which of the following is the *most* important factor for the nurse to remember when planning how best to work with adolescent patients?
    ① Their general dislike of adults
    ② Their need to experiment with substances
    ③ Their level of cognitive ability to consider consequences
    ④ Their natural mistrust of health-care providers

127. Laboratory reports reveal that a patient has leukopenia. Specific nursing interventions will include:
    ① Avoiding injections or rectal temperatures
    ② Provisions for adequate periods of rest
    ③ Protecting from infections
    ④ The liberal use of antiemetics

128. The nurse is explaining to her patient that the communicable disease that affects the parotid glands near the ear and jaw is called:
    ① Measles
    ② Mumps
    ③ Scarlet fever
    ④ Chicken pox

129. A patient complains of severe chest pain, and the nurse prepares to administer his *first* dose of nitrate. The nurse should follow which of these procedures?
    ① Take his pulse and blood pressure, then administer a transdermal patch
    ② Take his pulse and blood pressure, then administer sublingual nitrate
    ③ Administer sublingual nitrate immediately, then take his pulse and blood pressure
    ④ Before administering the nitrate, obtain a detailed medical history to be sure the pain is related to angina

130. The nurse should teach a new mother that the *best* way to ensure the infant has an adequate supply of breast milk is for her to:
    ① Follow a daily exercise program
    ② Drink generous amounts of milk each day
    ③ Eat a high-protein diet
    ④ Allow the infant to empty each breast at each feeding

131. In planning nursing care for a child with whooping cough, the nurse needs to consider that the child with whooping cough:
    ① Is severely ill
    ② Usually has to be hospitalized in the intensive care unit
    ③ May become physically exhausted from coughing
    ④ Does not require medical treatment

132. Bladder retraining is to be started because the patient developed incontinence as a result of a stroke. Which of the following actions is usually included in a training program?
    ① Limit fluid intake during the day
    ② Offer the urinal q2h
    ③ Check for residual urine after each voiding
    ④ Use disposable adult diapers to protect the skin

133. A patient's family asks when her symptoms of depression are going to get better. What is the nurse's *best response*?
    ① "As soon as she makes up her mind to get better."
    ② "There is no way to tell how long she will be depressed."
    ③ "We need more information to determine how long she might be ill."
    ④ "We will know better in another week."

134. Assessment of the patient admitted with a history of a stroke reveals a right hemiplegia. To avoid aspiration, the patient would be instructed to *avoid*:
    ① Sitting up for meals
    ② Lying down immediately after meals
    ③ Swallowing with his head slightly flexed
    ④ Placing liquids in the left side of the mouth

135. A patient in active labor requests medication for pain, and the physician orders meperidine (Demerol) 50 mg IM. The nurse should know that:
    ① This is not a correct dose
    ② The newborn infant will require Narcan
    ③ Meperidine is given only orally
    ④ Meperidine is a narcotic analgesic

136. A 5 year old was admitted to the hospital for diagnostic studies and heart surgery for repair of tetralogy of Fallot. The nurse should expect a child with tetralogy of Fallot to exhibit which of the following clinical manifestations?
    ① Skin with a bluish tint; favoring of squatting position
    ② Skin with a natural pink color; clubbing of the fingers and toes
    ③ Retarded growth, but usually normal in intelligence
    ④ Hypertension in the upper extremities and hypotension in the lower extremities

137. Before administering the bronchodilator metaproterenol sulfate (Alupent), the nurse should obtain a relevant nursing history, note the character of the sputum, and obtain which of the following?
    ① Baseline temperature
    ② Baseline heart rate
    ③ Sputum specimen for culture
    ④ Blood specimens ordered

138. A patient asks the nurse if he can "have a date" after his discharge from the hospital. The *best response* by the nurse would be:
① Nothing; ignore the question
② Nothing; she shouldn't speak to him again until discharge
③ To go over the goals of their relationship
④ To tell him she is upset by his request

139. Which of the following nursing diagnoses addresses the *highest priority* for a patient hospitalized with symptoms of depression?
① Anxiety related to unfamiliar environment
② Fluid volume deficit related to limited intake
③ Nutritional deficit related to limited intake
④ Ineffective family coping related to hospitalization

140. A patient has been scheduled for a stat cesarean delivery because of abruptio placentae. As the nurse assists in transporting her to the delivery room, she should expect to observe:
① Profuse vaginal bleeding
② A tense, painful abdomen
③ Strong, spasmodic contractions
④ Painless, bright red vaginal drainage

141. The nurse finds her patient huddled in his room with a frightened look on his face. He says, "The voices are back, telling me to do bad things." The nurse's *best response* is:
① "Listen to my voice, not to what they are telling you."
② "We'll put you into seclusion until the voices stop."
③ "I don't hear anything like that."
④ "Let's go find something for you to do."

142. According to experts who have studied its incidence and occurrence, rape is *best* defined as:
① An act of sexual frustration
② An act of sexual aggression
③ An act of sexual dominance
④ An act of sexual ambivalence

143. A child is seen in the pediatric clinic for iron deficiency, and the physician prescribes an iron supplement. Home care instructions for the patient include teaching the mother to:
① Mix the iron product with the child's milk to disguise the flavor
② Use a dropper to drop the medication directly into the child's mouth
③ Place the medication on a cookie and have the child eat the cookie
④ Mix the iron product with juice to disguise the flavor and have the child use a straw

144. A patient has a generalized seizure. After the seizure activity ceases, the nurse should implement which nursing action *first?*
① Insert an airway
② Position him on his side
③ Take vital signs
④ Begin oxygen administration

145. A 55-year-old patient is admitted for observation. The history reveals changes in level of consciousness and a possible cerebrovascular accident (CVA). The plan of care includes assessment of the patient's level of consciousness using the Glasgow Coma Scale. With this tool, the nurse assesses the patient's:
① Emotional reactions
② Intellectual functioning
③ Best motor and verbal responses
④ Lower extremity strength and gait

146. Which of the following immunizations should the nurse recommend to the mother of a child before he starts kindergarten?
① Diphtheria-pertussis-tetanus (DPT) injections only if he did not receive them during infancy
② DPT booster, even if he had the injection during infancy
③ Active immunization against chicken pox
④ Immunization against cholera

147. After receiving a narcotic for incisional pain, a patient's vital signs are blood pressure 100/60, pulse 68, and shallow respirations at 8/min. The physician is notified and orders the narcotic antagonist naloxone [Narcan]. After administering naloxone, the nurse should assess for return of the pain and:
① A further drop in blood pressure
② A drop in the pulse rate
③ An increase in respirations in about 15 to 20 minutes
④ A decrease in respirations in about 15 to 20 minutes

148. Which of the following responses by a mother indicates her understanding of discharge instructions for her baby, born with Down syndrome?
① "The baby should be fed a little more often in order to gain weight."
② "The baby should be dressed very warmly to prevent colds."
③ "The baby should not have visitors for several weeks."
④ "The baby has a higher risk of upper respiratory infections than do other babies."

149. A frightened patient comes to the emergency room for treatment after coming home from class to find a man in her apartment who raped her. The nurse knows that rapists and their victims come primarily from which population group?
① Poor and lower-class whites
② Young blacks between 25 and 35 years of age
③ All ethnic and socioeconomic groups
④ Single urban Latinos

150. As the emergency room nurse interviews a rape victim, she finds the patient to be calm, able to answer questions without hesitation, and in apparent control, with no evidence of anger, fear, or tearfulness. What is the *most likely* explanation for her behavior?
① She has calmed down since being raped
② She is in a state of emotional shock
③ She agreed to have sex with her assailant
④ She is using intellectualization to cope

151. A 2-year-old girl is brought into the well-baby clinic for a checkup. The average vital signs for a 2 year old should be:
    ① Heart rate 110; respirations 25, blood pressure 96/68
    ② Heart rate 120, respirations 35, blood pressure 70/50
    ③ Heart rate 88, respirations 19, blood pressure 110/70
    ④ Heart rate 100, respirations 21, blood pressure 105/70

152. After administering one nitroglycerin tablet sublingually to a patient, a nurse evaluates his condition and finds that he is still complaining of pain and has a blood pressure of 80/50. The nurse would *first:*
    ① Wait another 3 minutes and take the blood pressure again before giving another dose of nitroglycerin
    ② Call the physician immediately and withhold the second dose of nitroglycerin
    ③ Elevate his feet (unless contraindicated) and give another dose of nitroglycerin
    ④ Elevate his feet (unless contraindicated), withhold the medication, and notify the physician

153. When checking the head dressing following intracranial surgery, the nurse notes the presence of clear drainage from the ear. The patient is also complaining of a postnasal drip. Which nursing action is *most* appropriate?
    ① Notify the physician
    ② Circle the drainage, noting the date and time
    ③ Recognize that this is normal mucus drainage
    ④ Reinforce the dressing until the physician arrives

154. After being admitted to the psychiatric unit, a patient refuses to get out of bed to shower, have breakfast, or join in unit activities. The *best action* for the nurse to take is:
    ① Ignore the patient's lack of participation
    ② Set small goals and stay with the patient while she completes them
    ③ Encourage the patient to be active but do not force her
    ④ Restrict the patient's phone calls until she follows the rules

155. A patient receiving external radiation therapy is concerned about being "radioactive." The nurse tells the patient that:
    ① The external radiation effects are generalized to all body systems
    ② He is radioactive only while he is receiving the therapy
    ③ Only his urine and bodily secretions are radioactive
    ④ He is not radioactive

156. The nurse administered a theophylline preparation PO to a 3 year old with asthma. Vital signs are temperature 100.1° F (37.8° C) axillary, apical pulse 90, respirations 28. One hour after the administration of theophylline (Theo-Dur), the nurse notes the patient has a pulse of 110. The nurse identifies this as:
    ① An expected outcome
    ② A side effect
    ③ The desired effect
    ④ A toxic effect

157. Which of the following characteristics should the nursery nurse observe for when Down syndrome is suspected in an infant?
    ① Blue hands and feet; irregular respirations at birth
    ② The presence of inner epicanthal folds; small ears
    ③ Head circumference larger than chest circumference
    ④ The infant's arms and legs are flexed on the chest and abdomen

158. An 83-year-old man has a history of congestive heart failure and beginning renal failure. The nurse should be *most* concerned about which principle of drug action?
    ① Absorption
    ② Distribution
    ③ Metabolism
    ④ Excretion

159. The nurse is caring for a patient who has had intracranial surgery. A possible pituitary problem is suspected when the nurse notes which of the following?
    ① An increased temperature
    ② Sluggish pupil reaction to light
    ③ Clear drainage on the head dressing
    ④ Increased output of low-specific-gravity urine

160. In reviewing breast self-examination (BSE) information, the nurse instructs the patient to:
    ① Conduct the examination before her menstrual period
    ② Check the breast while positioning herself in both supine and erect positions
    ③ Perform the examination on a weekly schedule
    ④ Use the palm of the hand for the examination

161. A patient who is admitted with a threatened abortion has symptoms that include cramping with moderate bleeding. In addition to bed rest and vital sign assessment, the nurse's *major* goal for the patient should be to:
    ① Prepare for immediate surgery
    ② Replace electrolytes promptly
    ③ Provide supportive emotional care
    ④ Prepare for oxytocin administration

162. A patient who is 1 day postpartum and not breastfeeding tells the nurse she has noticed a significant increase in bleeding, as she has saturated several pads. The nurse's first action should be to:
    ① Assess vital signs including blood pressure
    ② Turn her on her side
    ③ Encourage fluids PO
    ④ Palpate her fundus and massage until firm

163. A patient whose newborn has been diagnosed with Down syndrome asks the nurse, "How retarded will my baby be? What will he be able to do?" Which of the following statements is the *best response* by the nurse?
    ① "Only genetic counseling can determine the extent of the disability."
    ② "Most children with Down syndrome eventually become self-sufficient."
    ③ "Children with Down syndrome are generally severely retarded."
    ④ "It is not possible to determine the extent of the disabilities at this time."

164. A patient is scheduled for a right modified radical mastectomy. The patient tells the nurse that she is anxious and afraid of the surgery. She is fearful that she might even die during the procedure. What would be the nurse's *best* response?
① "Why are you afraid of the surgery?"
② "Try to get as much rest as possible before surgery."
③ "Those must be frightening feelings. Tell me more about them."
④ "Don't worry, you won't die. That type of procedure is quite perfected and is done often."

165. The nurse explains to a patient that German measles are also known as:
① Red measles
② Roseola
③ Scarlet fever
④ Rubella

166. An 11-year-old girl is admitted to the hospital with severe abdominal pain, vomiting, and a temperature of 101° F (38.3° C). The physician diagnosed her as being in sickle cell crisis. The nurse knows that sickle cell anemia results from:
① An infection in the blood
② Failure to follow a correct diet
③ Malformed cells clumped together
④ White blood cells attacking red blood cells

167. The nurse administers the same medication to a patient that he has been taking at home. He states that the medicine still works, but lately it seems to take more of the drug to be effective. The nurse should consult the physician after suspecting which of the following:
① Tolerance
② Additive effect
③ Idiosyncratic reaction
④ Psychologic dependence

168. The 16-year-old patient is having his annual sports physical before the start of the football season. He has had all of his childhood immunizations. The nurse recognizes that the patient needs which of the following vaccines at this time?
① Diphtheria and polio
② Diphtheria and tetanus
③ Tetanus and pertussis
④ Polio and pertussis

169. A patient, pregnant with her first child, asks the nurse about where conception takes place. The nurse notes this as an opportune teaching moment and responds that conception takes place in the:
① Uterus
② Corpus luteum
③ Vagina
④ Fallopian tubes

170. Which of the following possible nursing interventions for a victim of rape should be implemented *first?*
① Discuss evaluation for sexually transmitted diseases
② Discuss the possible need for postcoital contraception
③ Discuss community resources and possible referrals
④ Discuss and identify her immediate needs and concerns

171. The test that is used to determine if a breast lump is benign or malignant is:
① Biopsy
② Ultrasonography
③ Xeroradiography
④ Computed tomography (CT)

172. While doing discharge planning for the patient, the nurse stresses the importance of taking the prescribed dose of interferon at bedtime with acetaminophen (Tylenol). Why is this important?
① To decrease nausea and vomiting
② To lower fever
③ To treat associated sore throat
④ To minimize flu-like symptoms

173. On the third day of hospitalization, a patient voices several complaints. The complaint that should alert the nurse to possible digitalis toxicity would be:
① "My back hurts today."
② "I'm so nauseated and I have no appetite."
③ "I feel like I've put on 5 pounds."
④ "I'm too tired to sleep well at night."

174. In caring for a patient in the early period after vaginal delivery, which of these measures by the nurse is *most essential?*
① Keep environmental stimulation at a minimum
② Offer her frequent sips of water
③ Be certain that the uterus remains contracted
④ Take her temperature q4h

175. A 16 year old is brought to an outpatient clinic for alcohol counseling. She admits to drinking but denies she has a problem, stating that she hates her parents. According to Erickson, the developmental issue facing this patient is:
① Autonomy vs. shame and doubt
② Industry vs. inferiority
③ Intimacy vs. isolation
④ Identity vs. identity diffusion

176. A 39 year old, scheduled for a tubal ligation tomorrow, has a health history that reveals that she smokes two packs of cigarettes a day, is overweight by 50 lb, and is a borderline hypertensive. Following surgery, the *priority* nursing diagnosis for this patient is:
① Ineffective individual coping related to lack of support system
② Impaired physical mobility: ambulation related to abdominal discomfort
③ Potential ineffective airway clearance related to smoking
④ Alteration in nutrition: greater than body requirements, related to excessive caloric intake

177. Which of the following is an appropriate goal for a psychiatric patient to increase his socialization?
① Join a singles dating service
② Join a social skills outpatient group
③ Volunteer in his local community
④ Become more involved in his church

178. A 16 year old has been diagnosed with anorexia nervosa. She has lost 24 pounds in 3 months. She weighs 102 pounds and is 5 feet 4 inches tall. The patient tells the nurse that she is still overweight until her hands and feet get smaller. The *priority* nursing diagnosis for this patient is:
    ① Altered nutrition: less than body requirements related to lack of interest in eating
    ② Body image disturbance related to distorted perceptions
    ③ Impaired social interactions related to manipulative behavior
    ④ Potential for violence: self-directed, related to suicidal feelings

179. A nursing intervention in the plan of care for a patient with hypothyroidism should include:
    ① Providing a calm, nonstimulating environment
    ② Providing high-calorie dietary supplements
    ③ Providing a warm environment
    ④ Testing urine for glucose

180. A 19-year-old male is hospitalized for an appendectomy. Nursing history reveals that he has a seizure disorder and that he has seizures when he is sick. The patient has a generalized seizure when the nurse is in the room. Which of the following nursing actions is appropriate during the seizure?
    ① Insert a padded tongue blade
    ② Notify the physician immediately
    ③ Remain with the patient
    ④ Restrain his extremities if possible

181. During a patient's admission assessment, she tells the nurse that she has not been eating, has been unable to sleep through the night for the past 3 months, and cannot seem to concentrate on any task long enough to finish it. The symptoms that the patient is describing are *most likely* a result of:
    ① An affective disorder
    ② A personality disorder
    ③ A substance abuse disorder
    ④ A thought disorder

182. When Down syndrome is suspected, the nursery nurse should carefully assess which of the following?
    ① Heart sounds
    ② Cognitive deficits
    ③ Visual impairments
    ④ Hearing impairments

183. A patient has admitted that he does not take the prescribed fluphenazine (Prolixin) every day. What is the *best way* for the nurse to increase the likelihood that he will be more compliant about taking his medication following discharge?
    ① Ask his family to administer his medication
    ② Ask him to come to the clinic to get his medication
    ③ Ask him when the best time is for him to take his medication
    ④ Inform him that his physician can prescribe an injectable long-acting form

184. Immediately after returning to his room from the recovery room, a patient complains of severe pain at his incision site. He has a narcotic analgesic ordered for pain q4h prn. The nurse should withhold the medication if:
    ① Vital signs were equal to or within the range before surgery
    ② Oxygen was still being administered and respirations were 18
    ③ Pain medication was administered in the recovery room an hour before returning to the room
    ④ Proper positioning and preparation of a quiet environment did not provide relief

185. Which of the following is the most important aspect of the relationship of the nurse to the patient in crisis?
    ① The nurse provides primary emotional support for the patient
    ② The nurse identifies the most appropriate resources for the patient
    ③ The nurse assists the patient to regain equilibrium
    ④ The nurse supports the patient's significant others

186. When collecting admission information from a patient diagnosed with hypothyroidism, the nurse should expect the patient to complain about:
    ① Exophthalmos
    ② Fine tremors
    ③ Heat intolerance
    ④ Facial puffiness

187. A congenital disorder characterized by protrusion of the abdominal organs through an abnormal opening in the abdominal wall, forming a sac lying on the abdomen, is otherwise known as:
    ① Esophageal atresia
    ② Omphalocele
    ③ Hirschsprung's disease
    ④ Pyloric stenosis

188. Combination intravenous chemotherapy is planned for a patient with cancer. The patient asks why there are numerous side effects associated with the administration of the medications. The nurse's response is based on the knowledge that:
    ① Side effects are limited to single-agent chemotherapy
    ② Rapidly dividing normal and abnormal cells are destroyed
    ③ Chemotherapeutic drugs administered intravenously have less side effects
    ④ Side effects will be minimal if the medications are given as a one-time dose

189. Which of the following agents is (are) used to promote fertility?
    ① Rho-gam
    ② Ergot alkaloids
    ③ Androgens
    ④ Human chorionic gonadotropin

190. A 13 month old is admitted to the hospital with a fracture of the right femur. She is accompanied by both parents, each of whom provides a different story. Child abuse is suspected. The nurse knows that legal aspects of child abuse require that she:
① Report her findings to a physician
② Report this as a known or suspected case of child abuse
③ Exercise caution; reporting does not grant immunity from civil suits
④ Exercise caution; this is considered privileged communication

191. Postoperative care following a right modified radical mastectomy will include:
① Limiting movement of the right arm
② Keeping the right arm below heart level
③ Instructions to use her left arm for such activities as hair brushing
④ Posting signs warning against taking blood pressure or drawing blood from the right arm

192. When administering nose drops to an infant, the nurse should:
① Hold the infant in a sitting position during and after the procedure
② Place the infant on his abdomen after instilling the drops
③ Hold the infant with his head down lower than his body, maintaining this position for several minutes
④ Place the infant on his side during and after the procedure

193. Codeine is available in vials containing 30 mg/ml. If gr ¾ is ordered q4h prn, how many milliliters should be administered per dose? (Use 1 gr = 60 mg)
① 1.5 ml
② 2 ml
③ 2.5 ml
④ 3 ml

194. The nurse monitors the postoperative intracranial surgery patient for signs of increased intracranial pressure. An early indication is:
① Drowsiness
② Elevated temperature
③ Decreasing pulse rate
④ Irregular respirations

195. A patient admitted with weakness and pain in the left leg is placed on bed rest. The nurse should inform the nursing assistants to avoid which of the following?
① Bathing the patient's legs
② Turning the patient on the left side
③ Turning the patient on the right side
④ Massaging the left leg during the bath

196. The physician has ordered fluid restriction for a patient. The order reads "Limit fluid to 1400 ml/24 hrs." The nurse would inform the patient and place a sign in the room indicating which of the following distributions?
① Day shift, 700 ml; evening shift, 300 ml; night shift, 400 ml
② Day shift, 700 ml; evening shift, 700 ml; night shift, 0.0 ml
③ Day shift, 1000 ml; evening shift, 200 ml; night shift, 100 ml
④ Day shift, 700 ml; evening shift, 500 ml; night shift, 200 ml

197. A 25-year-old woman has been transferred from the ICU, where she has been receiving thrombolytic therapy for 2 weeks due to a blood clot in her leg. On entering the patient's room, the nurse finds her upset and crying. An appropriate nursing intervention would be to:
① Call her physician and suggest an antidepressant prn
② Allow her time to cry and express her feelings, while providing her with support
③ Call her family to bring her make-up, gowns from home, and a depilatory to remove the hair from her legs
④ Ask her family to talk to her and find out why she is crying

198. When the patient returns from the postanesthesia unit following a craniotomy for a frontal lobe tumor, his wife asks about the swelling around his eyes. Which of the following is the *most* appropriate action by the nurse?
① Notify the physician immediately
② Keep the bed in a flat position at all times
③ Ask the patient's wife to bring dark eye glasses for her husband
④ Reassure the wife that the edema is normal and will subside in a few days

199. A woman is admitted to the hospital with a diagnosis of threatened abortion. She is on complete bed rest. Which of the following nursing actions would be a *priority* in caring for this patient?
① Save any tissue passed vaginally
② Place the patient in semi-Fowler's position
③ Provide a nonstimulating environment
④ Force fluids

200. Phenobarbital is ordered gr s̄s̄ per feeding tube bid. An elixir of 30 mg/7.4 ml is supplied. Using the conversion 1 tsp = 5 ml and 1 gr = 60 mg, how many tsp should the nurse give?
① 1 tsp
② 1.5 tsp
③ 2 tsp
④ 2.5 tsp

201. A new mother is breast-feeding her baby. The nurse should teach her that at the end of a feeding session, she should release the baby from the nipple by putting gentle downward pressure on the infant's:
① Lips
② Nose
③ Chin
④ Forehead

202. A patient complains of the following symptoms at 22 weeks of pregnancy. Which is cause for *immediate* concern?
    ① Absence of fetal movement
    ② Swelling in the feet and ankles
    ③ Weight gain of 3 lb over the last month
    ④ Clear watery discharge from the vaginal area

203. A 16 month old, admitted to the hospital with dyspnea, looks slightly cyanotic and has a temperature of 103° F. The physician has diagnosed him as having a severe upper respiratory infection and orders a Croupette with oxygen. A Croupette is *best described* as:
    ① An aerosol therapy that deposits medication into the airway
    ② A plastic tent designed to provide cool, moist air and oxygen for the patient to breathe
    ③ Prepared by placing a blanket over the sides of the crib and placing a steam pot nearby
    ④ A plastic tent designed to keep air warm and moist inside the tent

204. The patient has an order for chlorothiazide (Diuril) each morning. What patient teaching would be appropriate?
    ① Urine output will be decreased
    ② The need to eat foods high in potassium
    ③ The need to measure urine output
    ④ The need to strain all urine

205. To determine if a mother understands the instructions concerning her infant's immunizations and feeding, the nurse should:
    ① Ask the mother to repeat the instructions
    ② Link sensory perceptions
    ③ Interpret all medical terms for the mother
    ④ Check for communication barriers between herself and the mother

206. The *most appropriate* short-term goal for the patient to work on in a situational crisis is:
    ① To improve her relationship with her own family
    ② To return her to her precrisis level of function
    ③ To decrease her incidence of physical symptoms
    ④ To explore her feelings about her losses

207. The nurse is helping a patient figure her expected date of confinement (EDC). The first day of her last menstrual period (LMP) was October 4. Using Nägele's rule, the nurse would conclude the due date to be:
    ① March 7
    ② July 11
    ③ August 7
    ④ January 8

208. For the nursing diagnosis "ineffective airway clearance related to increased secretions," a nursing intervention is to "assess respirations and sputum." This nursing intervention statement is:
    ① Incomplete without a physician's order
    ② Appropriate for the nursing diagnosis
    ③ Inappropriate for the nursing diagnosis
    ④ Too general to be effective in giving care

209. It is essential that the nurse observe the postpartum patient closely for hemorrhage after delivery, because excessive bleeding is most likely to occur:
    ① During the first hour after delivery
    ② About 8 to 10 hours after delivery
    ③ About 10 to 24 hours after delivery
    ④ About 24 to 72 hours after delivery

210. The charge nurse starts an aminophylline drip (1 g in 500 ml) as ordered at 30 gtt/min. The nurse wants to chart the milligrams of aminophylline the patient is receiving per minute. In calculating the milligram per minute, if the drop factor is 60 gtt/ml, which of the following is correct?
    ① 0.05 mg/min
    ② 1 mg/min
    ③ 2 mg/min
    ④ 3 mg/min

211. While taking a patient's medical history during admission, the nurse discovers that he is an alcoholic taking disulfiram (Antabuse) prescribed by the treatment center he has been attending. In providing patient teaching to a patient taking the drug disulfiram, the nurse would explain that it is important to avoid any medications in which of the forms listed below?
    ① Tinctures
    ② Oral solutions
    ③ Enteric coated tablets
    ④ Sustained-release action tablets

212. As a pregnancy progresses, normal changes in hemoglobin and hematocrit occur. The nurse expects:
    ① Hemoglobin to increase and hematocrit to decrease
    ② Hemoglobin to decrease and hematocrit to increase
    ③ Hemoglobin and hematocrit to become slightly lower
    ④ Hemoglobin and hematocrit to become slightly higher

213. In planning nursing care for a patient in sickle cell crisis, the nurse knows that the treatment plan will include:
    ① Chemotherapy
    ② Supportive therapy for presenting symptoms
    ③ Fluid restriction
    ④ Active range-of-motion exercises

214. A 27 year old is admitted to short-stay surgery for an inguinal hernia repair. Which of the following factors *does not* predispose a patient to hernia formation?
    ① Congenital defects
    ② Obesity
    ③ Appendicitis
    ④ Defect in the muscular wall

215. Which one of the following menus would be *most appropriate* for a patient with diverticulitis?
    ① Turkey on whole-wheat bread and an apple
    ② Ham omelet and ice cream
    ③ Cream of shrimp soup and canned pears
    ④ Strawberry yogurt and chocolate chip cookies

216. The nurse has been evaluating a patient's understanding of the physician's health teaching during the prenatal period. Which statement made by the patient indicates a need for further teaching?
① "I can get calcium from milk, cheese, and yogurt."
② "I can continue to have sexual intercourse throughout the pregnancy."
③ "I will eliminate my alcohol intake."
④ "I will decrease my smoking to a pack a day."

217. A patient returns from surgery, having had a cholecystectomy. Her postoperative orders include keeping her NPO and connecting her nasogastric tube to low intermittent suction. Ten hours after surgery, the patient's abdomen is distended. The *priority* nursing action should be to:
① Advance the position of the nasogastric tube 2 inches
② Irrigate the tube with 30 ml of normal saline solution
③ Check the suction equipment
④ Call the physician

218. While teaching a patient with symptoms of preeclampsia about high blood pressure, water retention, and weight gain during the last trimester of pregnancy, the nurse should instruct the patient about:
① Bed rest and decreasing her caloric intake
② Moderate exercise and decreasing her caloric intake
③ Bed rest and decreasing her salt intake
④ Moderate exercise and decreasing her salt intake

219. A patient visiting the OB-GYN office for the first time states she may be pregnant. Which of the following assessment areas are presumptive signs of pregnancy?
① Breast changes
② Goodell's sign
③ Positive urine pregnancy test
④ Darkened, vascular vaginal area

220. During a routine check on the newest addition to the nursery, the nurse notes that one of the babies has acrocyanosis. She knows that this means:
① The skin is reddish-blue in color
② Extremities are bluish in color
③ The skin has a mottled appearance
④ Extremities are covered with a bluish-white substance

221. A patient has a discharge order that includes a buccal tablet. The nurse knows the patient understands the correct method of administration when she says:
① "I will let the tablet completely dissolve in my mouth."
② "I will follow the tablet with 8 oz of water."
③ "I will allow the tablet to dissolve between my cheek and gum."
④ "I will place the tablet under my tongue."

222. A congenital disorder that occurs as a result of a chromosomal abnormality affecting chromosomes in the number 21 position is:
① Down syndrome
② Patau syndrome
③ Turner syndrome
④ Klinefelter syndrome

223. After teaching a patient about diabetes mellitus, the nurse knows he understands his condition when he states that diabetes mellitus is the result of:
① Eating too much sugar and carbohydrates
② Eating less sugar and carbohydrates
③ Decrease or no production of insulin
④ Increase or more production of insulin

224. A 5-month-old, 12-lb infant was brought to the pediatric clinic and diagnosed as having acute otitis media, which is most commonly secondary to:
① Mastoiditis
② Scarlet fever
③ Measles (rubeola)
④ Respiratory infections

225. Timolol maleate (Timoptic) is an agent used for long-term control of glaucoma. The nurse should know the action of this drug causes:
① Miosis
② Mydriasis
③ Diaphoresis
④ Diuresis

226. The nurse should be prepared to assist the patient with gout to accept a dietary modification that will restrict foods high in:
① Purines
② Fats
③ Carbohydrates
④ Calcium

227. The nurse would instruct the mother to instill ear drops in her 5-month-old child's ear by grasping the:
① Auricle and gently pulling down and back
② Auricle and gently pulling upward
③ Pinna and gently pulling backward and up
④ Pinna and gently pulling downward

228. In caring for a patient with pernicious anemia, the nurse evaluates the patient's response to therapy, which includes the patient's response to:
① Transfusions of whole blood
② Transfusions of packed cells
③ Injections of iron dextran (Imferon)
④ Injections of vitamin B_{12}

229. The nurse discusses motor skill development with a mother, explaining that at about 7 months of age her child will *most likely* be able to:
① Walk with assistance
② Feed herself with a spoon
③ Stand holding onto furniture
④ Sit alone using her hands for support

230. While observing a patient receiving a blood transfusion, the nurse must be prepared for a possible reaction. Which of the following differentiates a hemolytic reaction from an allergic or pyogenic reaction?
① Urticaria and pruritus
② Fever and chills
③ Hypertension and low back pain
④ Oliguria and hematuria

231. While planning for the patient's care, a rehabilitative approach is considered. To implement a rehabilitative approach, the nurse will consider:
    ① Consulting with physical and occupational therapy
    ② Consulting with a registered dietitian
    ③ Consulting with speech therapy
    ④ Actual and potential problems that may be encountered

232. The nurse is assigned to a patient who is to receive a unit of whole blood. The nurse observes the patient carefully for any signs of incompatibility during transfusion, which is indicative of an antibody and antigen reaction more commonly known as:
    ① Achromia
    ② Agnosia
    ③ Agglutination
    ④ Anticoagulation

233. A 5 year old is admitted to the emergency department. He is lethargic, is coughing and wheezing with nasal flaring, has moist breath sounds, and has an increase in respiratory and heart rates. The nurse's *first* intervention should be to:
    ① Elevate the head of the bed
    ② Administer oxygen as needed
    ③ Administer aerosol treatment
    ④ Monitor respiratory rate q2h

234. Rehabilitation of a patient with a myocardial infarction is flexible to meet the patient's needs. The nurse should anticipate the effect of activity and reevaluate the rehabilitation program if the patient:
    ① Complains of dyspnea on exertion
    ② Expresses denial of the condition
    ③ Refuses to accept dietary restrictions
    ④ Expresses lack of knowledge of prescribed medication

235. A physician has prescribed a monoamine oxidase inhibitor for his patient's depression. Which of the following should the nurse tell the patient regarding her medication?
    ① You will need to have frequent blood tests done
    ② You will experience some gastrointestinal distress
    ③ You will need to avoid chocolate and red wine
    ④ You will experience visual changes

236. When checking patient response to initial nitrate therapy, which of the following adverse reactions would the nurse commonly note?
    ① Hypertension
    ② Headache
    ③ Bradycardia
    ④ Drowsiness

237. The physician decides to give electroconvulsive therapy (ECT) to a patient who has not responded to medication. Which of the following is the *most appropriate* nursing action to take with a patient immediately following an ECT treatment?
    ① Give extra fluids because the patient has been NPO
    ② Encourage rapid ambulation
    ③ Reorient the patient to time, place, and person
    ④ Give the patient a small high-protein meal

238. The physician writes an order to weigh her patient, who has ankle edema, every day. The patient asks the nurse why she is being weighed every day. The *best* explanation is that:
    ① The physician wants to know her weight every day so she can change medication dosages if necessary
    ② It is necessary to determine if her low-calorie diet is effective
    ③ The physician wants to know if she has congestive heart failure
    ④ Comparison of daily weights is a good indication of whether she is losing excess fluids

239. The family of a patient admitted with depression asks if she "will ever get sick like this again." The *most appropriate* answer for the nurse to give them is:
    ① "No, she will not be sick like this again."
    ② "Her chances of having another episode are increased."
    ③ "No; if it happens again it will be worse."
    ④ "Not if she takes medications and has electroconvulsive therapy."

240. While teaching the patient about health promotion, an excellent tool to use is modeling. Which of the following would be the best example of modeling?
    ① The patient imagines troublesome situations and how she would deal with them
    ② The patient observes the behavior of others who are following a healthy life-style
    ③ The patient receives positive reinforcement for positive actions
    ④ The patient receives negative reinforcement for negative actions

241. A patient has experienced severe diarrhea for several weeks since being prescribed her drug regimen. The nurse should be *most* concerned about which of the following?
    ① Drug absorption
    ② Drug elimination
    ③ Drug metabolism
    ④ Drug distribution

242. If a duodenal ulcer perforates, which one of the following symptoms would the nurse *most likely* expect a patient to exhibit?
    ① Clay-colored stools
    ② Coffee-ground emesis
    ③ Boardlike abdomen
    ④ Distention after eating

243. While working as a staff nurse on the same unit for 5 days, the nurse notices that several of the patients on the unit have developed urinary tract infections after being catheterized by the same nurse. The nurse should do which of the following to convey her concerns?
    ① Report the incident to the physician on the next rounds
    ② Confront the nurse and suggest that she has used an inappropriate technique
    ③ Follow the proper chain of command and report the incident so that Quality Assurance personnel can follow up
    ④ Try to enter the room the next time this nurse performs a catheterization in order to observe her technique

244. Caffeine-containing beverages are avoided by patients with peptic ulcer disease because caffeine:
    ① Depresses the central nervous system
    ② Dehydrates the body
    ③ Delays production of gastric secretions
    ④ Stimulates gastric secretions

245. Which of the following statements is considered correct, factual recording of patient data in the nurse's notes?
    ① "Patient is aggressive and obnoxious today."
    ② "Patient stated something about wanting to die."
    ③ "Patient is hard to please and refusing any efforts to make him comfortable."
    ④ "Patient refused lunch and did not engage in conversation. Observed staring blankly at wall."

246. A patient is admitted with pain in the lower right quadrant and rebound tenderness. As symptoms indicate appendicitis, the nurse should also note an elevated:
    ① Red blood cell (RBC) count
    ② Hemoglobin level
    ③ Serum lipase level
    ④ White blood cell (WBC) count

247. A 23-year-old man was seen in the emergency room after falling into a hay bailer and suffering multiple lacerations. He was given a tetanus toxoid and discharged. He asked when he would need another tetanus shot. The nurse should tell him the injection he received is good for:
    ① 3 years
    ② 10 years
    ③ Lifetime
    ④ Until the next accident

248. A patient is admitted to the hospital with chest pain and has physician's orders to receive topical Nitro-Bid q8h. She is scheduled for several tests to determine the cause of her chest pain. What nursing intervention does the nurse take when administering Nitro-Bid to an ambulatory patient?
    ① Weigh the patient, because the dose is based on weight
    ② Check the most recent laboratory tests for nitrate levels
    ③ Obtain the blood pressure and pulse rate after the patient lies down
    ④ Monitor the ECG tracing

249. Which of the following patients is at greatest risk of developing an infection?
    ① A terminally ill child receiving care at home
    ② A nursing student rotating clinical areas within the agency
    ③ A pediatric patient receiving treatment for a simple laceration in the emergency department
    ④ An acutely ill elderly patient admitted to the intensive care unit

250. A nurse is caring for a patient who has been receiving a blood transfusion for about an hour. As the nurse assesses the patient's vital signs, he complains of the following. Which complaint demands priority intervention by the nurse?
    ① A "cool" sensation at the site
    ② The need to void
    ③ The need to sit up to "get his breath"
    ④ A slow-dripping IV

CHAPTER 6

Answers and Rationales
for Review Questions

All questions have been classified by cognitive level, nursing process, patient need, and level of difficulty. These classifications are provided following the question number.

The first word signifies the cognitive level of the questions: knowledge, comprehension, or application. The second word indicates the phase of the nursing process: assessment, planning, implementation, or evaluation. The third word indicates the type of patient need and is abbreviated as follows: environment = safe, effective care environment; physiologic = physiologic integrity; psychosocial = psychosocial integrity; health = health promotion/maintenance.

The letters in parentheses indicate the difficulty of the question. The letter *a* signifies that more than 75% of students should answer the question correctly; *b* signifies that between 50% and 75% should answer correctly; and *c* signifies that between 25% and 50% should answer correctly.

Rationales for all four answer choices for each question are provided. The rationale for the correct answer is listed first, followed by rationales for the incorrect answer choices.

MEDICAL-SURGICAL NURSING

1. Comprehension, assessment, physiologic (b)
    3 Pain and stiffness that is more severe in the morning and less at the end of the day are classic symptoms of rheumatoid arthritis.
    1 This is classic for osteoarthritis, not rheumatoid arthritis.
    2 The patient may experience a low-grade fever throughout the day, not only at night.
    4 This is classic of osteoporosis, not rheumatoid arthritis.
2. Application, implementation, health (c)
    3 Aspirin will reduce inflammation and decrease pain and stiffness in the morning.
    1 A warm bath would relax muscles and decrease pain and stiffness. A cool bath is contraindicated.
    2, 4 This type of exercise is too strenuous for rheumatoid arthritis.
3. Application, implementation, physiologic (a)
    2 When the patient is in the prone position, he/she cannot flex the hips or knees; therefore, flexion deformities would be prevented.
    1 High-Fowler's position could actually cause flexion deformities of the hip.
    3 Sims' position could cause knee and hip deformities.
    4 Trendelenburg's position is not used in rheumatoid arthritis because it is not a comfortable position, and it will not prevent flexion deformities.

4. Comprehension, implementation, environment (b)
    4 Active/passive exercising allows continued movement of the joints to prevent complications and assists in reducing pain.
    1 Bed rest limits activity and contributes to complications even with range-of-motion exercises.
    2 Balanced, rather than limited, activity with rest is needed to prevent complications even if it does tire her.
    3 Immobility leads to joint damage and deformity.
5. Application, implementation, environment (a)
    2 Medication is given with meals so that food in the stomach can help prevent gastric irritation.
    1 Gastric irritation occurs when no food or milk products coat the stomach lining.
    3 There is an increased risk of irritation of the gastric lining at bedtime, when no food or milk coats the stomach lining.
    4 This is an inappropriate response; medication is needed on a regularly scheduled basis.
6. Comprehension, assessment, physiologic (a)
    2 Chronic inflammatory reaction in the synovial membrane affects freely movable joints.
    1 This is characteristic of osteoarthritis.
    3 This is characteristic of osteoporosis.
    4 This is characteristic of osteomyelitis.
7. Comprehension, planning, environment (a)
    4 This restores and maintains function of the affected parts while preventing further debilitating complications.
    1 Bed rest increases the opportunity for further debilitating complications.
    2 Feeding meals encourages patient dependency rather than maximal functioning.
    3 Total care not only promotes dependency but decreases the needed stimulation of doing things for herself and feeling a useful purpose in life.
8. Application, implementation, psychosocial (b)
    3 This encourages the patient to talk about the cure, to express her feelings about her diagnosis, and to keep her physician informed.
    1 There is danger in following programs that promise false cures.
    2 This response does not allow her to express her feeling.
    4 This response does not allow her to share the information she has found and logically discuss the implications of the "cure."
9. Comprehension, planning, physiologic (a)
    1 The accumulation of uric acid is a result of the body's inability to metabolize purines.
    2 This is the pathologic cause of diabetes.
    3 This is the pathologic cause of arthritis.
    4 This is the pathologic cause of colitis.

10. Knowledge, assessment, physiologic (a)

    3 Acute pain results from the accumulation of uric acid salts deposited in a joint, most frequently in the great toe.

    1 This is an objective symptom; gout does not necessarily affect all joints at the same time.

    2 These are subjective symptoms of scleroderma.

    4 This is a subjective symptom associated with osteoarthritis.

11. Application, implementation, environment (b)

    4 Organ meats are high in purines, which break down into uric acid.

    1 These are avoided by lactose-intolerant patients.

    2 Lean meats are not high in purines.

    3 Potatoes, breads, and sugars are carbohydrates, not high in purines.

12. Knowledge, planning, physiologic (a)

    1 Allopurinol inhibits the formation of uric acid.

    2 Corticosteroids are antiinflammatory agents and would be used in treatment of lupus erythematosus.

    3 Acetaminophen (Tylenol) is an analgesic.

    4 Estrogen replacement is recommended for osteoporosis.

13. Comprehension, assessment, physiologic (b)

    1 A herniated intervertebral disk can occur suddenly (from lifting, twisting, or trauma) or gradually (from degenerative changes).

    2 These are signs and symptoms of a fracture.

    3 These signs and symptoms may indicate osteogenic sarcoma.

    4 These signs and symptoms may indicate multiple myeloma.

14. Comprehension, assessment, physiologic (c)

    2 Magnetic resonance imaging (MRI) uses magnetic forces to image the body structures. Computed axial tomography (CT or CAT scan) provides a three-dimensional picture of the structures being studied. A complete history and physical examination are essential.

    1 These are tests indicated for seizure disorders.

    3 These are tests indicated for various tumors of the bone.

    4 These are tests indicated for degenerative joint disease (osteoarthritis).

15. Application, implementation, health (c)

    3 Laminectomy involves excision of the ruptured portion of the nucleus pulposus.

    1 This is the surgical procedure for diskectomy.

    2 This is the surgical procedure for spinal fusion.

    4 This drug dissolves the nucleus pulposus; the procedure *cannot* be performed on patients with nerve involvement.

16. Comprehension, implementation, physiologic (c)

    4 Assessment should be completed for erythematous purulent exudate from the wound. Because ventilation is vital, the nurse should assist the patient to turn, cough, and deep breathe q2h. In transferring the patient out of bed, the nurse should limit the sitting position to a period of time; the straight back chair allows for greater comfort in and out of the sitting position. The patient may be permitted to walk as much as possible.

    1 This is nursing care for cardiovascular accident (CVA).

    2 This is nursing care for spinal cord injury.

    3 This is nursing care for fractures and fractured hip.

17. Comprehension, implementation, health (a)

    1 The nurse should review with the patient the physician's orders. After discharge information has been discussed, the nurse should evaluate the patient's comprehension by asking questions. Patient teaching, patient's condition, and method of discharge should be charted.

    2 These are dismissal instructions for patients with dislocations.

    3 This is nursing care for patients with total knee replacement.

    4 This is nursing care for a patient with Parkinson's disease.

18. Comprehension, assessment, physiologic (b)

    4 White females are at higher risk of developing osteoporosis than any other group.

    1 Females have a higher risk of osteoporosis.

    2 People of Hispanic origin have a lower risk of osteoporosis than do Caucasian women.

    3 African-Americans have a lower risk than do Caucasian women.

19. Knowledge, assessment, physiologic (b)

    3 Osteoporosis results from bones losing calcium and phosphorus faster than they can be replaced.

    1 Size of bones does not relate to bone density.

    2 Estrogen protects the bones from losing calcium.

    4 This is greater than the recommended daily allowance for calcium.

20. Comprehension, implementation, environment (b)

    2 Nonpharmacologic pain relief measures should be implemented first unless contraindicated. Nursing interventions should move from least to most invasive.

    1 Giving a patient an analgesic does not always guarantee removal of pain; nonpharmacologic interventions should be implemented first.

    3 The response of the nurse to the patient is inappropriate; nurses are to provide care that is competent, compassionate, and timely.

    4 There is nothing in the stem to indicate that lying in the bed is the cause of the patient's pain.

21. Application, implementation, physiologic (c)

    3 The patient has symptoms of a slipped disk and needs to seek medical help immediately.

    1, 4 Self-care for a slipped disk is not recommended.

    2 Ice packs will probably decrease the swelling, but the patient needs to see a physician.

22. Comprehension, implementation, environment (b)

    1 This position stretches the muscles of the lower back, relieving spasms.

    2 This position would be very uncomfortable.

    3 This position would be appropriate for relieving rectal pain.

    4 This position is helpful for examining the pelvic area.

23. Comprehension, assessment, physiologic (b)

    3 This can be done when checking vitals and other assessments.

    1 This is not often enough; the patient may lose vascular status to the leg.

    2 Data gathering should be done frequently enough to provide comparison readings.

    4 Too-frequent assessments can make a patient more anxious and waste nursing time.

24. Application, evaluation, physiologic (c)

    4 There may be significant loss of blood during surgery or immediately afterward.

    1 Symptoms of osteomyelitis will not occur for at least 48 hours.

    2 Rejection of a metallic prosthesis is extremely rare.

    3 Confusion is abnormal following surgery.

25. Application, implementation, environment (b)
    4 The abductor pillow helps keep the new prosthesis in alignment.
    1 Crossing the legs at the ankles or knees could cause dislocation.
    2 Turning the patient every 2 hours will help prevent skin breakdown, but it will not affect her hip.
    3 The hip should not be flexed more than 90 degrees.

26. Application, implementation, physiologic (c)
    4 This area would be a safe place to administer heparin.
    1 Subcutaneous injections should not be given in a muscle.
    2 This site would be safe to administer an intramuscular injection.
    3 Injections should be avoided within a 2-inch radius of the umbilicus.

27. Comprehension, evaluation, physiologic (b)
    3 Regular exercise can help relieve tension, which will help decrease TMJ pain. By stating that he is limiting exercise, the client must not understand the relationship between stress and TMJ pain.
    1 Grinding the teeth needs to be avoided. Many times patients are not aware that they are grinding their teeth and must have someone remind them not to.
    2 Braces can help the pain if the client's bite is uneven.
    4 Stress can aggravate the pain of TMJ. The client needs to be encouraged to practice stress relievers.

28. Knowledge, planning, physiologic (a)
    1 The tibia articulates with the femur above and talus below, supporting the entire body.
    2 The tibia is located at the lower aspect (medial side) of the leg.
    3 The tibia is surrounded by a lot of muscular tissue.
    4 The distal end of the fibula is connected to the tibia.

29. Knowledge, assessment, physiologic (a)
    4 This describes a complete-type fracture in which the break is all the way through the bone.
    1 The torsion fracture coils around the bone.
    2 This describes a comminuted-type fracture.
    3 The telescoped fracture is an impacted-type fracture.

30. Application, implementation, psychosocial (b)
    3 The nurse should be factual and supportive, encouraging him to talk about his concerns.
    1 This response gives false assurance.
    2 This response gives inaccurate information.
    4 This comment stops the patient from asking questions and leaves him unsupported.

31. Comprehension, implementation, physiologic (b)
    2 This provides good alignment and support for calcification and healing to the fracture.
    1 This is not a major goal.
    3 This is not an appropriate response.
    4 This is not applicable to this situation.

32. Application, implementation, environment (a)
    1 This decreases pressure on the skin when elevating the body.
    2 The nurse should not put anything between the cast and the skin that may increase pressure on the skin.
    3 This adds pressure in the groin area by the cast edge.
    4 This causes potential for disproportionate pressure by the cast.

33. Application, implementation, environment (c)
    4 The nurse should use a new sterile 4×4 pad for each area and move from the center of the wound outward to prevent contamination of the wound from organisms on the skin surface.
    1 The nurse is moving from a dirty area and will contaminate the wound; see No. 4.
    2 The nurse should use different pads/wipes to prevent cross-contamination; see No. 4.
    3 The nurse will not be moving the debris from the wound with this technique and will only cross-contaminate with use of a circular motion; see No. 4.

34. Application, planning, environment (c)
    4 Patients are often immunosuppressed and have decreased resistance; strict asepsis is needed to minimize exposure to microorganisms.
    1 Preparing supplies is important, but most important is to prevent contamination of supplies.
    2 Drainage tubes will be checked as part of the assessment, but reducing the spread of microorganisms takes priority.
    3 Attention will be paid to the patient's needs, but most important in planning wound care is to avoid a wound infection.

35. Application, implementation, environment (c)
    4 The nurse should begin at the lowest point (distal part) and bandage in a direction toward the heart to prevent venous congestion and swelling in the unbandaged area.
    1, 3 Not bandaging toward the heart will result in venous congestion.
    2 The distal part (hand) will swell as a result of uneven compression on tissue and blood vessels.

36. Application, assessment, health (c)
    2 A patient with a new cast should be assessed at least every hour for 24 hours.
    1 Less frequent assessment of a cast may be safe in some situations and is not necessary q15min.
    3, 4 The cast is assessed q4h for another 2 or 3 days after the first 24 hours.

37. Application, implementation, health (c)
    4 Petals are trimmed strips of tape inserted over the edges of a cast that smooth and repair cast edges temporarily to protect the integrity of the skin.
    1 Petaling will not keep the cast from becoming wet.
    2 Petaling will not keep the cast from becoming too tight; it only stops the irritation that results when the cast is too tight.
    3 Petaling will not keep debris from getting under the cast.

38. Comprehension, planning, physiologic (a)
    1 The abducted position keeps the prosthesis in the appropriate alignment.
    2 The adducted position would dislodge the prosthesis from alignment.
    3 The flexed position is contraindicated; the hip should not be flexed.
    4 The prone position is inappropriate because just the leg alone could not be positioned in this manner.

39. Application, implementation, health (a)
    2 The patient should be placed on the unaffected side with appropriate supports to maintain proper alignment of the prosthesis.
    1 It is contraindicated to place a patient on the affected side because this may cause the prosthesis to become dislodged.
    3, 4 These are inappropriate because it could cause flexion of the hip.

40. Comprehension, planning, physiologic (a)
    4 This is the usual time allowance for a hip prosthesis.
    1 This applies to a hip pinning.
    2 The patient is not allowed full weight bearing until 4 weeks.
    3 Partial weight bearing is in 10 to 14 days; it may not be necessary to use crutches in 3 to 6 months.
41. Application, implementation, psychosocial (b)
    1 This statement allows the patient to express his feelings more fully.
    2, 3 These responses provide false assurance.
    4 This statement avoids the patient's feelings and does not allow him to express himself.
42. Application, planning, psychosocial (b)
    4 Patients frequently have body image disturbances following an amputation. The patient may feel less whole and need a lot of emotional support to get over the trauma of losing a body part.
    1 The patient's self-esteem will be altered, but the disturbance of body image is the cause.
    2 Skin integrity may be impaired on the limb to be amputated, but the amputation will remove the problem.
    3 Problems with tissue perfusion may be the reason for the BKA, but the amputation will improve the problem.
43. Comprehension, assessment, physiologic (b)
    1 Assessment of pain characteristics, including location, is the most important factor before considering the administration of any pain medication.
    2 This is an assessment for cardiac status.
    3 This is an assessment for renal status.
    4 This is an assessment for gastrointestinal status.
44. Comprehension, evaluation, physiologic (c)
    3 The main purpose of the compression bandage is to reduce edema and promote venous return.
    1 This indicates healing is occuring.
    2 This indicates the wound is free from infection.
    4 This indicates there is adequate circulation to the area.
45. Comprehension, evaluation, environment (b)
    1 Alcohol is drying and will promote skin breakdown on the residual limb.
    2 This is a good exercise to toughen the residual limb.
    3 Good hygiene with mild soap and water is appropriate skin care.
    4 Range of motion to the joints above and below the residual limb is important to prevent contractures.
46. Application, implementation, environment (c)
    4 The tripod position, with the crutches 6 inches apart and 6 inches from the feet, is the beginning position for all gaits.
    1 The crutch and the unaffected leg must ascend first to afford greatest support.
    2 The major part of the weight is maintained with the hands. Weight on the axilla can lead to brachial injury or paralysis.
    3 If the patient constantly looks down, he will lose his balance and fall.
47. Comprehension, planning, health (b)
    2 Frequent turning decreases the incidence of complications, provides good circulation, and maintains good skin integrity.
    1 Referring to an adjustment period produces anxiety and fear.
    3 The patient may experience phantom pain.
    4 This increases the incidence of complications, poor circulation, and poor skin integrity.
48. Comprehension, assessment, physiologic (b)
    4 This action assesses the arterial blood flow to both legs; Doppler pressure measurements can also be implemented.
    1 There is a need to increase the collateral circulation to the leg; elevation is not recommended.
    2 Blood work will not directly provide this information.
    3 Movement is needed to increase the collateral circulation to the leg.
49. Comprehension, implementation, environment (b)
    3 If bleeding does occur, it will drain down under the residual limb.
    1 This will cause discomfort. Elevating the foot of the bed slightly should assist circulation and decrease bleeding.
    2 This causes flexion of the hip, which can further cause contractures.
    4 There is no therapeutic advantage to this procedure.
50. Comprehension, assessment, physiologic (c)
    1 Because of the level of amputation, the flexor muscles get stretched when the hip is flexed.
    2 Because of the location of the incision, strong sutures and a pressure dressing are usually in place to decrease chances of hemorrhage.
    3 Because of the type of surgery, antibiotics are usually given both before and after surgery, decreasing the incidence of infection.
    4 Good preventive postoperative care decreases the incidence of this.
51. Application, implementation, health (c)
    2 Elastic wraps shape the residual limb into a cone to facilitate proper fitting of the prosthesis.
    1 Because of the location of the incision, strong sutures, not the use of elastic wrap, decrease the chance of hemorrhage.
    3 This is not a primary consideration.
    4 This is an inappropriate response; there is no direct relationship between elastic wraps and decreasing the chance of infection.
52. Application, implementation, physiologic (a)
    3 Epistaxis is the term used for nose bleed. The first emergency action the nurse can perform is to try to control the bleeding by applying pressure to the bridge of the nose.
    1 This is not an immediate action of the nurse because information can be obtained from a family member by another health care worker.
    2 Fear and anxiety are not life threatening; however, these should be alleviated as quickly as possible.
    4 Assessing vital signs and level of consciousness is usually done q15min, however, control of bleeding takes priority until the nurse can be relieved by another person.
53. Application, implementation, environment (a)
    3 Fowler's position with the head leaning forward prevents the patient from swallowing the blood draining from the nose that could cause nausea and vomiting.
    1, 2, 4 These are contraindicated because they would not allow the patient to expectorate the blood; they could cause blockage of the airway.
54. Comprehension, implementation, physiologic (a)
    4 After total laryngectomy, the patient breathes through a permanent tracheostomy stoma.
    1 Because of removal of the entire larynx, the patient's breathing pattern is altered, and breathing is through a permanent tracheostomy stoma.
    2 The patient's breathing pattern is altered as a result of extensive surgery.
    3 The tracheostomy is permanent following a total laryngectomy.

55. Application, implementation, physiologic (b)
    1 The suction is turned off as the catheter is inserted to avoid irritation of the trachea and additional loss of oxygen.
    2 Suctioning does not relate to blocking of the catheter.
    3 Having the suction on or off does not relate to an infectious process.
    4 Having the suction on or off does not relate to "kinking" of the catheter.

56. Comprehension, assessment, physiologic (b)
    3 Increasing respirations and use of accessory muscles to facilitate breathing indicate the need for suctioning due to blockage of the tube by mucus.
    1 Pulse and respiratory rate would increase rather than decrease.
    2 Increased swallowing and moisture on the neck dressing may indicate bleeding.
    4 Pain and a dry, hacking cough are more indicative of lower airway infection.

57. Application, implementation, physiologic (b)
    2 Prolonged suctioning may cause mucosal damage.
    1 Continuous suctioning may cause mucosal damage.
    3 If suction is applied, the catheter may "grab" mucosa and cause damage.
    4 The patient should be placed in semi-Fowler's position.

58. Comprehension, implementation, physiologic (b)
    2 This position best minimizes the risk of aspiration in the immediate postoperative period.
    1 The supine position does not promote maintenance of a patent airway in the immediate postoperative period.
    3 Positioning the patient with the head down does not promote maintenance of a patent airway in the immediate postoperative period.
    4 In the immediate postoperative period, the patient is partially anesthetized, and in this position the patient would be at increased risk for aspiration.

59. Application, planning, health (b)
    1 Because water could easily enter the stoma during showering, the patient will need to wear some type of protection.
    2, 3, 4 Resuming and continuing these daily activities would contribute to the healing process.

60. Knowledge, application, physiologic (b)
    3 These are classic symptoms.
    1 Joint pain is not usually seen.
    2 Heart irregularities are not common primary symptoms.
    4 Neither of these is a primary symptom.

61. Application, planning, physiologic (c)
    4 Normally, excessive levels of carbon dioxide stimulate breathing in a healthy individual, but in chronic lung disease the stimulus is hypoxia. If high levels of oxygen are given, the patient will stop breathing.
    1 Too much oxygen will cause the patient to stop breathing.
    2 Narcotics may decrease the respirations even more.
    3 The bed needs to be in high Fowler's position, which is at a 90-degree angle.

62. Application, implementation, health (a)
    2 Lying on the affected side helps to splint the chest and assist in coughing.
    1 Because it is painful to breathe, the patient will avoid deep breathing.
    3 Coughing increases the pain if there is no chest support.
    4 In this position the patient will be unable to give support to the affected side. This will not help the amount of pain the patient is experiencing.

63. Comprehension, planning, physiologic (b)
    1 Increased fluids increase output and filtration of body wastes through the kidneys.
    2 Fluids alone will not contribute to proper nutrition.
    3 Waste products are not diluted but are excreted from the body.
    4 This is an indirect contributory factor; not the main purpose of forcing fluids.

64. Knowledge, planning, health (a)
    3 These tests are microscopic examinations to determine which organisms are present.
    1 This confirms existence of disease; it does not determine causative organisms.
    2 This obtains stomach contents.
    4 This is a diagnostic test of lung tissue.

65. Comprehension, evaluation, physiologic (a)
    3 Acetaminophen (Tylenol) is an antipyretic medication that relieves fever by central action in the hypothalamic heating regulating center.
    1 Acetaminophen has no direct effect on kidney function.
    2 Acetaminophen has no direct effect on sputum reduction.
    4 Acetaminophen has no effect of fluid retention.

66. Knowledge, assessment, physiologic (a)
    4 Pulse rate would increase.
    1 This indicates lack of oxygen to the tissues.
    2, 3 This indicates the lungs are working harder to obtain needed oxygen.

67. Comprehension, assessment, physiologic (a)
    1 On the affected side, there will be little or no movement of the chest wall; on the unaffected side, breathing will appear normal.
    2 This is a symptom of infection.
    3 Pain is a symptom, but position is not an aggravating factor.
    4 These are symptoms of asthma or infection.

68. Application, assessment, physiological (b)
    1 The patient has classic symptoms of a pneumothorax. A pneumothorax can be life threatening and needs to be treated immediately.
    2 The patient needs to be treated immediately.
    3 Since the doctor will not be there for 2 more hours, it would be best to send the patient to the emergency room.
    4 The nurse cannot order chest x-rays and angiograms.

69. Comprehension, evaluation, health (b)
    3 To prevent the backflow of drainage from the collection system, the system should be kept below the chest level.
    1 The drainage chamber is never emptied; the chest tube should be removed before this chamber is filled.
    2 This is not necessary. A patient must lie on the affected side only if he has a lobectomy.
    4 This is not necessary. As long as the drainage system is below chest level, the patient may be out of bed as the physician allows.

70. Application, implementation, physiologic (b)
    1 The most important initial action is to prevent air from entering the chest cavity and disturbing negative pressure balance.
    2 No. 1 must be done before notification of the team leader.
    3 This is not necessary at this point.
    4 This is never done; it is not within a nurse's scope of practice.

71. Knowledge, planning, physiologic (a)
    1 Pneumothorax occurs when air or gas accumulates within the pleural cavity. This leads to partial or complete collapse of the lung.
    2 Pneumonia is inflammation of lung tissue.
    3 Epistaxis is the term for a nose bleed.
    4 Hemothorax is the term for blood in the pleural space.
72. Comprehension, assessment, physiologic (a)
    2 Bright-red frothy sputum is indicative of a punctured lung because air is entering the chest and lung tissues.
    1 This is usually indicative of congestive heart failure.
    3 This is usually indicative of an infectious process within the pulmonary system. This could also indicate other disease processes. The word *purulent* indicates infection.
    4 This is not an appropriate symptom regarding lung injury.
73. Comprehension, planning, physiologic (a)
    3 This is the space between the visceral lining and the pleural lining. The tubes allow drainage of secretions, blood, and air.
    1, 2, 4 This is inappropriate placement of tubes; it would not facilitate lung expansion.
74. Comprehension, planning, physiologic (c)
    1 Chest tubes are inserted between the ribs into the pleural space to allow drainage of secretions, blood, and air.
    2 The negative pressure within the thoracic cavity is restored when the lung is expanded.
    3 Atmospheric pressure rushing into the thoracic cavity causes the lung to collapse.
    4 The thoracic cavity pressure is normally negative as opposed to the atmospheric pressure. The pressure is not equal.
75. Comprehension, implementation, physiologic (b)
    2 This bottle is used to allow the flow of secretions and air by gravitation.
    1 Suction is possible by a second or third bottle and sometimes may be connected to a suction machine.
    3, 4 Measurement is not the purpose of the closest bottle.
76. Comprehension, implementation, environment (b)
    2 This allows for drainage of secretions, blood, and air via gravity
    1 This is contraindicated because the drainage would flow back into the thoracic cavity, causing further complications.
    3 This is contraindicated because drainage would re-enter the pleural space.
    4 The level is of primary importance to prevent complications and respiratory distress.
77. Knowledge, implementation, physiologic (a)
    4 Close observation of both the patient for respiratory distress and the underwater-seal drainage for proper functioning is the primary responsibility of the nurse.
    1 This is contraindicated; the drainage system is kept below the patient to facilitate proper drainage.
    2 This does not apply.
    3 The drainage chamber is not emptied. The chest tube should be removed before the chamber is filled.
78. Application, implementation, physiologic (b)
    4 Unless contraindicated, this should be done to prevent spontaneous pneumothorax and further complications.
    1 This can be done, but it is not the *first* action.
    2 This should be done after clamping the chest tubes.
    3 This should be done if the patient exhibits signs of respiratory distress.

79. Knowledge, assessment, physiologic (b)
    1 Dyspnea, chest pain, and decreased movement of the involved chest wall are usual clinical manifestations.
    2 Pain is not relieved with leaning forward. Insertion of a chest tube is usually required.
    3 Breath sounds are usually decreased on the affected side.
    4 Breath sounds may be absent on the affected side.
80. Comprehension, implementation, physiologic (b)
    2 Marking the level of drainage and noting the time should be done according to prescribed protocol. Changes in the amount or characteristics of drainage can be noted and reported.
    1 The practice of "stripping" chest tubes is controversial and needs a specific order. It is not usually necessary when chest tubes are used to drain air.
    3 Lifting the bottle(s) would allow air and/or fluid to be pulled back into the pleural cavity.
    4 The bottle(s) should be placed below the level of the patient's chest so air and/or fluid is not pulled back into the pleural cavity. Drainage is also facilitated.
81. Application, assessment, physiologic (c)
    3 Fluctuations in rising with inspiration and falling with expiration should be observed in patients who are breathing spontaneously.
    1 When the system is working effectively, intermittent bubbling is seen in the water seal.
    2 Continuous and constant bubbling usually indicates an air leak. The source should be determined; retaping all connections may be necessary.
    4 Fluctuation of the fluid in the water-seal chamber should remain constant.
82. Application, implementation, safety (c)
    3 Forced expiratory efforts against a closed airway help to create positive pleural pressure and decrease the likelihood that air will enter the pleural space.
    1 This does not facilitate creation of positive pleural pressure. Air could enter the pleural space on tube removal.
    2 Air could enter the pleural space as the tube is removed.
    4 Pursed-lip breathing involves slow exhalation. Chronic obstructive pulmonary disease patients are frequently helped with this type of breathing.
83. Comprehension, assessment, physiologic (b)
    1 A productive cough with rust-colored sputum (indicating slight bleeding in the respiratory tract) is a common symptom.
    2 Fever is usually normal during the day, but it elevates in the late afternoon and evening.
    3 This is a symptom of poor circulation in the lower limbs.
    4 This is a symptom of allergy or dermatitis.
84. Comprehension, assessment, physiologic (b)
    3 Coughing from the diaphragm will generate sputum as deeply as possible from the respiratory tract.
    1 Abdominal breathing is too shallow to encourage the expectoration of sputum.
    2 This will destroy bacteria that are an important part of the specimen.
    4 A high-Fowler's position is preferable to encourage the expectoration of sputum.
85. Comprehension, planning, physiologic (c)
    4 This is the most realistic goal because it takes about 2 weeks for therapeutic blood levels of medication to develop.
    1, 2, 3 These would be unrealistic because the therapeutic blood levels of medication are not reached.

86. Application, implementation, health (c)
    3 This is an expected reaction. The drug should not be discontinued because of this.
    1 The dose should not be increased without the physician's order.
    2 This is unnecessary in relationship to the drug.
    4 The physician must be notified before this is done.

87. Comprehension, assessment, physiologic (b)
    1 The *Mycobacterium tuberculosis* in the system may be in either an active or an arrested state.
    2 The Mantoux test does not necessarily mean an active case of TB, because exposure can cause a positive test reaction.
    3 The Mantoux test does not rule out TB.
    4 Being exposed to TB does not necessarily mean active disease is present.

88. Comprehension, planning, physiologic (b)
    4 With less movement, secretions are not coughed up and are not contaminated with food and fluids.
    1 Procedures should not be planned based on staff convenience.
    2 Coughing does occur during the day.
    3 Assignments are made based on good patient care, not arbitrarily.

89. Comprehension, planning, environment (a)
    2 These procedures decrease the spread of the infection.
    1 Contact with people is important for the patient.
    3, 4 These are important but not primary.

90. Application, implementation, health (b)
    1 These medications inhibit the enzyme needed for the growth of the bacilli.
    2, 4 The treatment regimen is usually 9 months or longer.
    3 These drugs nearly, but never completely, eliminate viable bacilli.

91. Comprehension, evaluation, environment (b)
    3 The lesion will heal by fibrosis and calcification but remains in an arrested or inactive state.
    1 The disease becomes arrested or inactive.
    2 This is not necessarily so, because disease in an arrested or inactive state can reactivate.
    4 Reinfection can occur, giving rise to a progressive form of the disease.

92. Knowledge, assessment, physiologic (a)
    3 Elevated temperature and night sweats are symptoms characteristic of tuberculosis.
    1 This is characteristic of asthma.
    2 This is characteristic of cerebral anoxia.
    4 This is a term meaning blood in the pleural space.

93. Knowledge, assessment, physiologic (b)
    3 Koch's bacillus is the causative organism of tuberculosis. AFB stands for acid-fast bacillus.
    1 *Shigella* is a bacterium that causes bacillary dysentery.
    2 The gas bacillus is a spore-forming type of organism that is responsible for gas gangrene.
    4 The Epstein-Barr virus is responsible for infectious mononucleosis.

94. Application, implementation, physiologic (a)
    1 A 15-degree angle of the needle allows insertion just under the skin.
    2 A 25-degree angle is not the proper angle for administration of this test.
    3 This is an appropriate angle for a subcutaneous injection.
    4 This is an appropriate angle for an intramuscular injection.

95. Comprehension, implementation, physiologic (a)
    3 The site of injection should not be rubbed; it should be marked to be read in 48 hours.
    1, 2 The area should not be massaged at all.
    4 The site should not be rubbed with an alcohol swab.

96. Comprehension, implementation, environment (a)
    2 A positive tuberculosis (TB) skin test indicates exposure to the TB organism and is not diagnostic in itself.
    1 A positive TB skin test does not indicate infection or necessitate admission to the hospital.
    3 This is not correct because a positive TB skin test does not ensure immunity. To tell the relative not to worry gives false assurance.
    4 A positive TB skin test is not the same as an allergic reaction; however, it should not be repeated. It should be followed by an x-ray examination.

97. Knowledge, planning, physiologic (a)
    3 Asthma involves recurring episodes of increased tracheal/bronchial responsiveness to various stimuli.
    1 This is the definition of emphysema.
    2 This is the definition of bronchiectasis.
    4 This is the definition of pulmonary tuberculosis.

98. Knowledge, assessment, health (a)
    2 Cigarette smoking is the highest risk factor for the development of emphysema.
    1 Although pneumonia can precipitate severe hypoxia in a patient with emphysema, it is not a risk factor.
    3 Air pollution can be a risk factor for the development of emphysema, but smoking is a greater risk factor.
    4 This is not a risk factor for emphysema.

99. Comprehension, implementation, physiologic (a)
    1 Theophylline (Theo-Dur) relaxes smooth muscle in the bronchi so that ventilation becomes easier.
    2 Bronchoconstriction would make breathing more difficult.
    3 This drug does not act on secretions.
    4 Vasoconstriction of major vessels is not an action of this medication.

100. Knowledge, assessment, environment (a)
    2 Aminophylline, because it relaxes smooth muscle, may cause hypotension as a side effect.
    1 Tachycardia is a side effect.
    3 Restlessness is a side effect.
    4 Nausea and anorexia are side effects; weight gain is not.

101. Comprehension, assessment, physiologic (b)
    4 Because of chronic hypoxia and labored breathing, the chest develops a barrel-like configuration and the fingertips become blunted and clubbed.
    1 Pigeon chest is a congenital deformity; it is not usually the result of a chronic respiratory disease.
    2 The hair would become dry and sparse as a result of conditions other than emphysema.
    3 Moist shiny skin is not a manifestation of emphysema.

102. Application, planning, physiologic (c)
    2 Isuprel is a bronchodilator and is used as an inhaler in respiratory distress.
    1 Morphine will depress respirations.
    3 Inderal slows and strengthens the heart.
    4 Mannitol is given for cranial edema.

103. Comprehension, planning, environment (b)
    3 After the procedure, the patient is not allowed oral fluids until the gag reflex has returned. A topical anesthetic is used before the bronchoscope is introduced.
    1 Sputum collection is not part of the standard postoperative bronchoscopy orders.
    2 The procedure allows for a direct visualization of the larynx, trachea, and bronchi. A flexible fiberoptic bronchoscope is usually used. No surgical incisions are necessary.
    4 Voice restriction is associated with laryngoscopy.

104. Application, implementation, environment (c)
    2 A local anesthetic is applied to the throat before the bronchoscopy is done. The anesthetic removes the gag reflex. The patient should not have anything by mouth until the gag reflex returns to guard against choking.
    1 Bed rest is not necessary unless a sedative was given.
    3 No fluids should be given until the gag reflex returns.
    4 A bland diet is not usually necessary.

105. Knowledge, planning, physiologic (a)
    4 The entire lung is removed in a pneumonectomy.
    1 In a wedge resection, a specific diseased portion is removed.
    2 When one or more lung segments are surgically removed, the procedure is called a segmental resection.
    3 Removal of one lobe of the lung is termed a lobectomy.

106. Comprehension, implementation, physiologic (b)
    2 The remaining lung can expand better in the semi-Fowler's position.
    1 Chest drainage tubes are not usually used. These permit serous fluid to accumulate in the space.
    3 Anticoagulant medications are not usually indicated following lung surgery.
    4 Lungs can expand better in the semi-Fowler's position than in the supine position.

107. Comprehension, assessment, physiologic (c)
    4 There is an accumulation of serous fluid in interstitial lung tissue.
    1 This is characteristic of arterial respiratory distress.
    2 This is characteristic of chronic obstructive pulmonary disease.
    3 This is characteristic of pulmonary emboli.

108. Comprehension, assessment, physiologic (b)
    3 Bronchial structures become engorged with fluid as a result of interstitial edema.
    1 Pulmonary means lungs; therefore, there is accumulation of fluid in the lungs.
    2 Edema means swelling; therefore, there is an increase, not a decrease, of fluid.
    4 Edema means swelling, and pulmonary refers to lungs.

109. Application, implementation, environment (b)
    2 Body weight indicates the effectiveness of a diuretic used to reduce alveolar and systemic edema by increasing urinary output.
    1 Monitoring intake and output alone does not indicate reduction of alveolar and systemic edema.
    3 These procedures will not remove the fluid in body tissue.
    4 These procedures alone will not accurately indicate fluid reduction in body tissue.

110. Application, implementation, psychosocial (c)
    1 To assist the patient in good oxygen/carbon dioxide exchange, the nurse should implement nursing measures to decrease the patient's anxiety and inform the charge nurse.
    2 Medication can assist respirations to a point; anxiety reduction treats the major cause of distress.
    3 Such a direct response may increase her anxiety even more.
    4 This does not provide the immediate assistance needed.

111. Comprehension, planning, health (a)
    4 The nasal cannula allows her more freedom to move around, eat, and talk while getting the oxygen needed.
    1 The face mask fits too snugly, is too confining, and adds to her feeling of suffocation.
    2 The oxygen tent is too constricting and anxiety-producing.
    3 The nasal catheter traumatizes nasal mucosa.

112. Application, evaluation, health (c)
    4 These symptoms indicate a decrease in potassium, a side effect of too much fluid loss.
    1 Hematuria is not a side effect of this medication.
    2 These are side effects that bear watching, but they are not significant.
    3 Diarrhea by itself is not indicative of a problem.

113. Application, assessment, physiologic (c)
    4 Persons with diabetes are at risk for the development of coronary artery disease.
    1 An active lifestyle is a preventative factor.
    2 Familial history of cancer does not increase the risk of coronary artery disease.
    3 This cholesterol level is within normal limits.

114. Knowledge, assessment, physiologic (b)
    1 Anatomically, the tricuspid valve is located between the right atrium and right ventricle.
    2 Anatomically, the bicuspid valve is located between the left atrium and left ventricle.
    3 The aortic valve guards the opening between the left ventricle and the aorta.
    4 The mitral valve is also known as the bicuspid valve.

115. Application, implementation, physiologic (b)
    2 Smoking increases any cardiac risk.
    1 Smoking alone does not cause heart attacks.
    3 Women have four times the risk of heart attack than nonsmokers or men.
    4 Risk reduction from smoking cessation takes up to 3 years.

116. Comprehension, planning, environment (b)
    1 A plan of scheduled exercises will maintain adequate circulation through musculoskeletal activity; position changes diminish orthostatic hypotension events, and adequate fluid intake maintains fluid volume.
    2 Unless contraindicated, patients should have a schedule of exercises and be out of bed every shift. Kilocalories are usually increased to facilitate the healing process, and fluid intake is maintained or slightly increased to maintain fluid and electrolyte balance.
    3 Strenuous exercise may not be indicated, but a reasonable level of exercises should be decided on by the patient and other health care team members; a supine position will precipitate postural hypotension, and continuous hemodynamic monitoring is not necessary if the patient is stable.
    4 Appropriate exercise and socialization should be a part of the patient's plan of care.

117. Comprehension, evaluation, physiologic (b)
    3 There could be a clot causing an interruption in blood flow.
    1, 2, 4 These are all expected findings.
118. Knowledge, implementation, physiologic (c)
    2 Injury to the heart causes increased permeability of the cell membranes, releasing the cardiac enzymes into the serum.
    1 The cardiac enzymes are found in all living tissue.
    3 Enzymatic action is not required for the conductive system.
    4 There are no enzymes specific to measure damage in the heart valves.
119. Knowledge, implementation, physiologic (b)
    4 Wall motion abnormalities are detected with an echocardiogram.
    1 An arteriogram or angiogram views the coronary arteries.
    2 The veins of the heart are insignificant.
    3 An electrocardiograph (ECG) provides information about the electrical activity of the heart.
120. Knowledge, assessment, physiologic (a)
    2 The sinoatrial node is located in the wall of the right atrium.
    1 The left atrium does not contain a primary conduction node, but it does contain conduction fiber.
    3 The left ventricle does not contain a primary conduction node, but it does contain conduction fibers.
    4 The right ventricle does not contain a primary conduction node, but it does contain conduction fibers.
121. Comprehension, assessment, physiologic (a)
    4 Angina pectoris is the result of insufficient oxygen to the myocardium and is usually related to stress, exercise, or heavy meals.
    1 This is the definition of arteriosclerosis.
    2 This is the causative factor in a myocardial infarction.
    3 This is related to congestive heart failure.
122. Comprehension, assessment, physiologic (b)
    2 Angina pectoris usually occurs during exertion and usually subsides with rest and vasodilators.
    1 This is typical of pain with a myocardial infarction.
    3 Although this may be present with angina, it is typical of pain with a myocardial infarction. The key is to distinguish between the two conditions.
    4 Radiating pain is typical for both angina and myocardial infarction; however, this kind of pain seems more common with angina.
123. Comprehension, assessment, physiologic (b)
    2 Sharp, burning substernal pain radiating to the jaw, shoulder, or left arm is the most common description of anginal pain.
    1, 4 These are not descriptive of anginal pain; wrong location.
    3 This is more descriptive of a myocardial infarction.
124. Comprehension, evaluation, health (c)
    3 A burning sensation under the tongue is an expected reaction and means that the medication is effective. These pills should not be destroyed.
    1 Nitroglycerin may be taken prophylactically to prevent the onset of angina before physical activity.
    2 This is proper storage of nitroglycerin.
    4 Nitroglycerin must be taken in this manner, 5 minutes apart.
125. Comprehension, assessment, physiologic (b)
    4 Angina means pain, and pectoris refers to the chest.
    1 This symptom most likely occurs in a heart attack.
    2 Cyanosis is not necessarily a symptom of angina.
    3 Elevated blood pressure is not related to anginal pain.

126. Application, planning, physiologic (a)
    1 Although the patient takes the nitroglycerin as needed, the amount taken must be documented on the record.
    2 It is not necessary to take the blood pressure q6h.
    3 This is not necessarily a dependency drug.
    4 It is the nurse's responsibility to monitor nitroglycerin use.
127. Application, implementation, physiologic (b)
    3 This would most accurately and completely document an anginal episode. It is especially important to document activity in relation to the anginal episode.
    1 This is not complete. Vital signs and patient activity at the time of the attack must be included.
    2 Recording must include onset and duration of pain.
    4 Recording must include vital signs and time of onset of pain.
128. Application, implementation, environment (a)
    1 This includes all aspects that would be considered for patients with angina pectoris.
    2 It would be impossible to *avoid* emotions; it is more accurate to learn to deal with emotions of anxiety. Avoiding exercise would not be appropriate for most conditions.
    3 This does not include all aspects to be considered for angina pectoris; patients are also cautioned to avoid extreme changes in temperature and eating heavy meals.
    4 This does not include all areas necessary for follow-up.
129. Knowledge, assessment, physiologic (c)
    3 Angina pectoris is characterized by the inability of the coronary arteries to meet the oxygen demand of the myocardial muscle, a condition leading to pain (angina).
    1 Necrosis would be indicative of myocardial infarction, not angina.
    2 Although the friction of an enlarged epicardium rubbing against the pericardial sac may cause pain, it is not typical of anginal discomfort.
    4 Vasospasm of a coronary artery is transient and reversible; it is not generally relieved by decreasing activity, as it is in the case of angina.
130. Comprehension, assessment, physiologic (b)
    3 Although the exact cause of hypertension is not known, heredity plays an important role because of familial tendencies.
    1 This has no effect on hypertension.
    2 Overweight is a predisposing factor to hypertension.
    4 Parents with hypertension would more directly predispose a patient to this disease, because they were a much closer relation to the patient.
131. Comprehension, assessment, physiologic (b)
    1 Nosebleed is commonly associated with hypertension.
    2 This may indicate a problem but not a blood pressure problem.
    3, 4 These are not associated with blood pressure problems.
132. Comprehension, assessment, physiologic (b)
    4 There are few symptoms associated with the disease, so the patient does not feel ill. Patients find side effects of the medication to be too bothersome.
    1 This is becoming true, but No. 4 is more accurate.
    2 With hypertension, there are not very many symptoms present.
    3 Because the patient was taking the medication, she most likely received instructions from the prescribing physician or her nurse.

133. Application, implementation, physiologic (c)
     1 Constriction of the arterioles occurs in these patients. The heart exerts more pressure to circulate; thus an elevation of systolic/diastolic pressure occurs.
     2 Caffeine does not contribute to increased cholesterol.
     3 Caffeine does not harden the vessels.
     4 Caffeine constricts; it does not dilate.
134. Comprehension, implementation, environment (a)
     2 The patient has a borderline blood pressure reading for hypertension. Smoking increases his risk of coronary artery disease by causing arterial vasospasm.
     1 The normal adult will require 8 hours of sleep to maintain health.
     3 This is not an appropriate suggestion; it is not physiologically necessary.
     4 An exercise program would be helpful to this patient.
135. Comprehension, assessment, physiologic (a)
     2 A typical sign of primary hypertension is a chronically elevated diastolic pressure. Usually a diastolic pressure of 90 mm Hg is the cutoff.
     1 This is not assessed specifically for essential hypertension.
     3 Diastolic pressure is primarily involved.
     4 Pulse pressure is the difference between systolic and diastolic pressures.
136. Application, planning, physiologic (a)
     2 Pretzels are high in sodium content.
     1, 3, 4 These are low in salt.
137. Comprehension, planning, physiologic (a)
     1 The purpose in treating hypertension is to minimize the damage that has occurred to the blood vessels.
     2 This is not applicable at this time.
     3 It is not advisable to lower blood pressure below normal level.
     4 Because there are no early symptoms, some damage has already occurred and cannot be repaired.
138. Comprehension, implementation, health (b)
     2 A gradual weight loss program, with a loss of no more than 2½ lb per week, is the most effective.
     1 A very rapid weight loss is not recommended.
     3 A vegetarian diet is not necessary.
     4 1000 calories per day is not sufficient for an adult male.
139. Comprehension, evaluation, physiologic (c)
     1 Chronic hyperglycemia can damage the lining of blood vessels, allowing atheromatous material to aggregate.
     2 Elevated uric acid levels will cause gout.
     3 Tingling indicates a problem with nervous function.
     4 Keeping the blood sugars consistent is easier on the tissues.
140. Application, assessment, physiologic (c)
     2 These are all risk factors for developing cardiovascular disease.
     1 A patient in this category would be considered at low risk for CVD.
     3 This patient has two risk factors: over 40 and not enough exercise. Although some risk factors are present, this is still not as serious as No. 2.
     4 This patient displays two risk factors: over 40 and diabetic.
141. Application, implementation, physiologic (b)
     1 Thromboembolic stockings promote venous blood return.
     2 Clots usually form in the veins where blood pools.
     3 The stockings prevent venous stasis.
     4 The muscles aren't moving during surgery, so they aren't able to facilitate venous return.

142. Comprehension, assessment, physiologic (a)
     1 Intermittent claudication results from inadequate circulation to the muscles as a result of decreased blood supply to the extremities.
     2 This is a temporary cause of symptoms if the blood supply is cut off; it has no relationship to intermittent claudication.
     3 This causes other health problems, but not intermittent claudication.
     4 The amount of rest has no bearing on intermittent claudication.
143. Knowledge, assessment, physiologic (b)
     3 Angina is the most frequent presenting symptom of coronary artery disease in women.
     1 Mitral valve prolapse occurs more frequently in women, but it is not a sign of coronary artery disease.
     2 Endocarditis usually has fever, chest pain, and shortness of breath as symptoms.
     4 Myocardial infarction is the most common indicator in men of coronary artery disease.
144. Application, assessment, physiologic (c)
     1 Hypertension and diabetes both affect the arteries.
     2 Obesity is a controllable factor.
     3 Smoking and alcohol use increase the risk but are controllable factors.
     4 Postmenopausal women are at increased risk for an MI, but these are additional risk factors.
145. Application, implementation, physiologic (c)
     3 An occlusion of the coronary artery leads to tissue death as a result of oxygen deprivation.
     1 The blockage is in the coronary arteries, which feed the heart muscle.
     2 Injury to valves does not result in death of heart muscle.
     4 Inability to pump fluid is a sign of congestive heart failure or cardiogenic shock.
146. Knowledge, evaluation, physiologic (c)
     3 The Reserpine may be the cause. Impotence is a common side effect of this drug. The physician can switch the patient to another medication to see if it helps.
     1 If a drug change does not help, the patient may then want to see a psychologist.
     2 This may be an option if the drug change does not work.
     4 If the drug change does not work, the nurse can discuss other options for the patient.
147. Knowledge, assessment, physiologic (b)
     2 These symptoms, accompanied by cyanosis, are suggestive of a myocardial infarction.
     1, 3, 4 With these conditions, the patient usually does not have cyanosis, a condition that indicates lack of oxygen to the tissues.
148. Knowledge, assessment, physiologic (a)
     1 These are subjective data because the patient must express these to the nurse. They cannot be observed by the nurse.
     2, 3, 4 These are objective data that can be observed by the nurse.
149. Comprehension, planning, physiologic (b)
     4 The primary goal is to provide complete bed rest to promote healing of the damaged myocardium.
     1 This is important, but immediate attention should be to provide rest for the damaged myocardium.
     2 A gradual increase of activities may begin the second day, but initially bed rest is most important.
     3 To provide diversional activity is not a primary goal; this is, however, included as part of the nursing care.

150. Comprehension, implementation, physiologic (b)
    4 The description of the type of chest pain is significant to assist in diagnosing a myocardial infarction, angina pectoris, or congestive heart failure.
    1, 2, 3 These relate to symptoms of congestive heart failure.
151. Application, planning, environment (b)
    2 Assessment of the patient's knowledge is always the first step in health teaching.
    1 The patient should be assessed for knowledge of nutritional needs before patient teaching.
    3 The patient's knowledge level should be assessed first.
    4 The patient may not know what to ask concerning his illness.
152. Application, assessment, physiologic (b)
    3 The patient should be on a low-fat diet to help lower his cholesterol level.
    1 Some foods may not contain cholesterol (found in animal foods) but may have a high level of fat content such as vegetable oil. A low-fat diet best reduces cholesterol levels.
    2 This would have no effect on serum cholesterol.
    4 This is not specific to the patient's dietary needs.
153. Comprehension, planning, physiologic (a)
    2 A low- to moderate-sodium diet is recommended because of tendency to retain fluids.
    1 A bland diet is more often associated with gastric problems.
    3 A low-fat diet is recommended for healthy living.
    4 This is not recommended for any diagnosis.
154. Knowledge, implementation, physiologic (b)
    1 Nitroglycerin tablets are only effective when administered sublingually.
    2 Liquids should not be taken with nitroglycerin.
    3 Nitroglycerin is not taken with food. It is inactivated in the stomach.
    4 It is not necessary to take nitroglycerin at bedtime, unless the patient is experiencing angina.
155. Comprehension, assessment, environment (c)
    2 The pain associated with an acute myocardial infarction is usually not relieved with rest, nitroglycerin, or changes in position.
    1 The pain of a myocardial infarction is typically not relieved with rest.
    3 Pain is often described as severe, squeezing, or crushing.
    4 The pain of a myocardial infarction is usually not relieved with the administration of nitroglycerin.
156. Comprehension, assessment, physiologic (c)
    1 Symptoms of acute pulmonary edema include rapid onset of severe dyspnea, coughing, and orthopnea. This is often followed by the production of frothy, pink-tinged sputum. Heart failure is a potential complication following a myocardial infarction.
    2 Findings of cardiogenic shock include falling blood pressure; tachycardia; weak pulse; cool, clammy skin; and decreasing urinary output.
    3 With pulmonary embolism, signs and symptoms usually include onset of shortness of breath with or without pleuritic chest pain.
    4 Right-sided failure is characterized by pitting edema, distended neck veins, fatigue, and increase in the size of the abdomen.

157. Comprehension, implementation, physiologic (b)
    1 In an upright position, full expansion of the lungs is facilitated. Decreasing venous return reduces the cardiac workload.
    2 Rest is important in reducing oxygen requirements, but relieving the dyspnea would not be helped by placing the patient in the supine position.
    3 Measures to decrease, not increase, venous return should be implemented.
    4 With the patient's head down, additional respiratory distress would occur.
158. Comprehension, assessment, environment (b)
    4 Echocardiography is a noninvasive test that is used to evaluate changes in the heart's structure and function.
    1 The chest x-ray examination provides information about respiratory disorders.
    2 The electrocardiogram (ECG) provides specific information about the electrical forces of the heart.
    3 Serial blood cultures provide information about infections.
159. Application, planning, physiologic (c)
    4 The goal for these nursing interventions is that the patient will adjust to changing energy levels and will learn to conserve energy.
    1 These are the nursing interventions for a patient with depression.
    2 These are the nursing interventions for hypertensive crisis (a sudden, severe elevation of blood pressure with systolic greater than 200 mm Hg and diastolic greater than 120 mm Hg).
    3 These are the nursing interventions for secondary polycythemia. This is a compensatory response to hypoxemia, which may result from chronic obstructive pulmonary disease (COPD) or congenital heart disease.
160. Comprehension, implementation, physiologic (b)
    4 Decreased cardiac output causes blood to dam up in the left side of the heart; blood can't be pumped effectively, resulting in lung congestion.
    1 This may be a contributing factor, but it is not the primary cause.
    2 This is not a primary cause. Etiologic factors associated with congestive heart conditions are coronary occlusion, myocardial infarction, vascular heart disease, and pericardial inflammatory condition. The underlying mechanism in congestive heart failure involves failure of the heart's pumping mechanism to respond to the body's metabolic changes. Congestive heart failure is also attributed to hypertension, stress, hyperthyroidism, hemorrhage, anemia, or fluid-replacement therapy.
    3 This may be a result; however, it is not a primary cause.
161. Knowledge, assessment, physiologic (a)
    2 Paroxysmal nocturnal dyspnea (waking up at night with shortness of breath) is a common sign of early congestive heart failure as a result of decreased cardiac output.
    1 These are signs of pulmonary edema, a life-threatening complication of CHF.
    3 These are symptoms of emphysema.
    4 These are symptoms of pulmonary tuberculosis.
162. Knowledge, planning, physiologic (b)
    3 This results from the inability of the heart to function as a pump.
    1 This is a symptom of myocardial infarction.
    2 This is a symptom of endocarditis.
    4 This is a symptom of an aneurysm; an aneurysm can result from trauma, congenital weakness, arteriosclerosis, or infection.

163. Application, assessment, physiologic (c)
    2 This is most characteristic when the lungs are congested.
    1 These sounds are associated with pneumothorax.
    3 These are sounds of chronic obstructive pulmonary disease.
    4 This is not expected when auscultating.
164. Comprehension, assessment, physiologic (a)
    1 Inflammation is the body's reaction to injury or irritation, not to an invasion of pathogenic microorganisms.
    2 Allergy is an antigen-antibody reaction of the body to a substance, causing the body to be hypersensitive to that substance.
    3 Infection occurs when the body is invaded by microorganisms and illness develops.
    4 Immunity is the body's ability to have a resistance to a specific disease. Resistance can be the result of either active or passive immunity.
165. Application, implementation, health (a)
    3 Exercise and support hose help reduce the complication and possibility of clots in the lower extremities.
    1 Exercise usually increases rather than decreases circulation.
    2 Exercise does not prevent abdominal edema.
    4 Exercise does not necessarily reduce edema of the extremities.
166. Knowledge, assessment, physiologic (a)
    2 Citrus fruits in their natural state are least likely to contain large amounts of sodium.
    1 Baking soda has a high sodium content.
    3 These choices contain sodium.
    4 Canned meats are high in sodium.
167. Knowledge, planning, physiologic (a)
    4 Digitalis strengthens and tones the heart muscle.
    1 Antianxiety drugs are used to lessen the tension or anxiety when required.
    2 Coagulants are used to stop bleeding.
    3 This is used to stimulate breathing.
168. Comprehension, assessment, physiologic (b)
    4 These symptoms are the results of pulmonary congestion in the interstitial spaces and alveoli.
    1 Dyspnea is experienced, but not necessarily on exertion.
    2 Orthopnea, not necessarily angina, is experienced.
    3 Sputum is frothy, not tenacious.
169. Comprehension, planning, physiologic (a)
    2 The gain or loss of body weight usually indicates a gain or loss of body fluid.
    1 This is not an indication for daily weights.
    3 Body fat is not a factor in weight loss of a patient with congestive heart failure.
    4 Loss of appetite does not necessarily mean a loss of weight.
170. Comprehension, assessment, physiologic (c)
    1 This causes a backup of blood into the lungs.
    2 This does not affect the backup of blood into the lungs.
    3, 4 There is no backup of blood flow into the lungs.
171. Comprehension, assessment, physiologic (c)
    4 Increased pulmonary pressure occurs with fluid buildup in the lungs (pulmonary edema).
    1 Fatigue does occur, but it is not a significant indication of complications.
    2 Restlessness may occur without indicating a major problem.
    3 This is not indicative of the diagnosis.

172. Comprehension, planning, environment (b)
    3 Maintaining skin integrity, rest, and position for easier breathing are important considerations.
    1 This is not commonly considered.
    2 Stabilization of the condition is needed first, before ambulation.
    4 The nurse must avoid increasing the strain on the heart; increasing fluid intake will also increase fluid buildup in the lungs.
173. Application, evaluation, environment (c)
    1 This provides for systematic monitoring of fluid intake and output.
    2 This is indicative, but daily weights are needed for closer monitoring.
    3, 4 Activity is not a factor in fluid balance.
174. Application, planning, environment (c)
    3 Patients with valvular disease need prophylactic antibiotic therapy before dental or surgical procedures to reduce their risk of developing endocarditis.
    1 Although activity may be restricted for a short time, the patient does not usually need to continue with a sedentary lifestyle.
    2 Dehydration is not an associated problem.
    4 The patient must watch for signs and symptoms of infection, but wearing a mask in crowds is not practical or appropriate.
175. Knowledge, planning, physiology (b)
    4 This results from an infectious process.
    1 This is a symptom of an aneurysm.
    2 This is a symptom of the inability of the heart to function like a pump.
    3 This is a symptom of myocardial infarction.
176. Knowledge, planning, physiologic (a)
    4 Rheumatic fever is seen in children between 5 and 14 years of age.
    1 It is more prevalent in children.
    2 It is no more prevalent in males than it is in females.
    3 It is no more prevalent in females than it is in males.
177. Application, implementation, health (b)
    2 The patient will be awake during the procedure and can view the monitor.
    1 There may be discomfort as a result of the procedure, but there should be no pain.
    3 The NPO order is for 6 to 8 hours before the procedure.
    4 Blood samples from the various chambers of the heart are obtained.
178. Comprehension, evaluation, physiologic (c)
    1 The P wave is caused by the atria, thereby recording the impulse from the sinoatrial node.
    2 The Q, R, S, and T waves are related to the contraction of the ventricles.
    3 It is not the P wave that diagnoses myocardial infarction.
    4 The P wave records impulses, not lesions.
179. Application, implementation, physiologic (a)
    3 This represents the pressure within the artery between beats.
    1 Refractory period refers to skeletal muscle fiber.
    2 Systole represents the ventricles contracting.
    4 Atrial systole refers to the contraction of the atria.
180. Comprehension, evaluation, physiologic (c)
    1 Scar tissue forms, affecting the functioning of these valves.
    2 The tricuspid valve is not affected.
    3 The pulmonary valves are not affected.
    4 These valves are not affected.

181. Comprehension, assessment, physiologic (b)
    1 Plaque formation occludes major coronary arteries, obstructing the blood supply to the myocardium.
    2, 3 ASHD does not affect the lungs.
    4 Endocarditis is a bacterial infection with no direct relationship to sclerotic vessels.

182. Application, implementation, physiologic (a)
    4 This artery provides the best pulsating sound and is easily accessible.
    1 The radial artery's pulsating sound is not clear and strong.
    2 This artery can be used but usually is not unless the brachial site is unavailable.
    3 The location of the femoral artery is not convenient for this procedure.

183. Application, implementation, safety (a)
    2 Bed rest assists in maximizing cardiac function; penicillin and aspirin are given to minimize the inflammatory process.
    1 Dietary implications are not a factor.
    3 Steroid therapy is used with complications such as arthritis or congestive heart failure.
    4 This is treatment for anginal pain; it is not applicable.

184. Knowledge, planning, physiologic (a)
    4 There is an obstruction or cutting off of the blood supply to the coronary artery or its branches.
    1 A seizure has no relation to coronary occlusion.
    2 Coronary refers to the heart.
    3 The coronary arteries can become occluded by a thrombus or embolus.

185. Comprehension, planning, physiologic (a)
    2 This grafts healthy vessels around the area of the occlusion.
    1 Coronary refers to the heart.
    3 No stimulation of the heart muscle is needed.
    4 This procedure is known as an endarterectomy.

186. Knowledge, assessment, physiologic (b)
    2 A cardiac catheterization is an invasive test using radiopaque dye to visualize the patency of the coronary vessels.
    1 The test will not determine the actual amount of blood entering the right atrium.
    3 Left ventricle pressure may be measured during the procedure, but is not the primary purpose of the test.
    4 Ventricle contractility may be measured in terms of an ejection fraction, but the most common purpose of catheterization is to determine blockage.

187. Knowledge, assessment, physiologic (c)
    4 Contrast medium contains iodine, which is also found in seafood.
    1 There is no correlation between the contrast medium and the intake of foods high in fat.
    2 Antihistamines do not affect the contrast medium.
    3 Weight gain or loss is not relevant to the use of a contrast medium.

188. Comprehension, implementation, physiologic (b)
    1 A potential complication is the formation of an arterial thrombus that is so large that it completely or partially occludes the artery. The pulse distal to the catheter entry site should be assessed frequently during the first few hours following the procedure.
    2 The extremity used for the catheter insertion is immobilized and kept in a straight position.
    3 Hyperextension and flexion of the extremity are to be avoided.
    4 Fluids are usually encouraged to aid in removing the contrast medium from the body, especially from the kidneys.

189. Application, assessment, psychosocial (b)
    4 Nicotine acts as a vasoconstrictor that results in poor circulation to the extremities.
    1 There is some connection that needs further explanation.
    2 This is not an accurate statement.
    3 Arteriosclerosis does not directly affect the lungs.

190. Knowledge, assessment, physiologic (b)
    1 Because of lack of blood supply to lower extremities, the patient with arterial insufficiency may experience loss of hair on the extremity.
    2 This would be a sign of varicose veins, not arterial insufficiency.
    3 This is normal.
    4 This is more likely a symptom of venous disease.

191. Knowledge, assessment, physiologic (c)
    4 Lack of pedal pulse means that there is a gross lack of blood supply to the extremity. This must be reported immediately.
    1 This is an indicator of arterial insufficiency, but it is not as severe as No. 4.
    2, 3 These are normal.

192. Comprehension, evaluation, physiologic (b)
    2 The temperature of the patient's leg gives an indication of blood supply to the leg.
    1 Vital signs should be taken more often initially to monitor for bleeding or hypovolemia.
    3 This is not relative to circulation assessment.
    4 This is not necessary immediately following surgery.

193. Comprehension, assessment, physiologic (b)
    3 Homans' sign is elicited by dorsiflexing the foot and is considered positive when pain is present.
    1 Platelets (thrombocytes) are necessary blood constituents of the clotting process, but they are not specifically elevated in thrombophlebitis.
    2 Chvostek's sign is a contraction of facial muscles in response to a light tap over the facial nerve in front of the ear.
    4 Anemia is a reduction in the number of erythrocytes and levels of hemoglobin and hematocrit; it is not a manifestation of thrombophlebitis.

194. Knowledge, planning, physiologic (c)
    2 The cardinal symptoms of a blood clot in a vein are pain, heat, redness, and swelling.
    1 Fever, nausea, and vomiting may be associated with an infectious process, but they are not specific for thrombophlebitis.
    3 These gastrointestinal symptoms are not related to venous obstruction.
    4 Anorexia may occur as a result of the pain involved in vascular obstruction. This answer, however, is not inclusive of the primary symptoms of thrombophlebitis.

195. Knowledge, implementation, physiologic (b)
    3 The inflammation and clot formation are associated with venous stasis.
    1 There is no ulcer present.
    2 There is inflammation, but the condition involves a clot.
    4 Phlebitis is an inflammation of the vein.

196. Application, evaluation, physiologic (b)
    1 Chest pain is exhibited if the embolism is lodged in the lungs. Severe pain can lead to shock and depletion of proper circulation.
    2 Areas involved would be cyanotic and cold; the patient would complain of a tingling sensation or numbness.
    3 The patient's pulse would be elevated.
    4 The patient would show apprehension and sudden onset of dyspnea.

197. Knowledge, implementation, physiologic (a)
    4 This is a blood clot that circulates in the blood and more commonly lodges in the lungs.
    1 An embolism travels.
    2 Most emboli arise from deep-vein thrombi.
    3 Emboli can lodge in different vital organs.
198. Knowledge, implementation, physiologic (a)
    2 Early ambulation and exercise promote circulation.
    1 This is not given in this situation.
    3 Massage helps to relax, providing some circulation; however, it is not the best choice.
    4 Encouraging movement in bed prevents venous stasis.
199. Application, implementation, physiologic (a)
    1 Massaging the legs could dislodge the thrombus that becomes an embolus, which can circulate in the blood to the vital organs.
    2 This could help circulation and relaxation.
    3 The patient has no limitation of activity in bed.
    4 Elevating the head does not affect this condition.
200. Application, implementation, health (a)
    1 Because circulation is poor, there is a good chance of burns to the extremities.
    2 Snug shoes will further impair circulation.
    3 Legs should be elevated periodically to improve circulation.
    4 Extreme cold weather should be avoided to prevent further constriction and impairment of circulation.
201. Comprehension, assessment, physiologic (b)
    1 Assessment of the patient's description of the pain would be the first step in the nursing process. Subjective data from the interview should be obtained first.
    2, 3, 4 These would be done after No. 1. They are based on objective data.
202. Comprehension, assessment, physiologic (b)
    4 Thrombophlebitis, as do other venous disorders, causes edema and redness of the lower extremity because of venous pooling.
    1, 3 These are signs of arterial, not venous, disease.
    2 Redness, not ecchymosis, would be present.
203. Application, implementation, environment (b)
    4 Elastic stockings support the leg and encourage venous blood return. They should be worn at all times.
    1 This is not necessary, because no wound is present.
    2 The affected extremity should not have range of motion. Inflamed parts must be at rest.
    3 Warm compresses are preferred to encourage venous circulation.
204. Comprehension, evaluation, health (a)
    3 Green leafy vegetables are a source of vitamin K, which enhances the clotting process and should be avoided.
    1, 2, 4 These are not good sources of vitamin K.
205. Comprehension, assessment, physiologic (c)
    2 When the valves are no longer able to function, the venous return of blood becomes sluggish and blood accumulates in the veins.
    1 There is no infection involved.
    3 This condition is not considered congenital.
    4 There is no deposit of materials in the veins.
206. Knowledge, planning, physiologic (b)
    1 Varicose veins are dilated and tortuous veins that are a result of a backflow of blood because of inadequate closure of valves.
    2 The increased amount of blood causes further dilation of the veins.
    3 Because of elasticity, the veins become longer as well as larger.
    4 There are no bacteria involved.

207. Application, implementation, physiologic (a)
    3 Thrombolytic drugs are used to promote the digestion of fibrin to dissolve the clot(s).
    1 Antibiotics are used to fight bacterial infection.
    2 Vitamins are used for vitamin deficiencies.
    4 Antineoplastic agents are used for chemotherapy.
208. Application, implementation, physiologic (c)
    1 The blood transfusion needs to be stopped immediately since the patient is experiencing early signs of a transfusion reaction. The doctor needs to be notified so further treatment can be given.
    2 Any blood the patient receives from the same transfusion bag will further the allergic reaction and could lead to an anaphylactic reaction.
    3 Benadryl cream will not help the systemic effects of the reaction.
    4 Treatment needs to be started immediately to prevent severe complications or even death.
209. Application, assessment, physiologic (c)
    4 Iron is a component of hemoglobin. A deficiency of iron affects the ability of the red blood cells to carry oxygen to the tissues. The red blood cells contain decreased levels of hemoglobin.
    1 Impaired production of blood-forming elements is associated with aplastic anemias.
    2 White blood cells protect the body against disease.
    3 Platelet destruction and bleeding are related to coagulation disorders.
210. Application, planning, physiologic (b)
    4 Fatigue is a common symptom associated with iron-deficiency anemia. Because of chronic tissue hypoxia, the patient has an activity intolerance.
    1 Pain is not associated with iron-deficiency anemia.
    2, 3 These are not specific for iron-deficiency anemia.
211. Application, planning, physiologic (b)
    4 Nursing interventions focus on balancing activity and rest periods.
    1 Absolute bed rest is not needed.
    2 This is not a specific intervention for iron-deficiency anemia.
    3 The patient needs more rest periods rather than increased periods of exercise.
212. Comprehension, evaluation, environment (b)
    4 Green leafy vegetables are a good source of iron.
    1 These are not a problem for iron-deficiency anemia.
    2 Although eggs do contain some iron, green vegetables are a better source.
    3 Milk does not contain iron. A quart of milk is unnecessary for adults.
213. Knowledge, assessment, physiologic (c)
    4 Sickle cell anemia is a hereditary trait that occurs mostly in the black population.
    1 Sickle cell anemia is not a viral disease.
    2 It is not a bacterial disease.
    3 The disease is not caused by blood transfusions.
214. Comprehension, assessment, physiologic (b)
    1 In acute leukemia, there is an abnormal overproduction of a specific white blood cell, usually at an immature stage.
    2 Decreased T-lymphocytes are associated with immune disorders.
    3 A marked increase in hematocrit is associated with the blood disorder polycythemia vera.
    4 A low level of hemoglobin is associated with iron-deficiency anemia.

215. Comprehension, planning, environment (c)
    2 Because of the thrombocytopenia (lower-than-normal number of platelets), the patient is at risk for bleeding. Patient should be taught about bleeding precautions.
    1, 3, 4 These choices address precautions to be taken when the patient is at risk for infection because of neutropenia or leukopenia.

216. Application, implementation, physiologic (c)
    2 Patients with leukopenia are at increased risk for infection. When the WBC count is low or there are large numbers of immature white cells, the usual signs of infection (redness, heat, swelling) are not manifested. The presence of fever is very significant, and efforts must be made to find the source of the infection.
    1 Rectal temperatures are not necessary. Patients receiving chemotherapy are also at risk for thrombocytopenia, and rectal temperatures are not recommended.
    3 Bleeding is associated with thrombocytopenia.
    4 Although fluids are important, on the basis of the situation this is not the action that is most warranted.

217. Application, implementation, environment (b)
    3 A vial of medication, even if new, should be cleansed with an antiseptic before inserting the needle for withdrawal.
    1 To prevent further contamination to broken skin, sterile gloves would be best during a dressing change.
    2 An IV site that is red and warm should have the IV discontinued, not slowed down.
    4 A new isolation gown should be worn every time a nurse enters the patient's room.

218. Comprehension, planning, physiologic (b)
    3 The human immunodeficiency virus (HIV) attacks the immune and nervous systems.
    1 This virus causes mononucleosis.
    2 This virus causes cold sores.
    4 This virus causes hepatitis.

219. Comprehension, planning, environment (b)
    1 The major source of HIV transmission is via blood and body fluids.
    2 This is not medically necessary, nor is the social isolation good for the patient psychologically.
    3 This is not medically indicated.
    4 This is not medically necessary because transmission is from blood and body fluids.

220. Comprehension, planning, environment (c)
    3 Oral poliovirus is made from live attenuated virus culture.
    1 Tetanus and diphtheria are inactivated for the vaccine.
    2 Diphtheria and pertussis may not be caught from the vaccine.
    4 Polio may not be caught from this vaccine.

221. Knowledge, assessment, environment (b)
    4 These are the major routes of AIDS transmission.
    1, 2, 3 Although HIV has been isolated in these routes of transmission, the primary routes remain sexual, blood, and transplacental.

222. Comprehension, assessment, health (c)
    2 The enzyme-linked immunosorbent assay (ELISA) is an AIDS virus antibody test that detects the organism causing the disease. For most persons, this test could detect marker antibodies at or about 10 to 12 weeks after exposure. Some persons may not experience marker antibodies for as long as 6 months after exposure.
    1, 3, 4 Although these diseases are often *associated* with AIDS, the ELISA is not specifically for them.

223. Comprehension, assessment, physiologic (c)
    4 Karposi's sarcoma, which manifests as purplish skin lesions, is a common symptom in homosexual men with AIDS.
    1 Patients with AIDS usually have chronic diarrhea, not constipation.
    2 This is not a usual symptom of AIDS.
    3 The temperature of AIDS patients is usually elevated, not subnormal.

224. Comprehension, assessment, physiologic (b)
    3 Oral candidiasis causes painful lesions in the mouth and throat.
    1, 2, 4 These are not signs of candidiasis.

225. Application, implementation, environment (a)
    4 Chlorine bleach is the best disinfective against the AIDS virus, which could be found in body fluids.
    1, 2 These are not necessary. Blood and body fluids are the infective material. Gloves, gown, mask, or goggles should be used only when there is danger of contact with body fluids.
    3 AIDS patients may be in semiprivate rooms and share bathrooms because blood and body fluids are the only modes of transmission.

226. Knowledge, implementation, physiologic (b)
    3 A residual of more than 50% of previous feeding indicates slow gastric emptying time. The feeding needs to be withheld and the physician called. The gastric contents are returned to prevent fluid and electrolyte imbalance.
    1 The gastric contents should not be discarded; this would cause fluid and electrolyte imbalance.
    2 Having too much stomach contents will cause nausea.
    4 Gastric contents should be returned.

227. Knowledge, assessment, physiologic (a)
    3 A strangulated hernia is an emergency situation in which the blood supply of the protrusion is eliminated, resulting in potential gangrene.
    1 An incarcerated hernia is edema of the protruding structures, which eliminates the possibility of returning the structures to the involved cavity.
    2 An incisional hernia occurs through the scar of a surgical incision when healing has been impaired.
    4 An umbilical hernia usually occurs because the umbilical orifices fail to close after birth. Obesity and prolonged abdominal distention can also result in an umbilical hernia.

228. Comprehension, implementation, environment (b)
    4 The appropriate preparation for a barium enema is to keep the patient NPO and to give enemas until clear, to visualize the lower colon.
    1 The patient is to be NPO after midnight.
    2 This is the preparation of a patient for oral cholecystography.
    3 This is part of the procedure for a liver biopsy.

229. Application, planning, environment (a)
    3 An endoscopy is considered an invasive procedure; preparation is similar to preparing a patient for surgery.
    1 This refers to an oral cholecystography.
    2 This refers to a T-tube cholangiography.
    4 This applies to noninvasive procedures such as ultrasounds and computed tomography (CT) scans.

230. Comprehension, implementation, physiologic (a)
    2 The patient's gag reflex is temporarily anesthetized; therefore, the patient is to be NPO until the gag reflex returns.
    1, 4 This is contraindicated until the gag reflex returns.
    3 There is no time limit as to when the patient can have food or liquids. The only criterion is to wait for the gag reflex to return.

231. Comprehension, assessment, physiologic (b)
    1 Gastric ulcer pain is more frequent when the stomach is empty and hydrochloric acid is secreted. Food relieves this.
    2 Pain in gastric ulcer disease is relieved by vomiting because hydrochloric acid is expelled.
    3 Food relieves the pain of gastric ulcers.
    4 Pain may occur during the night but also when the stomach is empty during the day.

232. Comprehension, evaluation, physiologic (c)
    4 Sudden onset of intense abdominal pain is a sign that the ulcer has perforated and peritonitis is developing.
    1 Body temperature may rise.
    2 This is not a sign of perforation.
    3 Vomitus would be grossly bloody, not blood tinged.

233. Application, implementation, safety (c)
    3 Nasogastric tubes must always be connected to low intermittent suction. High suction would disturb acid/base balance.
    1 Fluids are not given with a nasogastric tube.
    2 Normal saline only must be used as an irrigant to preserve acid/base balance.
    4 Cantor tubes, not nasogastric tubes, are advanced hourly.

234. Comprehension, evaluation, environment (c)
    4 Carbohydrates, particularly refined carbohydrates, are contraindicated in a postgastrectomy patient because they are absorbed quickly, causing an increase in dumping syndrome symptoms. Fats delay absorption.
    1, 2, 3 These will prevent premature emptying of the stomach.

235. Application, implementation, safety (b)
    3 The warm moist urine could foster growth of microorganisms, resulting in an inappropriate diagnosis and treatment for the patient.
    1 A urine specimen does not need to be warm when it arrives in the laboratory.
    2 The specimen could be spilled, but this would not be the most important concern.
    4 The microorganisms will continue to grow instead of dying.

236. Comprehension, planning, safety (b)
    1 The endoscope will be passed into the stomach; no food or fluid should be present to obstruct the view.
    2, 3, 4 These are not needed; it is the stomach that will be viewed.

237. Application, implementation, physiologic (b)
    2 Drug therapy will decrease or neutralize the normal gastric acidity.
    1 After medication therapy, a high-fat, high-carbohydrate diet is needed.
    3 A high-fat, high-carbohydrate diet is needed for gastric juices to digest over a longer period of time and thus decrease gastric acidity.
    4 The diet should be low in protein and milk products to decrease the need for high levels of gastric juices.

238. Comprehension, planning, physiologic (c)
    3 This decreases acid production by the parietal cells of the stomach.
    1 This procedure, known as an antrectomy, is not necessary.
    2 This procedure, known as a gastric resection, is not necessary.
    4 This procedure, known as a gastrectomy, is not necessary.

239. Comprehension, planning, physiologic (c)
    4 Rapid gastric emptying is the result of a bolus of hypertonic food that increases motility and peristalsis and thus changes blood glucose levels.
    1 This is only a partial causative factor.
    2, 3 These are not caused by the amount of hydrochloric acid in the stomach.

240. Application, implementation, physiologic (c)
    1 This decreases or slows the emptying time of the stomach.
    2 Reclining before meals is not helpful to the condition.
    3 The nurse should teach the patient to avoid fluids during meals to decrease motility and peristalsis after eating.
    4 A decreased amount of carbohydrates will slow the emptying time of the stomach.

241. Comprehension, assessment, physiologic (b)
    4 It is not uncommon for the ulcerative colitis patient to experience 10 to 12 bloody stools per day.
    1 Constipation is not a symptom.
    2 Bright dark-red bleeding is more common than tarry stools.
    3 Pain is located in the lower abdomen.

242. Comprehension, evaluation, physiologic (b)
    1 Oatmeal and orange slices are high in fiber. Most ulcerative colitis patients have a lactose intolerance; milk should not be included.
    2, 3, 4 These are low-residue foods.

243. Comprehension, assessment, physiologic (a)
    1 Because the feces is coming from the ileum, the consistency is semiliquid with mucous shreds from the lining.
    2 Blood should not be present. Semiformed feces would come from an ascending colectomy.
    3 This would be characteristic of a sigmoid colectomy.
    4 Blood should not be present in the stool after an ileostomy.

244. Knowledge, planning, physiologic (a)
    1 Histamine is normally present in the body, but when given it stimulates the production of gastric secretions.
    2 Belladonna inhibits gastric secretions, which is contrary to the purpose of a gastric analysis.
    3 Atropine blocks vagal effect rather than stimulates it as the diagnostic test requires.
    4 Paregoric diminishes digestive secretions, which is contraindicated in this test.

245. Comprehension, planning, psychosocial (a)
    3 The disease is managed on an outpatient basis with sedatives, tranquilizers, antispasmodics as indicated by the individual patient's need.
    1, 2, 4 With today's managed care forces, this condition is treated on an outpatient basis.

246. Application, assessment, physiologic (b)
    2 A liquid light-brown stool is expected from a transverse colostomy in the immediate postoperative period.
    1 Bloody stool with clots is not a normal expectation of a colostomy, even in the postoperative period.
    3 A semisolid stool is expected after the patient has a normal food intake.
    4 A solid stool is not normally produced by a transverse colostomy. Blood is also not a normal expectation.

247. Comprehension, evaluation, physiologic (a)
    1 This would indicate less irritation or active disease process within the colon.
    2 Hardening is not a factor in the disease process.
    3 Normal stools are not present in the disease process.
    4 A decrease is indicative, but a decrease in pus, blood, and mucus is also a factor.

248. Application, assessment, physiologic (c)

    4 A purple discoloration may indicate inadequate circulation to the stoma; therefore the physician should be notified.

    1 The nurse's notes may not be immediately read by the physician; this may leave the patient's problem untreated for some time.

    2 A purple discoloration on the stoma does not necessarily indicate simple bruising; it may indicate inadequate circulation to the stoma.

    3 A petrolatum dressing will do nothing to treat the problem.

249. Comprehension, assessment, physiologic (c)

    4 Stool is passed through the narrowed colon to form a thin stool before exiting through the rectum.

    1, 2, 3 These are not the appropriate locations for such a stool.

250. Comprehension, planning, physiologic (a)

    2 This will clean out the lower bowel for visualization of the lower colon.

    1 This will not clean out the lower bowel

    3 This is not appropriate for this procedure.

    4 Both methods are not needed.

251. Comprehension, assessment, physiologic (c)

    1 The sigmoid colostomy removes the specific area involved.

    2 This is not appropriate; it involves the small intestine.

    3 The colectomy is removal of the area that is not involved.

    4 This is not the area where the involvement is located.

252. Knowledge, evaluation, physiologic (a)

    4 Cramping does occur when fluid is first introduced.

    1 The level of the container does not affect cramping.

    2 Cramping normally occurs so there is no need to discontinue the procedure.

    3 This will not allow irrigation and will not change the cramping effect.

253. Comprehension, implementation, safety (a)

    2 This is adequate placement for the solution to reach the stool.

    1 This is not in far enough; the solution will drain out.

    3, 4 This is too far in for the solution to irrigate the colon.

254. Knowledge, evaluation, psychosocial (a)

    2 This indicates denial of both the colostomy and the need for self-care.

    1 It is not unusual to have not gained full appetite back yet.

    3, 4 This is appropriate after having such a procedure.

255. Knowledge, assessment, physiologic (a)

    1 Chole (gall) lithiasis (stone) is the correct term.

    2 Cholecystitis is the term for inflammation of the gallbladder.

    3 Nephrolithiasis is the term for renal calculi.

    4 Glomerulonephritis is the term for inflammation of the nephrons of the kidneys.

256. Knowledge, assessment, physiologic (a)

    4 Bile is essential for the breakdown of fats; therefore the inability to digest fats properly is noted, along with the accumulation of bile, causing jaundice.

    1 This is indicative of hepatitis.

    2 This is indicative of peritonitis.

    3 This is indicative of cirrhosis.

257. Comprehension, planning, physiologic (a)

    2 This is a specially designed tube resembling a T that is placed in the common bile duct to facilitate drainage of bile.

    1 This is appropriate for a thoracotomy.

    3 This is appropriate for wound drainage.

    4 This is appropriate to provide an artificial airway.

258. Knowledge, planning, environment (a)

    4 These choices offer the least fat content.

    1, 2, 3 These choices offer more fat content than choice No. 4.

259. Application, assessment, physiologic (b)

    2 Nausea, bloating, and vomiting may occur due to impaired fat digestion and impaired bile flow.

    1 Bile pigments may be present in urine, giving it a very dark color.

    3 Stools may become grayish or "clay-colored" because of the absence of bile pigments.

    4 Abdominal pain may occur after eating fatty foods, not carbohydrates.

260. Application, implementation, physiologic (b)

    4 To prevent damage to the gastric mucosa, low intermittent suction should be used.

    1 Irrigation is not necessary unless the nasogastric tube is clogged.

    2 Wrapping the tube will serve no purpose in preventing postoperative nausea and vomiting.

    3 The patient will be NPO following surgery.

261. Application, implementation, physiologic (b)

    1 The dressing will need to be changed because even small amounts of bile leakage around the T-tube will irritate the skin.

    2 Reinforcing the dressing can still leave bile drainage on the skin.

    3 This is inappropriate general postoperative care.

    4 The patient will need appropriate analgesia, not usually sedation.

262. Application, planning, environment (b)

    3 This position will prevent the backflow of bile into the common bile duct.

    1 Tight clothing or a binder can cause pressure and irritation of the wound site.

    2 Showers are preferred because running water will prevent the possibility of bacteria entering the wound.

    4 Without clarification of this statement, the patient may consider all signs of redness and tenderness normal, even those associated with a developing infection, and so may not report the symptoms to the physician.

263. Knowledge, assessment, environment (b)

    1 Usually someone contracts hepatitis A from another person with unwashed hands.

    2 Hepatitis B may be spread through the sharing of body fluids.

    3 Intravenous drug users are at high risk for Hepatitis B.

    4 Hepatitis A is usually spread when there is poor hygiene.

264. Comprehension, assessment, physiologic (b)

    3 This indicates the inability of liver cells to remove bile pigment from circulating blood.

    1 This is a cause of diabetes.

    2 This is intestinal involvement, which is not connected to the biliary system.

    4 This is untrue; the cause *is* known.

265. Comprehension, planning, safety (b)

    1 This is a disease transmittable through direct contact with body fluids and secretions.

    2 IV antibiotics are not generally ordered unless severe infection is present.

    3 Universal precautions are a higher priority.

    4 This is contrary to treatment because altered nutrition usually occurs and increased fluid intake will be needed.

266. Comprehension, planning, physiologic (c)
    2 This indicates the inability of the liver to metabolize bile, which causes the elevation of bilirubin, SGOT, and serum glutamic pyruvic acid (SGPT).
    1 These results measure red blood cell values.
    3 An elevation of aspartate aminotransferase (AST) is noted, but there is a decrease in serum albumin.
    4 A decrease is noted in the serum albumin, but there is no direct relationship to hemoglobin noted in the test results.

267. Comprehension, planning, physiologic (b)
    2 Bed rest is necessary to decrease physical debilitation.
    1 Diet of choice is low in fat.
    3 This is an inappropriate response; diet is an integral part of the treatment plan.
    4 This would increase physical debilitation.

268. Knowledge, assessment, physiologic (a)
    3 Stool is clay-colored as a result of poor metabolism by the affected liver.
    1 This is usually the color of a normal stool.
    2 Black stool could be indicative of bleeding, but it is also noted in patients who are taking iron preparations.
    4 This could be indicative of a disease process, but not in this case.

269. Application, implementation, health (b)
    2 Providing six small meals with high-calorie in-between snacks promotes nutritional intake while maximizing energy and enhances the healing process of the liver.
    1 This is related to a nursing diagnosis of knowledge deficit.
    3 This is related to a possible diagnosis of injury related to bleeding.
    4 This is related to possible bleeding disorders associated with hepatitis B.

270. Comprehension, assessment, physiologic (b)
    3 The liver is primarily responsible for various drug metabolism and involves two processes.
    1 The liver is the most important organ in drug metabolism.
    2 The liver plays a major role in drug metabolism.
    4 The cardiovascular system is important in drug distribution. The liver is the major organ responsible for metabolism of drugs.

271. Comprehension, assessment, psychosocial (b)
    2 Codependency is defined as a set of maladaptive and/or immature responses, behaviors, and feelings experienced by someone closely associated with an actively chemically dependent person. Commonly reported symptoms include a self-esteem that relies heavily on feeling needed by others, the need to control others, and the tendency to develop complicated relationships with chemically dependent people.
    1 He may feel he is doing this as a caring husband; however, he may in fact be contributing to the problem itself.
    3 This behavior demonstrates acting on the problem.
    4 This behavior demonstrates awareness of the problem.

272. Knowledge, assessment, physiologic (c)
    3 A sign of acute pancreatitis is an elevated serum amylase level. Serum amylase levels increase within 24 to 48 hours of the onset of the condition and can range from 300 to 800 Somogyi units, although there is no apparent relationship between the severity of the disease and elevation of enzyme levels.
    1 The abdomen becomes hard and rigid.
    2 Bloody urine is not a usual sign.
    4 Elevated serum creatinine is indicative of poor kidney function, not poor pancreatic function.

273. Comprehension, evaluation, environment (b)
    3 Steamed vegetables and skimmed milk are fat-free foods.
    1 Tuna salad is made with mayonnaise, which is a fat.
    2 Hamburger is usually a high-fat meat.
    4 Cheese is a high-fat food. Usually butter or margarine is added in the grilling process.

274. Comprehension, planning, physiologic (b)
    3 Leukocytosis indicates an abnormal increase in the number of circulating white blood cells, a condition that often accompanies bacterial, but not usually viral, infections.
    1 Agranulocytosis is an abnormal condition of the blood characterized by a severe reduction in the number of granulocytes.
    2 Leukopenia is an abnormal decrease in the number of white blood cells to fewer than 5000 cells/ml³.
    4 Aplastic anemia is a deficiency of all of the formed elements of the blood, representing a failure of the cell-generating capacity of the bone marrow.

275. Comprehension, evaluation, physiologic (a)
    1 Peritonitis is an inflammation of the parietal and visceral surfaces of the abdominal cavity caused by bacterial infection.
    2 Ileitus is an inflammation of the ileum.
    3 Colitis is an inflammatory condition of the large intestine.
    4 Diverticulitis is an inflammation of one or more diverticulae; penetration of fecal matter through the thin-walled diverticula causes inflammation and abscess formation in the tissues surrounding the colon.

276. Comprehension, planning, safety (b)
    4 An ice bag to the abdomen is ordered to safely relieve the pain.
    1 Narcotics mask symptoms, especially of a ruptured appendix.
    2 Heat on the abdomen increases circulation to the area and can contribute to a ruptured appendix.
    3 A cleansing enema contributes to rupture of the appendix.

277. Knowledge, planning, physiologic (a)
    1 There is speculation that acute appendicitis is from a hardened mass of stool or foreign body.
    2, 3, 4 These bear no relationship to appendicitis.

278. Knowledge, implementation, psychosocial (a)
    3 This provides the patient with information about what he should expect after surgery, thereby decreasing his anxiety level and soliciting his assistance.
    1, 4 These are not immediate concerns.
    2 The pain caused by the appendicitis should be gone.

279. Comprehension, evaluation, environment (b)
    1 Typing and working on the computer aggravates the condition and should be avoided until symptoms subside. Then frequent rest periods need to be taken.
    2 Exercise needs to be continued, particularly movement of the fingers and wrists. Frequent rest periods are important.
    3 Calcium does not affect carpal tunnel syndrome. It is caused by compression of the median nerve.
    4 Rich foods can aggravate gout, but there is no indication that they will affect carpal tunnel syndrome.

280. Application, implementation, physiologic (b)
    2 Loss of sensation in the periphery may cause the person to not notice an injury.
    1 Postural hypotension is usually not associated with diabetic peripheral neuropathy.
    3 Waterlogged tissues are more prone to injury.
    4 A podiatrist should remove any calluses. Small breaks in the tissue may become infected.

281. Comprehension, implementation, physiologic (c)
    2 Reglan decreases the effect of gastric paresis found with autonomic neuropathy.
    1 Reglan doesn't affect blood pressure.
    3 Damage to nerves is not reparable.
    4 Reglan cannot generate new tissue.
282. Application, implementation, physiologic (c)
    1 Chocolate and citrus fruits have been identified as triggers for migraines. Both of these foods, along with red wine, chicken livers, and aged cheese, need to be avoided.
    2 Caffeine-containing beverages are also considered to be a trigger. These should be limited, although some studies have indicated that by taking two aspirins along with a caffeine-containing drink at the first sign of an attack may actually limit the pain.
    3 The patient needs to lie down in a dark room at the first sign of an attack. Exercise will only make it worse.
    4 Sleeping only 4 to 5 hours per night has not been shown to be effective in limiting migraines.
283. Comprehension, assessment, physiologic (c)
    1 Change in level of responsiveness is the earliest sign.
    2, 3, 4 These are signs of increased intracranial pressure but not the earliest.
284. Application, assessment, physiologic (c)
    4 Forceful vomiting is a sign of increased intracranial pressure.
    1 Hematoma formation is common with this type of injury.
    2 Headache is a frequent complaint when the head receives a blow.
    3 Hematoma formation and blackened eyes are common if the temporal area is injured.
285. Application, implementation, environment (a)
    4 The supine position with the head elevated 30 degrees allows for proper drainage of cerebral edema and will help reduce intracranial pressure (ICP).
    1, 2 These will not help reduce ICP.
    3 This will increase ICP.
286. Comprehension, assessment, physiologic (a)
    3 Vital sign changes with intracranial pressure (ICP) include elevated blood pressure, bradycardia, slow irregular respirations, and elevated temperature.
    1 Temperature is elevated.
    2 These signs alone do not indicate an increase in intracranial pressure.
    4 Bradycardia, elevated temperature, and hypertension are signs of increased intracranial pressure.
287. Knowledge, assessment, physiologic (c)
    2 The Glasgow Coma Scale has been designed to quantitatively relate consciousness to motor, verbal and eye-opening responses. Higher scores indicate increased degrees of arousal. A score of 14 or 15 indicates a patient is not neurologically impaired.
    1 Depending on the system used, scores of 9 or more do not qualify as coma; however, it is the examiner who determines the best response the patient can make to a set of standardized stimuli.
    3 Depending on the system used, a score less than 7 is accepted to indicate a coma.
    4 Determining a patient's orientation via a "best" verbal response is only one of the three responses tested using the Glasgow Coma Scale.
288. Comprehension, assessment, physiologic (a)
    1 These are subjective in that the patient would have to tell the nurse these symptoms.
    2, 3, 4 These are objective in that they are seen and measurable.
289. Application, assessment, physiologic (b)
    2 Rechecking ensures equipment is functioning, and reporting to the immediate supervisor (charge nurse) brings prompt attention to the changes; these changes indicate increased intracranial pressure.
    1, 3 Delay of reporting could have serious consequences, and therefore these are not correct procedures.
    4 These changes are significant and need to be reported.
290. Comprehension, planning, environment (a)
    4 Trendelenburg's (shock position) is contraindicated because it would increase the flow of blood to the cranium.
    1, 2, 3 These positions may be permitted.
291. Comprehension, planning, psychosocial (b)
    4 Although all of the answers could cause anxiety before the surgery, the patient's fear of the unknown would be the priority concern and could be relieved by the nurse explaining all procedures.
    1, 2, 3 These are not priority concerns.
292. Comprehension, assessment, physiologic (c)
    1 Dilated fixed pupils are the most ominous sign of neurologic damage and increased intracranial pressure (ICP).
    2 Widening pulse pressure is a sign of increased ICP.
    3 This is not the most critical sign.
    4 These are normal vital signs.
293. Comprehension, assessment, physiologic (c)
    2 This could mean injury to the spinal cord and leakage of cerebral spinal fluid.
    1, 4 These are not common complications of craniotomies.
    3 This would be a normal sign.
294. Application, implementation, physiologic (c)
    1 Determining if the patient is having airway difficulty should always be a first priority.
    2 The supine position could cause the patient to aspirate any secretions.
    3 Ice would be a good way to cool the patient, but airway management is always a top priority.
    4 After airway, breathing, and circulation are evaluated, obtaining assistance would be recommended.
295. Application, implementation, environment (b)
    4 Priority interventions during a seizure would be to remove harmful objects and protect the patient from injury.
    1 It is not necessary to monitor vital signs during a seizure.
    2 The nurse would be unable to open the patient's jaws; nothing but airways should be used in the mouth.
    3 Although a side-lying position is important, safety is the priority.
296. Comprehension, evaluation, environment (c)
    2 Gingival hyperplasia is a side effect of phenytoin (Dilantin) and should be reported to the physician for treatment.
    1 Weight loss is a side effect of phenytoin.
    3 Pink urine is a common, harmless side effect of Dilantin. It does not mean that the drug should be stopped.
    4 The patient must be stabilized on the drug for 2 years before driving a car or participating in hazardous activities.
297. Application, assessment, physiologic (c)
    1 This seizure activity is associated with complex distortion of thinking and feeling, as well as partially coordinated motor activity.
    2 This seizure activity is characterized by peculiar generalized tonelessness.
    3 This seizure activity may or may not be progressive.
    4 This seizure activity is characterized by mild or rapid forceful movements.

298. Application, assessment, safety (b)
    3 A complete health history is necessary to document any history of seizures.
    1 A skull series of x-ray examinations is a diagnostic study and not a nursing assessment; it will not provide necessary data because most seizures are not the result of musculoskeletal injury.
    2 The neurologic examination is not a nursing assessment; it is rather a diagnostic study. A complete neurologic examination will not demonstrate necessary information to diagnose seizure activity.
    4 This is a laboratory study, not a nursing diagnosis. It will not provide pertinent information for accurate diagnosis.

299. Comprehension, assessment, physiologic (b)
    4 Status epilepticus is a medical emergency and requires medical and nursing intervention to prevent death from brain damage that is a result of prolonged hypoxia and exhaustion.
    1 Grand mal seizure activity is characterized by loss of consciousness for several minutes.
    2 Psychomotor seizures are characterized by a sudden change in awareness associated with a complex distortion of feelings and thinking and partially coordinated motor activity.
    3 Petit mal seizures are characterized by sudden impairment in or loss of consciousness, with little or no tonic-clonic movement.

300. Application, implementation, physiologic (b)
    4 This is the result of prolonged hypoxia and exhaustion.
    1 Status epilepticus does not cause toxic disturbances.
    2 Status epilepticus does not cause metabolic problems.
    3 Status epilepticus does not cause hypertension.

301. Comprehension, implementation, health (b)
    3 Most states now require medical proof that seizures are under control.
    1 Driving during daylight hours does not decrease seizure activity.
    2 Driving laws vary concerning specific regulations. This is not the most common requirement
    4 It is recommended that the patient carry an identification card; however, this is not legally required.

302. Application, planning, health (b)
    4 The warning feelings some people experience are odd sensations such as unpleasant odors, spots before their eyes, flashing lights, vertigo, tingling, or numbness.
    1 This occurs during the recovery stage, in the postictal period. During this time there are common complaints of headaches and muscle aches.
    2 This is sometimes reported postictally.
    3 Hallucinations are not reported in most seizure activities.

303. Knowledge, assessment, physiologic (a)
    2 Complaints of headache are common.
    1, 4 These are not typically associated with seizures.
    3 This is not typical postictally.

304. Comprehension, implementation, physiologic (c)
    4 Most seizure disorders can be controlled partially or completely with anticonvulsants. These drugs also act to raise the seizure threshold. The choice of medication depends on the type of seizures.
    1 Digitalis preparations and atropine are examples. They are used to slow and strengthen the heartbeat and increase the heart rate.
    2 Anticonvulsants are central nervous system (CNS) depressants.
    3 Antispasmodics are used to treat muscle spasms and are *not* anticonvulsants.

305. Comprehension, assessment, health (b)
    3 Hypertension is a major risk factor associated with a cerebrovascular accident (CVA) or stroke. Other risk factors are emboli, intracranial hemorrhage, diabetes mellitus, increased blood viscosity, and cardiac disease.
    1, 2, 4 These individuals do not have known risks.

306. Comprehension, assessment, physiologic (b)
    2 Transient ischemic attacks may be a warning of an impending stroke.
    1 He is normotensive.
    3 Cigarette smoking causes vasoconstriction sytemically; chewing snuff causes a local reaction.
    4 Gardening alone is not a risk factor for stroke.

307. Application, planning, environment (b)
    4 Environmental assessment involves assessing the physical environment for potentially hazardous conditions. The following is a list of environmental concerns: poorly lighted stairwells, halls, or bathrooms; stairs with weak or absent banisters; absence of grab bars in the bathtub; glare in hallways; absence of a working smoke alarm; wet and/or waxed floors, poorly placed extension cords; throw rugs, clutter, inappropriate footwear, high beds; improper use of walking aids; and restraining and protective devices
    1 This addresses general considerations that are not all specific to environmental concerns.
    2 This addresses needs relevant to safe transportation, not the physical environmental concerns of the home.
    3 This addresses the availability of resources rather than environmental concerns.

308. Comprehension, planning, physiologic (b)
    1 An EEG tests brain wave activity.
    2 An ECG tests the heart.
    3, 4 MRI and CT scans are used to locate tumors.

309. Knowledge, assessment, physiologic (b)
    2 Ataxic refers to a clumsy gait.
    1 Otic refers to conditions of the ear.
    3 Apneic refers to periodic absences of breathing.
    4 Aphasic refers to the inability to speak.

310. Application, implementation, physiologic (c)
    3 The patient has left-sided neglect.
    1 The patient is unaware of food that is placed out of sight.
    2 The patient should be allowed to maintain his independence.
    4 Actually seeing the food rather than hearing about it will make him more likely to eat it.

311. Comprehension, planning, physiologic (b)
    3 Multiple sclerosis is a progressive degenerative disease in which the myelin sheath of the brain and the spinal cord is destroyed.
    1 This is characteristic of a type of seizure in epilepsy.
    2 This is characteristic of Parkinson's disease.
    4 This is characteristic of Ménière's syndrome.

312. Comprehension, implementation, physiologic (c)
    2 The Glasgow Coma Scale rates the best speech, ability to follow commands, and level of consciousness.
    1 Pain scale rating is not a part of a typical neurologic exam.
    3 Vital signs are taken and reviewed, but there is no scale to rate changes.
    4 Level of consciousness is examined, not level of orientation.

313. Comprehension, assessment, physiologic (b)
    2 Loss of muscular activities is a result of interference of nerve impulses.
    1 This is characteristic of a grand mal seizure.
    3 This is characteristic of a head injury.
    4 This is characteristic of Parkinson's disease.

314. Application, planning, health (a)
    1 The patient should remain active as long as possible and continue daily activities without becoming fatigued.
    2 This is recommended in Parkinson's disease.
    3 The patient is not to assume complete bed rest until complete loss of muscular function necessitates it. The drug therapy of choice is corticosteroids, which are anti-inflammatory agents, not antibiotics.
    4 The diet recommended is high calorie, high vitamin, and high protein.

315. Knowledge, implementation, psychosocial (a)
    3 Independence is always encouraged for the patient's well being.
    1 The patient should be encouraged to maintain social activities as long as possible. Occupational activities may have to be changed if necessary. Appropriately trained persons would best meet these needs of the patient.
    2 The patient should be encouraged to avoid treatments that promise a cure, because there is no cure.
    4 The patient should avoid complete bed rest unless absolutely necessary. The patient should be encouraged to be independent for as long as possible.

316. Application, implementation, health (b)
    1 At the present time there are no drugs that can stop the degenerative process of multiple sclerosis.
    2, 3, 4 These are included in the education for patients with multiple sclerosis.

317. Comprehension, planning, environment (b)
    4 This provides necessary exercise that is recommended for patients with Parkinson's.
    1 This does not provide exercise.
    2 In this activity, dexterity may be a problem; also, it does not provide needed exercise.
    3 This does not provide needed exercise.

318. Comprehension, planning, physiologic (a)
    3 The nurse should encourage daily exercise as tolerated to prevent pneumonia and to maintain joint mobility. Participation in previous work, as well as social and diversional activities, should be encouraged; this will avoid social withdrawal.
    1 Many patients with Parkinson's disease live for years.
    2 At this time there is no known way to stop the progression of this disease.
    4 There is no known cure at this time.

319. Comprehension, planning, environment (c)
    1 This is the nursing diagnosis for low back pain. Pain in the lower back may be caused by a variety of diseases.
    2 There is a potential for powerlessness imposed by progressive physical deterioration, loss of body control, and/or threat to physical integrity. The goal is for the patient to demonstrate an optimal level of mobility.
    3 The goal with this nursing diagnosis is to meet the patient's self-care needs by such measures as encouraging self-care as tolerated; promoting adequate pulmonary function by encouraging coughing and deep-breathing exercises; maintaining a well-balanced soft diet; and providing small feedings as indicated.
    4 This is an appropriate nursing diagnosis for Parkinson's disease. The goal is for the patient or significant other to demonstrate understanding of home care and follow-up instructions through interactive discussions and actual return demonstration.

320. Knowledge, assessment, physiologic (a)
    4 This is the disorder in adults that results from excessive secretion of the growth hormone.
    1 This is the disorder of hypopituitarism.
    2 This is the disorder of hyperthyroidism.
    3 This is the disorder of excessive production of the growth hormone in children.

321. Comprehension, assessment, health (b)
    1 These features are typical in an adult as a result of closure of the epiphyses of the long bones.
    2 These are subjective symptoms, not observations.
    3, 4 These are objective symptoms of gigantism.

322. Comprehension, implementation, psychosocial (b)
    4 Coarse facial features and broad hands, fingers, and feet may make one avoid social contacts.
    1 These are observations after a thyroidectomy if the parathyroids have been accidentally removed.
    2 These are dietary changes for hypoparathyroidism patients.
    3 These are observed with adrenalectomy patients.

323. Comprehension, assessment, physiologic (b)
    1 Hyperactivity and excitability are some of the classic signs of hyperthyroidism.
    2, 3 These are signs of hypothyroidism.
    4 This is not a sign of thyroid dysfunction.

324. Application, implementation, environment (b)
    3 This position will prevent stress on the suture line and prevent postoperative bleeding.
    1 This position would cause too much stress on the suture line.
    2 The head must be kept straight after surgery to prevent bleeding. A side-lying position is contraindicated.
    4 The prone position would cause stress on the suture line.

325. Comprehension, implementation, physiologic (b)
    4 This is to be prepared in case of excessive swelling of the throat that may occur, resulting in an emergency situation.
    1 This is not needed because in most cases the patient would be too warm (not of an emergent nature), and the blanket would cool off rapidly at the bedside.
    2 These are not used, and seizures are unlikely.
    3 This is not commonly needed for a thyroidectomy patient postoperatively (not of an emergent nature).

326. Application, implementation, environment (a)
    2 Iodine stains the teeth.
    1, 4 Iodine can be irritating to an empty stomach.
    3 Iodine should be diluted well.

327. Knowledge, evaluation, physiologic (a)
    2 This indicates elevated blood flow over the thyroid.
    1 This indicates blockage in the carotid arteries.
    3 T_3 resin uptake would be high.
    4 This indicates diabetes.

328. Application, planning, physiologic (c)
    1 The symptoms manifested by a hyperthyroid patient are the result of an accelerated metabolism and a speeding up of all physiologic processes. Signs and symptoms are weight loss, nervousness, weakness, insomnia, tachycardia, palpitations, exertional dyspnea, and ankle edema.
    2, 3, 4 Refer to option No. 1 for rationale.

329. Application, implementation, health (b)
    3 Keeping the head straight after surgery prevents stress on the suture line and prevents bleeding.
    1 The patient should be able to swallow right after surgery.
    2 This is not a priority in the early postoperative period.
    4 Coughing is contraindicated right after surgery because it could cause bleeding.

330. Comprehension, implementation, environment (b)
    2 The patient is instructed not to cough because it could cause bleeding.
    1 Fluid intake is necessary and can be given in spite of sore throat.
    3 This fails to facilitate breathing for the patient and does not allow for easier observation of respiratory complications.
    4 Caution must be exercised with morphine because it depresses respirations.
331. Comprehension, assessment, physiologic (b)
    4 Tetany manifested by involuntary tremors may be a sign of decreasing calcium levels.
    1, 2, 3 These are signs of hypercalcemia.
332. Comprehension, evaluation, physiologic (b)
    1 The medication actually blocks the production of thyroid hormones, thus decreasing the activity of the gland.
    2, 3 The medication decreases, rather than increases, the activity of the gland.
    4 Activity has no effect on the pancreas.
333. Knowledge, planning, health (a)
    4 Graves' disease is a disorder characterized by pronounced hyperthyroidism; it is usually associated with an enlarged thyroid gland and exophthalmos.
    1 Myxedema is the most severe form of hypothyroidism. It is characterized by swelling of the hands, face, feet and periorbital tissues and may lead to coma and death.
    2 Cretinism is a condition characterized by severe congenital hypothyroidism; it is often associated with other endocrine abnormalities.
    3 Colloid goiter involves a greatly enlarged, soft thyroid gland in which the follicles are distended with colloid.
334. Knowledge, implementation, physiologic (a)
    3 One of the functions of the thyroid gland is to regulate metabolism.
    1 This is not an endocrine gland but one of the largest pair of salivary glands that lie at the side of the face just below and in front of the external ear.
    2 The parathyroid gland is an endocrine gland that helps to maintain the level of blood calcium and ensures normal neuromuscular irritability, blood clotting, and cell membrane permeability.
    4 The pituitary gland is an endocrine gland supplying numerous hormones that govern vital processes such as growth and development, milk secretion, and contraction of smooth muscle.
335. Knowledge, planning, physiologic (a)
    2 Overproduction of the thyroid hormone thyroxin increases the activity of the thyroid gland.
    1 Lethargy occurs in hypothyroidism.
    3 Thyroxin levels would be high, not low.
    4 Thyroxin levels would be high.
336. Application, assessment, physiologic (b)
    2 Tetany can be caused by the parathyroid gland having been removed inadvertently or by excessive edema that can occlude parathyroid functioning.
    1 There is no direct relationship to the urinary system that would cause problems.
    3 This is to be expected as a result of edema in the throat.
    4 This could be a result of poor fluid intake because of edema of the throat; if observed, this should not become a major complication.

337. Application, planning, environment (a)
    1 Iodine can be irritating to the lining of the stomach and is difficult to absorb; additional fluids are necessary.
    2 An empty stomach has a high potential for irritation.
    3 The medication is being given for a purpose; giving it on a prn basis does not meet that purpose.
    4 Iodine preparations should not be given on an empty stomach because of irritability and poor absorption.
338. Application, evaluation, physiologic (b)
    1 Increased pulse rate is a result of a release of large amounts of thyroid hormone into the bloodstream.
    2 The pulse rate would increase.
    3 The large amount of thyroid hormone released should increase respirations.
    4 The increased amount of thyroid hormone released should elevate the temperature.
339. Application, implementation, environment (b)
    3 Regular insulin starts to work in ½ to 1 hour. When a mix of NPH and regular insulin is given in the morning, breakfast must be given within ½ hour of administration of the insulin.
    1 Regular insulin peaks in 2 to 3 hours. Not eating before this time could cause hypoglycemia.
    2 So that there is food for it to work on, regular insulin is always given before meals.
    4 Regular insulin peaks in 2 to 3 hours.
340. Application, implementation, environment (c)
    2 The American Diabetes Association recommends that if an individual is unable to eat the usual foods, appropriate liquids and/or soft foods should be substituted. Examples include ½ cup of apple juice, ½ cup of regular 7-UP, 1 cup of chicken noodle soup, ½ cup of sherbet, ½ cup of cooked cereal, 6 saltine crackers, or ½ cup fruit-flavored yogurt.
    1 Early self-care interventions may prevent the onset of nausea and vomiting. Nausea and vomiting require immediate reporting to the physician.
    3 If the patient is able to tolerate some foods and liquids and the illness does not progress, it is not necessary to immediately inform the physician.
    4 Insulin should be held only with the physician's order.
341. Knowledge, planning, environment (b)
    3 The individual diet is based on the patient's type of diabetes, weight, height, usual dietary intake, cultural preferences, exercise level, and daily schedule. Generally, meal plans comprise 55% to 65% carbohydrates, 12% to 15% proteins, and 20% to 30% fats, with limited amounts of concentrated sweets and adequate amounts of fiber.
    1, 2, 4 Refer to No. 3.
342. Comprehension, assessment, physiologic (b)
    2 Lethargy leading to coma develops because of metabolic acidosis (ketoacidosis).
    1, 4 These are not symptoms of ketoacidosis.
    3 This may be a symptom of hypoglycemia, not ketoacidosis.
343. Knowledge, implementation, physiologic (b)
    2 Cauterization by laser prevents blood from leaking into the vitreous humor.
    1 Detached retinas cause blindness.
    3 Serum glucose affects fluid balance, not the presence of glucose in the humor.
    4 Rods and cones are part of the nervous system and are unaffected by glucose levels.

344. Comprehension, assessment, physiologic (c)
    3 The autonomic nervous system regulates a man's ability to have an erection.
    1 The hemopoietic system regulates the amount of hemoglobin in the body.
    2 Low serum potassium levels are usually the result of fluid loss.
    4 Muscle cramps are usually the result of an electrolyte imbalance.

345. Knowledge, planning, environment (a)
    3 Annual examinations by the ophthalmologist can help prevent the visual problems associated with diabetes.
    1 Unless the person is experiencing significant visual problems, quarterly examination is unnecessary.
    2 Semi-annual visitation to an ophthalmologist is not recommended or cost effective.
    4 Five years is too long between examinations. Annual visits can help prevent blindness.

346. Comprehension, assessment, physiologic (c)
    2 Numbness and tingling indicate involvement of autonomic and peripheral nervous systems.
    1 Color changes indicate cardiovascular problems.
    3 Itching usually comes from dry skin.
    4 Loss of fine motor skills indicates progressive peripheral neuropathy.

347. Comprehension, assessment, physiologic (c)
    4 Blindness results as fluid fills the macula.
    1 Blind spots are usually a result of retinal hemorrhages.
    2 The tear ducts are external parts of the eye.
    3 Pain is usually acute as it is part of the eye's protective warning system.

348. Application, implementation, psychosocial (b)
    3 This option allows the person to reestablish and maintain control over her life and allows the older adult to adapt to change with assistance.
    1 This is an inappropriate response from the nurse; clearly the patient is seeking assistance from a health care provider. This response places the sole burden of care on the patient.
    2 This response does not address the patient's question.
    4 The answer is ambivalent and non-caring. The nurse should proactively pursue the available options in this situation.

349. Application, planning, physiologic (b)
    1 Bearing down while defecating increases the intraoccular pressure, therefore increasing the risk of hemorrhage.
    2 Exercises for the eye are usually for the purpose of strengthening eye muscles.
    3 Allergies do not cause proliferative retinopathy.
    4 Wearing sunglasses may protect the eye from exposure to ultraviolet rays that may cause cataracts.

350. Application, implementation, physiologic (c)
    4 Capillary blood glucose should always be tested before strenuous activity. Because exercise burns glucose and lowers blood glucose levels, it is important to assess the blood glucose level before exercising so that food and insulin could be adjusted to prevent hypoglycemia.
    1 Although testing the blood glucose level after exercise could be done, it is not the most important time to do this.
    2 Two hours after meals, blood glucose levels would be at their highest; this is not the best time.
    3 Although the level could be taken before lunch, this is not the best time.

351. Application, implementation, physiologic (a)
    4 As blood glucose levels fall, the first symptom that the patient develops is hunger.
    1 Flushed face may be a sign of hyperglycemia.
    2 Diplopia is not a symptom of hypoglycemia.
    3 Slurred speech is not an early symptom of hypoglycemia; it may be a sign of hyperglycemia.

352. Knowledge, evaluation, physiology (a)
    4 Lack of insulin from the pancreas causes diabetes.
    1 The liver aids in the process of digestion.
    2 The ileum is the distal portion of the small intestine and is considered a primary organ in the GI system.
    3 The stomach acts as a reservoir for food and allows for continuation of the digestive process.

353. Application, implementation, psychosocial (b)
    4 This response gives the patient the opportunity to talk more about what is bothering him.
    1 Putting him off doesn't help his concerns or the stress they may be causing.
    2 Making such a decision for him is inappropriate.
    3 This is an inappropriate, judgmental response.

354. Application, planning, psychosocial (c)
    2 This allows the patient input into decisions about his or her care.
    1 This doesn't allow for the patient's individual needs.
    3 This is not an important factor at this time.
    4 The patient is the primary focus at this point.

355. Comprehension, evaluation, health (b)
    2 Hamburger and peanut butter are both in the meat group. They may be exchanged.
    1 Fruit salad is in the fruit group.
    3 Tomato soup is in the vegetable group.
    4 Corn muffin is in the bread group.

356. Application, evaluation, physiologic (b)
    2 Minor structural damage is repaired with increased blood flow to the kidneys.
    1 Exercise decreases destruction of the renal pelvis.
    3 Osmotic pressure is reduced in the nephron.
    4 Blood flow is increased in the kidney.

357. Comprehension, evaluation, physiologic (c)
    1 Exercise burns glucose; therefore, insulin needs may decrease.
    2, 3 Less insulin is required (see No. 1).
    4 This is an untrue statement. Food alone cannot control diabetes or affect insulin requirements. The combination of food, exercise, and insulin is needed.

358. Application, planning, physiologic (c)
    2 NPH insulin peaks in approximately 4 to 12 hours after administration. Insulin reactions may occur at this time if there is not enough carbohydrate to maintain blood glucose levels within normal range. A split dose of NPH insulin before breakfast and at bedtime could lead to an insulin reaction at 4 to 5 PM and/or during the night.
    1 This is too soon for the morning NPH insulin to peak.
    3 One hour after breakfast is too soon for morning NPH insulin to peak; 1 hour after dinner is too soon for the afternoon NPH insulin to peak.
    4 One hour after lunch is too soon for morning NPH insulin to peak. Because the patient is still metabolizing carbohydrates from lunch, an insulin reaction at this time is unlikely.

359. Comprehension, assessment, health (b)
    1 Obesity and genetics are the primary risk factors in the development of type II diabetes.
    2 Eating many sweets does not cause diabetes.
    3, 4 These are symptoms of type II diabetes; they are not risk factors.

360. Application, implementation, health (b)
    4 Drinking alcohol when taking Micronase can make the drug more potent, increasing the risk of hypoglycemia.
    1 Insulin may be adjusted according to capillary blood glucose levels. Micronase is given in a standard dose.
    2 Exercise should be performed after meals, not after taking Micronase.
    3 Micronase should be taken before breakfast.
361. Comprehension, evaluation, physiologic (a)
    4 The action of Micronase is to stimulate the pancreas to produce more insulin and to increase the sensitivity of insulin receptors on the cell.
    1 Oral hypoglycemics are not insulin and cannot replace it.
    2 Oral hypoglycemics have no digestive action.
    3 Oral hypoglycemics have no effect on weight.
362. Application, implementation, health (b)
    2 Public health agencies and home health agencies provide this service.
    1 Without knowing how old the granddaughter is, this is unsafe to assume this may be done.
    3 In the future, this patient may need to mix doses; telling her never to do this will increase anxiety and doubt regarding nursing skills.
    4 Accuracy is very important when administering insulin.
363. Application, planning, physiologic (b)
    3 The most pressing problem with the patient is to heal the wound and decrease the blood sugar.
    1 The patient shows no sign of impaired adjustment.
    2 The ulcer will probably restrict activity, but the immediate concern is to heal the ulcer.
    4 No problem is apparent with breathing.
364. Comprehension, planning, health (b)
    2 Maintaining ideal body weight is essential in the control of type II diabetes.
    1 Insulin is not necessary. Achieving ideal body weight through diet and exercise would be the primary method of control.
    3 The ideal diabetic diet is 60% complex carbohydrates.
    4 This is unnecessary for a type II diabetic unless the condition is out of control. This is not a priority at this time.
365. Comprehension, planning, physiologic (b)
    3 There is a decreased production of insulin needed to metabolize carbohydrates.
    1 This condition does not interfere with the body's ability to absorb minerals.
    2 This condition does not interfere with the body's ability to absorb vitamins.
    4 Diabetes mellitus involves the pancreas and the lack of insulin secretion by the beta cells.
366. Comprehension, assessment, physiologic (c)
    4 This is the normal amount of glucose that is found in the bloodstream as an end product of digestion.
    1 Reading of 50-59 is below normal.
    2, 3 Reading above 110 is above normal.
367. Knowledge, planning, environment (a)
    3 Orinase stimulates the beta cells in the pancreatic islets to produce insulin so that glucose metabolism occurs.
    1 There is no medication classified as an "oral" insulin.
    2 The medication must be taken on a regular basis in order to be effective.
    4 There are different types of oral hypoglycemics; not all diabetics require the same type of medication or need them at all.

368. Comprehension, assessment, physiologic (a)
    4 An increase of acetone in the body accounts for fruity-smelling breath and hot, dry skin.
    1, 2 These are indicative of hypoglycemic reaction.
    3 The systolic blood pressure drops, and circulatory collapse may occur.
369. Application, implementation, physiologic (c)
    1 Oral hypoglycemic agents stimulate the pancreas to produce insulin; exercise and dietary control of metabolism are also needed.
    2 Adult-onset diabetes in overweight men needs exercise and dietary control, but the disease usually can be controlled without insulin.
    3 Insulin replacement is needed when diet and oral hypoglycemic agents can't control the disease.
    4 Weight loss is indicated, but stimulating insulin production is needed most at this point.
370. Comprehension, evaluation, health (c)
    2 Too little insulin causes ketoacidosis from high glucose level; coma may occur if the condition is untreated.
    1 This is an incorrect response. Too much insulin decreases the glucose level in the body and causes a hypoglycemic reaction.
    3 This is an incorrect response; there is a presence of ketone bodies.
    4 Absence of appetite usually occurs.
371. Knowledge, assessment, physiologic (a)
    2 An abnormally high glucose level in the blood and glucose in the urine are characteristic symptoms of diabetes mellitus.
    1 Hypoglycemia is an abnormally low glucose level in the blood, making this statement incorrect.
    3 Hypoglycemia is an abnormally low glucose level in the blood, and hypokalemia is an abnormally low potassium level in the blood.
    4 Hyperglycemia is correct, but glycogen is the product of the breakdown of carbohydrates; it is stored in the liver and muscles.
372. Comprehension, assessment, physiologic (b)
    3 The skin becomes dry and flushed, and the patient usually complains of extreme thirst with diabetic acidosis (coma).
    1 The skin is not moist, but dry; not pale, but flushed. A gradual loss of appetite, not extreme hunger, occurs with diabetic acidosis.
    2 The skin is dry, but not pale. Extreme hunger makes this response wrong. The patient usually has a gradual loss of appetite.
    4 The skin is flushed and anorexia may be present. The skin is dry, not moist, with diabetic acidosis.
373. Comprehension, assessment, physiologic (a)
    1 Increased levels of glucose in the blood are a result of insufficient insulin to help the body use glucose.
    2 This would be the result of excess insulin in the blood.
    3 This would result in hypoglycemia.
    4 Pancreatic juices play a role in digestion of foods, not in the body's use of glucose.
374. Knowledge, assessment, physiologic (b)
    2 These symptoms, along with Kussmaul's respirations and an increased pulse rate, are later symptoms of diabetic acidosis.
    1, 3, 4 These are symptoms of insulin shock.

375. Knowledge, assessment, physiologic (c)
     4 Ketoacidosis is the accumulation of glucose and waste products from the increased metabolism of fats and proteins.
     1 Insulin reaction occurs when the body has increased insulin in the blood.
     2 Hypoglycemia is an abnormally low level of glucose in the blood.
     3 Diabetic retinopathy is a severe complication of diabetes in which there are pathologic changes involving the optic nerve that can lead to blindness.

376. Comprehension, assessment, physiologic (b)
     2 Fragile skin that is prone to breakdown is a classic symptom of Cushing's syndrome.
     1 Cushing's syndrome usually causes weight gain from retention of sodium and water.
     3 Cushing's syndrome causes hypertension because of retention of sodium and water.
     4 Cushing's syndrome causes hyperglycemia and can induce diabetes.

377. Comprehension, planning, health (c)
     3 Depression is a sign of Cushing's syndrome. Increased mental stability would be an appropriate goal.
     1 Patient's with Cushing's syndrome need to be on a low-sodium diet.
     2 Because they retain fluids, patients need fluid restriction.
     4 Weight loss is a more appropriate goal.

378. Comprehension, planning, health (b)
     1 Because sodium and water are retained as a result of the increase in corticosteroid levels, a low-sodium diet is an important intervention in Cushing's syndrome.
     2 High protein intake is not necessary; calcium should not be decreased because of bone softening from the disease.
     3 This would irritate skin that is prone to breakdown.
     4 Monitoring blood glucose levels is important, but testing urine glucose levels is unnecessary and inaccurate.

379. Comprehension, planning, physiologic (b)
     1 Overstimulation by the pituitary hormone ACTH produces an overabundance of the hormone in the cortex of the gland.
     2 This is caused by increased production of ACTH.
     3 This is a cause of diabetes mellitus.
     4 This is a cause of Graves' disease.

380. Comprehension, assessment, physiologic (b)
     3 Muscle weakness is a result of muscle wasting; osteoporosis is a result of abnormal calcium absorption.
     1 Hypertension is more the case with peripheral edema and weight gain.
     2 Increased appetite and weight gain are more usual. Muscle weakness does occur.
     4 Moon face does occur from overabundance of the hormone, but hypertension is indicated because of weight gain and edema.

381. Comprehension, planning, physiologic (b)
     1 This procedure is necessary to maintain fluid balance.
     2, 4 These are not a primary concern.
     3 Sugar is not excreted in urine.

382. Comprehension, planning, physiologic (b)
     3 Adrenocorticotropic hormone (ACTH) is released by the anterior portion of the pituitary gland, which regulates functional activity of the adrenal cortex.
     1 The adrenal cortex secretes cortisol and androgens; the adrenal medulla secretes the catecholamines epinephrine and norepinephrine.
     2 Growth is a factor related to the thyroid hormone.
     4 ACTH stimulates growth of the adrenal cortex and the secretion of corticosteroids.

383. Application, implementation, environment (c)
     4 Accurate records of intake and output provide information about fluctuation and instability of the adrenocortical hormones, thus preventing complications.
     1 This is always included for postoperative management but is not most significant in this case.
     2, 3 These are not the highest priority in this case.

384. Comprehension, evaluation, physiologic (c)
     1 Addison's disease is adrenocortical insufficiency when the adrenal glands do not secrete adequate amounts of ACTH.
     2, 3 These do not directly involve the parathyroid.
     4 This does not involve the thyroid gland.

385. Application, implementation, health (c)
     2 Stress is the major precipitating factor in adrenal crisis.
     1 Salt intake should be restricted.
     3 Moderate activity with some rest periods is required.
     4 There is no interference with insulin production from the pancreas.

386. Comprehension, implementation, physiologic (b)
     4 Cystoscopic examination allows visualization of the inside of the bladder.
     1 The size, shape, and location of the kidneys are usually determined by an intravenous pyelogram.
     2 The prostate gland is usually not visualized with contrast media and cannot be seen on cystoscopic examination.
     3 Visualization of the ureters requires the use of a contrast medium. A cystoscopic examination does not require the use of a contrast medium.

387. Application, implementation, physiologic (c)
     1 Voiding on a routine prevents the bladder from becoming too full.
     2 Increasing fluids increases bladder distension.
     3 Spices do not affect the functioning of the bladder.
     4 Wearing an incontinence pad promotes the loss of dignity for the patient.

388. Application, implementation, physiologic (c)
     4 A low-protein diet facilitates renal functioning.
     1 A low-fat diet is recommended for diabetes, but renal function is not optimized.
     2 A sodium-restricted diet is more important with cardiovascular disease.
     3 A high-protein diet may adversely affect renal functioning.

389. Knowledge, planning, physiologic (a)
     1 The examination of the kidneys, ureters, and bladder (KUB) provides proper visualization of the structures to confirm the suspected diagnosis.
     2 The cystourethrogram is a radiograph of the urinary bladder and urethra; it is insufficient to confirm this diagnosis.
     3 Cystometry is a study of bladder function.
     4 Proctoscopy is an examination of the rectum with an endoscope.

390. Comprehension, evaluation, physiologic (b)
     3 The nurse should not be concerned about the color since the patient is on Pyridium. Pyridium turns the urine a reddish-orange color.
     1 There is no need to report to the doctor since this is a normal occurrence when taking Pyridium.
     2 This action should be done only if the doctor requests it.
     4 The nurse can check specific gravity to see if the urine is concentrated, but the color is from the drug.

391. Knowledge, planning, health (a)
    3 The purpose of the urine culture is to identify the organisms in the genitourinary (GU) tract and to determine which antibiotics they are sensitive to.
    1 This would be a routine urinalysis.
    2 This would be a urine cytology test.
    4 This is not a purpose of the urine culture and sensitivity.

392. Knowledge, planning, physiologic (a)
    3 Urine is strained to detect if a stone or clot is passed.
    1 No tests are routinely done on strained urine.
    2 No tests are done routinely.
    4 It is not measured unless there is a specific order to do so.

393. Knowledge, implementation, physiologic (b)
    2 A scope is inserted to visualize the inside of the bladder.
    1 The patient is not catheterized.
    3 The kidneys are not studied in this examination.
    4 The prostate is not studied.

394. Knowledge, planning, physiologic (b)
    2 Blood in the urine is common after this examination.
    1 This should not affect the level of consciousness.
    3 The patient should not be nauseated.
    4 This examination does not affect bowel function.

395. Application, assessment, physiologic (b)
    3 Allergy to the dye is common.
    1 This is not the most important information.
    2 The patient should have had enemas.
    4 This is not important.

396. Application, planning, physiologic (b)
    4 Vigorous exercise and sexual intercourse should be avoided for 2 to 3 weeks.
    1 Fiber intake should be increased to prevent straining with bowel movements.
    2 Sitting in hot water may increase the pain.
    3 Fluids should be increased to increase bowel motility.

397. Knowledge, assessment, physiologic (a)
    2 Overflow incontinence occurs when the bladder is distended.
    1 Functional incontinence refers to the inability to get to bathroom facilities.
    3 Stress incontinence is caused by increased intraabdominal pressure.
    4 Urge incontinence occurs when there is a sudden urge to void but an inability to get to facilities.

398. Comprehension, assessment, physiologic (b)
    4 The urge to suddenly void and having lack of bladder control is called urge incontinence.
    1 Functional incontinence results when the person is physically unable to reach the bathroom facilities in the time needed to void.
    2 Stress incontinence results because of increased intraabdominal pressure.
    3 Overflow incontinence results from overdistension of the bladder.

399. Comprehension, assessment, physiologic (b)
    3 Stress incontinence is the loss of bladder control as the result in sudden increases in intraabdominal pressure.
    1 Functional incontinence refers to the inability to get to the bathroom.
    2 Overflow incontinence results from the bladder becoming too distended.
    4 Urge incontinence results from the sudden urgency and inability to get to the bathroom.

400. Application, implementation, environment (a)
    4 To properly collect a 24-hour urine specimen, the patient discards the first void. Timing begins when the patient collects the total amount of voiding for 24 hours.
    1 This is not a 24-hour specimen; separate containers are not necessary.
    2 This is not a 24-hour specimen; all urine is to be collected after the patient discards the first void.
    3 This is not a 24-hour specimen; this is the procedure for maintaining strict intake and output.

401. Knowledge, assessment, health (b)
    3 Intravenous urogram (pyelogram) is the test that allows for visualization of the size, shape, and structure of the kidney, ureters, and bladder. It also determines if the bladder empties sufficiently in a post-void film.
    1 Cholecystography is an x-ray examination using a contrast substance to evaluate the functioning of the gallbladder and to detect disease or gallstones.
    2 Cystography is an examination of the urinary bladder using a contrast medium introduced through a urethral catheter.
    4 Retrograde pyelography is a more sophisticated test of the urinary system whereby a contrast medium is injected directly into the ureters through catheters introduced through cystoscopy; this test is generally used to confirm findings suspected on the intravenous urogram.

402. Knowledge, assessment, physiologic (a)
    2 Severe flank pain and hematuria are cardinal symptoms of renal calculi.
    1 These may be symptoms of incontinence and/or infection.
    3 Frequency and dysuria are indicative of cystitis.
    4 Urgency and polyuria may be associated with an endocrine disorder.

403. Comprehension, assessment, physiologic (b)
    1 Severe, colicky flank pain, radiating to the testes, is a common symptom of renal calculi in male patients.
    2 This is not a symptom of renal calculi.
    3 These are more common symptoms of urinary tract infection.
    4 This may be a symptom of bladder cancer.

404. Knowledge, planning, physiologic (a)
    4 Renal colic is a spasm in the tubular structure of the ureter that causes pain.
    1 The kidney moves from its normal bed of fat but does not produce the symptoms described in this case.
    2 Hardening of the kidney does not present the symptoms described.
    3 Collection of urine in the kidney does not present the symptoms described.

405. Application, planning, physiologic (a)
    2 Straining urine allows observation of passage of the stone(s).
    1 On the contrary, fluid should be encouraged to flush out the stone(s).
    3, 4 These are not medically necessary.

406. Application, implementation, safety (a)
    4 2 mg per 1 ml (cc); desired is 5 mg; have 2 mg per 1 ml; dose is 2.5 ml.
    1, 3 This is too low a dose.
    2 This is too high a dose.

407. Comprehension, evaluation, environment (b)
    2 Peristalsis is activation of wavelike motion that assists in forcing food through the digestive tract.
    1 There has not been sufficient time for the digestive process to begin working.
    3 There could be insufficient time for the digestive process to begin working or the IV could be maintained long after the digestive process has been restored.
    4 There is no direct relationship.
408. Knowledge, planning, health (a)
    2 These foods are high in calcium.
    1 These foods are high in protein.
    3, 4 These foods are most noted for their vitamin and fiber content.
409. Comprehension, evaluation, health (b)
    2 This combination of foods contains very little calcium.
    1 Cheese and green salad are high sources of calcium.
    3 Yogurt and broccoli are high sources of calcium.
    4 Spinach and skim milk are high sources of calcium.
410. Knowledge, assessment, physiologic (b)
    3 Painless hematuria is the most common early symptom of cancer of the bladder.
    1 Suprapubic pain may be present in cancer of the bladder, but it is not the most common early symptom.
    2 Elevation of temperature is usually a symptom of an infection or inflammatory disease; it is not necessarily an early sign of cancer of the bladder.
    4 Dysuria may be a symptom of cancer of the bladder, but painless hematuria is the earliest symptom.
411. Knowledge, assessment, physiologic (b)
    4 Urinary retention is not a common symptom of an enlarged prostate.
    1 This is not usually seen.
    2 This is not usually a problem.
    3 This is not common.
412. Comprehension, assessment, physiologic (b)
    4 Urinary retention due to enlargement of the prostate is a classic symptom of benign prostatic hypertrophy (BPH).
    1, 2, 3 Bleeding and pain usually do not occur with BPH unless there is an infection present.
413. Application, implementation, physiologic (a)
    2 To obtain the urinary output, subtract the amount of solution from the total urinary drainage in the bag.

    $$\begin{array}{r} 3800 \text{ ml} \\ -2000 \text{ ml} \\ \hline 1800 \text{ ml} \end{array}$$

    1 This amount is too much.
    3, 4 These amounts are too little.
414. Application, implementation, environment (b)
    3 Assessing for urinary retention resulting from blockage would be the priority initial intervention at this time.
    1 Mild spasms are normal. A feeling of having to void could indicate urinary blockage and must be assessed further.
    2 This is not to be done if the bladder is already full.
    4 Assessment of the bladder must be done first and findings reported to the team leader.
415. Application, planning, physiologic (b)
    1 The nurse must be sure there are no kinks or obstructions.
    2 The catheter already has continuous irrigation.
    3 This is not necessary.
    4 The patient cannot use a urinal; he has a catheter.
416. Comprehension, implementation, health (b)
    4 Kegel exercises can strengthen the perineal muscles and help control bladder function.
    1, 2, 3 These will not promote urinary control.

417. Comprehension, assessment, physiologic (a)
    3 Because of blockage as a result of the neoplasm, the patient has had increasing problems passing urine through the urethra.
    1 Urine is blocked, not creating urgency.
    2 Urine is not able to pass, so there is no frequency.
    4 There is no burning sensation when blockage is the problem.
418. Knowledge, planning, physiologic (b)
    2 This condition is a common occurrence with the over-55 male group.
    1 Recurrent infection is not a predisposing factor.
    3 Sitting on the job is not a contributory factor.
    4 Sexual inactivity is not a predisposing factor.
419. Comprehension, planning, physiologic (a)
    4 The incision is made through the abdomen; the bladder is opened and the gland is removed from above.
    1 This is a perineal prostatectomy.
    2 This is a transurethral prostatectomy.
    3 This is a retropubic prostatectomy.
420. Application, implementation, environment (b)
    3 It is important to observe for bleeding, clots, concentration of the urine, and for satisfactory amount of urine output.
    1 This is important, but it is not a major consideration.
    2 This is an incorrect response; increased fluid intake is important to not only hydrate the patient but to flush the system.
    4 This may be indicated, but it is not a major consideration.
421. Application, planning, environment (b)
    1 This is an indication that the tubing is not patent and that there may be blockage preventing the flow of urine.
    2 As long as the urine is flowing there is no need for irrigation.
    3 This is an inappropriate response; judgment must be based on clinical indications.
    4 Pain is not always an indicator of problems with urinary flow.
422. Application, implementation, health (b)
    2 It is important to use sterile techniques with the presence of urine to avoid infection and skin irritation.
    1 This is an incorrect response; the sterile technique must be followed.
    3 This is an inappropriate response; appropriate care of the wound and skin needs to be maintained.
    4 This is an inappropriate response; the analgesic will not decrease or stop spasm or urine flow.
423. Application, implementation, physiologic (b)
    3 Bowel sounds should be present in all four abdominal quadrants before the patient is given food.
    1 Food may be given when bowel sounds are present. Food intake may help the patient expel flatus.
    2 This is not necessarily true.
    4 IV fluids are usually continued until the patient is able to retain at least a clear liquid diet.
424. Application, implementation, physiologic (b)
    1 Under normal circumstances, the patient should be able to stand beside the bed to void. This facilitates bladder emptying for men.
    2 Applying pressure over the bladder is contraindicated for a herniorrhaphy.
    3 Noninvasive interventions should be tried before catheterization is done.
    4 Notify the physician if noninvasive measures have not been successful. The physician usually orders a catheterization prn.

425. Application, implementation, health (b)
     3 After a herniorrhaphy, the patient should avoid lifting or straining for 6 weeks. Using a book as an example gives the patient a reference weight.
     1 After a herniorrhaphy most patients can return to work as soon as they feel they are able, as long as they understand that they may not lift or strain.
     2 A soft diet is not necessary. Roughage should be increased to avoid constipation and straining.
     4 A shower is the best method of bathing because running water keeps the incision clean. Tub bathing is not the best method of bathing.

426. Comprehension, assessment, physiologic (b)
     4 Because of the retention of waste products, including sodium, hypertension is an expected result of acute renal failure.
     1, 2, 3 These are not signs of acute renal failure.

427. Application, implementation, environment (c)
     3 Elevating the head of the bed to high-Fowler's position would be the first nursing action for a patient who is experiencing dyspnea.
     1, 2, 4 Elevating the head of the bed is the priority action to ease the patient's dyspnea.

428. Comprehension, assessment, physiologic (b)
     4 Hearing a bruit indicates that blood is rushing through the shunt and the shunt is functioning properly.
     1, 2, 3 It is not conclusive that the shunt is patent.

429. Comprehension, evaluation, health (b)
     3 Applesauce and raisins contain no protein.
     1 Custard is made with milk and eggs, which contain protein.
     2 Yogurt is made with milk.
     4 Gelatin contains protein, and cream also has a small amount of protein.

430. Application, implementation, health (a)
     4 Diagnosis is confirmed by a Gram-stained smear of the discharge from the penis.
     1 A blood test is used to diagnosis syphilis, not gonorrhea.
     2 This is used to determine the organisms in the colon.
     3 This is used to determine the types of organisms present in the throat.

431. Comprehension, implementation, health (a)
     2 Her age category places her at high risk for cervical cancer, so early detection is imperative.
     1 This is an incorrect response; irregular periods are caused by a variety of reasons.
     3, 4 These are incorrect responses; she is in a high-risk category, and early detection is imperative.

432. Knowledge, implementation, physiologic (a)
     2 Lying on her back with thighs flexed on the abdomen allows for easier accessibility to the perineal area; this position allows for easier visualization of the reproductive organs.
     1 Lying on her side with a knee drawn up does not allow for easy access to the perineal area.
     3 Lowering the head with the feet elevated does not allow for easy access to the perineal area.
     4 Lying down with moderately flexed, outward-rotated extremities does not provide easy access to the perineal area.

433. Comprehension, implementation, environment (a)
     2 Handwashing, when done correctly, is the most effective of all procedures recommended for the prevention of the spread of infectious agents.
     1 Wearing gloves is indicated if there is a high probability of contact with body fluids.
     3 Wearing a gown is indicated if soiling or contact with body fluids is likely.
     4 Surgical asepsis is required for specific procedures, such as opening a sterile tray, but it is not required for all patient contact.

434. Knowledge, planning, environment (a)
     1 This allows for comfort, safety, visualization of the uterus, and a decrease in pressure caused by a full bladder that lies just behind the uterus.
     2 This has no direct relationship to the examination.
     3 It is unnecessary to restrict fluid because there is no direct relationship to the examination.
     4 An increased amount of urine in the bladder affects comfort, safety, and visualization of the uterus.

435. Knowledge, planning, health (a)
     4 Scrapings of secretions and cells from the cervix are analyzed for the presence of cancer cells.
     1 Blood tests are used to determine ovarian function.
     2 There is no test available to do so; the length of the cervix is not really important.
     3 The pH of vaginal secretions is determined by use of nitrazine sticks.

436. Knowledge, implementation, psychosocial (b)
     4 The brain allows enjoyment of the sexual experience, but it can also prevent satisfaction. If the person is thinking about problems or work, satisfaction may be difficult.
     1 The penis is obviously important for sexual satisfaction, but the brain can cause other thoughts to interfere with satisfaction.
     2 The female genitalia are important, but the brain plays an even more important part.
     3 The ovaries are important because of the hormones secreted.

437. Knowledge, assessment, physiologic (a)
     2 Menorrhagia is defined as abnormally heavy or long menstrual periods that occur occasionally during most women's reproductive years.
     1 This is the absence of menstruation.
     3 This is uterine bleeding other than that caused by menstruation.
     4 This is painful menstruation.

438. Application, implementation, psychosocial (b)
     3 This response indicates recognition and understanding by the nurse and allows the patient the opportunity to discuss her feelings in greater detail.
     1 With this response the nurse does not recognize the patient's concern and assumes too much specific to the relationship between the patient and her husband.
     2 This response, although a possibility, does not offer recognition or understanding by the nurse.
     4 This response by the nurse does not address the patient's concern, nor does it indicate understanding of the patient's feelings at this time.

439. Comprehension, planning, health (b)
    3 A physical activity that does not cause strain is swimming, which is often helpful for both physical and emotional well-being.
    1 Resuming sexual activities is permitted within 4 to 6 weeks following surgery; 2 weeks is too soon.
    2 Strenuous activities such as jogging, dancing, and fast walking cause congestion of blood in the pelvis; such activity should be avoided for several months.
    4 Heavy lifting and strenuous physical activity should be avoided for several months.

440. Knowledge, planning, physiologic (b)
    2 This is an abnormal condition characterized by ectopic growth and function of endometrial tissue.
    1 This is an inflammatory condition of the endometrium, usually caused by bacterial infection.
    3 This is an inflammatory condition of the internal eye, in which the eye becomes red, swollen, painful, and sometimes, filled with pus.
    4 This is an infection of the intestine or liver by a species of pathogenic amebas.

441. Application, implementation, psychosocial (c)
    2 The patient has a legal right to request that a nurse be present during the examination.
    1 Although the physician can be trusted, the patient has a legal right to her request.
    3 The nurse should not assume that the patient will feel better with her husband present, and the patient has a legal right to her request.
    4 Nervousness about an examination does not require psychologic help.

442. Application, implementation, physiologic (b)
    1 Maintaining the patient in a low-Fowler's position or flat in bed will prevent increased intraabdominal pressure strain on the suture line.
    2 A laxative and several enemas are given 24 hours before surgery to ensure a relatively empty bowel. Clear fluids are given 24 hours before surgery to reduce the contents of the bowel. For 5 days after surgery only liquids are permitted by mouth.
    3 Camphorated tincture of opium (paregoric) is administered to further inhibit bowel function.
    4 Enemas to relieve flatus and cleanse the bowel are withheld for at least 1 week following surgery.

443. Application, implementation, physiologic (a)
    3 Treatment of choice for stage I cervical cancer is a radical hysterectomy with pelvic lymph node dissection.
    1 This is stage II of cervical cancer; it does not involve the lower third of the vagina.
    2 This is stage 0 of cervical cancer.
    4 Cervical cancer stage IV is all-inclusive; the cancer extends outside the cervix, involving the pelvic wall, the lower third of the vagina, and the bladder and rectum. Metastatic spread may also be indicated.

444. Comprehension, planning, physiologic (c)
    3 A decrease in the systolic pressure causes cessation of glomerular filtration. The body at this point is unable to rid itself of fluid and nitrogenous wastes. Treatment for shock usually is done by fluid replacement and vasoactive drugs. Response to treatment assists urinary output to return to normal.
    1 Activity tolerance is an expected outcome; pulse increase should be no more than 20 beats per minute.
    2 This is an expected outcome, but not necessarily for toxic shock syndrome.
    4 This is an expected outcome, but it is not a greater priority than No. 3.

445. Knowledge, assessment, physiologic (b)
    3 The vaginal discharge is as described and in most instances the vulva is inflamed, edematous, and often excoriated as a result of scratching. Similar white and curd-like patches seen in the newborn are known as thrush.
    1 A white vaginal discharge normally occurs in varying amounts and consistency during the course of the menstrual cycle and is not indicative of disease.
    2 This describes the vaginal discharge from a patient with bacterial vaginosis.
    4 This describes the vaginal discharge from a patient with trichomoniasis.

446. Application, implementation, health (b)
    4 Nurses are vital in the role as patient educators; for this patient the nurse's teaching includes aspects of self-care, prevention, transmission, and ways to prevent recurrence of the disease.
    1 This is not the most appropriate response. The patient is 18 years of age and not usually concerned about infertility. No. 4 is priority in the prevention of infertility.
    2 It is strongly recommended that both the patient and all sexual partners be treated individually. Sharing medication would reduce effectiveness of the treatment and could possibly lead to unwanted complications (an allergic response to the medication).
    3 The condition in and of itself is not life-threatening.

447. Application, implementation, health (a)
    3 Breast self-examinations done on a regular basis are the most accessible tool to detect early breast lesions. Although statistics indicate that 90% of all breast cancers are discovered by self-examinations, many detections are not reported immediately because of fears of mutilation and death.
    1 This is currently being evaluated for use in detecting lesions in dense breasts of younger women. Its value as a diagnostic tool for breast cancer is still being determined.
    2 Annual mammography is recommended for all women over 50 years of age, according to the American Cancer Society.
    4 This is an important aspect of prevention; however, this does not replace the necessity of doing regular breast self-examinations.

448. Application, implementation, physiologic (a)
    4 A sign should be made indicating that blood pressure checks, injections, and blood tests are not to be done on the affected side because these would increase potential for impairment of circulation and infection. Lymphedema is a very real concern for this patient.
    1 This may be so, but it is not the most appropriate response.
    2 Although a quiet and comfortable environment is a goal, patient observation is an absolute must. A dimly lit room may not be the best environment, especially immediately following surgery.
    3 This is true, but it is not the most appropriate response.

449. Comprehension, assessment, environment (b)
    4 Bleeding from a mastectomy can trickle down the side to the back of the patient. Turning the patient and feeling her side will detect such bleeding.
    1 This would miss bleeding on the side. Dressings are usually removed by the physician immediately after surgery.
    2 Every 4 hours would be too long to wait to check the patient.
    3 This is unnecessary and could lead to the development of infection. Dressings are usually removed by the physician initially after surgery.

450. Application, implementation, environment (b)
   3 This position elevates the extremity high enough to prevent lymphedema.
   1, 2 Abduction and adduction of the affected arm are contraindicated after a mastectomy. The arm should not be suspended.
   4 The patient's arm is not elevated high enough in this position.
451. Application, implementation, psychosocial (a)
   4 This statement reflects on the patient's feelings, allowing for open communication.
   1 This is giving advice, closing communication between the nurse and patient.
   2 Silence would not be an appropriate method of fostering communication at this time.
   3 Commenting on how everyone else feels does not help the way the patient feels; this blocks communication.
452. Application, implementation, physiologic (b)
   3 To prevent damage to the lymphatic circulation, this is most important for the patient to understand.
   1 The diet should be high in protein and vitamin C to ensure wound healing.
   2 Exercises should be performed at least three to four times a day; once is not enough.
   4 Although this is important, No. 3 is more important.
453. Comprehension, assessment, psychosocial (b)
   3 She is denying a need for additional treatment.
   1 This is daydreaming.
   2 She isn't explaining it away.
   4 She has not attributed her behavior to anyone else.
454. Comprehension, evaluation, health (b)
   1 This step is important to assess for symmetry of the breasts.
   2 The pillow should be under the right shoulder when examining the right breast.
   3 The patient must be in a supine position when examining the breasts.
   4 To flatten breast tissue, her right arm must be over her head when examining her right breast.
455. Comprehension, implementation, physiologic (b)
   3 Frequent changes in position promote circulation to pressure areas; cleanliness is extremely important in the prevention of skin breakdown; gentle massage promotes circulation to the affected area; and adequate nutrition promotes healing.
   1 Maintaining proper body alignment is important; however, a supine position without frequent changes will promote pressure area development, and having the bed in low position does not affect impact the development of decubitus ulcers.
   2 The maximum allowed time between position changes is 2 hours regardless of whether the patient is in the bed or the wheelchair.
   4 Adequate measures should be taken to prevent friction when moving patients; protein requirements are increased in the presence of wounds; and strict bed rest promotes decubitus formation.

456. Comprehension, assessment, physiologic (c)
   4 A stage II decubitus is described as an area that is blistered, cracked, or abraded; the area surrounding the damaged skin is also reddened.
   1 A stage I decubitus is described as an area of skin that is deep pink, red, or mottled. Digital pressure on the area will cause temporary blanching for up to 15 minutes after the pressure is released.
   2 A stage III decubitus is described as an area of skin that is ulcerated and has a crater-like sore, with underlying tissue involvement.
   4 A stage IV decubitus is described as a deep ulceration and necrosis involving deeper underlying muscle and possibly bone tissue.
457. Application, assessment, physiologic (c)
   2 18% for the chest, 4.5% for one inner arm, and 4.5% for the other inner arm.
   1, 3, 4 These are incorrect totals.
458. Comprehension, planning, physiologic (b)
   1 Fluid replacement is based on the combination of body surface area burned and body weight.
   2 The patient's usual intake has no relationship to fluid lost from the burned surface.
   3 The standard requirement does not take into consideration body surface area burned and weight.
   4 This is part of the formula to determine the amount of fluid replacement, but the patient's weight is needed as well.
459. Comprehension, planning, physiologic (a)
   4 This monitors renal functioning on an hourly basis.
   1 The bedpan is difficult and painful to use, and it decreases the chance of accurate measuring of output.
   2 This is not a significant factor.
   3 This has no relationship to caring for burn patients.
460. Comprehension, implementation, environment (b)
   4 Burn patients are highly susceptible to transmitted infection.
   1 This is the purpose of isolation precautions.
   2 Isolation precautions are taken to protect hospital personnel.
   3 This protects the patient from microorganisms being transmitted to him by visitors.
461. Knowledge, assessment, environment (a)
   3 Protective or reverse isolation is used for burn patients because they are more susceptible to infections.
   1 Enteric precaution is for illnesses that transmit microorganisms through excreta.
   2 Drainage or discharge precaution is for illnesses that transmit microorganisms through the drainage or discharge from a wound.
   4 Respiratory isolation is for illnesses that transmit microorganisms through the respiratory tract.
462. Knowledge, assessment, physiologic (a)
   3 A homograft is done primarily to help prevent fluid loss from the burn site and to prevent infection.
   1 Pain is only decreased through narcotic or analgesics in first- and second-degree burns.
   2 A homograft will aid in improving circulation at the burn sites, but it is used primarily to prevent fluid loss and infection.
   4 The patient's diet will assist the body in healing itself and in rebuilding lost tissue.

463. Knowledge, assessment, environment (a)
    4 There is pain associated with first- and second-degree burns, and a narcotic is given.
    1 Meperidine hydrochloride (Demerol) is given preoperatively to allay anxiety; it is given in this situation for pain.
    2 Meperidine hydrochloride does not prevent nausea, which is an adverse effect of this drug.
    3 Meperidine hydrochloride is not used to promote sleep, but dizziness and drowsiness are adverse effects of this drug.

464. Application, planning, health (c)
    1 Cheese and nuts are high in protein content. A diet rich in protein helps to rebuild tissue destroyed by burns.
    2 Cheese spread contains protein, but the potato chips contain little or no protein.
    3 Jello with cream contains little or no protein. Milk is a complete protein.
    4 Popcorn and pretzels contain little or no protein.

465. Comprehension, implementation, physiologic (b)
    2 Exposed skin area and burned skin increase the incidence of infection significantly.
    1 This may be secondary, depending on the patient's past health history and heart condition.
    3 Close monitoring of urinary output decreases the incidence of this being a causative factor.
    4 This is an inappropriate response.

466. Comprehension, evaluation, health (b)
    1 The condition of the burns and the patient's total well-being are major factors.
    2 This is included in her total well-being.
    3 Self-care is included in her total well-being.
    4 This is important, but the patient is the primary factor.

467. Knowledge, assessment, physiologic (a)
    3 Ultraviolet radiation comes from sunlight.
    1 Ionizing radiation is associated with exposure to sources of radiation such as uranium.
    2 There is no such thing as de-ionizing radiation.
    4 There is no such thing as superviolet radiation.

468. Knowledge, planning, environment (b)
    3 The abbreviation ou means both eyes.
    1 The abbreviation for the right eye is od.
    2 The abbreviation for the left ear is as.
    4 The abbreviation for the mouth is po.

469. Knowledge, implementation, physiologic (c)
    4 Compromised night vision is very common following laser surgery.
    1 Corneal sensation is not affected; therefore tears help protect the eye.
    2 Depth perception is unaffected by laser surgery.
    3 Pinkeye is contagious if careful handwashing is not done, however, it doesn't affect the laser surgery.

470. Comprehension, implementation, environment (b)
    1 This avoids introducing any contaminants into the ducts.
    2 This option could introduce a chemical into the ducts and cause more damage.
    3 This option would not let the irrigant drain and rinse the conjunctiva.
    4 This would be ineffective, cause more damage, and be uncomfortable and messy.

471. Application, assessment, physiologic (c)
    2 Hyperglycemia alters the serum osmotic pressure and results in fluid being shifted out of the lens. This alters the shape of the lens, which causes the blurred vision.
    1 Cataracts may form from chronic glucose fluctuations.
    3 Conjunctivitis is caused by infection.
    4 Double vision does not usually occur with diabetic visual problems.

472. Application, planning, physiologic (a)
    3 The otoscope is the instrument used to visualize the internal structures of the ear.
    1 The ophthalmoscope is used to examine the eye.
    2 The laryngeal mirror is used to examine the throat.
    4 The Pomeroy syringe is used to irrigate the ears.

473. Application, planning, physiologic (a)
    2 The laryngeal mirror is used to visualize the throat.
    1 The Schioetz tonometer is used to measure intraocular pressure.
    3 The ophthalmoscope is used to visualize the internal structures of the eye.
    4 The otoscope is used to examine the ear.

474. Comprehension, assessment, physiologic (a)
    4 A characteristic symptom of a developing cataract is progressive blurring of vision that seems like a film over the eye. This is a result of partial or complete opacity of the crystalline lens or its capsule. There is an eventual loss of vision.
    1 Refractive errors indicate a condition in which the light rays do not appropriately focus on the retina.
    2 Glaucoma is a result of increased intraocular pressure.
    3 Retinal detachment occurs when the retina is dislodged; the usual symptoms are spots and bright flashes of light.

475. Application, planning, health (a)
    1 The ophthalmologist is a medical physician who specializes in diagnosis, treatment, and surgery of the eyes. The physician may also prescribe corrective lenses if necessary.
    2 The optometrist prescribes corrective lenses for refractive errors. This person does not diagnose disease, prescribe medication, or treat diseases of the eyes.
    3 The optician fills prescriptions for corrective lenses and makes adjustments of glasses for proper fitting.
    4 The neurologist specializes in the diseases and treatment of the nervous system.

476. Knowledge, assessment, physiologic (b)
    1 Trauma, infection, or disease process is the most likely cause of a cataract developing in a person under the age of 40.
    2 It is common for cataracts to develop as a result of the aging process; but this is not the correct answer for this question.
    3 Weight is not a factor that leads to the development of a cataract.
    4 Cataracts are not related to any occupational factor or how much the eyes may be used in working or reading.

477. Knowledge, assessment, physiologic (a)
    4 Spots (floaters) and flashes of light are indicative of retinal detachment.
    1 This is not indicative of retinal detachment, but it could be an adverse reaction to medication.
    2 This is not indicative of retinal detachment or other complications related to cataract extraction.
    3 Myopia (nearsightedness) and purulent drainage are not appropriate responses. Myopia is a refractive error, and purulent drainage could be infection.

478. Comprehension, assessment, physiologic (a)
    2 There is a gradual opacification of the lens as a result of the aging process.
    1 This is a symptom of glaucoma.
    3 This is an incorrect response.
    4 This is a separation of the retina from the choroid in the posterior area of the eye.

479. Comprehension, planning, environment (a)
   3 It is important to ensure the proper technique of hand-washing, administration of the medication, and application of the eye patch.
   1 There is no need for lengthy bed rest.
   2 This is not needed, except in the bright sunlight.
   4 This is an inappropriate response.
480. Application, implementation, psychosocial (b)
   4 This response allows the patient to talk about her feelings and raise questions that need to be addressed.
   1 This response cuts the patient off and does not allow her to state what is really bothering her.
   2 This gives false reassurance.
   3 This response doesn't address the patient's concerns.
481. Comprehension, implementation, physiologic (a)
   1 These symptoms indicate complications such as internal bleeding, increased fluid, or internal pressure in the eye.
   2 This is a common occurrence with retinal detachment.
   3 This is an inappropriate response.
   4 This is not the best response; blurred vision is to be expected.
482. Knowledge, assessment, psychosocial (a)
   2 It is not necessary to speak in a louder voice because the patient does not have a hearing problem.
   1 Orientation to the room is particularly important to this patient.
   3 It is important to encourage the patient to express his needs.
   4 This is important for all patient admissions.
483. Application, planning, physiologic (b)
   3 It is important to medicate the patient promptly if nausea occurs because vomiting may place undue pressure on his eyes.
   1 Coughing and deep breathing may cause pressure on the patient's eyes and should not be done.
   2 The patient should be able to move freely. He will need some ambulation assistance initially to regain his sense of balance.
   4 There is no reason why the patient cannot have visitors.
484. Application, implementation, safety (a)
   4 The nurse should orient the patient to where the food is located on his plate. Using the clock position as an example is very helpful.
   1 Assuming that he will need to be fed will hurt his sense of self-esteem.
   2 There is no reason to chop the food into small pieces. It may be helpful to ask if he would like any of his food cut up.
   3 The patient will need some assistance. Managing the meal by himself may be frustrating.
485. Knowledge, assessment, physiologic (a)
   3 Tonometry involves indirect measurement of intraocular pressure. The patient with glaucoma has increased intraocular pressure.
   1 This checks for color blindness.
   2 This checks for refraction errors.
   4 This tests for infectious processes.
486. Comprehension, implementation, environment (a)
   4 The medication should be placed in the pocket of the lower lid for easier distribution.
   1 Dropping it into the center of the eye will make the patient blink and receive less medicine.
   2 The medication will drain from the eye through the tear ducts with this technique.
   3 Pulling the upper eye lid away to deliver the medication on the upper conjunctiva is difficult to do.

487. Knowledge, assessment, physiologic (a)
   2 The Snellen chart is used to check refraction errors.
   1 The ophthalmoscope is used to visualize the internal structures of the eye.
   3 The otoscope is used to examine the ear.
   4 The tonometer is used to measure intraocular pressure.
488. Comprehension, assessment, physiologic (a)
   2 Increased intraocular pressure is a result of a blockage of the aqueous humor fluid in the anterior chamber of the eye.
   1 The vitreous humor is in the posterior chamber of the eye.
   3 An increase, not a decrease, of aqueous fluid is what causes glaucoma.
   4 In glaucoma there is an increase, not a decrease, in the intraocular pressure.
489. Knowledge, assessment, physiologic (b)
   3 Acute glaucoma and closed-angle glaucoma are the same. The symptoms are sudden and require immediate attention.
   1 This refers to chronic glaucoma.
   2 This term indicates increased ocular pressure without symptoms.
   4 Chronic glaucoma symptoms are slow and progressive. Often the patient is not aware of damage until vision is lost.
490. Knowledge, assessment, health (a)
   4 The incidence of glaucoma increases after age 40.
   1, 2, 3 These are not related to the incidence of glaucoma.
491. Knowledge, assessment, physiologic (a)
   4 The tonometer is used to measure intraocular pressure.
   1 The ophthalmoscope is used to visualize the internal structures of the eye.
   2 The Snellen chart is used to check for refraction errors.
   3 The otoscope is used to examine the ear.
492. Comprehension, assessment, physiologic (b)
   2 Loss of peripheral vision is a sign of open-angle glaucoma.
   1 This could be a sign of infection, not glaucoma.
   3 Pain is not a symptom of open-angle glaucoma; it is a sign of closed-angle glaucoma.
   4 A reddened eye is a sign of closed-angle glaucoma, not open-angle.
493. Comprehension, evaluation, physiologic (a)
   4 Timoptic is a beta blocker that directly reduces the production of aqueous humor.
   1 There is no action on the pupil.
   2 Timoptic decreases the production of aqueous humor.
   3 There is no effect on the muscles of the eye.
494. Comprehension, assessment, physiologic (c)
   1 Timolol (Timoptic) could cause hypotension, so blood pressure readings are important before administering the drug. Acetazolamide (Diamox) is a diuretic and could cause a loss of potassium; therefore, it is important to assess electrolyte balance.
   2 Timolol could cause bradycardia, but blood levels of these drugs are not significant.
   3 Blood pressure readings are important; urinalysis is not necessary.
   4 These readings would not be effected by timolol or acetazolamide.
495. Comprehension, planning, environment (b)
   1 Antihistamines could contain atropine, which increases intraocular pressure.
   2 Patching the eye is not necessary.
   3 This would be dangerous because visual activity is affected.
   4 Medications for glaucoma must be taken for life.

496. Knowledge, assessment, physiologic (b)
    2 Flashes of light are a symptom of a detached retina.
    1 Detached retina is painless.
    3 This could be a symptom of cataracts or glaucoma, not detached retina.
    4 This is a symptom of acute open-angle glaucoma, not detached retina.

497. Comprehension, planning, environment (a)
    1 Bed rest is indicated preoperatively to prevent further tearing and bleeding of the retina.
    2 Coughing is contraindicated because it increases intraocular pressure and could cause further bleeding.
    3 Irrigation is not necessary in detached retina.
    4 Both eyes are patched to prevent ocular movement.

498. Application, implementation, physiologic (b)
    4 Laughing will not cause an increase in intraoccular pressure.
    1 Sneezing increases intraoccular pressure.
    2 Coughing should be avoided as it increases intraoccular pressure.
    3 Bending, stooping, and lifting are to be avoided because of the risk of increased pressure.

499. Comprehension, assessment, physiologic (a)
    1 These are symptoms of Ménière's disease. Usually only one ear is affected. The patient experiences recurrent episodes of vertigo with associated nausea and tinnitus and sometimes hearing loss. During these attacks vomiting, diaphoresis and nystagmus may occur. Sudden movements aggravate symptoms.
    2 Ménèire's disease is a *chronic* disease of the middle ear in which there is an increase in endolymph fluid either from increased production or decreased absorption. Although there is no specific therapy for this disease, fluid restriction, diuretics and a low-salt diet are usually prescribed in an attempt to decrease fluid pressure.
    3 This is most common in women between the ages of 50 and 60.
    4 The diagnostic testing includes an audiologic tuning fork that shows a sensorineural deficit. Vestibular testing reveals lack of balance.

500. Knowledge, assessment, physiologic (a)
    4 High heat and humidity increase the risk of heat exhaustion because they slow the dissipation of the heat.
    1 Either sex may suffer from heat exhaustion.
    2 Young adults have heat exhaustion more frequently. This may be because a person becomes more sedentary with age.
    3 Strenuous activity may contribute to heat exhaustion if the person is not acclimatized to the heat.

501. Application, implementation, physiologic (b)
    2 Strenuous exercise may cause the loss of potassium, sodium, and glucose. Fluids will correct hypovolemia caused by sweating.
    1 Oxygen may be needed if his condition worsens.
    3 Loosening the clothing will promote heat dissipation, but it is not the first thing that should be done.
    4 Elevating the feet may help correct any hypotension, but the first thing is fluid volume replacement.

502. Comprehension, assessment, physiologic (b)
    4 In heat stroke the body becomes overheated, but the cooling mechanism of perspiration does not operate, causing the body to store excessive heat.
    1 These are symptoms of food poisoning.
    2 These are symptoms of heat exhaustion.
    3 These are symptoms of frostbite.

503. Application, implementation, physiologic (b)
    2 A low blood pressure in one arm can be misleading, especially if the patient feels well and has no symptoms. The nurse should always compare the pressure in both arms before other interventions are initiated.
    1 The physician may suggest that the pressure also be assessed in the other arm; two phone calls will have to be made instead of one.
    3 It is safe practice to verify an abnormal reading with another nurse, but only after the assigned nurse has assessed the situation thoroughly.
    4 This blood pressure warrants further investigation; this procedure alone would be unsafe.

504. Application, implementation, physiologic (b)
    2 Applying ice to neck, groin, and axillary areas promotes heat loss because of the nearness to the skin of the larger blood vessels.
    1 Cool cloths alone will not significantly cool this patient.
    3 In high humidity a fan alone will not relieve the patient's hyperthermia.
    4 Loosening or removing clothing alone will not significantly reduce hyperthermia.

505. Comprehension, planning, physiologic (a)
    3 Establishing and maintaining an airway is a priority nursing intervention. It is important to cool the person as quickly as possible.
    1 This is the intervention for frostbite.
    2 This is the intervention for insulin reaction.
    4 This is the intervention for heat exhaustion.

506. Knowledge, assessment, physiologic (c)
    1 These symptoms are consistent with loss of fluid volume.
    2 Cardiogenic shock results from the heart's inability to pump fluid.
    3 Damage to the nervous system may cause a temporary paralysis.
    4 Septicemia usually presents with a fever and flushed, dry skin.

507. Application, implementation, physiologic (c)
    4 Wound management follows the stabilization of hemodynamics.
    1 Control of bleeding prevents further fluid loss.
    2 Additional oxygen helps support tissues.
    3 Fluid replacement helps correct hypovolemia.

508. Application, evaluation, physiologic (c)
    4 Normalization of vital signs indicates improvement of clinical status.
    1 Improvements in mentation indicate physiologic stabilization.
    2 Urine output >30 ml/hr indicates sufficient renal blood flow.
    3 Hypotension is consistent with hypovolemia.

509. Comprehension, planning, environment (b)
    2 This is a vasodilator that increases blood circulation and relieves bronchospasms in respiratory distress.
    1 This drug is for hypotensive conditions not associated with respiratory distress.
    3 Neosynephrine produces local vasoconstriction; it comes in drops or spray form.
    4 This is a slower-acting bronchodilator that is given by mouth.

510. Knowledge, evaluation, physiologic (b)
    4 A sudden release of histamines decreases the amount of blood available for circulation, thereby causing capillary hyperpermeability.
    1 This is the reaction of the nervous system to an emotional stimulus.
    2 Neurogenic shock is the result of failure of the nervous system to maintain normal contractions of the blood vessels.
    3 Anaphylactic shock is the result of poor heart function caused by various cardiovascular abnormalities.

511. Comprehension, assessment, physiologic (b)
    1 This indicates a systemic reaction to increased histamine, which decreases the amount of blood for circulation.
    2 These are not symptoms presented with increased histamine in the body. Pulse increases and blood pressure decreases.
    3 Cold and clammy skin accompanies shock.
    4 Lowered respiratory symptoms occur.

512. Comprehension, assessment, health (b)
    2 Patients often use denial and attribute the pain to something like indigestion. They will commonly use some form of home remedy before they realize the seriousness of the situation.
    1 Calling for help immediately is usually not the first action.
    3 Calling the physician is not usually the first action.
    4 Most patients will first try some form of remedy.

513. Application, assessment, health (a)
    4 The first rescuer should ascertain the presence of breathing and pulse. If it is not necessary to start cardiopulmonary resuscitation (CPR) immediately, the rescuer should call for help.
    1 The patient should not walk; he should lie down wherever he is.
    2 CPR is never initiated when the patient is still breathing and has a pulse.
    3 In the event of a heart attack, the rescuer should call for help rather than driving the victim to the hospital because there is no other person in the vehicle to offer assistance if it is needed for CPR.

514. Comprehension, implementation, environment (b)
    1 Airway patency commands primary consideration. If the airway is not patent, all ventilatory attempts will be futile and vital organs will quickly become oxygen-deprived.
    2 Breathing is definitely imperative, but as above, if the airway is not patent, oxygen/carbon dioxide exchange cannot occur.
    3 Promotion of circulation is another important consideration. However, it will be ineffective if the circulating blood is not properly oxygenated.
    4 Definitive therapy follows once the arrest state has been corrected.

515. Comprehension, assessment, physiologic (c)
    3 Sinus tachycardia is a regular rhythm with a P wave for every QRS complex and a rate of 100 to 160 beats/min.
    1 Complete heart block indicates no impulses from the atria being conducted to the ventricles; the atria and ventricles contract independently of one another.
    2 Atrial fibrillation is characterized by a total disorganization of atrial electrical activity without effective atrial contraction. The atrial rate may be as high as 300 to 400 beats/min, while the ventricular rate is 100 to 160 beats/min.
    4 Sinus bradycardia is a regular rhythm with a P wave to every QRS complex and a rate of 40 to 60 beats/min.

516. Knowledge, planning, physiologic (b)
    4 Elective cardioversion is a procedure in which electrical voltage is emitted via defibrillator paddles to restore normal electrical activity of the heart and thus eliminate rapid rhythms.
    1 Elective cardioversion is not the choice when ventricular conduction is in disharmony. This situation calls for *immediate* action, not elective.
    2 Cardioversion does not directly affect the pump action of the right ventricle or of any of the other chambers of the heart.
    3 Heart block is typically characterized by a disruption of electrical impulses through the atria and ventricles. Cardioversion may make the disturbance worse.

517. Knowledge, implementation, physiologic (c)
    2 Immediate defibrillation is the first choice to correct ventricular fibrillation.
    1 From a cardiac perspective, atropine's main action is to increase the heart rate; therefore it would be contraindicated in the treatment of ventricular fibrillation.
    3 Endotracheal intubation does not affect the electrical activity of the heart. However, the situation may warrant intubation once the fibrillatory state is corrected.
    4 Cardioversion is used for terminating rapid, less lethal dysrhythmias, not ventricular fibrillation.

518. Knowledge, planning, physiologic (b)
    3 An electrocardiogram is a graphic measurement of electric currents generated by the conduction within the heart.
    1, 2 Echocardiography is a noninvasive technique that evaluates the internal structures and motions of the heart and great vessels. It shows internal dimensions of the chambers, size and motion of the intraventricular septum and posterior left ventricular wall; valve motion and anatomy; and direction of blood flow.
    4 Arterial blood gas studies provide information on the diffusion of gas across the alveolar capillary membrane and the adequacy of oxygenation of tissues.

519. Application, assessment, psychosocial (c)
    2 Anxiety and fear of dying are not unusual when a person has suffered a heart attack.
    1 The nurse is not giving the husband reassurance.
    3 This feeling is not typical.
    4 The heart attack does not necessarily affect the mind.

520. Knowledge, assessment, physiologic (c)
    1 Oxygenated blood flows from the ascending aorta to nourish the heart muscles.
    2 The left subclavian artery carries blood to the upper left extremities.
    3 The carotid arteries carry blood to the head.
    4 The intercostal arteries carry blood to the chest wall.

521. Comprehension, assessment, physiologic (b)
    2 These enzymes are found mainly in the heart muscle and are released into the bloodstream when there is injury to the myocardium.
    1 This is not applicable in damage to the myocardium.
    3 These are signs/symptoms of other conditions.
    4 Enzymes would be increased, not decreased.

522. Knowledge, planning, health (a)
    2 Legally, the nurse should obtain an account in her own words.
    1 Legally, this is not a requirement. The patient may feel more safe and secure if the nurse stays with her.
    3 Legally, this is not a requirement. In addition, the patient may not prefer to be alone.
    4 This would be preferable for the patient; however, it is not a legal requirement.

523. Knowledge, assessment, environment (a)
    4 It is important to prevent the further transmission of venereal disease by early diagnosis and treatment.
    1 Painful urination may occur; however, a urinalysis is needed.
    2 Dysmenorrhea is painful menstruation; it is not a key reason for a physical examination.
    3 This would be too early to detect pregnancy. A prophylaxis can be given if a method of contraception is not already in use.

524. Comprehension, assessment, physiologic (b)
    1 The effects of a drug in the elderly are related to an alteration of absorption/metabolism, structural and physiologic changes, diminished immune system, and polypharmacy.
    2 Forgetfulness, cost of medications, decreased sex drive, and a greater reliance on faith are considered influencing factors in terms of medication compliance, but none have an effect on the pharmacokinetics of a drug.
    3 The renal system undergoes significant changes throughout the aging process, which causes problems with drug effects. The central system undergoes changes at varying rates and does affect pharmacokinetics; however, No. 1 is the most complete response.
    4 This is an incomplete response. Renal system deficits will affect pharmacokinetics; however, the musculoskeletal system does not have a direct effect on pharmacokinetics.

525. Knowledge, implementation, psychosocial (a)
    1 The major need is personal and body functioning.
    2 This is an inappropriate response; they need to have a purpose in life.
    3 Isolation with only some group contact is unacceptable. It causes a mere state of existence rather than as full a life as possible.
    4 This is an unacceptable approach. These residents should be involved in making as many decisions as possible to maintain a sense of self-worth.

526. Knowledge, planning, physiologic (a)
    2 Body fluid that is lost is not normally replaced by intake of food and fluids.
    1 Edema, not dehydration, occurs.
    3 Uremia, not dehydration, occurs.
    4 Incontinence, not necessarily dehydration, occurs.

527. Knowledge, assessment, physiologic (b)
    4 The normal aging process results in a decrease of total body water and muscle mass, with an increase in total body fat.
    1 There is a decrease in total body water.
    2 There is a decrease in muscle mass.
    3 There is a decrease in total body water and muscle mass.

528. Application, implementation, psychosocial (c)
    2 Patients with Alzheimer's disease frequently wander off and cannot find their way back. It is very important to be sure the patient cannot leave the building so he will not get hurt.
    1 A patient with this disease does need to eat a well balanced diet, but just because he has been diagnosed with Alzheimer's does not mean he cannot feed himself.
    3 A patient with Alzheimer's does not usually recognize himself as he appears today. A picture taken when the patient was young is much more effective.
    4 A patient should not be restrained unless absolutely necessary to prevent him from harming himself or the staff. A doctor's order must accompany this action.

529. Comprehension, assessment, psychosocial (b)
    1 Recent memory loss is common with neurologic disorders.
    2 Memory for past events is usually unaffected.
    3 The question asked about a neurologic disorder.
    4 This does not answer the question.

530. Knowledge, assessment, physiologic (b)
    2 Newer, better, and more potent medications are developed daily, which increases the availability of medications, and patients are much more educated regarding health care today, which affects patient expectations. The elderly frequently seek medical assistance from primary care physicians and specialists, which increases the risk of double-prescribing a medication. Changes within the health care system further enhance polypharmacy.
    1 Medications are expensive, and many elderly struggle to fill prescriptions; the use of a primary care physician could decrease polypharmacy. The elderly purchase approximately 40% of all over-the-counter products.
    3 Availability of medication has increased.
    4 The elderly are no more likely to seek a second opinion than is a younger adult. Many elderly people live with health problems and seek medical intervention only if the condition becomes serious.

531. Comprehension, evaluation, physiologic (b)
    2 Diarrhea is a common side effect.
    1 This is not usually seen.
    3 The opposite is true.
    4 This is not common.

532. Comprehension, planning, environment (b)
    1 Physiologic changes direct the goal of therapy in terms of achieving maximum therapeutic effectiveness while administering the smallest amount of medication possible to achieve maximum results.
    2 The goal of medication administration in all populations is to achieve maximal therapeutic effectiveness at the smallest possible dosage.
    3 Achieving maximal therapeutic effectiveness is the goal of medication administration.
    4 Physicians make mistakes; a nurse is responsible for verifying the physician's orders before administering any drug.

533. Knowledge, planning, health (a)
    3 Studies and evidence do not support this idea; creativity and intelligence do not change with age.
    1 This statement is true.
    2 This statement is true, although elderly people generally do not limit their ability to manage their households.
    4 The majority of elderly people have at least one weekly contact with family and a network of friends.

534. Knowledge, assessment, health (a)
    2 The myth is that most older people *are* isolated and alone. The majority of elderly people have at least weekly contact with family, and many have developed a network of friends who provide support and relationships
    1 This is a myth because in reality, studies and evidence indicate the decline is not inevitable. Creativity and intelligence do not appear to decline. Serious decline in mental capabilities is generally the result of a disease process, not age.
    3 This is a myth because only 5% of the elderly reside in hospitals or nursing homes. The majority own and live in their own homes.
    4 This is a myth. Although most elderly people have at least one chronic condition, these conditions generally do not limit their ability to manage their households and activities on a day-to-day basis.

535. Comprehension, planning, environment (c)
    3 MDS clearly identifies areas that need to be addressed in planning resident care.
    1 This is not true. It is a valuable tool in planning care.
    2 This is incorrect. It is comprehensive information pertinent to the resident as a total person and his needs.
    4 This is not necessarily true. Some states have been given permission to use an alternate version.
536. Comprehension, planning, environment (c)
    4 RAPs are a tool that identifies problems and specific interventions to address in care plans.
    1 This is untrue because it is a valuable tool in planning care and possible changes as needs change.
    2 This is incorrect because this tool generates comprehensive information pertinent to the resident as a total person and his needs.
    3 This is incorrect because this tool provides the specific care needs.
537. Comprehension, assessment, health (c)
    1 U.S. Congress sought federal approval to ensure quality of care.
    2, 3, 4 These are incorrect because these requirements are for both Medicare and Medicaid.
538. Comprehension, assessment, health (c)
    3 Assessments must be conducted or coordinated by RNs along with appropriate participation of other health-care professionals.
    1, 2, 4 All health care personnel can participate, but the RN is the designated coordinator.
539. Comprehension, assessment, psychosocial (b)
    3 Adjusting to changes in one's health, family relationships, and such problems as the loss of a job are normal characteristics for a middle-aged adult.
    1 Although the patient may be having trouble adjusting to the hospital, help from a social worker is premature at this time.
    2 If the patient has always provided for his wife, this is not an abnormal reaction to his illness.
    4 It *is* important to recognize that growing older is difficult for some, and adjusting to a loss of children and possibly a job is frightening to anyone, whether ill or not.
540. Knowledge, implementation, environment (a)
    1 Narrative charting describes events in sequence throughout the course of a nursing shift.
    2 SOAP charting is problem-oriented in nature; the S stands for subjective data; the O for objective data; A addresses the assessment or analysis of the problem; and the P relates to the plan.
    3 Focus charting is a modification of the SOAP charting method and uses a DAR format; the D stands for data; A represents action; and R is response.
    4 PIE is a problem-oriented form of charting; PIE is the acronym for problem, intervention, and evaluation.
541. Knowledge, implementation, environment (a)
    2 The S in SOAP charting is representative of what the patient states.
    1, 3, 4 These are examples of objective data.
542. Knowledge, implementation, environment (a)
    4 A Kardex is not a permanent part of the record and is altered frequently; therefore, using a pencil is appropriate.
    1 The flow sheet is part of the permanent record and the use of a pen is legally required for making entries.
    2 The discharge summary is a permanent part of the chart and therefore requires the use of a pen.
    3 The medication record is part of the permanent record, and the use of a pen is required.

543. Application, implementation, physiologic (c)
    4 This documentation provides specific objective information about the patient's neuromuscular status.
    1 "Limited" response is neither objective nor specific.
    2 "Decreased" strength is broad and subjective.
    3 "At intervals" and "most of the time" are subjective assessments since they are nonspecific.
544. Comprehension, implementation, psychosocial (c)
    2 The use of reassuring clichés is a barrier to therapeutic communication because these responses tend to convey to the patient that the nurse feels the patient is worrying needlessly or that the nurse does not understand the problem.
    1 The nontherapeutic technique of disagreeing with the patient implies that what the patient said is not acceptable. Disagreeing may serve to threaten the patient.
    3 In belittling the patient's feelings, the nurse devalues them by implying they are commonplace and insignificant. Belittling serves to lower the patient's self-esteem.
    4 The technique of giving approval creates a block by shifting the focus to the nurse's values. The nurse now becomes judgmental.
545. Application, implementation, psychosocial (b)
    3 People differ in personal hygiene practices. These practices are affected by culture and socioeconomic class. The patient's wishes need to be considered.
    1 The nurse is being aggressive and trying to force her desires on the patient. The patient's desires must be considered.
    2, 4 It is not necessary to bring the supervisor or doctor in on the matter.
546. Application, implementation, psychosocial (b)
    4 The patient always has the final say on whether to have treatment or not. Many times the patient is just frightened and after talking with the nurse will agree to have the surgery. If the patient continues to refuse surgery, the surgeon needs to be informed. Surgery must not be done against the patient's wishes.
    1 Even after premedication has been given, the patient still has the right to refuse surgery.
    2 It is illegal to do surgery against the patient's wishes. The patient could bring assault and battery charges against the nurse and surgeon.
    3 The nurse should not cancel the surgery until speaking with the surgeon.
547. Application, implementation, psychosocial (b)
    4 This is the best choice because the nurse is restating what the patient has said and allowing the patient to rethink what he said. Many times something else is upsetting the patient and he will use a statement such as this to start a conversation. By restating what the patient has said, the nurse may keep him talking.
    1 It is unwise for the nurse to defend the doctor or staff member. This statement would end the conversation and the nurse would not discover what was really bothering the patient.
    2 This statement will also end the conversation. The nurse is confrontational and the patient may feel threatened. The goal is to keep the patient talking.
    3 The nurse is giving advise to the patient, which is always unwise.

548. Comprehension, assessment, psychosocial (b)
    2 Use of an open-ended question gets her to tell the nurse more about what she is thinking.
    1 This is an inappropriate response; it prevents establishing an effective relationship with the patient.
    3 This does not allow her to express her concerns.
    4 This response prevents establishing therapeutic communication.
549. Knowledge, implementation, psychosocial (b)
    1 The use of direct eye contact is one of the characteristics of attentive listening, conveying an attitude of caring and interest.
    2 The overuse of personal experiences focuses on the nurse and not the patient.
    3 The misuse of social graces implies that the nurse is not attentively listening.
    4 Providing privacy is an appropriate action to the situation; however, the use of direct eye contact *best* indicates that the nurse is interested in what the patient is saying.
550. Comprehension, implementation, psychosocial (b)
    3 Denial is subconscious blocking of anxiety-producing events. Reality is distorted or transformed.
    1 Rationalization is a defense mechanism that transfers the self-responsibility to a person or an object.
    2 Regression is defined as a coping strategy that produces behaviors associated with an earlier developmental stage.
    4 Compensation as a defense mechanism means making up for a deficiency in one aspect of self-image by focusing on a feature that is considered to be an asset.
551. Comprehension, implementation, psychosocial (c)
    1 Patients with expressive aphasia have difficulty in speaking and writing. Associating words or providing pictures of physical objects assists the patient in communicating his needs.
    2 The patient with expressive aphasia can communicate, but he will need assistance.
    3 To best help the patient with expressive aphasia, the nurse should not supply the correct word immediately. The patient should have a longer time in which to respond.
    4 The patient should be encouraged and stimulated to talk.
552. Comprehension, assessment, physiologic (b)
    4 Gastric analysis examines gastric secretions to determine the presence of malignant cells.
    1 The cholecystogram is diagnostic for gallbladder disease.
    2 The gastroscopy procedure involves the use of an illuminated scope to visualize the stomach and surrounding structures.
    3 Fluoroscopy is an x-ray examination of the stomach that could reveal pathology.
553. Knowledge, assessment, physiologic (a)
    1 Blood urea nitrogen (BUN) is one of the significant tests done to measure kidney function; it is elevated in renal disease.
    2 BUN is elevated in renal disease.
    3 BUN is directly related to kidney disease.
    4 This is one of the most significant tests for determining renal function, particularly when correlated with blood creatinine levels.
554. Knowledge, assessment, physiologic (c)
    3 CK-MB, isoenzymes LDH_1 and LDH_2 specifically measure the amount of myocardial tissue damage (necrosis).
    1 Although SGOT and SGPT may elevate in cardiac necrosis, these enzyme tests are more specific for liver dysfunction.
    2 CPK enzyme elevation may occur in cardiac necrosis; however, it may also elevate in musculoskeletal and/or cerebral injury. Therefore it is not specific for measuring cardiac damage. SGPT is more specific for determining liver dysfunction.
    4 Neither of these exist as a laboratory enzyme study.
555. Application, assessment, physiologic (b)
    3 The presence of protein in the urine indicates the kidneys are beginning to show signs of damage.
    1 Blood urea nitrogen indicates difficulty with protein metabolism.
    2 Hemoglobin indicates the percentage of oxygen-carrying protein in the blood.
    4 Ketones in the urine are a late sign of prolonged hyperglycemia.
556. Application, assessment, physiologic (b)
    4 Urine should be slightly aromatic. After standing, it begins smelling like ammonia from the bacterial action.
    1 Urine should be clear and straw-colored.
    2 Normal pH of urine is 4.6 to 8.0.
    3 Normal specific gravity of urine is 1.010 to 1.025.
557. Knowledge, assessment, physiologic (b)
    4 Amylase is an enzyme secreted by the pancreas. It is necessary for digestion.
    1 Glucose is specific for diabetes.
    2 Glycosylated hemoglobin is used in the diagnosis of diabetes.
    3 Blood urea nitrogen is helpful in determining kidney disorders.
558. Application, evaluation, physiologic (c)
    1 Respiratory alkalosis is the most likely result of hyperventilation. The patient is blowing off carbon dioxide, which is converted to carbonic acid in the body.
    2 The patient is blowing off so much carbon dioxide that it is unlikely that the pH will remain within normal limits unless the buffer systems are working extremely well.
    3 A patient with respiratory acidosis may begin to breathe faster in order to blow off excess carbon dioxide to act as a buffering system to stabilize the pH. Since this patient has been breathing so rapidly for several hours, it is unlikely that the pH would still be acidic. The patient is exhaling too much carbon dioxide for the pH to be acidic. The more likely occurrence would be respiratory alkalosis.
    4 Tachypnea will affect the respiratory system first. If respiratory distress continues long enough, it may lead to metabolic acidosis or alkalosis.
559. Knowledge, implementation, physiologic (a)
    3 Left Sims' is believed to straighten the colon and enhance the cleansing ability of the enema.
    1 Prone is uncomfortable for the patient.
    2 Supine is difficult for the nurse but possible if necessary for the patient's comfort.
    4 Left side is more effective.

560. Application, implementation, environment (b)
    2 When a 24-hour specimen is disrupted, a new container should be obtained and the collection should be restarted. Documentation of the reason for starting again and the time the new collection was started should be made in the nurse's notes.
    1 The specimen collection could be inaccurate if all the urine for 24 hours was not collected.
    3 Adding to the urine already collected would result in some of the specimen being more than 24 hours old, which could give false readings.
    4 There is no justification for waiting until the next morning unless the physician prefers to wait.

561. Comprehension, assessment, physiologic (a)
    4 Once food is digested, gastric juices needed for digestion have no more food to work on and can irritate the stomach lining, forming ulcerations.
    1 Symptoms do not occur when food is in the stomach.
    2 Symptoms are less severe or absent when food is in the stomach.
    3 Gastric juices are stimulated by introduction of food.

562. Comprehension, implementation, physiologic (b)
    3 Having the patient take deep breaths will relax the external sphincter, allowing for easier passage of the catheter.
    1 Coughing would constrict the urinary meatus and sphincter.
    2 This technique would contaminate the catheter and increase the risk of introducing microorganisms into the bladder.
    4 This approach also increases the risk of contamination of the urinary tract.

563. Knowledge, assessment, physiologic (a)
    2 Residual urine is defined as the urine that remains in the bladder after urination.
    1 Reflex incontinence is an involuntary loss of urine occurring at predictable intervals when a specific urinary volume is reached.
    3 Urge incontinence is an involuntary passage of urine after a strong sense of urgency to void.
    4 Retention is an accumulation of urine in the bladder because the bladder is unable to empty.

564. Knowledge, assessment, physiologic (a)
    3 Residual urine measures the amount of urine left in the bladder after the patient voids.
    1 This methodology only measures urine output in an 8-hour period.
    2 This procedure does not relate to any urine testing method.
    4 This is not an appropriate method to test for residual urine. However, it may be used in urine glucose testing.

565. Knowledge, implementation, environment (a)
    2 It is suggested that 50 to 100 ml of urine be sent to the laboratory if possible, so that a thorough assessment can be performed.
    1 The size of the container has nothing to do with the suggested amount of urine to be collected.
    3 Water is contraindicated because it may dilute and/or contaminate the specimen.
    4 A routine urinalysis does not require the use of a sterile container; however, urine for culture and sensitivity does.

566. Comprehension, implementation, physiologic (a)
    2 Reporting potential complication symptoms is an accountable nursing action. The vital signs are imperative for baseline assessment data.
    1 This is appropriate, but the patient needs first-priority assessment.
    3 This selection indicates poor clinical judgment; it does not address the immediate potential complication symptoms.
    4 This could be done simultaneously in the assessment phase; however, No. 2 is the more complete nursing action, given the situation.

567. Knowledge, planning, physiologic (a)
    3 The oil-retention enema softens and lubricates to ease defecation for a patient with this condition.
    1 A Fleet enema would be safe, but it is not the best answer for this patient. Straining may still occur if the stool is hard and difficult to pass.
    2 Saline is not recommended in cardiac patients because of the possibility of electrolyte and fluid changes.
    4 The amount and type may place too much of a strain on an already weakened heart.

568. Application, implementation, physiologic (c)
    2 This noninvasive method of a tight face mask will produce a range of 40% to 65% O_2 within the mask with the flow rate at 6 to 12 L/min.
    1 The nasal cannula will produce an oxygen range of 24% to 40% and will not usually be adequate for anesthesia recovery. The rate of 1 to 4 L/min is also inadequate.
    3 This method produces only varying amounts of O_2 to the patient.
    4 Rebreathing CO_2 in a paper bag will not provide O_2 levels to support increased tissue perfusion.

569. Application, implementation, physiologic (b)
    1 Removing as much mucus as possible allows more air to reach the smaller air passages.
    2 If the patient breathes as rapidly as possible, he may feel dizzy and hyperventilate.
    3 The patient should sit up as much as possible to allow for better use of the diaphragm.
    4 Some postoperative patients may not want to try the spirometer because of fear or postoperative discomfort; they must be encouraged.

570. Application, implementation, physiologic (c)
    2 Clean gloves are permissible to remove the dressing, which should be removed one layer at a time to avoid dislodging the Penrose drain.
    1 Removing the dressing all at once may dislodge or pull out the Penrose drain.
    3 The entire dressing should be changed.
    4 It is normally necessary to touch the clean gauze during a dressing change; therefore, clean, nonsterile gloves may be used to remove the old dressing, and sterile gloves may be used to apply a clean dressing.

571. Application, implementation, psychosocial (a)
    2 An interpreter must be found to explain the surgery to the patient so she can give informed consent.
    1 It is much too soon to give preoperative medication.
    3 An enema would be contraindicated. It could cause the aneurysm to rupture.
    4 The nurse cannot get a medical history until an interpreter is found.

572. Application, assessment, physiologic (b)
    3 Redness and swelling are common signs of a wound infection after surgery.
    1 An oral temperature of 101° F (38.3° C) is more indicative of an infection.
    2 A small amount of clear yellow drainage may be a normal part of the healing process. Cloudy, yellow/green drainage is not normal.
    4 A sudden drop in blood pressure on the day of surgery is more indicative of hemorrhage.

573. Application, assessment, physiologic (b)
    3 Dorsiflexing the patient's foot is a good postoperative nursing action for the possible complication of emboli. The nurse should report any complaints of pain (Homans' sign).
    1 Patients ambulate or do passive exercises as soon as possible after surgery to prevent the formation of emboli.
    2 If used, elastic stockings should be worn constantly. They may be removed for a bath.
    4 The patient's legs should never be rubbed. This can stimulate the movement of a clot forming in the leg.

574. Knowledge, implementation, environment (a)
    3 100° F (37.7° C) to 105° F (40.5° C) is warm to the body.
    1, 2 These options are cooler than body temperature and will defeat the goal of warmth to the perineum.
    4 This temperature is hot enough to endanger skin integrity.

575. Knowledge, assessment, health (b)
    3 The goal is to help the nurse reenter nursing in a systematic, planned, and safe way. This may include restriction on narcotics for a period of time.
    1 If a colleague is suspected, it is important to notify the supervisor, who will often notify the state nursing association or board of nursing.
    2 Before peer assistance programs, often nurses would be fired or be free to move to other facilities where the abuse could continue.
    4 The basis of peer assistance programs is one nurse helping another nurse.

576. Comprehension, implementation, environment (b)
    4 The urine in the Foley bag should never be allowed to flow back into the bladder. Urine in the bag could harbor microorganisms that could cause a urinary infection.
    1 The overbed table is designated for eating and would probably be above the bladder.
    2 In the patient's lap, the urine could flow back into the bladder.
    3 The Foley catheter should be maintained as a closed system and does not need to be disrupted for this reason.

577. Application, implementation, physiologic (a)
    3 When suctioning a patient, it is important to give oxygen before and after because suctioning removes oxygen as well as secretions. The length of time to suction would be 10 to 15 seconds. At least 5 minutes should elapse between each suctioning.
    1 Thirty seconds is too long; this would remove oxygen from the system.
    2 Coughing and deep breathing should not be performed as part of the suctioning procedure. Oxygenation is the last step.
    4 Twenty-five seconds is too long and would remove oxygen from the system. The last step is to oxygenate.

578. Knowledge, assessment, environment (a)
    1 The inflatable cuff prevents saliva and foreign objects from going through the trachea by sealing the tube against the tracheal wall.
    2 The trach tube does not stop bleeding.
    3 The trach tube itself increases oxygen exchange, but the cuff does not.
    4 If the trach tube is pulled on, the tube will still come out even if the cuff is inflated.

579. Comprehension, planning, physiologic (b)
    1 The esophagus undergoes smooth muscle weakness with age. Foods and liquids of moderate consistency are more easily swallowed and passed into the stomach.
    2 This should be considered but only to the extent that the food or beverage choice could lead to an aspiration episode.
    3 The hospital's dietary department is fully capable of offering therapeutic diets for all patients.
    4 The physician's order must clearly be followed; however, it is certainly within the nursing function to ensure that patients with dysphagia get appropriate meals based on the patient's problem.

580. Application, planning, psychosocial (a)
    3 The patient is confused and will not understand the importance of not getting out of bed alone. The patient must be watched carefully to prevent falls. It would be best if someone would stay with the patient at all times.
    1 At this point the patient will be unable to comprehend or remember instructions.
    2 The patient is confused and will not remember instructions. Before discharge the nurse can instruct the patient if she is more alert, but the nurse also will need to involve the family to assist the patient.
    4 Visitors could be of great benefit to monitor the patient when the nurse is not able to be in the room. Visitors that the patient knows well could also help orient the patient.

581. Application, evaluation, environment (b)
    4 The main purpose for the incident report is to refresh the nurse's memory of the events which occurred.
    1 The incident should not be put in the patient chart and no mention should be made of the report in the chart. In some states, an attorney can get access to the report, but in most it is considered privileged information.
    2 An incident report would not prevent a lawsuit.
    3 An incident report would not prevent a reoccurrence.

582. Application, implementation, environment (b)
    4 Assault is an unlawful threat to harm another physically. Battery is the carrying out of bodily harm such as touching without authorization. By doing the surgery without consent, the surgeon, hospital, and staff can be charged with battery.
    1 An invasion of privacy charge would stem from sharing information in the patient's medical records without the patient's consent.
    2 The doctrine of *res ipsa loquitor* means "the thing speaks for itself." This doctrine applies to injuries sustained by patients while in the hospital.
    3 Under the corporate negligence doctrine, the facility may be liable for failing to ensure that an acceptable level of care is provided.

583. Application, planning, environment (b)
 1 The case must be canceled until the Versed has worn off and the patient can sign her own consent form.
 2 A patient's spouse cannot sign the operative permit unless the patient has been legally declared incompetent.
 3 A patient's children cannot sign the consent unless they have legal power of attorney.
 4 A patient cannot legally sign an informed operative consent while she is under the influence of medication.

584. Comprehension, evaluation, health (b)
 3 The best indication that learning has taken place is when a change in behavior is noted.
 1 The nurse can facilitate learning by having the client repeat the instructions, but this is not necessarily an indicator that learning has taken place.
 2 Videos are a good instructional tool but do not necessarily guarantee learning has occurred.
 4 The patient is displaying interest by asking questions. This will help in the learning process.

585. Application, assessment, physiologic (c)
 4 Weight loss, fatigue, and lack of appetite are classic symptoms of cancer. The physician will need to order tests to determine the location and type of cancer.
 1 Anorexia nervosa usually occurs in a teenaged girl or a patient in the early twenties. It would be unlikely to start in a 45 year old who had never had an eating disorder before.
 2 There was no mention of coughing or other symptoms of TB.
 3 No abdominal pain or bleeding was mentioned.

586. Comprehension, implementation, environment (c)
 4 Controlled substances must be accounted for.
 1 This is a safe practice to ensure the right patient receives the right drug, but it doesn't relate to the Controlled Substance Act.
 2 This is another safe practice, but it doesn't relate to the handling of controlled substances.
 3 Documentation of medications is required, but this is not specified in the Controlled Substance Act.

587. Application, implementation, psychosocial (c)
 1 A clock is very good to orient the patient. A calendar or wrist watch would also be helpful.
 2 Visitors need to be encouraged; this will provide social stimuli for the patient.
 3 The nurse should do morning care slowly while talking to the patient. This is an excellent way to provide stimulus to the patient.
 4 The patient needs hearing aids and eyeglasses to assist in receiving environmental stimuli.

588. Comprehension, planning, environment (b)
 4 Restraints should be removed as soon as the patient regains control.
 1 Restraints should be checked several times during each shift.
 2 Restraints should not be too tight.
 3 Minimal staff should be required.

589. Application, implementation, physiologic (b)
 3 Simple nursing measures should be tried first.
 1 Pain medication is not called for in this situation.
 2 A physician's order is required for a catheter.
 4 Positioning probably has no bearing in this situation.

590. Application, implementation, physiologic (b)
 4 If simple nursing measures fail, a catheter order may be needed.
 1 This will not stimulate urination.
 2 This will not solve the problem.
 3 8 hours is long enough if the patient is uncomfortable.

591. Comprehension, evaluation, physiologic (a)
 1 The BMR decreases each decade, and consequently fewer calories are needed to maintain weight. Therefore the food intake needs to decrease.
 2 Many adults over 30 are still quite active.
 3 Food intake can remain the same, and weight will still increase because of the decrease in BMR.
 4 There is not necessarily an increase in carbohydrates and fats after the age of 30. Elderly adults tend to eat increased carbohydrates because they are easier to digest than proteins. This high carbohydrate intake can lead to nutritional problems.

592. Application, assessment, physiologic (b)
 1 Thirst and increased body temperature are common symptoms of hypernatremia. The nurse needs to look for abnormal loss of fluid or low intake. Drugs such as Alka-Seltzer can also cause an increase in the sodium content.
 2 Muscle twitching occurs with hyponatremia.
 3 These are symptoms of hypokalemia or hyperkalemia.
 4 These are symptoms of hypocalcemia.

593. Comprehension, implementation, physiologic (b)
 4 The elderly are prone to hypothermia, and special measures must be followed to preserve normal body temperature.
 1 An infant is also susceptible to hypothermia, but by the time a child is 10 years old the risk has diminished greatly.
 2, 3 Both of these patients would be in the lowest risk group for hypothermia unless they had a chronic illness.

594. Comprehension, implementation, physiologic (b)
 3 The orthopneic position promotes oxygen transport into the lungs.
 1 This position is used when exposure of the rectal area is needed.
 2 Lithotomy position is helpful when exposure of the perineum is required.
 4 Supine positioning would increase the patient's dyspnea.

595. Application, evaluation, physiologic (b)
 1 Obesity predisposes the patient to hypertension, increased heart rate, varicose veins, and osteoarthritis.
 2 There is no indication that obesity leads to hypotension or asthma. Also, the pulse rate of an obese patient is usually higher.
 3 Hypovolemia is not caused by obesity. There is also no indication of obesity being a predisposing factor for hypoglycemia. In fact, obese patients are prone to get diabetes mellitus, which is hyperglycemia.
 4 Hypervolemia is not caused by obesity even though obesity can cause some edema in the extremities. Obese patients are not prone to become hypothermic easier than thin patients.

596. Comprehension, implementation, physiologic (b)
 2 This measure will help keep the patient mobile.
 1 The patient has a right to refuse therapy.
 3 This will not prevent immobility.
 4 This will not improve mobility.

597. Comprehension, implementation, physiologic (b)
 1 Vomiting or aspiration during anesthesia could be deadly.
 2 Being NPO does not affect anesthesia.
 3 Having an empty stomach will not affect the bowel's ability to function.
 4 Having something in the stomach does not affect the sensation of nausea.
598. Application, evaluation, environment (b)
 3 Disclosure of information is limited to certain individuals.
 1 This deals more with not exposing the patient.
 2 This has to do with releasing the name.
 4 Rules are made based on the necessity of keeping information confidential.
599. Application, implementation, environment (b)
 2 Shaking the canister will mix the drug with the inhalant.
 1 This is unnecessary and will not affect the dosing or usage.
 3 Rinsing the mouth between different drugs is important to prevent drug interaction.
 4 Ten seconds is long enough to hold the breath. This is the time necessary to get the drug into the lungs.
600. Application, evaluation, physiologic (c)
 2 This is a normal finding.
 1 Normally, diastolic blood pressure lowers when the person moves from supine to erect.
 3 Activity may increase the heart rate.
 4 Urine output volume should not be affected by short-term position changes.
601. Application, implementation, physiologic (b)
 2 The patient needs to be assisted into the position in which it is easiest to breathe. Proper air exchange is the main concern.
 1 Chest x-rays will be ordered later.
 3 The patient must be made comfortable first; sedatives may depress respiration even further.
 4 The patient will be unable to answer questions until the gas exchange improves.
602. Application, implementation, psychosocial (b)
 4 A patient in isolation often feels lonely and frightened. The patient needs supportive measures by the nurse.
 1 The patient needs to be allowed visitors to help relieve the feelings of loneliness. The visitors need to be instructed on donning the hat, gown, and mask and must be shown good handwashing technique.
 2 The isolated patient is at risk for sensory alteration, so the clocks need to remain in the room.
 3 A high-calorie diet including carbohydrates needs to be encouraged for the patient undergoing chemotherapy. Cancer increases the metabolism, and the patient will have difficulty keeping on weight.

603. Application, implementation, psychosocial (b)
 2 Part of a nurse's job is to care for all patients without discrimination. A nurse cannot pick and choose her patients. It is the nurse's responsibility to care for all patients using universal precautions. The nurse could seek counseling to assist with the fear.
 1 The nurse cannot refuse to care for a patient unless for religious or ethical reasons. Even then the nurse needs to have discussed the issue with the supervisor before the issue arose. An HIV-positive patient would not fall under the category of religious or ethical reasons.
 3 The supervisor will be very upset to receive a phone call such as this at home. Caring for the patient is the professional responsibility of the nurse.
 4 It would be unethical and unkind to approach the patient in this way. The patient needs caring and understanding, and it is the nurse's responsibility to give those things unconditionally.
604. Application, planning, environment (b)
 3 A face shield would protect the nurse from getting splashed in the face or eyes.
 1 Lab coats are not impervious to liquid penetration.
 2 Paper shoe covers may help keep the floor clean from cross contamination, but they are unnecessary in this situation.
 4 Another pair of gloves will give additional protection from exposure to blood or body fluid.
605. Knowledge, assessment, environment (b)
 4 The correct definition of cachexia is chronic protein malnutrition.
 1 Osteomalacia is a condition characterized by demineralization of the bone matrix.
 2 Obesity is defined as being 20% or more over ideal body weight.
 3 Gastritis is a condition characterized by gastric mucosal irritation.
606. Knowledge, evaluation, environment (a)
 2 UTIs are the most common nosocomial infection in the United States and Canada. Breaks in aseptic technique while catheterizing the patient may result in serious and even fatal consequences.
 1 Respiratory tract infections are the most frequently occurring infections that bring the patient to the hospital, but UTIs are the most frequently occurring nosocomial infections.
 3 Because of the adherence to strict aseptic technique, surgical wound infections do not occur frequently.
 4 The patient usually enters the hospital with gastrointestinal infections rather than contracting them once in the hospital.
607. Application, implementation, environment (b)
 1 The first action should be to explain the procedure to the patient. If the patient knows what is going to happen, sometimes he can assist.
 2 The procedure needs to be explained first before anything else is done so the patient will not become anxious.
 3 Closing the door is necessary to maintain the patient's privacy, but it is not really a safety measure.
 4 The nurse cannot raise the side rails until the patient has been moved.
608. Knowledge, assessment, psychosocial (a)
 3 Confabulation is used to fill in gaps of information.
 1 Lying is not a part of a neurologic disorder.
 2 Remote memory is usually better than current memory.
 4 This is not related to memory loss associated with aging.

609. Comprehension, assessment, physiological (b)
    1 Subjective data are verbal data obtained from the patient and/or significant other.
    2, 3, 4 These are objective data.
610. Application, implementation, environment (b)
    4 In the presence of an actual infection, the patient and/or family members should be taught how to prevent the spread of infection to others and to prevent further spread of infection within the patient.
    1 A balance of rest and activities is recommended during times of healing, with an increase in nutrient-dense foods and fluid intake to facilitate the healing process. Returning to work too soon may lead to a relapse and slow healing.
    2 Patients cannot monitor their own blood work.
    3 It is appropriate to teach the signs and symptoms of local inflammation, but it is also necessary to recognize signs and symptoms of systemic infection. The statement is soliciting information specific to prevention of the spread of infection.
611. Comprehension, assessment, psychosocial (b)
    1 The nurse must assess her own feelings about working with an alcoholic.
    2 This is not what she needs to do first.
    3 This is not appropriate in multidisciplinary treatment planning.
    4 This is not a first action.
612. Application, implementation, physiologic (b)
    4 Increased fluids will aid bowel function.
    1 Increased exercise is good for the bowels, but this could cause increased shoulder injury.
    2 A diet high in fiber aids the bowels. High protein aids wound healing.
    3 Narcotic analgesics are highly constipating.
613. Comprehension, planning, physiologic (b)
    1 Finger foods require gross motor control and promote independence.
    2 Patients should be allowed to chew food if they can.
    3 This option promotes a loss of independence.
    4 A bib is not going to ensure that the patient has enough food, and it may humiliate him.
614. Application, implementation, physiologic (b)
    3 Suction should not be applied as the catheter is being introduced because it can cause trauma and remove needed oxygen.
    1 The catheter should be lubricated with sterile saline. Mineral oil is not water soluble and can cause aspiration pneumonia.
    2 Suction should be applied 10 to 15 seconds at a time. Longer than that will remove too much oxygen.
    4 Never force the catheter; it will cause trauma.
615. Application, planning, physiologic (c)
    3 Daily weight is a much more accurate reflection of the patient's fluid balance. The patient should be weighed before breakfast every day wearing the same type of clothing and on the same scale.
    1 I & O is not very accurate because of the many errors that can occur when the nurses and the patient are trying to remember to document everything taken in or eliminated. It is difficult to accurately measure how much fluid is lost through a bowel movement or respirations.
    2 Abdominal girth is used to assess ascites.
    4 Mental status may or may not change with changes in fluid volume.

616. Comprehension, assessment, health (a)
    3 An illness that develops from an invasion of microorganisms is termed an infection.
    1 Inflammation is the body's reaction to injury or irritation, not to an invasion of pathogenic microorganisms.
    2 Allergy is an antigen-antibody reaction of the body to a substance, causing the body to be hypersensitive to that substance.
    4 Immunity is the body's ability to have a resistance to a specific disease. Resistance is the result of either active or passive immunity.
617. Application, implementation, environment (a)
    1 If the oxygen is not attached to a water reservoir, the oxygen will dry out the mucous membranes.
    2 Nasal prongs are frequently used.
    3 Powder is contraindicated around the face; the patient can aspirate the powder.
    4 The doctor orders the flow rate. High levels of oxygen can be dangerous to the patient.
618. Application, implementation, environment (c)
    3 Oxygen administration is unnecessary with metered-dose inhalation.
    1 This method would safely deliver the drug.
    2 This method would provide adequate inhalation of the medication.
    4 This method could be used to effectively deliver the drug dose.
619. Application, assessment, physiologic (b)
    1 The problem may simply be a result of the patient turning, causing kinks and blockage in the tubing.
    2 The nurse should assess for other problems before alerting the physician.
    3 The patient may feel fine even though the Foley is not draining well. This action may yield little help in solving the problem.
    4 This should not be done first of all unless an order is obtained. Secondly, an increase in fluids may produce severe discomfort for the patient if the Foley is not working properly.
620. Comprehension, implementation, physiologic (c)
    1 It is recommended to instill no more than 5 ml of irrigating solution into the ureters because of their small diameter and the close proximity to the kidney; more would allow for a greater risk of infection.
    2, 3 This is too large an amount. It may flow directly into the kidneys, thus increasing the risk for infection.
    4 This is not a sufficient amount of fluid for irrigation.
621. Knowledge, implementation, physiologic (a)
    4 Perineal exercises strengthen the muscles of the perineum that support the urinary bladder; this helps reduce incontinence.
    1 Perineal exercises do not affect the formation or amount of residual urine.
    2 Urinary retention is not relieved by perineal exercises.
    3 Dysuria usually indicates a bladder infection; perineal exercises may not be prescribed.
622. Knowledge, implementation, physiologic (a)
    3 Massage increases circulation to the affected area, thereby supplying nutrients to promote tissue health.
    1 Alcohol causes drying, and rubbing the area may promote tissue destruction.
    2 Semi-Fowler's position would cause direct pressure to the coccyx region.
    4 Heating increases vasodilation; this measure is suggested when dealing with an open wound.

623. Comprehension, assessment, environment (a)
    3 Assessment involves gathering, verifying, and communicating data about a patient, which is the first phase of the nursing process.
    1 The implementation process includes the nurse's performing or assisting in the achievement of patient-centered outcome. However, this is step No. 3 in the overall process.
    2 The evaluation component measures the patient's response to outcomes. In this process, the nurse may need to alter the plan of care.
    4 Nursing diagnosis follows the assessment phase and is the responsibility of the registered nurse.

624. Knowledge, assessment, physiologic (a)
    2 A reduction in the volume of packed red blood cells per 100 ml of blood or in hemoglobin or in the number of circulating red blood cells may indicate an anemic condition.
    1 This is the term used to designate a malignant neoplasm of blood-forming organs.
    3 Hemolysis designates the breaking down or destruction of red blood cells.
    4 Leukocytosis refers to an abnormally high white blood cell count (leukocytes).

625. Knowledge, assessment, physiologic (a)
    3 Edema of the fingers is indicative of Na^+ retention.
    1 Heartburn is not a symptom of fluid imbalance.
    2 Skin rash is not a symptom of fluid imbalance.
    4 Excessive tearing, when not related to crying, is usually indicative of a disorder of the lacrimal glands.

626. Knowledge, assessment, physiologic (a)
    4 The term "syndrome" designates a group of symptoms, which may be subjective or objective, as in a nephrotic syndrome, which is another name for nephrosis.
    1 This is the type of symptom that the patient describes to the nurse.
    2 This is the type of symptom that the nurse observes.
    3 A sign is a term that detects objective evidence. An example of an objective sign would be the "finding" following use of an instrument such as a percussion hammer or blood pressure cuff.

627. Knowledge, assessment, physiologic (a)
    3 A sign is objective evidence that is obvious and definitive as well as separate from the patient's impression (e.g., blood pressure reading).
    1 This is the type of symptom that the patient expresses to the nurse.
    2 This is the type of symptom that the nurse observes.
    4 The term "syndrome" designates a group of symptoms, such as in a nephrotic syndrome.

628. Knowledge, assessment, environment (a)
    2 Nausea is a subjective experience reported by the patient.
    1 Temperature is measurable; therefore it is an objective finding.
    3 Blood pressure results are an objective finding.
    4 Rapid shallow respirations are a visual quantitative finding.

629. Knowledge, assessment, environment (a)
    4 Temperature measurement is an objective finding that is obtained by the nurse.
    1 Loss of appetite is a subjective experience determined by the patient.
    2 Pain is a subjective experience reported by the patient. It may also include objective findings.
    3 Nausea is a subjective sensation reported by the patient.

630. Application, planning, physiologic (c)
    3 The patient is at increased risk of delayed wound healing due to her obesity, which impairs circulation to damaged areas secondary to the surgery.
    1 The statement lacks appropriate assessment data to formulate a fluid volume deficit diagnosis.
    2 The statement lacks sufficient data to support activity intolerance as a diagnosis.
    4 The statement lacks sufficient data to support impaired gas exchange as a diagnosis.

631. Comprehension, planning, physiologic (b)
    3 Patients undergoing surgery lose large amounts of fluid through bleeding and loss of other body fluids. Since the patient was NPO at least 8 hours before surgery, she was low on fluids before the surgery began.
    1 This can be a concern following surgery, but it is not a main concern.
    2 Surgery is usually viewed as a positive treatment to assist the patient to a more normal lifestyle. Hopelessness is usually a diagnosis for a patient who is facing impending death.
    4 The surgical patient is not usually restricted in socializing after the initial healing has taken place.

632. Comprehension, evaluation, environment (b)
    1 Care plans should be workable, flexible, and individualized to promote optimal health and functioning. The process to ensure the care plan is meeting the needs of an individual is to routinely review and revise the plan of care.
    2 The plan of care should be reviewed when a major health change has occurred and also regularly reviewed for necessary changes and modifications.
    3 All goals may not be met; therefore, the importance of reviewing the plan of care cannot be understated.
    4 The plan of care must be flexible.

633. Application, planning, physiologic (c)
    4 The NPO status, nasogastric tube, and IV fluid require frequent monitoring of the patient's fluid and electrolyte status.
    1 This goal is related to pain, not alteration in nutrition.
    2 This goal is related to infection as opposed to alteration in nutrition.
    3 This goal is related to tissue perfusion as opposed to alteration in nutrition.

634. Application, implementation, environment (a)
    2 These interventions will promote circulation and healing and will decrease pressure to areas prone to breakdown secondary to unrelieved pressure.
    1 These interventions protect the patient from possible falls.
    3 These interventions enhance physical mobility and adequate lung expansion but do not adequately prevent pressure sore development.
    4 This protects the patient from possible falls.

635. Knowledge, assessment, physiologic (b)
    1 The health history and physical assessment are the two key elements of the nursing assessment. The history should be done first, followed by a head-to-toe assessment by the nurse.
    2 The cultural history will be a part of the health history. The care plan will be done during the planning stages.
    3 Blood work is not a part of the nurse's assessment.
    4 The emotional status of the patient will be part of the physical assessment.

636. Comprehension, assessment, physiologic (b)
3 In this way the nurse will transmit the organisms from her hands to her eyes.
1, 2 Coming in contact with the person is not enough to transmit the disease.
4 Transmission will not occur through a third person.

637. Application, implementation, environment (a)
3 This follows universal precaution guidelines to decrease the possibility of needlestick injury.
1 This action is a violation of the Centers for Disease Control and Prevention's (CDC) guidelines for universal precautions.
2 This maneuver is in violation of CDC standards and has been linked to an increased incidence of needlestick injury.
4 This action is not recommended and is not regarded as safe practice.

638. Knowledge, planning, health (b)
3 The vaccine provides resistance to and decreases the severity of the disease if it is contracted.
1 The vaccine is to provide resistance to the organism before the possibility of contracting the disease.
2 Human blood plasma is not used; the vaccine does not spread the disease.
4 This is an incorrect response because different organisms cause these diseases and vaccines are organism-specific.

639. Comprehension, assessment, physiologic (b)
2 Suggested oral intake is approximately 1500 ml/24 hours; 800 to 1000 ml would be a moderate restriction given no further directions.
1 This is too restrictive; it could result in dehydration.
3, 4 These amounts are not restrictive in nature.

640. Application, implementation, physiologic (b)
3 Mouth care will relieve thirst and provide comfort to a patient who is NPO and who has a nasogastric tube for suction.
1 The patient is NPO; he cannot have sips of water.
2, 4 These will not relieve thirst.

641. Knowledge, planning, environment (a)
3 Ice cream does not come from a clear liquid and is therefore not included in the diet.
1 Tea and coffee without milk or cream is permitted.
2 Popsicles and gelatin come from clear liquids.
4 Chicken and beef broth or bullion are clear liquids.

642. Comprehension, planning, nutrition (b)
2 This is the most complete group of foods representing complex carbohydrates, with 15 grams of carbohydrates each.
1, 3, 4 These are not high in complex carbohydrates.

643. Comprehension, planning, physiologic (b)
3 Vitamin D enables the body to process calcium from dietary sources.
1 Vitamin A is necessary for night vision.
2 Vitamin C is necessary for wound healing.
4 Vitamin K is needed for proper coagulation.

644. Comprehension, planning, environment (b)
3 Whole milk contains 290 milligrams of calcium, green leafy vegetables contains 400 milligrams, and cottage cheese contains 170 milligrams of calcium.
1 Canned salmon contains approximately 60 milligrams of calcium; ribeye steak, peanuts, and eggs have a high protein content.
2 Beef liver and chicken liver have high protein content, yeast rolls have complex carbohydrate, and green beans have both calcium and carbohydrate content in significant amounts.
4 These foods are primarily associated with complex carbohydrates.

645. Knowledge, planning, nutrition (b)
4 Puddings are usually made with whole or skim milk.
1 Fresh pineapple's main nutrient value is a high vitamin C content.
2 Fish is high in protein and low in fat.
3 Potatoes are high in vitamin B and carbohydrates.

646. Knowledge, implementation, nutrition (a)
1 Sherbet is made without milk and can be included on a clear-liquid diet.
2 This contains milk. It may be included on a full-liquid diet.
3 Oatmeal is considered a soft food, not a clear liquid.
4 Skim milk makes this a full liquid.

647. Comprehension, implementation, nutrition (b)
3 Avocado is very high in fat content.
1 Sweet potato is allowed, but the patient should not use much butter.
2 Lima beans are okay.
4 Blueberries are okay.

648. Comprehension, planning, environment (b)
2 Congestive heart failure (CHF) causes fluid volume overload; therefore, an individual with CHF should follow strict dietary guidelines to prevent excess fluid accumulation.
1, 3, 4 Refer to No. 2.

649. Comprehension, assessment, environment (b)
1 Nutrition supplies energy and sustains life; it is considered to be the primary basis for promoting health and disease prevention throughout the life span.
2 This option addresses influences on eating habits, not fundamental elements.
3 Foods contain some fluid content; however, the primary source of fluid is liquid. Fluid intake and renal function influence urinary output. This is not a primary basis for nutrition.
4 A primary basis for nutrition is not to maintain appetite or the sleep/wake cycle.

650. Comprehension, assessment, environment (b)
2 The enjoyment and intake of food depends on the individual having an appetite. Physical causes for a loss of appetite are poorly fitting dentures, stomatitis, decaying teeth, and halitosis. A psychologic factor of diminished or altered mental status will affect an individual's appetite.
1 These are related to good eating habits.
3 These are related to digestion/absorption, with the exception of eating alone. Eating alone can diminish one's appetite.
4 These are related to poor, unhealthful eating habits.

651. Application, planning, environment (c)
3 This is the most appropriate healthful menu based on the physician's order. The food selections are low in saturated fat, low in cholesterol, and contain the appropriate amount of calories for one meal.
1, 2 The meal selection is high in saturated fat, cholesterol, and calories.
4 The meal selection is high in fat, calories, and cholesterol.

652. Application, assessment, environment (c)
1 This represents the best selection of protein requirements for women based on the 0.8 gm/kg of body weight and the fact that if 12% to 15% of total calories come from protein, there is usually enough to meet daily protein needs.
2, 3 These exceed daily protein requirements.
4 This far exceeds daily protein requirements.

653. Application, planning, physiologic (c)

2 This is the best selection because the meal offers a variety of foods from the food groups and adds extra protein needed for the healing process to take place.

1 This is not a nutritionally sound diet because it has a high fat content, lacks variety, and lacks added protein.

3 This offers high calories with high fat content, and high simple sugar content, and it lacks added protein to facilitate healing.

4 This offers nutritional variety but lacks added protein to enhance the healing process.

654. Comprehension, assessment, psychosocial (c)

4 Food plays an important part of many family and social rituals and ceremonies. Older adults especially will not eat what they do not like nor will they eat a food if it is against their religious beliefs.

1 Feelings of insecurity may lead to undereating or overeating.

2 A self-reported history of poor eating requires collection of more data in order to intervene.

3 This is not a valid response.

655. Knowledge, assessment, physiologic (b)

1 Nutrition for the elderly is similar to that of the younger adult in terms of total fat, saturated fat, refined carbohydrates, and sodium levels. The elderly require a decrease in kilocalories but an increase in nutrient-dense foods.

2 Physiologic changes in the elderly include a decrease in metabolism; therefore, kilocalories should decrease. Because of loss of lean muscle mass, nutrient-dense foods should be increased.

3 Dietary patterns are not opposite those of the younger adult; they are similar with slight variations.

4 Dietary calories in the elderly should be decreased, fat intake should be no more than 25% to 30% of total dietary intake, protein intake should be slightly increased in the elderly, and vitamin and mineral supplementation depends on daily nutritional intake and presence or absence of disease.

656. Knowledge, planning, environment (b)

3 The major essential nutrients that sustain physiologic processes are protein, carbohydrates, fat, minerals, vitamins, and water.

1 Protein and carbohydrates are major essential nutrients; however, iron and iodine are trace elements.

2 Protein, carbohydrates, and fat are major essential elements; amino acids are the building blocks of protein, of which nine are considered essential; and lipoproteins are a class of proteins that contain a lipid.

4 Protein is an essential nutrient; however, the other items listed in this option are food groups and represent a form of an essential nutrient.

657. Knowledge, assessment, environment (a)

4 Breads, cereal, pasta, starchy vegetables, and prepared foods are found in the bread category.

1 These foods are found in the milk category.

2 These foods are found in the vegetable category.

3 These foods are found in the meat category.

658. Comprehension, implementation, health (b)

1 Nutritional prevention strategies in the treatment of hypoglycemia are to eat meals 4 to 5 hours apart, including a prescribed snack, and to eat extra food for extra exercise to prevent hypoglycemia.

2 The attention of a physician is not required in the absence of hypoglycemia. The listed measures should prevent hypoglycemia and therefore eliminate the need for a physician.

3 This is the strategy to prevent hyperglycemia.

4 See No. 1.

659. Knowledge, planning, physiologic (b)

4 This intervention will prepare the patient for the painful dressing change.

1, 2 These measures promote comfort, but the use of pain medication before the procedure is the more appropriate nursing measure.

3 Diversion therapy is an appropriate nursing measure but does not take priority in alleviating the pain.

660. Comprehension, assessment, physiologic (a)

4 Pain is a subjective experience. It is helpful if the patient can freely describe his perception of the pain.

1 Leaving the patient unattended may elevate anxiety and increase pain perception.

2 This is nontherapeutic; it challenges his perception of the pain.

3 This is supportive but does not address the nature of the pain.

661. Comprehension, planning, health (c)

4 Before teaching is begun, the patient must realize he has a problem. Then he must work with the nurse to set his own goals for behavior change.

1, 2 These will be done later.

3 Both the patient and his wife must be involved in this.

662. Knowledge, implementation, psychosocial (a)

1 Attentive listening promotes emotional well-being.

2 This measure does not necessarily promote emotional well-being.

3 This procedure may be promoting only physical well-being.

4 The promotion of emotional well-being usually implies some contact between the patient and the nurse; avoidance behavior may not necessarily do this.

663. Knowledge, assessment, physiologic (a)

1 This is one of the most common side effects of narcotic analgesics and a common problem for the terminally ill patient. Other contributing factors are poor dietary intake and inactivity.

2 Anorexia may be caused by nausea, vomiting, constipation, dysphagia, stomatitis, and infections.

3 Nausea can be caused by narcotic analgesics; however, this is not the most commonly reported cause. Anxiety and constipation can also be causes.

4 This is not a reported side effect.

664. Comprehension, implementation, environment (b)
   1 The licensed practical nurse or licensed vocational nurse works under the supervision of a physician and registered nurse. Bedside nursing interventions appropriate to the terminally ill are provided.
   2 This is the responsibility of the primary nurse who is usually a licensed registered nurse. The primary nurse evaluates the patient's response to treatment and is an advocate between patient, family, physician, and an interdisciplinary team.
   3 The hospice volunteer usually assumes these duties. The volunteer has completed volunteer training of at least 24 hours and continues support throughout the bereavement period.
   4 These functions are through the primary pastor who supports the patient and family in coping with their fears and uncertainties.

665. Knowledge, assessment, environment (a)
   4 Palliative care is alleviating or controlling symptoms, but it does not produce a cure.
   1 Although support to the patient is provided, this is not the definition of palliative care.
   2 Palliative care is *not* curative in nature, nor is it centered in curative measures.
   3 Palliative care is just one part of holistic care. The holistic care approach focuses on numerous aspects that may include physical, psychosocial, and spiritual issues using the disciplinary team.

666. Comprehension, planning, psychosocial (b)
   1 According to the Patient Bill of Rights, the patient has autonomy in the course of his care whenever possible.
   2 According to the Patient Bill of Rights, the patient has the right to informed consent or to refuse treatment. The physician can act independently only in emergency situations or when the patient is unable to respond.
   3 The nurse is regarded as the patient advocate and thus facilitates the wishes of the patient.
   4 A relative is able to make only minor decisions regarding treatment or care when the patient is unable to do so.

667. Comprehension, implementation, psychosocial (c)
   4 A recently enacted law requires residents to have a legally designated person to make decisions about his health care in the event that he is not able to do so.
   1 This does not have to do with financial decisions.
   2 This is not intended to take away the decision-making power from residents who are able to make such decisions.
   3 This does not have to do with health-care financing.

668. Comprehension, implementation, psychosocial (c)
   2 These are all aspects related to his physical and mental health while a resident is in the nursing home.
   1 This does not have to do with personal finances.
   3, 4 These do not have to do with responsibilities after death.

669. Application, planning, environment (b)
   2 Pain medication needs to be given early in the cycle so it will reach its peak effectiveness as the pain begins to worsen. If she has not been relieved of pain for the interval between medication, this information should be reported.
   1 If she has no pain she does not need to inform the nurse, nor would the nurse wish to promote scheduled drug administration without need.
   3 If pain is already severe, medication may not be as effective.
   4 The nurse wants patients to inform her if their pain medication is not having a long enough duration. The nurse may need to replan.

670. Application, implementation, environment (b)
   2 If blood is aspirated, a new needle and syringe should be prepared, and an alternative site used.
   1, 3 The nurse should never proceed, because there is danger of injecting the medication directly into the bloodstream.
   4 The needle and syringe are contaminated and need to be changed before injecting in an alternative site.

671. Comprehension, planning, physiologic (c)
   3 Decreased metabolism and excretion of drugs occur in the aged; therefore it is prudent to give smaller doses, farther apart.
   1 Smaller doses may not achieve a desired effect, and because metabolism is decreased in the aged, there is a risk for the accumulation if doses are given too close together.
   2 Larger doses closer together are never given, as metabolism and excretion are decreased in the normal aging process.
   4 Larger doses could potentially lead to toxicity because metabolism and excretion are slowed in the aged.

672. Comprehension, implementation, physiologic (b)
   2 Pulling the tissue taut reduces resistance to the needle's entry through the skin.
   1 This is for disinfection.
   3 This is a safety measure to prevent intravenous administration.
   4 Medication should be injected slowly to decrease tissue discomfort.

673. Knowledge, implementation, physiologic (a)
   2 Medication labels should be checked when retrieving the medication from the shelf or drawer, before pouring, and when replacing the container or discarding.
   1 Checking the order is to be sure it was transcribed correctly.
   3 The medication should be checked before it is poured, not after.
   4 The medication has already been given. The right drug should have already been verified.

674. Application, implementation, environment (b)
   4 Immunizations should be stored inside the refrigerator and maintained at 35° to 46° F and may become toxic or ineffective if frozen or if they become too warm.
   1 This is unsafe; the pharmacy may not check on the agents until the refrigerator has cooled down again, and the vaccines may mistakenly be used by others.
   2 This is unsafe; another employee may not notice the defect and may use the vaccine.
   3 Agents should never be used once warmed to 80° F. Some of the agents may become virulent or inactive.

675. Application, implementation, environment (c)
   2 Unless she actually witnessed the action, a nurse should refuse to sign any record concerning scheduled drugs. She could be held liable in a court of law.
   1 Although nurses may trust each other, the nurse is legally accountable for anything signed.
   3 Forgetting the incident does not correct the situation; this could present a problem later.
   4 Initials are as legally binding as a signature.

676. Application, implementation, environment (b)
4 The nurse should be consistent with the practice of the patient at home to ensure delivery of the same dose of insulin. Using an air lock allows all the medication to clear the needle shaft. Lack of an air lock may allow some of the medication to remain in the needle.
1 Although use of an air lock may or may not be taught with a subcutaneous injection, the nurse's preference is not the best answer in this situation.
2 The length of the needle or the size of the patient does not change the use of an air lock for subcutaneous injections.
3 Neither frequency of administration nor age influences the decision to use an air lock.

677. Comprehension, planning, environment (b)
1 Because the deltoid muscle is a small muscle, 1 cc is safe to administer.
2 This volume could cause tissue irritation.
3 This is too much fluid for the muscle to safely absorb.
4 5 cc injected into the deltoid muscle could cause tissue necrosis.

678. Application, planning, physiologic (c)
4 The nonoperative side is preferred for injections.
1 This would require the injection to be given into the operative hip.
2 It is contraindicated to give injections into the operative hip.
3 Giving injections into limbs where there is an intravenous needle should be avoided.

679. Comprehension, implementation, environment (a)
4 The abdomen is the preferred site for a heparin injection because of the large amount of fat tissue.
1, 2, 3 These are not sites for subcutaneous administration of heparin.

680. Knowledge, implementation, environment (a)
1 The wrist band check is the most accurate means of patient verification.
2 Calling the patient by name is not a method to ensure accuracy, because the patient may respond to any name.
3 Bed cards may not be updated; this method does not ensure accuracy.
4 Patients are frequently moved from room to room, and their medication record may not reflect this occurrence.

681. Application, implementation, physiologic (b)
4 This is the correct dosage. The nurse would use the formula $\dfrac{\text{Desire}}{\text{Have}} \times \dfrac{\text{Milliliter}}{1}$

Example: $\dfrac{250,000 \text{ U}}{100,000 \text{ U}} \times \dfrac{1 \text{ ml}}{1} = 2.5 \text{ ml}$
1, 2, 3 These amounts would be less than what the doctor ordered.

682. Application, implementation, environment (a)
3 $\dfrac{\text{Desire}}{\text{Have}} \times \dfrac{\text{Milliliter}}{1}$

Example: $\dfrac{500 \text{ mg}}{125 \text{ mg}} \times \dfrac{5 \text{ ml}}{1} = 20 \text{ ml}$
1, 2 These doses are too low.
4 This dose is too high.

683. Application, implementation, physiologic (a)
1 $\dfrac{D}{H} \times \dfrac{5000}{10,000} = 0.5 \times 1 \text{ ml} = 0.5 \text{ ml}$
2, 3, 4 These are incorrect calculations.

684. Application, implementation, physiologic (a)
3 60 mg = 1 gr
1½ gr = 90 mg, or 1½ tablets
1 ½ tablet = ½ gr or 30 mg
2 1 tablet = 60 mg or 1 gr
4 2 tablets = 120 mg or 2 gr

685. Application, implementation, environment (b)
3 $15 \times \dfrac{6 \text{ ml}}{100U} = \dfrac{15 \times 6}{100} = \dfrac{90}{100} = 0.9 \text{ ml}$
1, 2 These dosages are too low.
4 This dosage is too high.

686. Comprehension, implementation, physiologic (a)
4 100 : 2 ml = 75 : X ml
100 X = 150 ml
X = 1.5 ml
1, 2, 3 These are not a sufficient amount.

687. Application, implementation, environment (a)
4 $\dfrac{1000 \times 1\cancel{0}}{8 \times 6\cancel{0}} = \dfrac{1000}{48} = 20.8 = 21 \text{ gtt}$
Drops are always rounded to the nearest whole number
1, 2 These calculations are incorrect.
3 This calculation is rounded incorrectly.

688. Application, implementation, environment (b)
4 Patients may refuse medication, but nurses who are responsible for the patient's safety, the plan of care, and the legal status of their license will provide and document the teaching provided to the patient regarding the actions of the drug and reasons for its use.
1 The response discounts the patient's right to participate in and decline treatment if desired.
2 This answer is true, but it is less complete than No. 4.
3 This response does not allow the patient to make her decision now; it is bargaining with the patient to avoid a problem.

689. Comprehension, planning, physiologic (b)
3 Stool softeners are more gentle to the gastrointestinal tract and promote regularity.
1 Oil-retention enemas are usually used for a fecal impaction.
2 Strong laxatives are not routinely administered to relieve constipation, and they are not given on a regular basis.
4 Saline enemas are only occasionally used to relieve constipation because there is the risk of inducing an electrolyte imbalance.

690. Application, implementation, physiologic (b)
4 Standard protocol for management of anginal pain is to use sublingual nitroglycerin at 5-minute intervals to total no more than 3 to 5 doses. The patient should seek emergency care if pain continues.
1 This answer is nontherapeutic and ineffective.
2 This answer is incorrect; the medication may be used more frequently.
3 A decrease in severity of pain usually occurs within 1 to 3 minutes; this may require as many as 3 tablets.

691. Comprehension, planning, physiologic (b)
3 The Maalox would be given 1 hour pc and not at the same time as the digitalis.
1 An antacid and digitalis preparation should not be given together because of interference with absorption.
2 The time of administration of the Maalox does not comply with the order.
4 Although this would probably be acceptable in most agencies because it is given within 30 minutes before or after the specified time, it is still close to the administration of digitalis and could result in interference.

692. Comprehension, implementation, environment (c)
3 The order for the Fiorinal, which contains aspirin, should be changed to a pain medication without aspirin.
1 This could result in unsafe practice; another nurse may not see the note or notice the combination of drugs.
2 This would be appropriate only if the patient had no complaints of pain. This is not implied.
4 Heparin and aspirin should not be given together.

693. Comprehension, assessment, environment (c)
2 The laboratory work could have been drawn after the 9 AM dose and given a false high reading. Checking this first could save time.
1 The physician should be notified if the results are truly correct. All other areas of concern should be monitored first.
3 The vitamin K will be required if bleeding occurs, but this is not the first step.
4 Protamine sulfate is the antidote for heparin.

694. Comprehension, assessment, physiologic (c)
3 This stimulates diruresis by preventing the antidiuretic from functioning.
1, 2, 4 Alcohol is not directly connected to these.

695. Application, implementation, physiologic (b)
1 This indicates decrease in myocardium contraction and buildup of fluid in the lungs.
2 This is not indicative of holding the medication.
3 This is a positive sign that is sought.
4 This is not indicative of a problem by itself.

696. Application, implementation, environment (b)
3 This order is incomplete, and the medication should not be given until clarified. The order should not have been transcribed onto the medication record sheet as written.
1 Nurses should never assume if medications are involved.
2 The nurse is taking the legal responsibility for the dosage given.
4 The dosage could be different from the standard two tablets and should be clarified first.

697. Comprehension, evaluation, physiologic (b)
2 Wheezing would signify that the bronchioles are constricted and that the medication is ineffective.
1 Bronchodilators dilate the bronchiole and do not change fremitus.
3 Crackles could be present even if the bronchodilator is effective.
4 The characteristics of the sputum may not change because of the bronchodilator.

698. Knowledge, planning, health (a)
3 Antibiotics, especially tetracyclines, lower the effectiveness of oral contraceptives. Patients often need to use other forms of contraception in addition to pills while on tetracycline products.
1 Birth control pills do not interact with antithyroid medications.
2, 4 These medications do not interfere with oral contraceptives.

699. Knowledge, planning, health (a)
3 Body temperature is the measurement for determining ovulation when using the rhythm method of birth control.
1 Weight does not directly affect ovulation.
2, 4 These are not altered during ovulation.

700. Application, implementation, environment (a)
1 All medications should be clarified with the physician if the method of administration must change.
2 Medication should not be held without notifying the RN or physician.
3 Enterically coated medication should not be crushed because it will lose its ability to protect the stomach, resulting in delayed absorption.
4 Swallowing tablets with a nasogastric (NG) tube in place can endanger the airway and may conflict with the reason the NG tube was originally placed.

701. Comprehension, assessment, environment (a)
2 Allergies to medication are common, and many drugs such as cephalosporins may have cross-allergies with penicillin products.
1, 3, 4 All of these facts are good to assess; however, these have a lower priority than allergies.

702. Comprehension, assessment, health (b)
3 Most frequently there is a loss of appetite. Newer *therapeutic* implications are associated with marijuana. THC has been used to combat nausea and vomiting associated with cancer chemotherapy. Current scientific studies are being completed.
1, 2, 4 In addition to these symptoms, she may also experience diarrhea and sleep disturbances.

703. Application, implementation, physiologic (b)
3 Diuretics given after 5 PM may work effectively but may keep the patient up all night. Scheduling the drugs early in the morning would allow the action to occur during waking hours.
1 The action of diuretics is to decrease sodium reabsorption.
2 Osmotics are used to decrease intraocular pressure.
4 Carbonic anhydrase inhibitors are weak and infrequently used today.

704. Comprehension, evaluation, environment (a)
1 A soft toothbrush will not injure the gums and will therefore prevent bleeding.
2 Green leafy vegetables contain vitamin K, which interferes with the action of warfarin (Coumadin).
3 Aspirin interferes with clotting time and will increase bleeding tendencies.
4 This is not necessary.

705. Comprehension, planning, health (a)
2 Vitamin K is the antidote for an overdose of warfarin (Coumadin).
1 This is an antidote for heparin.
3, 4 These are not antidotes for warfarin.

706. Knowledge, planning, physiologic (a)
3 Antiemetics act on the trigger zone located in the medulla, controlling nausea/vomiting responses.
1 Antispasmodics decrease vagal stimulation and motility; they are not related to the control of nausea and vomiting.
2 Anticholinergics affect the parasympathetic nervous system by blocking the action of acetycholine; this leads to decreased gastrointestinal secretions and peristalsis.
4 Cathartics increase peristalsis and water content of the feces, promoting elimination.

707. Knowledge, implementation, physiologic (a)
2 Antipyretics are agents that reduce the body temperature.
1 Antibiotics are used when an infection is identified.
3 Antiemetics are used to control nausea and vomiting.
4 Antihistamines are used to control symptoms of allergy.

708. Application, implementation, physiologic (b)
  3 A diuretic is usually given in the morning so the patient can urinate while awake.
  1 A diuretic given at 6 PM would require the patient to urinate frequently during the night.
  2 Any medication, including diuretics, that is ordered daily is usually given in the morning hours.
  4 A diuretic given at 4 PM would interfere with visitation and sleep.

709. Knowledge, implementation, physiologic (a)
  2 Spironolactone (Aldactone) is a potassium-sparing diuretic.
  1 Furosemide (Lasix) is a potassium-eliminating diuretic.
  3 Sulfisoxazole (Gantrisin) is classified as an antiinfective.
  4 Methenamine (Mandelamine) is classified as a urinary antiseptic.

710. Knowledge, evaluation, environment (a)
  1 Heparin is an anticoagulant and therefore may increase bleeding potential.
  2 The side effects of heparin do not include numbness.
  3, 4 The side effects of heparin do not involve the central nervous system.

711. Comprehension, assessment, physiologic (a)
  3 Cimetidine (Tagamet) specifically inhibits the production of hydrochloric acid by blocking the histamine receptor sites.
  1 Cimetidine does not have a direct healing effect on the ulcer site.
  2 Tagamet is not a neutralizing agent.
  4 Tagamet does not affect peristalsis.

712. Knowledge, assessment, physiologic (a)
  3 Cocaine is usually sniffed by inhalation through the nostrils; this is likely to cause red, irritated nostrils.
  1, 2, 4 These are not signs of cocaine use.

713. Application, implementation, environment (c)
  3 This is the best answer because these measures are helpful in overcoming thirst and a dry mouth.
  1 That is untrue; this is a common side effect.
  2 Sucking on hard candies will increase thirst and predispose the patient to dental caries.
  4 Rinsing the mouth with plain water may be beneficial. This should *not* include salt water because many elders also have conditions such as congestive heart failure or kidney disease, and this would cause fluid retention.

714. Comprehension, assessment, health (c)
  2 Anticoagulants such as heparin or warfarin (Coumadin) are given to reduce chances of clotting; analgesic drugs such as morphine are given to control pain; and antidysrhythmics such as lidocaine (Xylocaine) IV are used to treat ventricular dysrhythmias.
  1 These are frequently used medications for rheumatoid arthritis.
  3 These are medication therapy for congestive heart failure.
  4 These are medications for pheripheral artery disease.

715. Application, implementation, environment (b)
  4 The amount, route, place, and reason are all listed in this description.
  1 Although the description of the discomfort is good, the notes do not state where the injection was given.
  2 This charting does not indicate that the injection was given Z-track.
  3 This charting does not designate on which side the injection was given.

716. Knowledge, planning, environment (a)
  4 Flurazepam (Dalmane) is a sedative/hypnotic of the benzodiazepine group.
  1 Nalbuphine (Nubain) is a narcotic analgesic.
  2 Magaldrate (hydroxymagnesium aluminate) is an antacid.
  3 Indomethacin (Indameth) is a nonsteroidal antiinflammatory agent.

717. Knowledge, planning, environment (a)
  3 Acetazolamide (Diamox) is a carbonic anhydrase inhibitor and as such promotes diuresis.
  1 Acetazolamide has no effect on light sensation.
  2 Acetazolamide has no effect on sugar levels.
  4 Acetazolamide has no cardiac effects.

718. Application, planning, environment (b)
  3 The patient has a fresh open line to the central venous system and is beginning immunosuppressive medication; there is an increased risk for infection.
  1 She has no communicable disease process requiring isolation.
  2 The site will need only daily care.
  4 If stomatitis occurs, this would be true. At this time the nurse must optimize the patient's nutritional intake in an effort to prevent skin breakdown.

719. Application, assessment, environment (b)
  4 Patients receiving corticosteroids often retain fluid and have a blood pressure elevation as the therapeutic levels are attained. Nurses must monitor and report these changes.
  1 Although bone demineralization may occur with long-term steroid use, this is not a routine nursing assessment.
  2 Steroids may cause insomnia, but this is a lower priority than fluid and electrolyte balance.
  3 Steroid use may redistribute fat stores, but this can be visually observed and is not as high a concern as fluid retention and hypertension.

720. Comprehension, implementation, environment (b)
  1 Preoperatively, atropine is primarily used for its anticholinergic effects to decrease peristalsis and suppress GI secretions.
  2 The atropine may slightly effect an increase in heart rate, but it is not given for this reason. Atropine IV is used to increase the cardiac rate.
  3 Atropine has no effect on pain or anxiety.
  4 Atropine has no effect on the anesthetic.

721. Application, implementation, environment (a)
  3 All medication orders in question should be clarified with the physician as soon as possible, especially orders for medications that need to be given immediately.
  1 The vocational/practical nurse does not have authority to prescribe and therefore may not independently alter a physician's order.
  2 If the medication is out of the therapeutic dose range, the nurse is responsible to ensure the safety of her patient by clarifying the order and not giving a potentially dangerous dose.
  4 Holding a "now" order of medication until the physician makes rounds may have deleterious effects on the patient and is personal nursing judgment.

722. Application, planning, environment (b)
    2 Stat orders, especially if the order is for cardiac-related medication, should always receive high priority. Control for strong pain is also a high priority. Most institutions have a time range in which routine medication can be safely given.
    1 A routine antibiotic is not as high a priority as a stat order for nitrates, which can be life sustaining.
    3 Pain control, although highly important, is in this case a prn order that is lower priority than a stat order, which indicates *immediately.*
    4 This places the stat order in lowest priority and could cause a worsening of a potentially dangerous disorder.

723. Knowledge, implementation, physiologic (a)
    1 Morphine is given to patients with chest pains that are a result of coronary occlusion.
    2 Morphine does not relieve nausea.
    3 Morphine does not relieve vomiting.
    4 Morphine helps to relax and improve breathing, but this is not its primary use in this case.

724. Knowledge, implementation, physiologic (c)
    3 Warfarin (Coumadin) is an anticoagulant. *Anti* means against; coagulation refers to blood clotting.
    1 An anticoagulant used in excess would cause bleeding.
    2 Warfarin is not used for blood infections.
    4 This is not an action of Warfarin.

725. Comprehension, planning, physiologic (a)
    1 This interferes with the transmission of impulses from the thalamus to the cortex of the brain, causing sedation.
    2 An antiepileptic (anticonvulsant) drug such as phenytoin (Dilantin) decreases convulsions/seizures.
    3 An antidepressant is a substance such as amitriptyline that decreases depression.
    4 A tranquilizer is a substance used to calm anxious or agitated people without decreasing consciousness.

726. Comprehension, planning, psychosocial (b)
    1 Tranquilizers depress the central nervous system for antianxiety effects.
    2, 3 Major tranquilizers such as derivatives of phenothiazine, butyrophenone, and thioxanthene are generally used in the treatment of acute and chronic psychoses.
    4 Epilepsy is treated by use of anticonvulsant drugs such as phenytoin (Dilantin).

727. Application, implementation, physiologic (b)
    3 The first priority is to keep the patient safe from harm.
    1 A seizure is controlled by medications ordered by the physician.
    2 The patient is never restrained; fractures may occur if she is restrained.
    4 Oxygen may be ordered to increase circulation to the brain, but the first priority is to protect the patient.

728. Knowledge, evaluation, psychosocial (a)
    3 The action of this drug would be to relieve the apprehension, thus inducing sleep.
    1 This is the action of an antitussive.
    2 This is the action of an analgesic.
    4 This result, along with a decrease in respirations, is an adverse reaction to this medication.

729. Knowledge, planning, environment (a)
    2 This is a schedule II drug, a synthetic narcotic analgesic that is less potent than morphine.
    1 This is hydromorphine, a potent synthetic compound that maximizes analgesic effects and minimizes some of the common side effects of morphine.
    3 This is the trade name for the anticonvulsant phenytoin.
    4 This is an anticoagulant prescribed for prophylaxis and treatment of thrombosis and embolism.

730. Application, implementation, physiologic (b)
    2 Site rotation allows better absorption of the medication.
    1 One site is as painful as the next.
    3 This should not be a problem.
    4 This should not be more of a problem at one site than another.

731. Application, implementation, health (b)
    3 Aged cheeses can cause hypertensive crisis.
    1 Caffeine is contained in beverages that act as vasopressors, but it is not as great a problem as the aged cheese.
    2 This medication should be taken with food to avoid GI upset.
    4 Addiction is not a primary concern with these drugs.

732. Application, implementation, environment (b)
    3 0.6 ml is the correct answer.
    1 250 mg needs to be changed to 0.250 gm in the equation. 25 ml is too much to be given IM.
    2 The decimal point is in the wrong place.
    4 This is an incorrect calculation.

733. Application, implementation, physiologic (b)
    1 Metamucil is the best choice for long-term use. This type of laxative is bulk forming and stimulates peristalsis. Bulk-forming laxatives are considered the safest for long-term use.
    2 Magnesium citrate is safe for occasional use but should not be used daily. Frequent use leads to laxative abuse.
    3 Daily enemas will upset fluid and electrolyte balance.
    4 Mineral oil can cause decreased absorption of fat-soluble vitamins and some drugs.

734. Comprehension, planning, physiologic (b)
    4 Regular exercise has many benefits, including improving digestion and elimination. Intestinal tone will be increased with regular exercise.
    1 Fluids should be encouraged to at least 1000 ml per day. If the patient is constipated, increasing fluid intake can alleviate the problem.
    2 An increase in fat intake can cause digestion problems, particularly if the patient has gallbladder problems, but limiting fat intake to 20% per day is drastic. With 20% of calories coming from fat intake per day, the patient will lose weight. The American Heart Association recommends 30% to 35% of calories be from fats.
    3 An increase in carbohydrates will not necessarily solve the problem. An increase in fiber would be more beneficial.

735. Application, planning, physiologic (c)
    2 Zocor is indicated in patients with high cholesterol when diet and exercise have been unsuccessful in treating it.
    1 Lasix is a diuretic, and there is no indication in the information provided that the patient will be discharged with this medication.
    3 Atarax is an antianxiety agent, and there is no indication that this would be ordered for this patient.
    4 Tagamet reduces gastric acid secretion; the patient did not have this problem.

736. Application, implementation, physiologic (b)
    2 A side effect of morphine is nausea and vomiting. Changing to another pain medication may allow the nausea to pass without further treatment.
    1 The medication for vomiting can be given, but the underlying cause of the nausea needs to be treated.
    3 The patient needs fluids following surgery and should not be NPO.
    4 The patient needs to be up as ordered to prevent pneumonia.

737. Knowledge, implementation, environment (b)
    4 qod means every other day; in order to receive the correct dose, three pills must be taken.
    1, 3 This would not provide enough medication for the patient.
    2 The order reads every other day; the patient would be overdosed.
738. Comprehension, evaluation, environment (b)
    2 Inverting the chamber will allow air to fill the chamber again.
    1 This is not a cost-effective remedy.
    3 Squeezing the chamber alone will cause more fluid to enter the chamber.
    4 Inserting a needle into the chamber will contaminate it and cause it to leak.
739. Comprehension, implementation, environment (b)
    3 Intramuscular injections provide for rapid drug absorption.
    1 Intramuscular injections are less irritating to the tissues.
    2 Subcutaneous injections provide a slow, even rate of absorption.
    4 Intramuscular injections allow for larger volumes of fluid to be injected.
740. Application, planning, environment (b)
    3 This length would deliver the medication into the muscle.
    1 This needle length would be appropriate for an intradermal injection.
    2 This needle length is safe for a subcutaneous injection.
    4 This length of needle would be safe for an extremely obese person.
741. Comprehension, planning, environment (b)
    2 Methylprednisolone will help decrease the inflammatory response of allergens.
    1 Albuterol is in the beta-agonist category of drugs.
    3 Terbutaline is an injectable beta-agonist.
    4 Theophylline is in the antispasmodic category of methylxanthines.
742. Comprehension, planning, physiologic (b)
    3 The acromion forms the top part of the shoulder region.
    1 This landmark would be helpful in locating the gluteus medius muscle.
    2 This landmark would be helpful in locating the ventral gluteal site.
    4 The greater trochanter is a part of the femur.
743. Knowledge, planning, physiologic (b)
    3 The subcutaneous space is located under the skin but above the muscle.
    1, 2 This would be the intradermal area.
    4 This would be the correct place to administer an intramuscular injection.

744. Knowledge, planning, environment (a)
    2 This provides the correct dosage of laxative.
    1 The patient would not receive enough medication.
    3 The patient would be overmedicated.
    4 This is double the recommended dosage.
745. Knowledge, assessment, physiologic (b)
    2 Diuretic use may cause the person to lose fluids and electrolytes in addition to fluid lost from diaphoresis.
    1 Cardiac glycosides are not affected by heat.
    3 Heat does not affect the action of the antianxiety medications.
    4 Antibiotics do not affect the thermoregulation of the body.
746. Comprehension, implementation, physiologic (b)
    3 This patient is at high risk for clot formation.
    1 This dose will not provide enough analgesia to last all day.
    2 Aspirin will not prevent headache.
    4 Administering medication once a day is not enough to enhance narcotic action.
747. Application, implementation, environment (b)
    3 The correct action is to hold the medication and contact the physician to inform him that enteric-coated medications should not be crushed.
    1 Enteric-coated medications should not be crushed because the action of the drug is altered as a result.
    2 The medication should be withheld only until the order can be clarified.
    4 The nurse may not administer medications except as prescribed by the physician. The nurse needs order clarification from the physician.
748. Comprehension, assessment, physiologic (b)
    2 Digoxin is a positive inotropic drug that slows the heart rate and decreases conduction through the atrioventricular node. The frequent signs and symptoms of digoxin toxicity are abdominal pain, anorexia, nausea, vomiting, visual changes, bradycardia, ECG changes, arrhythmias, headaches and seizure.
    1, 3 These responses are not signs and symptoms associated with digoxin toxicity.
    4 Third-degree heart block is possible with digoxin toxicity, but hypertension and tachycardia are not signs and symptoms associated with digoxin toxicity. Hypokalemia can potentiate digoxin toxicity.
749. Comprehension, assessment, physiologic (b)
    4 Constipation is a side effect of antacids.
    1, 2, 3 This is not a common side effect.
750. Knowledge, planning, environment (b)
    2 Protamine sulfate 1 mg. will neutralize 100 U of heparin.
    1 This is used with Coumadin.
    3, 4 This thins the blood.

MATERNAL-CHILD HEALTH NURSING

1. Knowledge, implementation, health (b)
   2 Fetal lungs do not function as organs of respiration. Oxygenated blood enters fetal circulation through the umbilical vein.
   1 Arterial blood is brought to the fetal liver via the umbilical vein.
   3 The fetal brain receives oxygenated blood via the ascending aorta.
   4 The fetal kidneys receive oxygenated blood via the abdominal aorta. Small amounts of urine are being secreted by week 12.

2. Knowledge, implementation, health (a)
   3 Volume of amniotic fluid increases at the rate of 25 ml/week during the first trimester, 50 ml/week during the second trimester and reaches a total of about 1000 ml at full term; it is replaced every 3 hours.
   1 300 ml or less is considered abnormal and is called oligohydramnios. It is usually associated with fetal anomalies or disease.
   2 This amount is low for a full-term pregnancy and is bordering on being an abnormal amount.
   4 2000 ml or more would be considered abnormal and is called hydramnios, which is often associated with diabetic or cardiac conditions in the mother; it can also be indicative of fetal abnormalities such as cardiac defects.

3. Comprehension, planning, health (b)
   4 In normal pregnancy, some clotting factors, including fibrinogen, are increased.
   1 The RBC count increases, but later in the pregnancy, and is less than plasma volume.
   2 Hemoglobin values are decreased because of an increase in the ratio of plasma to red cells.
   3 A decreased white blood cell count could indicate compensation in bone marrow function; this is not a normal occurrence.

4. Knowledge, planning, health (a)
   3 This is the "true" female pelvis.
   1 This is the male pelvis.
   2 This type resembles the pelvis of anthropoid apes.
   4 This is the type classified as a flat pelvis.

5. Knowledge, implementation, health (a)
   3 By the fifth month of the pregnancy the fetus is fully developed and the fetal heart rate is heard by the examiner using a fetoscope.
   1, 2 These are too early.
   4 From the sixth through the ninth months the fetus grows in size and weight.

6. Knowledge, implementation, health (a)
   4 Fertilization of the ovum can occur only while the ovum is in the distal third of the fallopian tube.
   1 The ovum matures within the ovary and is released into the fallopian tube, where fertilization occurs.
   2 The fertilized ovum normally implants in the upper third of the anterior uterine wall.
   3 After being deposited in the vagina, sperm rapidly move into the cervix, then to the uterus and into the fallopian tube, where fertilization takes place.

7. Application, implementation, health (a)
   3 Demonstration and explanation are the most appropriate response.
   1, 2 Showing a picture of these with no explanation does not answer the patient's question in a satisfactory manner.
   4 Use of a chart is recommended, but the information is incorrect.

8. Knowledge, implementation, health (a)
   3 The umbilical vein carries oxygenated blood and nutrients to the fetus; the two umbilical arteries carry metabolic wastes to the maternal circulation.
   1, 2 A single umbilical artery is associated with congenital anomalies.
   4 There is only one umbilical vein.

9. Knowledge, implementation, health (a)
   3 Because it contains all essential amino acids, cheese is considered a complete protein; crackers are a source of carbohydrates.
   1 Cereal is a source of carbohydrates.
   2 Peanuts, although they contain protein, are considered to be an incomplete protein food.
   4 Although peanut butter contains protein, it is an incomplete protein food; an apple is a source of carbohydrates.

10. Comprehension, planning, physiologic (b)
    1 The calcium requirement is higher in adolescent girls than in adult women.
    2 The need for calcium is not lower; bones have not finished growing.
    3 The adult's need decreases because full growth is achieved.
    4 The calcium need is not always met; adolescents frequently eat junk food and fast food.

11. Knowledge, implementation, health (a)
    3 Raw fruits and vegetables with their high fiber content stimulate peristalsis.
    1 Milk and dairy products are low-residue foods that do not stimulate peristalsis; in some instances, cheese has been known to cause constipation.
    2 The process of refining cereals tends to lessen the amount of bulk or cellulose; this decreases peristalsis.
    4 Nonfibrous meats tend to decrease peristalsis; this in turn leads to constipation.

12. Knowledge, implementation, health (a)
    2 Milk and cheese products, especially hard cheeses such as cheddar, are excellent sources of calcium.
    1 Liver and organ meats are excellent sources of iron, not calcium.
    3 Dark yellow vegetables supply vitamin A.
    4 Enrichment usually provides nutrients such as B complex vitamins, not calcium.

13. Knowledge, implementation, psychosocial (b)
    2 WIC is a federally subsidized supplementary food program providing food for mothers as well as for infants and children under 5 years of age. Those in the program must meet certain criteria to be eligible.
    1 The patient asked for supplemental foods.
    3 WIC is not a full food program.
    4 The patient did not request information about welfare.

14. Knowledge, planning, physiologic (a)
    2 During gestation the fetus stores the iron necessary for the first 5 or 6 months of life, a time in which the infant's diet is lacking in iron because the principal food, milk, is lacking in iron.
    1 Prenatal iron reserves last longer than 3 months.
    3 Iron reserves are sufficient for only 5 or 6 months; a supplemental vitamin or food source of iron is needed after this time.
    4 Iron reserves sustain the infant for only the first 5 or 6 months of life.

15. Comprehension, implementation, health (a)
    4 These are a good source of low-cost protein.
    1 Red meats and fish, although high in protein, are also expensive.
    2 These are a good source of vitamins, especially vitamin A and vitamin C, but not protein.
    3 These contain carbohydrates and B-complex vitamins, but not protein.

16. Comprehension, evaluation, health (c)
    3 An infected mother can transmit the disease during or immediately after pregnancy. A woman who has been exposed to HIV has a 50% chance of producing a child infected with the virus.
    1 A C-section would not reduce the chance for the transmission of the disease.
    2 There are four modes of transmission for the virus:
    Having sexual contact with an infected person
    Sharing a contaminated hypodermic needle
    Receiving a contaminated blood transfusion
    A mother infecting her fetus/baby
    4 Blood transfusions can be a mode of transmission, but the mother is already HIV positive. If she needs blood during labor and delivery, it will not affect the virus.

17. Comprehension, implementation, psychosocial (b)
    2 A conductive oil or gel is spread on the skin to reduce friction from the transducer as it is moved across the abdomen.
    1 Ultrasound is a noninvasive procedure using ultrasound waves rather than dyes or radiation.
    3 The patient is positioned on her back.
    4 This is an explanation for amniocentesis.

18. Comprehension, planning, health (a)
    2 Abdominal ultrasound is not a routinely ordered examination. It may be used to confirm suspected pregnancy at an early date, to evaluate fetal development, or to evaluate placental placement.
    1, 3, 4 These are routinely done on the initial prenatal visit.

19. Comprehension, planning, health (b)
    2 The presence of antibodies to rubella indicates that the patient has had a rubella infection at some time in the past.
    1 An elevated titer can only indicate rubella in the past, not *when* in the past.
    3 Rubella titer drawn on the mother cannot indicate anything about the fetus.
    4 Only rubella vaccination can protect a patient.

20. Comprehension, assessment, environment (a)
    1 This is the most complete response; the original reason for these tests was to prevent pregnancy-induced hypertension.
    2 This is true, but it does not answer precise reasons for the tests.
    3 Urinalysis may be indicative of further testing for diabetes; however, this response does not include other complications that an increased blood pressure and weight gain would indicate.
    4 These tests would not be sufficient in detecting congenital anomalies.

21. Application, implementation, health (a)
    1 Add 7 days to the date her period started and count back 3 months—this is Nägele's rule.
    2 This added 7 days to when her period ended and counted back 4 months.
    3 This added 7 days to when her period ended.
    4 This counted back only 2 months.

22. Comprehension, assessment, environment (b)
    3 Presumptive signs of pregnancy include amenorrhea, fatigue, and urinary frequency. Chadwick's sign and positive pregnancy tests are probable signs of pregnancy. Fetal movements felt by anyone other than the mother are a positive sign of pregnancy.
    1 See above; quickening is a subjective symptom of presumptive signs that, combined with probable signs, strongly suggests pregnancy.
    2 See above; nausea and vomiting in and of itself can have other causes; however, morning sickness is considered a subjective symptom of presumptive signs of pregnancy.
    4 See above; breast changes can also be considered subjective symptoms of presumptive signs of pregnancy.

23. Knowledge, implementation, physiologic (a)
    3 Fetal heart tones heard by an examiner are a positive sign of pregnancy; other options listed are probable or presumptive signs.
    1, 2, 4 See response to No. 3.

24. Knowledge, planning, health (b)
    4 "Morning sickness" is a frequent problem for patients during the first few months of pregnancy. Receiving adequate rest and increasing carbohydrates in the diet help reduce this problem.
    1 This would not be a routine solution to the problem.
    2, 3 These would not resolve or reduce the problem.

25. Application, implementation, health (a)
    3 Questions should be answered honestly by giving information on the child's level of understanding.
    1 Putting off his questions may affect the way he relates to the new baby.
    2 Stork tales do not deal with reality.
    4 Avoidance and putting this off on his father does not give him satisfaction, nor does it guarantee the father will give him the answer.

26. Knowledge, planning, health (a)
    3 This is seen as a danger signal in pregnancy and should be reported immediately to the physician; other danger signals include visual disturbances, vaginal bleeding, constant headaches, dizziness, and constant vomiting. All are signs of impending danger, ranging from possible eclampsia to premature separation of the placenta. These danger signals should be reported to the physician immediately.
    1 Sexual intercourse is permissible as long as it is not uncomfortable and the cervix is closed; however, if a patient has had numerous miscarriages, the physician might suggest that the patient refrain from intercourse during the first 3 months to lessen the danger of a miscarriage.
    2 The recommended weight gain is about 25 lb; a weight gain slightly over that would not be considered excessive. It depends on the patient and what her weight was at the start of the pregnancy.
    4 Childbirth preparation classes are encouraged but not mandatory; this is not the best answer.
27. Comprehension, implementation, physiologic (b)
    4 The primary benefit would be to allow the mother to assist, if so desired, in as much of the birthing process as possible and to decrease the amount of actual medication used during labor.
    1 This may be true in some cases; rapidity of delivery and pain threshold vary with each individual.
    2 This may be true in some cases; pain threshold varies with each individual; small doses of medication are given and may actually facilitate the birthing process.
    3 This may also be true, but it is not considered to be the prime benefit of the classes.
28. Comprehension, implementation, health (a)
    3 This is the best explanation and advice.
    1 Wearing high heels during pregnancy should be discouraged for both health and safety reasons.
    2 Wearing lower heels may help, but this does not prevent varicose veins.
    4 This is good advice, but it does not explain consequences.
29. Knowledge, assessment, health (a)
    2 Colostrum is the thin, watery secretion from the breast that occurs during latter stages of pregnancy and after delivery.
    1 Lochia is the vaginal discharge that occurs following delivery.
    3 Chloasma is the pigmentary discoloration primarily found on the face during pregnancy.
    4 Chorion is a fetal membrane.
30. Application, planning, physiologic (b)
    2 Normal weight gain for the 9-month period is 25 to 30 pounds. The patient will probably gain at least another 4 pounds during the last 4 weeks, which will put her over the normal weight gain.
    1 She has already gained more than the optimal amount of weight.
    3 She has gained over the optimal amount.
    4 During the last 4 weeks it is normal for the mother to gain 4 pounds as the fetus grows.
31. Knowledge, planning, environment (a)
    1 The estimated date of confinement (EDC) is the estimated delivery date and is calculated by Nägele's rule.
    2 This is an incorrect response, as indicated above.
    3 This is some of the information necessary in using Nägele's rule.
    4 This is an incorrect response, as indicated above; it has no real significance.

32. Comprehension, planning, environment (a)
    2 This ensures optimal care of mother and baby.
    1 Lightening occurs before labor; this is late to ensure optimal care.
    3 Morning sickness varies in time; this is late to ensure optimal care.
    4 This usually occurs between 4 and 5 months of gestation; too late to ensure optimal care.
33. Comprehension, assessment, physiologic (b)
    3 The nonstress test is performed on the patient who is not in labor. It is based on the observation that acceleration of the fetal heart rate in response to fetal movement is a reliable indicator of immediate fetal well-being.
    1 The nonstress test is unable to view fetal position.
    2 The nonstress test is unable to determine gestational age.
    4 The nonstress test is unable to determine when labor will begin.
34. Knowledge, implementation, health (b)
    2 Pregnant women who contract German measles during the first trimester frequently give birth to children with cataracts, heart lesions, deaf-mutism, and microcephaly.
    1 German measles are very dangerous to the fetus and can cause many birth defects.
    3 There is a vaccine against German measles, but it cannot be given during pregnancy. If a mother needs the vaccine, it will be given just after delivery. It is best to wait at least 3 months after the vaccine is given before becoming pregnant.
    4 Antibiotics will not prevent German measles.
35. Knowledge, implementation, health (a)
    2 During pregnancy, progesterone is responsible for securing implantation, development of the placenta, and inhibiting uterine contractility.
    1 During pregnancy, estrogen is responsible for uterine growth, elasticity, and contractility; breast growth; and enlargement of external genitalia.
    3 Luteinizing hormone is responsible for the maturing of the graafian follicle and its release from the ovary (ovulation) during the menstrual cycle.
    4 Follicle-stimulating hormone stimulates the growth and development of ovarian follicles from about days 4 to 14 of the menstrual cycle.
36. Knowledge, evaluation, environment (a)
    1 The patient is correct to be afraid to use aspirin during pregnancy since it can cause bleeding and possible damage to the fetus.
    2 The patient has only stated her reservations about using aspirin. There is no indication of paranoia.
    3 The patient's statement shows a clear understanding of the danger of aspirin use during pregnancy.
    4 It is best not to use *any* drug during pregnancy, but if a drug is necessary for pain, Tylenol would be the safest choice.
37. Application, implementation, health (b)
    1 This is a normal occurrence as the pregnancy nears term; lightening occurs when the presenting part descends into the pelvis, accounting for greater pressure on the bladder.
    2 The patient did not indicate burning or other symptoms more commonly associated with a urinary tract infection.
    3 Restriction of fluids is not recommended and would not resolve the problem of urinary frequency.
    4 All complaints made by patients should be reported to the physician, but this one, as given in the situation, does not need immediate attention by the physician.

38. Knowledge, implementation, health (a)
    4 In the fourth month of antepartal growth and development, muscles are developed and movements of the fetus may be felt by the mother.
    1, 2 Movement is usual and expected during these months.
    3 It is too early to feel movements during this month.
39. Knowledge, assessment, health (a)
    3 Enlargement and tenderness of the breasts, amenorrhea, and frequency are all signs and symptoms of pregnancy that the nurse can assess.
    1 The physician usually assesses enlargement of the uterus during the physical examination.
    2 This requires an internal examination and is not the responsibility of the nurse.
    4 These signs and symptoms of pregnancy are usually not apparent during an initial prenatal visit, which most often occurs during the second or third month of pregnancy; fetal movements are usually felt by the mother during the fourth month, when quickening occurs.
40. Application, implementation, environment (a)
    4 Dependent edema occurs with decreased circulatory return and is relieved by elevating the legs.
    1 Dependent edema, which resolves after a night's sleep, does not require complete bed rest.
    2 Pregnancy-induced hypertension is characterized by hypertension, proteinuria, and edema.
    3 Sodium intake is not restricted for dependent edema. Reducing excessive sodium is encouraged for all.
41. Application, implementation, health (a)
    2 It is helpful to give the correct explanation using the word "uterus" instead of stomach, which connotes something being eaten.
    1 This is false information; eating is not the cause of growth.
    3 This is false information; the baby is not growing in the stomach.
    4 Emphasis on the baby can cause negative feelings.
42. Application, implementation, psychosocial (a)
    4 Involving him in the process gives him more positive attention.
    1 Avoidance doesn't solve the problem.
    2 This is false assurance.
    3 This is negative reinforcement.
43. Comprehension, planning, environment (c)
    3 If delivered vaginally, the baby will more than likely contract the disease. When delivered by a C-section, the baby does not enter the vaginal canal and will therefore not be exposed to the virus.
    1 Antibiotics could cross the placental barrier and cause damage to the fetus. Also there is no cure for genital herpes, so the antibiotics would have no effect.
    2 There is no cure for genital herpes.
    4 There is no immunization against genital herpes.
44. Application, implementation, health (c)
    1 Various hormonal changes tend to promote resistance to insulin, thus increasing the need for insulin.
    2 There is nothing to indicate a change in activity level.
    3 Prevention of urinary tract infections relies on frequent urine cultures, careful hygiene, and strict control of serum glucose levels.
    4 The fetus produces its own insulin.
45. Knowledge, planning, physiologic (a)
    3 Persistent, excessive vomiting accompanied by weight loss and fluid and electrolyte imbalance.
    1, 4 This is a condition of pregnancy characterized by hypertension, edema, and proteinuria.
    2 This is nausea and vomiting in pregnancy, usually subsiding by the twelfth week of gestation.

46. Knowledge, assessment, health (a)
    4 Untreated, this condition will cause death as a result of electrolyte, metabolic, and nutritional imbalances.
    1 This is not likely because the embryo or fetus would die as a result of severe starvation, resulting in hypoproteinemia and hypovitaminosis. Bleeding from mucosal surfaces occurs as a result of vitamin C and B complex deficiency and hypothrombinemia.
    2 This is completely unrelated.
    3 See response to No. 1.
47. Comprehension, implementation, physiologic (c)
    4 The symptoms presented are classic symptoms of an ectopic pregnancy. The patient requires immediate surgery to prevent rupture of the fallopian tube.
    1 An ectopic pregnancy is life threatening and requires immediate attention.
    2 Antibiotics would be of no use in an ectopic pregnancy.
    3 This action would further delay treatment.
48. Application, assessment, health (a)
    2 Elevated blood pressure (over 140/90) is a hallmark sign of preeclampsia.
    1 Fundal height is not affected by preeclampsia.
    3 Urine sugar and acetone are not affected.
    4 FHT will be abnormal only if the fetus is compromised, which is uncommon with the onset of preeclampsia.
49. Application, implementation, health (a)
    3 Flushing out the urinary tract reduces the amount of bacteria present.
    1 Fluid intake should be at least eight 8-oz glasses of fluid per day.
    2 Excessive carbohydrate and sugar intake may result in glycosuria, which promotes bacterial growth.
    4 Cotton underwear better absorbs moisture.
50. Application, implementation, physiologic (b)
    2 Bed rest reduces the effect of gravitational pull and reduces uterine activity.
    1 No routine salt restrictions are indicated.
    3 Good nutrition should be maintained.
    4 There is no indication to reduce fluids.
51. Comprehension, application, psychosocial (c)
    4 This stage is usually the most difficult. The patient may display irritability and unwillingness to be touched.
    1 Stage two is the expulsion of the infant.
    2 Stage three is the delivery of the placenta.
    3 This is the beginning of labor.
52. Application, implementation, physiologic (b)
    2 The strongest muscular contractions can be felt on the fundus, or top, of the uterus.
    1 This area is too low.
    3 This is not a suitable area.
    4 This is not applicable to the question.
53. Knowledge, planning, environment (a)
    1 This is true for most women delivering their first child; for subsequent pregnancies, the time is usually shorter.
    2, 3 Labor varies, yet the average is 14 to 16 hours.
    4 Labor varies; it is doubtful that the physician would permit a patient to be in true active labor for this period of time before evaluating for possible complications.
54. Knowledge, implementation, environment (a)
    4 Identification is legally validated in most states or areas by recording the infant's footprints and the mother's fingerprint.
    1 This is usual hospital policy and procedure and can be considered routine.
    2 This is not usual practice.
    3 This has nothing to do with legal identification of the infant; it is routine practice.

55. Comprehension, planning, physiologic (b)
    3 Clearing the airway of mucus will prevent aspiration.
    1, 4 This is usually done after breathing is established.
    2 This is usually done at 1 minute and 5 minutes after delivery.
56. Comprehension, implementation, psychosocial (a)
    1 This indicates recognition by the nurse that anyone the mother chooses can play a supportive role during labor.
    2 This ignores the patient's anxiety, which may be caused by her feeling "alone."
    3 This response ignores the feelings of this individual patient.
    4 Saying nothing in this situation excludes possibilities for reducing anxiety.
57. Application, planning, environment (a)
    2 Vaginal examinations should be done under conditions of strict cleanliness. The vulva should be washed well, and the examiner should use sterile gloves.
    1, 3, 4 These are not necessary to do a vaginal examination.
58. Comprehension, implementation, environment (a)
    4 This is the most common area to begin finding fetal heart tones.
    1, 3 These are correct but not precise.
    2 This is incorrect for the vertex position.
59. Comprehension, planning, environment (a)
    4 Providing for a clean delivery reduces the possibility of an infection.
    1 An enema does not prevent constipation during labor.
    2 An enema does not provide relief of pressure in case of episiotomy.
    3 This definitely does not ease contractions.
60. Knowledge, assessment, environment (b)
    3 True labor starts when uterine contractions occur regularly. There is complete effacement of the cervical canal, and the cervix dilates.
    1 Expelling the plug is a sign that labor is about to start.
    2 Membranes rupture before or after labor starts.
    4 Usually the fetus drops into the pelvis brim a week or two before delivery.
61. Comprehension, assessment, environment (b)
    4 This is a below-normal rate, which indicates fetal distress.
    1 Meconium is a potential problem; the nurse should check fetal heart tones frequently to determine fetal distress. This is not the best answer.
    2 Fetal inactivity itself is not a cause for alarm.
    3 This does not necessarily indicate danger; the nurse should note the time, amount, color, and odor.
62. Comprehension, implementation, environment (b)
    2 These are the correct instructions and posture for bearing down.
    1 Head back is the wrong position.
    3 The patient must hold her breath and push, or slowly let the breath out while pushing.
    4 Bearing down and pushing are impossible with this kind of instruction.

63. Comprehension, planning, environment (b)
    3 The physician is referring to the degree of dilation (opening) of the cervix as expressed in centimeters; the term "cephalic" refers to the part of the fetus, in this case the head, that is against the cervical opening and will be delivered first.
    1 The term denoting the thickness of the cervix is "effacement"; the term denoting the height of the presenting part in relation to ischial spines is "station."
    2 Although the fetal head may be against the cervix, there is no indication that the physician has determined effacement or thinning of the cervix.
    4 There is no indication that the physician has determined the station.
64. Application, implementation, environment (b)
    3 A prepared father or other support person should be allowed to assist in the mother's care; the nurse is responsible for monitoring the fetal heart tones and validating the pattern of contractions.
    1 In this option the nurse avoids nursing responsibilities.
    2 In this option the nurse assumes her responsibilities but can also increase the father's anxiety level.
    4 This option may be interpreted as discounting the father's preparation for the event.
65. Application, assessment, environment (a)
    3 The cord may have been compressed as the fluid left the uterus and the fetus settled into the pelvis. The fetal heart rate changes as a result of fetal distress.
    1 Nitrazine testing is done to confirm the presence of amniotic fluid.
    2 This is a part of assessment during labor, but it is not the priority after rupture of the membranes.
    4 Rupture of the membranes may result in fetal distress, not maternal distress.
66. Comprehension, planning, environment (b)
    2 In the early latent phase of the first stage of labor, the cervix dilates from 0 cm to 4 cm.
    1 False labor is characterized by irregular contractions that may stop with walking; there is little change in dilation or effacement of the cervix.
    3 True labor is characterized by regular contractions that are increasing in duration and intensity, spontaneous rupture of membranes, and bloody show; transition is the last phase of the first stage of labor.
    4 In the active phase of the first stage, the cervix dilates from 5 cm to 10 cm; the third stage is from delivery of the fetus to delivery of the placenta.
67. Application, implementation, environment (a)
    3 An enema may further enhance labor. In a multipara with a history of rapid labors, assessment of mother and fetus has priority.
    1 An external fetal monitor will not further stimulate labor; it will aid in fetal assessment.
    2, 4 These will not further stimulate labor; they will be of use in maternal assessment.
68. Knowledge, implementation, environment (b)
    1 The length of a contraction from beginning to end is called duration.
    2 The degree of hardness/firmness of the uterus is called intensity.
    3 Frequency is how often contractions occur, in minutes or seconds.
    4 The interval is the time from the beginning of one contraction to the beginning of the next.

69. Comprehension, assessment, environment (b)
    4 If the fundus becomes soft, the mother could hemorrhage.
    1 This is done during the first and second stage of labor.
    2 This is done during the third stage of labor.
    3 This can be done at any time after the baby is delivered, but it is much more important to ensure that the patient is not hemorrhaging.

70. Comprehension, assessment, environment (b)
    3 The third stage of labor is complete with the delivery of the placenta.
    1 This is usually noted as completion of the second stage of labor.
    2 This is usually done immediately following the birth of the baby.
    4 This is a dangerous complication in which the uterus is turned inside out so that the fundus intrudes into the cervix or vagina; it is caused by a too-vigorous removal of the placenta before it detaches from the uterine wall via the natural process of labor.

71. Application, implementation, physiologic (b)
    2 Shaking and chills are normal in the first hour after delivery; warmed blankets will provide comfort.
    1 An actual elevation of temperature is best identified by checking temperature after the chill has subsided.
    3 Shaking and chills are not indications for oxygen administration.
    4 The presence of a fever has not been assessed.

72. Comprehension, evaluation, physiologic (b)
    2 Oxytocic drugs are given to help strengthen contractions of the uterus and prevent excessive bleeding.
    1 The drug is not used for this purpose.
    3 The drug does not hasten this process.
    4 The drug does not prevent uterine inversion.

73. Comprehension, assessment, physiologic (b)
    3 The classic signs of preeclampsia are elevated blood pressure, proteinuria, and edema.
    1 Not necessarily; 2+ protein in urine is not normal.
    2 This is not an indication.
    4 This is not related to the situation.

74. Knowledge, planning, physiologic (c)
    3 The cocaine will, however, have an effect on the newborn.
    1, 2 Cocaine addiction does not affect labor.
    4 Because labor is not affected, the need for sedation is no different than for a nonaddicted mother; if withdrawal symptoms occur, the patient may have to be evaluated for relief or control.

75. Knowledge, planning, environment (a)
    3 Rubber gloves are worn and the hands are washed after each contact with the patient; care should be taken to prevent transfer of virus from vesicles to other skin or mucous membranes of the patient or any other individual.
    1 The condition does not warrant complete or strict isolation.
    2 This should be exercised at all times, not only when preparing the patient for delivery.
    4 This should also be done, but it is not the only consideration of the nurse, as noted in the rationale for the correct response.

76. Comprehension, implementation, environment (b)
    4 Pitocin, an oxytocin, is a strong uterine contractor and must be regulated so there are desirable intervals between contractions; tetanic contractions (very strong continual contractions) could jeopardize both the mother and the fetus.
    1, 2, 3 This may be so, but it is not the best answer.

77. Comprehension, evaluation, environment (c)
    3 Magnesium sulfate will reduce edema on the brain, thus reducing central nervous system symptoms. The plan of care should always include observing patient response to treatment.
    1 This has nothing to do with pulse rate; this drug is used to prevent seizures and can also be used as a cathartic.
    2 This drug is not an oxytocic.
    4 Any such outcome would be detrimental to the patient; this drug is not used for relief of epigastric pain.

78. Application, implementation, psychosocial (b)
    2 The patient needs information to help relieve her anxiety and to help her to understand treatment and procedures.
    1 The nurse should do this only after assessment, providing information, and treatments—if the patient so desires.
    3 Emergencies such as maternal shock and fetal distress can occur at any moment. The patient must not be left alone.
    4 Everything may not be alright. False reassurance is not appropriate.

79. Comprehension, assessment, environment (b)
    3 Abruptio placentae is the premature separation of a normally implanted placenta before birth.
    1 This is a pregnancy outside the uterus, usually in the fallopian tubes.
    2 Placenta previa is an abnormal implantation of a normal placenta.
    4 A complete abortion occurs when all of the products of conception are expelled.

80. Application, planning, psychosocial (a)
    2 A cesarean delivery is not a contraindication for breast-feeding. Assistance from staff will decrease anxiety and promote self-assurance for the mother.
    1 Encouragement will assist the patient in her decision to breast-feed.
    3 This is not necessary unless there is a physical problem.
    4 This response might discourage her; she needs a "listener."

81. Comprehension, evaluation, environment (b)
    1 The epidural block is safer for both mother and baby; it has minimal after-effects.
    2 A general anesthetic predisposes the infant to respiratory depression.
    3 The pudendal block is a regional anesthetic.
    4 Bier's block is a regional anesthetic; it has no effects on the abdomen.

82. Comprehension, implementation, environment (b)
    4 Maintaining the patient in this position for at least 8 hours is recommended as a means of preventing a spinal headache, which occurs as a result of loss of cerebrospinal fluid from the subarachnoid space and results in traction of the meninges on the pressure-sensitive intracranial structures.
    1 The fundus is palpated as with a normal vaginal delivery because hemorrhage is a very real possibility. This type of patient is really two patients in one, a surgical patient and an obstetric patient, neither of which should be overlooked.
    2 This may not be necessary because these patients are not usually given general anesthesia in addition to the spinal anesthesia.
    3 This is not necessary because the patient will usually have an indwelling catheter in place following the surgery.

83. Comprehension, assessment, physiologic (a)
    4 As the low-lying placenta separates during dilation or effacement, blood flows from the vagina.
    1 This is associated with the concealed bleeding present with abruptio placentae.
    2 This is associated with the bleeding occurring in abruptio placentae.
    3 Bleeding associated with placenta previa generally occurs before labor begins. Because the blood flows out of the vagina, the uterus does not become hard.
84. Application, implementation, environment (c)
    4 The risk of intrauterine infection associated with premature rupture of the membranes (PROM) is assessed by a close monitoring of maternal vital signs.
    1, 3 These are not a priority in assessment of PROM.
    2 Monitoring for a developing infection takes priority.
85. Application, implementation, environment (c)
    4 It takes about 72 hours for the danger of seizures to pass.
    1, 2, 3 The possibility of seizures lasts longer, about 72 hours.
86. Application, evaluation, environment (c)
    2 Respirations of less than 14, a decrease or absence of patellar reflexes, and urine output of less than 25 ml/hr are signs of magnesium sulfate toxicity.
    1 The nurse should record and monitor information, but she should also call the physician.
    3 The drug is discontinued immediately.
    4 This is not a normal result.
87. Comprehension, implementation, physiologic (b)
    1 Magnesium sulfate is a central nervous system depressant. It decreases nerve impulses from the brain to the muscles.
    2 This drug is not an analgesic.
    3 The drug does not increase blood pressure.
    4 The drug is not used for induction of labor.
88. Application, implementation, psychosocial (b)
    4 Siblings need to be a part of the care and attention given to the new baby.
    1, 2 Isolation keeps them apart from the care and attention given the baby.
    3 This response gives false assurance.
89. Comprehension, planning, psychosocial (c)
    4 Because sibling jealousy is related to competition for parents' love, their daughter will need special attention and time alone with her parents.
    1 Sibling jealousy relates to time, attention, and love rather than to material things.
    2 Their daughter will need help to deal with her jealousy rather than help in loving the new baby.
    3 Knowing that she is a big girl will not help in relieving their daughter's jealousy.
90. Comprehension, implementation, physiologic (a)
    4 Lochia rubra is bright or dark red, lasting 2 to 3 days.
    1 Lochia serosa is pinkish to brownish, lasting 2 to 5 days.
    2 Lochia alba is creamy and yellowish, lasting 5 to 10 days.
    3 This is not normal.
91. Knowledge, assessment, environment (a)
    4 When quick saturation and clots are involved, it is considered heavy.
    1 Moderate bleeding does not saturate pads quickly.
    2 This term is not used to describe lochia.
    3 This is the normal preferred amount of discharge after 24 to 48 hours.

92. Comprehension, planning, health (b)
    3 This amount provides necessary intake of nutrients and fluid within a 24-hour period.
    1 There is no set routine established to ensure adequate intake.
    2 This is an inadequate intake of nutrients and fluid.
    4 This is generally too much fluid for a 9-lb baby to tolerate.
93. Knowledge, implementation, physiologic (a)
    2 The warm water in a sitz bath promotes vasodilation, leading to increased comfort.
    1 Increased ambulation may cause additional discomfort because of increased engorgement and pressure.
    3 This technique serves no physiologic purpose in this situation.
    4 While this might be an appropriate intervention, non-medication therapy should be considered first.
94. Comprehension, implementation, psychosocial (a)
    4 Rooming-in allows mothers and new babies to share accommodations rather than being separated; ideally the maternity unit is designed so that the crib can be at the mother's bedside or in a nursery conveniently adjacent to the mother's room.
    1 The father may be present in the room, but this is not the true definition of the term "rooming-in."
    2, 3 These options are not applicable to the "rooming-in" situation.
95. Knowledge, planning, physiologic (a)
    3 Demand feeding is popular and allows the newborn to be fed at the time and in the amount desired.
    1 Crying does not always indicate hunger.
    2, 4 These are not considered part of the demand feeding method.
96. Knowledge, planning, health (b)
    2 Lactation produces an increased need for maternal energy, protein, minerals and vitamins; these aid secretion of milk, provide nourishment for the infant via the mother's milk, and protect the mother's stores of nutrients. A well-balanced diet with an extra 640 calories and extra fluids (as much as 3000 ml) is required for the breast-feeding mother.
    1 This is not sufficient fluid intake for a breast-feeding mother; see above.
    3 As long as the mother follows a well-balanced diet, there is no real need for supplements.
    4 See response to No. 3; milk can be considered part of the 3000 ml of fluids.
97. Application, implementation, psychosocial (a)
    3 This is the most appropriate response because the nurse fully responds to both concerns in a correct manner.
    1 This response is inadequate because it offers no reassurance to the patient; this is information the nurse should know.
    2 The first part of the response is correct; the second part of the response offers incorrect information.
    4 This is true, but it is not the most appropriate response because it does not respond fully to the patient's concerns.
98. Comprehension, implementation, physiologic (b)
    4 The nursing mother may have some breast engorgement as her milk comes in; nursing the newborn will often help relieve or reduce this congestion.
    1 This will not resolve the situation for the mother.
    2 This will not resolve the situation for the mother unless additional signs and symptoms of an infection are present.
    3 This action is taken only when the patient is known to be bottle feeding, not breast-feeding, her infant.

99. Application, implementation, environment (b)
    4 Following a spinal anesthetic the patient needs to remain flat in bed for 4 to 8 hours to prevent a spinal headache.
    1 Getting up too soon will cause a spinal headache; also the spinal anesthetic may not have worn off yet and the patient could hurt herself going to the bathroom.
    2, 3 Sitting up will cause a spinal headache.
100. Comprehension, implementation, health (b)
    2 Normal elimination patterns may be reestablished and constipation relieved by a well-balanced diet and ambulation.
    1, 4 These are irrelevant to the situation.
    3 These measures would not facilitate return to normal elimination patterns if used on a continual basis.
101. Application, implementation, physiologic (a)
    3 From eating little, there may be little bulk to stimulate bowel movement; fluids keep the stool moist and easier to pass.
    1 Ambulation is to be encouraged; an enema should be administered by the third day if the mother has not responded to the other measures.
    2, 4 Fecal impaction takes more than 2 days to develop.
102. Comprehension, assessment, physiologic (a)
    2 A full bladder causes the uterus to lie to either side instead of being centrally located.
    1 Stomach distention does not cause this.
    3 The uterus should be centrally located in the abdomen.
    4 This is not applicable.
103. Comprehension, planning, environment (a)
    3 An overdistended bladder leads to atony of the bladder wall, resulting in urinary distention, which provides an environment favorable to infection.
    1 A hematoma develops as a result of hemorrhage under the vaginal mucosa or in the connective tissue of the vulva; development of a hematoma is not related to an overdistended bladder.
    2, 4 These are not related to bladder distention.
104. Knowledge, implementation, health (a)
    4 In 1975 the American Academy of Pediatrics found no medical indication for routine newborn circumcision. Parents choose circumcision for personal reasons.
    1 Careful daily bathing provides adequate hygiene.
    2, 3 There is no scientific evidence to support this statement.
105. Comprehension, planning, physiologic (b)
    1 Petrolatum keeps the area from scabbing over and sticking to the diaper and thus prevents bleeding.
    2 Complications do not occur often because circumcision is a relatively minor procedure.
    3 Voiding is not frequently affected.
    4 Healing usually occurs quickly.
106. Knowledge, assessment, physiologic (a)
    1 Para indicates the number of live births.
    2 Gravida indicates the number of pregnancies.
    3, 4 These are incorrect numbers.
107. Application, implementation, health (a)
    4 The Norplant system is surgically implanted beneath the skin and leaks progesterone to stop the production of the follicle-stimulating hormone. The ovaries will not release an ovum for fertilization. It can be used on almost any healthy woman.
    1 Condoms are not as effective as the Norplant system and must be used every time intercourse occurs.
    2 Oral contraceptives are effective but have to be taken each day.
    3 The diaphragm is not as effective as the other three methods listed and must be used each time intercourse occurs.

108. Application, implementation, psychosocial (b)
    3 It is important to find out the patient's plans or ideas and explore possibilities with her.
    1 This reveals a judgmental attitude, which serves no purpose.
    2 The mother might not want to discuss the father.
    4 This would make her feel dependent, with no choices.
109. Comprehension, implementation, psychosocial (a)
    3 Knowing this is a normal response often decreases anxiety and encourages the patient to talk.
    1 This situation requires a nursing response.
    2 This response neglects an opportunity to teach the patient the normalcy of her feelings.
    4 Psychiatric intervention is not required at this point because postpartum blues are a normal response.
110. Comprehension, planning, environment (c)
    1 As a result of the overdistention of the uterus with two fetuses, the uterus may not contract sufficiently to control bleeding.
    2 Multiple gestation is not a risk factor for mastitis.
    3, 4 Multiple gestation is not a risk factor in these postpartum complications. Cesarean delivery greatly increases the risk of these complications.
111. Knowledge, planning, health (a)
    3 An antibiotic ointment effectively kills the gonococcal organism; silver nitrate eyedrops are also effective.
    1, 2 These do not cause blindness.
    4 Blindness is caused by high concentrations of oxygen.
112. Comprehension, planning, physiologic (a)
    2 If the newborn's body temperature drops, respiratory depression will develop.
    1 Weight can wait; every effort is taken to make sure the infant is breathing well and is stable.
    3 A bath will usually drop the newborn's temperature.
    4 This is done before discharge, not at birth; not all newborn males are circumcised.
113. Application, planning, environment (c)
    3 Vastus lateralis is the best-developed muscle in infants and is therefore the safest for intramuscular injections.
    1, 4 These are not suitable sites for injection.
    2 This might cause injury to the sciatic nerve.
114. Application, implementation, physiologic (b)
    2 Vitamin K helps the blood to clot.
    1 Vitamin K is not an anticoagulant.
    3 Antibiotics and antibiotic ointments help prevent STDs.
    4 Iron is needed to prevent anemia.
115. Comprehension, evaluation, physiologic (b)
    2 Ten (10) is the highest score an infant can attain. Each area evaluated is scored as 0, 1, or 2. The evaluation is ordinarily done 1 minute and 5 minutes after delivery.
    1 This score is not high enough to be the best.
    3, 4 These scores are not applicable; the highest attainable score is 10.
116. Application, implementation, environment (b)
    3 Wrapping the foot chosen for the heel stick in a warm wet cloth for 5 minutes and elevating the head of the crib to increase circulation to the extremity is the appropriate action.
    1 This is not so; see response to No. 3.
    2 Elevating the foot of the crib will decrease, not increase, circulation to the area.
    4 Saline solution would not affect circulation to the area and "soaking" would be difficult to accomplish with a newborn; there is no need to involve both feet.

117. Application, implementation, environment (b)
    3 The eyes of the newborn may initially be puffy and red as a result of the delivery and instillation of an antibiotic solution. Gentle cleansing of exudate is sufficient intervention at this time; purulent or odoriferous drainage should be reported.
    1, 2, 4 These are not appropriate at this time.
118. Knowledge, assessment, physiologic (a)
    2 (a)   8.0 lb (3632 g)   (b)   16.0 oz
    $$\begin{array}{ll} \underline{\times 10\%} & \underline{\times\ 0.8} \\ 0.8\ \text{lb} & 12.8\ \text{oz weight loss} \end{array}$$
    (c) 7 lb 16.0 oz—7 lb 12.8 oz = 7 lb 3 oz (3260 g)
    1, 3, 4 These are incorrect calculations.
119. Comprehension, planning, environment (b)
    4 Infection control is mandatory until all blood, amniotic fluid, and vernix are removed.
    1 Bath depends on temperature control, not PO intake.
    2 The nurse should begin with the eyes and wash the entire body.
    3 Cord care follows the bath.
120. Knowledge, assessment, physiologic (a)
    1 Discharge is normal because of maternal hormonal transfer across the placenta. At the time of delivery a greater exchange of hormones may occur, which causes a temporary increase of the infant's hormone level.
    2 Birth trauma does not usually occur in this area.
    3 The infant has not produced the increased hormonal level; see rationale No. 1.
    4 There is no such thing.
121. Comprehension, implementation, environment (a)
    4 The condition will disappear by itself.
    1 This will cause damage and may cause infection.
    2 Binders are used for engorged mothers.
    3 Hot packs are used by breast-feeding mothers.
122. Knowledge, planning, environment (a)
    1 Air swallowed during feeding most frequently causes regurgitation; therefore it is wise to burp the infant frequently during and following completion of the feeding.
    2, 3 These are inappropriate responses.
    4 This condition does not exist.
123. Comprehension, assessment, physiologic (b)
    1 This is a normal response in the newborn called the Moro reflex or startle reflex. It usually disappears by the sixth month.
    2 There is no need to call the doctor since this is a normal response.
    3 Restraining the baby may make the reflex worse and could harm the baby.
    4 Turning the baby will have no effect.
124. Knowledge, assessment, physiologic (a)
    1 This is the correct definition of the rooting reflex.
    2 This is a normal reflex noted in a young infant. It is elicited by a sudden loud noise that results in flexion of the legs, an embracing position of the arms, and a brief cry.
    3 It is a normal response in newborns to extend the arm and the leg on the side of the body to which the head is quickly turned while the infant is in the supine position, and to flex the limbs of the opposite side.
    4 This is the involuntary sucking movement of the circumoral area in newborns in response to stimulation; this reflex continues throughout infancy and often occurs without stimulation, even during sleep.

125. Knowledge, assessment, psychosocial (b)
    2 This is accurate information and the best nursing response.
    1 This response assumes that the information was covered in prenatal classes.
    3 This response is nontherapeutic.
    4 This response does not allay her fears.
126. Comprehension, assessment, physiologic (a)
    4 Respirations in the newborn may be irregular and range from 32 to 48 per minute. Respiratory distress evidenced by abnormal rate, cyanosis, substernal retractions, and flaring of the nares should be reported immediately.
    1 Respirations are often irregular; 36 is within normal range, but 24 is too low and would be evidence of respiratory distress.
    2 True respirations would probably be irregular; 40 is within the normal range, but 58 is too fast and would be evidence of respiratory distress.
    3 Respirations would most likely be irregular; 30 to 44 per minute falls within the normal range.
127. Application, implementation, environment (c)
    4 The newborn's temperature may rise when exposed to the heat produced by the phototherapy bulb.
    1 The infant's eyes are securely covered with patches.
    2 Fluids are encouraged to aid in excretion of bilirubin.
    3 The diaper is left on to protect genitalia.
128. Knowledge, assessment, physiologic (b)
    3 Physiologic jaundice between 48 and 72 hours of life is usually a result of the immature liver being unable to conjugate indirect bilirubin, the newborn's high red blood cell count, and hemolysis of fetal red blood cells.
    1 Pathologic jaundice associated with Rh incompatibility occurs within the first 24 hours of life.
    2 Pathologic jaundice associated with ABO incompatibility occurs with the first 24 hours of life.
    4 Biliary atresia is the obstruction of or absence of a portion of the bile duct. Jaundice is the earliest evidence of a problem. It may be apparent at birth, but it is not usually apparent until the child is 2 to 3 weeks of age.
129. Knowledge, assessment, physiologic (b)
    1 This is accurate information and the best nursing response.
    2 This response incorrectly accuses the mother.
    3 This response gives false information.
    4 This response can instill fear in the mother, and it is not within scope of nursing practice to make such a decision.
130. Comprehension, assessment, environment (b)
    4 This promotes safety and provides injury control.
    1 In this nursing response, there is no learning for the mother or safety for the baby.
    2, 3 In these responses by the nurse, there is no learning for the mother.
131. Application, evaluation, psychosocial (c)
    4 This response communicates findings of data collected.
    1, 2, 3 These nursing attitudes lack insight into the behavior exhibited.
132. Comprehension, assessment, physiologic (b)
    1 Vital signs are not stable in the newborn. Respirations can fluctuate from 30 to 60 per minute.
    2 This response can instill fear in the mother.
    3 The message to the mother is that she is not knowledgeable.
    4 Incomplete information is being offered.

133. Knowledge, assessment, physiologic (a)
    3 This is the most desirable heart rate for a newborn infant.
    1, 2 This heart rate is too low for a newborn at rest.
    4 This heart rate is too high for a newborn at rest.
134. Application, implementation, environment (b)
    4 A syringe against the interior aspect of the cheek will administer the medication far enough back to avoid spitting and will help to avoid choking.
    1 The results of mixing medication with formula are unpredictable; the newborn may not drink all the formula.
    2 Newborns have a protrusion reflex of the tongue that makes spoon-fed foods unreliable.
    3 As in Nos. 1 and 2, newborns will probably spit amounts of cereal out because of protrusion of the tongue. Giving cereal is not appropriate for the age of the baby.
135. Application, planning, physiologic (b)
    4 The fissure in the roof of the mouth and nasal cavities makes it very difficult for the infant to eat. It is best to hold the infant in an upright position and direct the milk against the side of the mouth.
    1 Although infection is a danger in the infant with a cleft palate, feeding is the most pressing issue.
    2 The parents may feel threatened by the defect, but the infant is too young to be affected.
    3 This will be a major concern following surgery to repair the cleft palate.
136. Comprehension, planning, environment (b)
    2 Infants should be fed upright to prevent aspiration. The nipple should be placed well back in the mouth to facilitate sucking.
    1 Parents must be permitted to verbalize their feelings to enable them to cope with their anxiety and guilt.
    3 When teaching parents about the outcome of the surgery, positive results should be emphasized to offer hope and decrease anxiety.
    4 Infants should be fed in the same manner as they were at home until NPO. Invasive feeding techniques are avoided except in severe cases of failure to thrive.
137. Knowledge, planning, environment (a)
    1 Down syndrome is a chromosomal abnormality characterized by varying degrees of mental retardation and multiple defects. It is also known as trisomy 21, mongolism, or trisomy G syndrome.
    2, 3 The condition is congenital and is not caused by an infection.
    4 Varying degrees of mental retardation are apparent in Down syndrome. This is directly related to the chromosomal abnormality and is not a result of oxygen deprivation at birth.
138. Application, implementation, psychosocial (b)
    2 Assuming a sitting position beside the father communicates concern and a willingness to help the person in emotional crisis.
    1, 3 These responses do not communicate concern; they create a closed situation.
    4 This action will discourage, not encourage, communication.
139. Comprehension, implementation, psychosocial (b)
    1 When responding to someone in crisis, it is better to respond to the questions and provide only the information asked for by the individual.
    2, 3 These are not appropriate at this time.
    4 This is an inappropriate nursing intervention; it shows lack of both concern and willingness to help. The individual must face the situation and find ways to cope.

140. Comprehension, assessment, physiologic (b)
    1 A complication of myelomeningocele is neurologic dysfunction at and below the site of the spina bifida; the parasympathetic and sympathetic nerve damage results in atonia of the bladder and the bowel.
    2, 3, 4 These are not relevant to the situation.
141. Comprehension, assessment, physiologic (a)
    1 Before, and especially after, surgery, the infant is observed for movement in the extremities and functioning of bowel and bladder to determine the extent of neurologic dysfunction.
    2, 3, 4 These are not relevant to the situation.
142. Comprehension, evaluation, physiologic (c)
    1 Because the newborn has been receiving cocaine on a continual basis throughout the pregnancy, it has become addicted to the drug and will undergo withdrawal symptoms if the drug is not resupplied.
    2 Prolonged use of drugs before conception may affect both the mother and the unborn child; prolonged use of the drug throughout the pregnancy will definitely lead to addiction in the newborn.
    3 Cocaine is dangerous; mixing it with other drugs could lead to problems of drug incompatability; the statement that the infant would be doubly addicted is incorrect.
    4 Cocaine does impair uterine growth, but it does not in and of itself give rise to RDS (respiratory distress syndrome).
143. Knowledge, assessment, health (a)
    3 This is infection of the newborn's eyes and is caused by gonococci.
    1, 2 These are not correct.
    4 Syphilis can cause congenital deformities.
144. Comprehension, planning, physiologic (c)
    2 A combination of a negative with a positive can produce a positive; if the infant is positive, the mother produces antibodies that cross the placenta barrier and damage the infant's red blood cells.
    1 Two Rh-negatives do not create an Rh-positive.
    3 This combination should not present any difficulties.
    4 Two Rh-positives do not create an Rh-negative.
145. Comprehension, evaluation, environment (b)
    1 Watery green stools result from extra bilirubin being excreted because of the phototherapy.
    2 This is the stool commonly noted in a baby that is being breast-fed.
    3 Meconium is formed during fetal life and is passed within the first 24 hours after birth in normal infants.
    4 This is the stool commonly noted in a baby that is being bottle fed.
146. Comprehension, planning, physiologic (c)
    4 ABO incompatibility involves type A or type B infants born to type O mothers.
    1 Physiologic jaundice occurs after the first 24 hours.
    2 Rh incompatibility occurs with an Rh-negative mother and an Rh-positive father.
    3 Jaundice in the infant with hepatitis B occurs after the fourth week of life.
147. Comprehension, assessment, physiologic (b)
    1 Within the first week of life, the newborn with congenital syphilis may develop a rash over the face, palms, and soles of the feet, as well as a purulent nasal discharge.
    2 These are not associated with congenital syphilis.
    3 These are signs of central nervous system damage associated with congenital syphilis that appears later in life.
    4 These are not associated with congenital syphilis.

148. Application, implementation, environment (b)
    3 Implementation of the standard precaution protocol is recommended in all health-care facilities when dealing with AIDS or HIV-positive patients.
    1 While this is still a procedure in the nursery, standard precautions are being used in health-care facilities when caring for AIDS or HIV-positive patients. In fact, whether or not an infant or its mother is tested for the virus, most health-care facilities recommend that nurses wear gloves during initial care of the newborn.
    2 It is not the responsibility of the nurse to report to the Centers for Disease Control and Prevention; the nurse is responsible to his or her supervisor, whose duty it is to report such cases.
    4 The mask, gown, and gloves at all times are not really necessary because most HIV-positive patients are not necessarily ill with the signs and symptoms of active AIDS. Use of masks, gowns, and gloves is for the patient whose immune system places him at risk.

149. Application, assessment, physiologic (b)
    2 An infant should double its birth weight in 6 months.
    1, 4 This is too much of a weight gain for a 6 month old.
    3 This is too little weight gain for a 6 month old.

150. Knowledge, implementation, psychosocial (c)
    2 The child realizes some measure of control over his surroundings and begins to test the extent of his power.
    1 This is Erickson's stage for school-age children.
    3 This is Erickson's stage for infants.
    4 This is Erickson's stage for preschoolers.

151. Comprehension, planning, psychosocial (c)
    2 Punishment should follow wrongdoing.
    1 This should not affect the consequence of wrongdoing.
    3 Punishment should not be used as an outlet for the parent's feelings.
    4 Punishment is not appropriate.

152. Knowledge, assessment, psychosocial (a)
    4 The time period to develop trust is the infancy period, birth to 1 year of age; psychosocial need, trust vs. mistrust (Erikson).
    1 This is the adolescence period, 12 to 19 years of age; psychosocial need, identity vs. role confusion (Erikson).
    2 This is the preschool period, 3 to 6 years of age; psychosocial need, initiative vs. guilt (Erikson).
    3 This is the school-age period, 6 to 12 years of age; psychosocial need, industry vs. inferiority (Erikson).

153. Comprehension, assessment, physiologic (b)
    4 At one month the infant can turn its head from side to side when placed on its abdomen.
    1 Between 3 and 4 months of age the infant can roll from back to side.
    2 At 4 months the infant can smile and laugh aloud when talked to.
    3 At 2 months the infant can hold a rattle for a brief period of time.

154. Knowledge, assessment, physiologic (a)
    2 At 4 months the infant is mastering these developmental tasks.
    1 At 2 months the infant cannot hold its head erect when in a sitting position.
    3, 4 At these ages the infant has mastered these developmental tasks and is trying to master other tasks appropriate for those developmental levels.

155. Knowledge, assessment, physiologic (a)
    4 The anterior fontanel closes between 15 and 18 months of age.
    1 The posterior fontanel closes between 2 and 3 months of age.
    2, 3 The posterior fontanel should have closed, but the anterior fontanel has not.

156. Knowledge, planning, health (a)
    1 Basic simple language is easily learned and understood.
    2 Many words are too new and not easy to understand.
    3 This prevents growth.
    4 This communication is beyond the child's level of comprehension.

157. Knowledge, implementation, physiologic (a)
    4 Physiologic development of the anal muscles and readiness for toilet training occurs at 2 years of age.
    1 The toddler can feed himself/herself with a spoon by 15 months of age.
    2 Walking with assistance occurs between 11 and 12 months.
    3 Manipulating building blocks occurs between 15 and 18 months. The toddler can build a tower of two blocks.

158. Comprehension, planning, psychosocial (a)
    3 Training pants are much like regular pants, but they have the absorbency in case he does wet accidentally.
    1 These are difficult to get off, and they do not provide a chance for developmental progress.
    2 The message is that it is okay to wet his diaper or pants.
    4 Overalls are difficult to get off quickly.

159. Comprehension, planning, environment (b)
    4 Toddlers are curious and continue to search out by feeling and tasting.
    1 Toddlers are too young to realize the concept of fear.
    2 Swallowing objects is not a usual means of getting attention for this age-group.
    3 Easy access, while a possible factor, is not the main motivating factor for children to act on their need to explore.

160. Comprehension, implementation, psychosocial (b)
    4 The child has no comprehension of sharing at this age; also common is "parallel play," a form of play among a group of children, usually toddlers, in which they each play independently, yet together, and are not influenced by one another nor share their toys/playthings.
    1 The child would not benefit from this.
    2 This is a very inappropriate answer.
    3 The mother should not encourage or push the child.

161. Application, implementation, health (b)
    3 A 14 month old is usually not physically mature enough to control the anal sphincter. Between ages of 18 and 24 months voluntary control becomes possible.
    1 The nurse could review these but should encourage the mother to wait several months before trying again.
    2 It is important that toilet training not be stressful on the child.
    4 Treats may also be effective once the child is mature enough to have voluntary control.

162. Knowledge, assessment, physiologic (a)
    1 Gross motor coordination involves the use of large muscles in the body, as in running and walking.
    2 Tying represents fine-motor coordination.
    3 Writing uses muscles in the hands and fingers, which is fine-muscle coordination.
    4 Sewing represents fine-muscle coordination and manual dexterity.

163. Knowledge, assessment, environment (a)
    2 90 to 100 beats/min for 2 to 6 years of age.
    1 76 to 90 beats/min for children over 10 years of age.
    3 110 to 140 beats/min for an infant, 1 month to 1 year of age.
    4 120 to 150 beats/min for a neonate, birth to 1 month of age.

164. Comprehension, implementation, psychosocial (c)
    3 Playing with other children the same age and giving and sharing are important to the socialization process.
    1 This will not necessarily change.
    2 This may not have a direct relationship.
    4 This may be an outlet but is not the focus.

165. Knowledge, assessment, psychosocial (a)
    2 Industry occurs during the school-age period, 6 to 12 years of age. Psychosocial need, industry vs. inferiority. Learning to win recognition by producing things (Erickson).
    1 This is the toddler period, 1 to 3 years of age. Psychosocial need, autonomy vs. shame. Trying out own (self) powers of speech (Erickson).
    3 Preschool period, 3 to 6 years of age. Psychosocial need, initiative vs. guilt. Questioning and exploring own body and development (Erickson).
    4 This is the young adulthood period, 20 to 40 years of age. Psychosocial need, intimacy vs. isolation (Erickson).

166. Knowledge, assessment, psychosocial (c)
    2 During the middle childhood period, 7 to 11 years of age, children engage in concrete operations. Reasoning is logical but limited to personal experience (Piaget).
    1 This is the period of "formal operations," a time during which the child, 11 to 16 years of age, acquires the ability to develop abstract concepts; becomes oriented to problem solving (Piaget).
    3, 4 The preoperational phase of cognitive development extends from age 2 to age 7 and is divided into two phases: the preconceptual phase, ages 2 to 4, during which the child is able to form general concepts but is not yet capable of reasoning; and the phase of intuitive thought, ages 4 to 7, a time during which perceptual thinking occurs and the child is capable of some reasoning but can concentrate on only one aspect of a situation at a time (Piaget).

167. Comprehension, evaluation, psychosocial (b)
    2 If trust vs. mistrust is not met, the baby will have problems developing relationships later in life.
    1 The baby will withdraw, and mistrust will develop.
    3 Lack of self-confidence will develop.
    4 Sense of purpose develops later in childhood.

168. Knowledge, planning, health (a)
    2 A baby has a total of 20 deciduous teeth.
    1 This is too few.
    3, 4 These are too many.

169. Application, assessment, health (c)
    1 24 Ounces is an appropriate amount for a toddler.
    2 Milk is an excellent source of protein and is recommended at 16 to 24 ounces per day.
    3 38 Ounces is too much and can result in inadequate intake of other foods.
    4 Toddlers are growing quickly and need adequate milk intake.

170. Knowledge, implementation, psychosocial (c)
    3 Children between the ages of 7 and 11 years are very concrete thinkers. They need to see and touch objects to understand.
    1 A child of 8 who has been well prepared for surgery should be able to be separated from the parent without too much anxiety.
    2 Children of this age are very concrete thinkers and cannot think in abstract terms.
    4 Explanations are very important and need to be directed toward the child, although the parents need to be included.

171. Knowledge, assessment, psychosocial (a)
    2 Although strong in our society, adolescent rebellion need not be inevitable. There is little evidence that a full-blown rebellion characterizes most relationships between teenagers and their parents.
    1 True. Many conflicts between parents and teens focus on sexuality and many adolescents have difficulty discussing sexual matters with their parents.
    3 True. Forty to fifty percent of today's 14-year-old girls will become pregnant in their teens if trends continue.
    4 True. There has been a steady trend by society in general toward acceptance of more sexual activity in more situations.

172. Comprehension, evaluation, psychosocial (b)
    2 Seclusiveness and moodiness are behavior characteristics of the 13 year old.
    1 Hormonal influences and uncertainty about self-identity make for very unpredictable behavior.
    3 The adolescent is usually not very accepting of parent's ideals; can be rebellious.
    4 The goal of the adolescent is to move from dependency to self-reliance, increasing autonomy.

173. Comprehension, planning, psychosocial (b)
    4 Adolescents, age 12 to 18, are at the stage in which they are searching for their own identity.
    1 This is the stage of school-age children, ages 6 to 12.
    2 This is the stage of infants, birth to 1 year of age.
    3 This is the stage of the child, 3 to 6 years of age.

174. Comprehension, planning, psychosocial (b)
    2 The adolescent is trying to become independent of parents and family.
    1, 3, 4 These are major developmental tasks during this period.

175. Knowledge, planning, physiologic (b)
    2 Active immunity is acquired through vaccination.
    1 Passive immunity is acquired through the body's immune system activation or at childbirth.
    3 There isn't an artificial immunity.
    4 Temporary immunity is not considered, although some vaccines provide short-term immunity.

176. Comprehension, evaluation, health (c)
    2 Immunizations have decreased the incidence of many communicable diseases, but some children are not receiving immunizations. This accounts for the fact that communicable diseases are still a major problem in children.
    1 Not all children have been immunized.
    3 Some communicable diseases are necessary to build up natural immunity.
    4 Some conditions are serious, and no immunization is available.

177. Comprehension, implementation, environment (a)
    1 The bevel of the needle should be up.
    2 Bevel down causes the injection to go into the subcutaneous layer.
    3 Injecting a drug with the bevel facing distally would cause a large hole for the fluid to leak from.
    4 The bevel of the needle should be parallel to the limb.
178. Comprehension, planning, health (c)
    2 This is the recommended schedule published in the *Morbidity and Mortality Weekly Report* by the U.S. Department of Health and Human Services.
    1, 3, 4 These are not the recommended schedule.
179. Application, planning, health (b)
    2 The American Academy of Pediatrics' Committee on Infectious Diseases recommends immunizations to begin at 2 months, except for the hepatitis B immunization, which can be given at birth.
    1 This is too soon to begin the immunizations. The infant's immune system needs to mature.
    3 4 Months is too long to wait to begin unless the infant has some health problems that prevent the immunizations from being given.
    4 By 6 months all 3 DTP shots should be completed along with 2 polios and the hepatitis vaccines.
180. Comprehension, evaluation, environment (b)
    3 Maternal antibodies can be present for up to 1 year, rendering this vaccine inactive.
    1 The side effects are unchanged by age.
    2 Children less than 1 year old are at risk for measles.
    4 No new strains of measles have been identified yet.
181. Comprehension, evaluation, physiologic (b)
    4 By the fourth month pureed foods should be added one at a time. The baby should be feeding itself by the seventh month.
    1 Breast milk or formula provides a complete diet until about the sixth month of life.
    2 Even vitamins will not be enough. The baby needs to be eating food.
    3 Breast milk is not enough after the sixth month of life.
182. Knowledge, implementation, health (a)
    3 Cereal is suggested at 5 months.
    1, 2 Breast milk or formula is suggested at these ages.
    4 Strained fruits, meats, and finger food are suggested at 7 to 8 months.
183. Knowledge, implementation, health (a)
    1 To avoid food allergies, the mother should introduce one food at a time.
    2, 3 This is important, but the concern of allergic reactions takes priority.
    4 Formula feedings are also supplemented with vitamins and iron.
184. Knowledge, planning, health (a)
    4 Citrus fruits are highly recommended as excellent sources of vitamin C.
    1 Milk, cheese, and eggs are sources of protein.
    2 Fats, oils, and sugar are not recommended as vitamin C sources, and all nutrition sources say this group should be used sparsely.
    3 Breads, cereals, rice is not a food group that provides a good source of vitamin C.

185. Knowledge, planning, health (a)
    1 A banana would be considered more nutritious, and it does not contain sodium.
    2 A candy bar would not be considered nutritious; it may contain some sodium.
    3 A ham sandwich would be omitted because ham contains sodium.
    4 Tuna salad would be omitted because tuna is found in salt water.
186. Knowledge, planning, physiologic (a)
    2 Carbohydrates provide fuel or energy for the body and should be increased when one has a temperature.
    1 Protein rebuilds and repairs body cells.
    3 Fats provide the padding for the vital organs.
    4 Fats insulate the body and help to control temperature.
187. Knowledge, evaluation, health (a)
    4 Vitamin A, vitamin K, and vitamin E are the fat-soluble vitamins. It is important for the nurse to identify these vitamins because it is possible for the patient to consume too much of these vitamins.
    1 Vitamin C and vitamin B_{12} are water-soluble vitamins. It is difficult to consume too much of these because they are excreted.
    2 Vitamin B_{12} and biotin are water soluble.
    3 Vitamin B_6 and folic acid are water soluble.
188. Knowledge, implementation, health (a)
    2 The complete proteins contain the eight essential amino acids required for growth and development.
    1, 3, 4 These foods provide incomplete protein.
189. Knowledge, implementation, health (a)
    4 This is the recommended procedure to prevent contamination of the vulvar area from organisms around the anal area. It is also recommended after bowel movements to avoid fecal contamination of the vulvar area.
    1 This may prove helpful for a time, but it is not sufficient to avoid further contamination over time.
    2 The situation does not indicate antibiotics were administered. In any case such advice is incorrect because antibiotics must be taken as ordered over a specified period of time, even after symptoms have subsided.
    3 Cranberry juice has no direct effect on bacteria. In any case, drinking only cranberry juice would not be a likely order.
190. Knowledge, assessment, physiologic (a)
    3 Head circumference should be checked until a child is 3 years old.
    1 Blood pressure is usually not checked until after 3 years of age.
    2 15 Months old is too young to include blood pressure.
    4 15 Months old is too young to do an oral temperature reading. Axillary, rectal, or tympanic readings are appropriate.
191. Comprehension, evaluation, environment (c)
    2 Valvular heart damage, especially mitral valve disease, is common following rheumatic fever.
    1, 3 These do not usually occur.
    4 There is no paralysis with this condition.
192. Knowledge, assessment, physiologic (b)
    4 The pathology of rheumatic fever is not clearly understood, but the disease tends to follow a recent infection with the beta-hemolytic *Streptococcus*.
    1 Virus is not a cause.
    2, 3 These are not applicable.

193. Comprehension, planning, physiologic (b)
    3 Aspirin is used for rheumatic fever primarily to relieve joint pain, inflammation, and fever.
    1 If carditis develops, corticosteroids are added to drug therapy.
    2 Aspirin is not used for this condition.
    4 Aspirin is not an antiemetic.

194. Comprehension, planning, environment (a)
    4 During the acute stage, the patient is on complete bed rest and must be turned.
    1 He needs a bed bath, not a shower.
    2 He should not be allowed to walk.
    3 This is not applicable to the situation.

195. Application, implementation, physiologic (c)
    1 Although cardiac catheterization usually has no complications, there can be some danger. The nurse should assess the catheter insertion site for bleeding or hematoma.
    2 The patient's peripheral pulses are checked every 15 minutes for an hour after the test and frequently after that for several hours. Monitoring must be more frequent than every 2 hours.
    3 Some physicians keep the patient in bed for the rest of the day. Place the child in a reclining position for several hours after the cardiac catheterization to avoid a drop in blood pressure and bleeding at the catheter insertion site.
    4 This should have been done preoperatively. The patient has returned to his room and requires postoperative assessment.

196. Application, implementation, environment (c)
    4 $\dfrac{60}{60} \times \dfrac{20}{1} = \dfrac{1}{1} \times \dfrac{20}{1} = 20$ drops/min
    1, 2, 3 These are incorrect calculations.

197. Knowledge, assessment, physiologic (b)
    4 The clinical signs and symptoms given indicate patent ductus arterious.
    1 Aortic stenosis is rarely symptomatic during infancy. In severe cases the infant will have decreased cardiac output. Older children will have chest pain, shortness of breath, and dyspnea.
    2 In pulmonary stenosis, the child is generally asymptomatic but may have decreased exercise tolerance and dyspnea and cyanosis with severe obstruction.
    3 In childhood, coarctation of the aorta is usually asymptomatic, and growth and development are normal.

198. Knowledge, assessment, physiologic (b)
    3 Patent ductus arteriosus (PDA) is an opening between the pulmonary artery and the aorta caused by failure of the fetal ductus arteriosus to close after birth.
    1 Atrial septal defect (ASD) is an abnormal opening in the septum between the left atrium and right atrium.
    2 Ventricular septal defect (VSD) is an abnormal opening in the septum between the right and left ventricles.
    4 This is anomalous venous return, in which oxygenated blood returning from the lungs is carried abnormally to the right side of the heart by one or more pulmonary veins into the right atrium.

199. Comprehension, planning, environment (a)
    3 The disease is considered a malignant neoplasm of the blood-forming organs; it is characterized by diffuse replacement of bone marrow with proliferating leukocyte precursors, and abnormal numbers and forms of immature white cells in circulation.
    1 Red blood cells and platelets are decreased; patients receive blood transfusions as part of their treatment.
    2 The opposite is true; weight loss, pallor, and fatigue are characteristic of the disease.
    4 The opposite is true; immature white blood cells are in circulation.

200. Knowledge, planning, physiologic (b)
    4 These, along with lethargy and fever, are all symptoms of the disease.
    1, 2 The white blood cell count is elevated in acute leukemia.
    3 The hemoglobin level is decreased in acute leukemia.

201. Application, evaluation, psychosocial (a)
    2 The nurse is allowing the child to express her feelings about dying. This response opens a line of communication.
    1 This response cuts the patient off from discussing her feelings.
    3 With this response, the child might think the nurse doesn't care.
    4 It is best not to avoid the issue; this response discourages the child from ventilating feelings.

202. Comprehension, planning, physiologic (c)
    1 In leukemia, the bone marrow is characterized by being hypercellular, lacking fat globules, and containing an increased number of immature white cells.
    2 Gastric analysis helps to determine some stomach conditions; it is not diagnostic for leukemia.
    3 ABGs determine oxygen needs and acid base balance; they are not diagnostic for leukemia.
    4 The cardiac echogram helps diagnose heart conditions; it is not diagnostic for leukemia.

203. Knowledge, planning, environment (a)
    3 Painful joints are a common symptom often relieved by bed rest. Exacerbated joint pain may be severe, especially in advanced stages.
    1 There is no cyanosis present.
    2, 4 These are not related to the situation.

204. Comprehension, assessment, physiologic (c)
    3 As leukemia progresses, membranes of the anal area tend to ulcerate and bleed.
    1 This is not applicable.
    2 Leukemia patients' skin is usually pale lemon-yellow.
    4 This is seen more commonly in heart or respiratory disease.

205. Knowledge, planning, physiologic (c)
    2 The combination of drugs helps induce remissions that may last for weeks, months, or even years.
    1 These drugs do not have analgesic actions.
    3 These are not antibiotics.
    4 This is not applicable.

206. Comprehension, assessment, physiologic (b)
    1 Petechiae, fever, weight loss, pallor, hemorrhages, and bone and joint pain are also symptoms due to accumulation of white cells in the bone marrow.
    2 Bleeding is not within the GI tract; it occurs under the skin. Nausea and vomiting are not usual symptoms.
    3 Fever does occur, but there is usually no accompanying rash or itchy skin.
    4 There is bleeding under the skin but not in the gastrointestinal tract. There is no rash.

207. Application, implementation, psychosocial (b)
   1 It is important for the nurse to be honest and truthful, and to explain procedures and answer questions as they come up.
   2, 3 These concerns may occur and can be handled better if her coping ability is developed.
   4 This is important but not a priority at this time; this is not the best response.

208. Comprehension, planning, health (b)
   4 These provide infection control and blood replacement for lost red blood cells and platelets.
   1 Once diagnosis is made and treatment is started, weight loss will stabilize.
   2 Weight loss is not a result of edema.
   3 Home care is not really necessary because the child is not home-bound in the early stages.

209. Knowledge, planning, physiologic (b)
   1 The pituitary gland is also called the hypophysis; therefore, the term for removal of the pituitary gland is hypophysectomy.
   2 This is the term for removal of the thyroid gland.
   3 This is the term for removal of the parathyroid glands.
   4 This is the term for removal of the adrenal gland.

210. Knowledge, implementation, health (b)
   2 The anterior pituitary gland produces the growth hormone, thyroid-stimulating hormone, adrenocorticotropic hormone, melanocyte-stimulating hormone, follicle-stimulating hormone, luteinizing hormone, interstitial cell–stimulating hormone, and prolactin.
   1 The thyroid gland produces thyroxin, triiodothyronine, and thyrocalcitonin.
   3 The posterior pituitary gland produces oxytocin and the antidiuretic hormone.
   4 The adrenal medulla produces adrenaline (epinephrine) and aldosterone.

211. Comprehension, assessment, physiologic (c)
   1 These are complications with removal of the anterior pituitary gland because of the other hormones produced by the gland.
   2 These complications should be observed with a thyroidectomy.
   3 These are complications that occur in diabetes mellitus.
   4 These are complications that occur with an adrenalectomy.

212. Comprehension, planning, health (b)
   3 Exchange lists for fast-food restaurants are available and enable the adolescent to be like his peers when eating out.
   1 This is an unrealistic expectation because adolescents do not want to be noticeably different from their peers. Lettuce-and-tomato salads should also be counted on the diabetic exchange list.
   2 A stable blood glucose level is desired. Varied fluctuations can lead to complications.
   4 Eating anything and ignoring the effects on blood glucose levels can lead to complications.

213. Comprehension, evaluation, physiologic (b)
   3 Short-acting insulin is always removed from the vial before long acting NPH to prevent displacing the short-acting into the long-acting insulin bottle, which would affect the onset, peak, and duration.
   1 Insulin is always refrigerated to prevent the breakdown of the medication.
   2 Vial is rotated gently to prevent the breakdown of the medication.
   4 Sites should be rotated to maintain proper absorption and prevent a complication known as lipodystrophy.

214. Knowledge, planning, physiologic (c)
   2 Hyperglycemia causes the red cells to clump easier and become more rigid. Therefore, the cells become trapped in the spleen.
   1 Hypoglycemia decreases the erythrocytes' affinity for oxygen through glycosolization.
   3 Elevated potassium levels will cause hypoglycemia.
   4 Lowered sodium levels do not affect cell morphology.

215. Comprehension, evaluation, physiologic (c)
   4 Consuming regularly scheduled meals is the best way to maintain serum glucose levels.
   1 An available glucose source is important but is needed only if a reaction occurs; it is not preventative.
   2 Increasing caloric intake is a prevention strategy, but maintaining glucose levels through proper nutrition throughout the day is of greater importance.
   3 When dietary intake is appropriate, risk of hypoglycemic episode is greatly decreased.

216. Application, planning, health (c)
   2 He should have a snack with him when he is driving in case he begins to feel hypoglycemic. This is a safety measure.
   1 If he understands that he needs to have a snack with him, there is no reason why he cannot drive.
   3 There is no reason to have another driver with him.
   4 A driver's license will be issued; however, his diabetes should be noted on the back of the license.

217. Comprehension, implementation, health (b)
   1 This syndrome is a metabolic defect precipitated by the ingestion of rye or wheat gluten.
   2, 3, 4 Lean meats, vegetables, and fruits are not contraindicated.

218. Knowledge, assessment, health (a)
   3 A soft diet of low-fiber, low-residue, bland foods that have a high protein and caloric content is ordered for patients with Crohn's disease.
   1 A full-liquid diet consists of only liquids and foods that liquefy at body temperature. There is no residue or fiber in this diet, which is usually ordered for patients unable to consume soft or semifluid foods after surgery.
   2 A clear liquid diet supplies fluids and provides minimal residue. The diet is nutritionally inadequate and is usually prescribed for a limited amount of time, such as 1 day, following surgery. Proteins are needed more than potassium.
   4 A soft diet is okay, but high-fiber foods are not permitted.

219. Knowledge, assessment, physiologic (a)
   2 These symptoms are commonly associated with UTI.
   1 This is not related to UTI.
   3 Urinary retention, not polyuria, is common.
   4 This is not usually seen unless UTI is well advanced.

220. Comprehension, planning, physiologic (c)
   4 Protein is usually limited in kidney disorders, but it is needed for replacement of urinary protein loss.
   1 Sodium and increased fluids tend to retain fluids in tissues.
   2 Protein is needed to maintain blood albumin levels.
   3 These are not relative to the situation.

221. Comprehension, assessment, physiologic (b)
   2 The urine reveals large amounts of proteinuria; blood is not usually present.
   1 No hematuria is revealed.
   3 This is not significant in this case.
   4 Albuminuria is abnormal in this case.

222. Comprehension, assessment, physiologic (b)
    1 Edema is the prime symptom of nephrosis. It may be so severe that the child reaches twice his normal weight.
    2 Proteinuria, not hematuria, is present.
    3 Petechial rash is not associated with this disease.
    4 This is not a prime symptom.

223. Comprehension, planning, physiologic (b)
    2 Immobilization of the recipient site prevents the possibility of dislodging the graft and destroying the tissue-building process.
    1, 3, 4 These actions do not necessarily facilitate acceptance of the graft.

224. Comprehension, planning, environment (b)
    1 During long periods of immobilization, calcium from bones and other tissues enters the circulatory system to be filtered and excreted by the kidneys; increased levels of calcium and urinary stasis in the renal pelvis predispose the child to renal calculi.
    2, 3, 4 These are inappropriate responses; these are not relevant to the situation.

225. Knowledge, assessment, physiologic (a)
    2 Second-degree burns are blistered and red. The patient has severe pain with these burns.
    1 First-degree burns do not blister.
    3 Third-degree burns appear as charred, black skin. Because the nerve endings are involved there is not as much pain as with a second-degree burn.
    4 Fourth-degree burns involve the skin and nerves completely through to the bone. These burns are very difficult to heal.

226. Comprehension, implementation, environment (a)
    2 To administer 20 mg of meperidine (Demerol) elixir, the nurse would convert the teaspoon measurement to milliliters and give 2 ml.
    1 Incorrect dose; too little.
    3, 4 Incorrect doses; too much.

227. Comprehension, evaluation, physiologic (b)
    1 This is the most likely choice since everyone in the family must be treated in order to prevent the child from becoming infected again.
    2 If used correctly the treatment would get rid of the infestation, but if the rest of the family is still infested, then the child will become reinfected.
    3 Infestations are not caused by lack of cleanliness; they are caused by contact with an infected person.
    4 There is no evidence of allergic reaction.

228. Knowledge, assessment, health (a)
    1 Ringworm is caused by a fungus and can occur on the scalp (tinea capitis), body (tinea corporis), or feet (tinea pedis).
    2 Pediculosis is an infestation of lice.
    3 Herpes is caused by a virus.
    4 Urticaria is more commonly known as hives, often caused by allergies to foods and animal furs.

229. Knowledge, assessment, physiologic (a)
    4 *Microsporum audouinii* is the major fungal pathogen that causes tinea capitis (ringworm of the scalp).
    1 A virus is a minute microorganism that can replicate only within a cell of a living plant or animal; it is not a fungus.
    2 This is a genus of aerobic, gram-positive, spore-producing bacteria in the family Bacillaceae; it is not a fungus.
    3 Bacteria are any of the small unicellular microorganisms of the class Schizomycetes; bacteria are not a fungus.

230. Application, implementation, physiologic (a)
    3 Keeping the skin clean and dry aids in the prevention of infection.
    1 The child's position should be changed frequently to avoid constant pressure to one area as well as severe itching.
    2 To reduce itching and subsequent scratching, a minimal amount of clothing is recommended.
    4 Warm, moist dressings would increase the itching; cool moist dressings should be used.

231. Knowledge, assessment, environment (b)
    3 Eczema occurs more commonly in winter months and tends to run in families.
    1 Impetigo is an infectious disease of the superficial layers of the skin; it is seen in infants and is caused by staphylococci.
    2 This is an abnormal chronic inflammatory disease of the sebaceous glands and hair follicles. It affects 90% of all adolescents in varying degrees.
    4 Dysplasia is an abnormal development of tissue.

232. Knowledge, planning, environment (b)
    1 The nurse should be knowledgeable of the type and purpose of traction to plan nursing care.
    2 The nurse must know more than function only.
    3 The nurse needs more information than this alone.
    4 The age of the patient is important to know in providing appropriate care.

233. Application, implementation, environment (a)
    2 Ropes, pulleys, and weights are equally important in maintaining correct traction.
    1 Weights set on the floor will defeat the purpose of pulling or tension.
    3 This is not applicable.
    4 The nurse should adjust the bed as necessary but should also maintain proper alignment and weight.

234. Application, implementation, physiologic (b)
    1 The nurse should check the skin condition for breakdown resulting from complete bed rest and limited movement.
    2 The nurse might check the left leg, but the right leg is affected.
    3 The child should have some kind of activity in bed to prevent complications.
    4 Although important, the mother's reaction is not included in the assessment.

235. Application, planning, physiologic (b)
    4 The nurse should encourage activity in bed to prevent complications such as calcification and atrophy during bed rest.
    1 The nurse should encourage activity; see No. 4.
    2 The nurse does not do this routinely or without an order.
    3 Not necessarily every 2 hours.

236. Knowledge, planning, environment (a)
    4 Alignment and immobilization allow the limb to heal.
    1 The fracture does not heal immediately.
    2 It is difficult to keep a child in bed without a reason.
    3 This is not necessarily true.

237. Comprehension, assessment, physiologic (b)
    1 Neurovascular assessment should be done in addition to an assessment of the musculoskeletal areas.
    2 Touch and wetness will not provide information about the extent of injury to the nerves or blood vessels.
    3 Sensation and ability to move the injured part are important, but touch is not.
    4 Stiffness and wetness are not part of an assessment that examines musculoskeletal and neurovascular injuries.

238. Comprehension, implementation, environment (a)
    1 Swelling and edema of the injured limb may increase after application of a cast; tightness of the cast should be determined to ensure that pressure areas that may constrict circulation are not present.
    2, 3, 4 These are definitely inappropriate statements and nursing actions.
239. Application, assessment, environment (c)
    1 The fact that the patient is a minor means parental consent must be obtained before treatment can be given.
    2 It would be more helpful to know what happened to the arm when wrestling.
    3 He felt, not heard, a snapping.
    4 It is the physician's responsibility to determine the diagnosis.
240. Comprehension, evaluation, psychosocial (b)
    4 This response informs the grandmother that bed-wetting is normal in children his age and that hospitalized children frequently regress into some behaviors that would not normally be seen at home.
    1, 2, 3 These are inappropriate nursing responses.
241. Knowledge, planning, physiologic (a)
    1 This is the definition of the term; scoliosis of the spine occurs because of rapid growth and is most often noted in girls.
    2 This is a disease of the kidneys, causing edema and proteinuria.
    3 This is a concave curvature of the spine, commonly known as swayback.
    4 This is a convex curvature of the spine, commonly known as hunchback.
242. Comprehension, evaluation, physiologic (b)
    4 The child attempts to maintain balance and an erect posture, resulting in a compensatory curve.
    1 Pain is rare in children with scoliosis, although some children experience chronic discomfort from continually sitting on their buttocks.
    2 If the deformity is uncorrected, it will result in respiratory compromise.
    3 Detection is simple by visual examination of the spine as the child bends from the waist.
243. Comprehension, assessment, physiologic (b)
    2 Changes in motion or sensation in the extremities are the most reliable determination of the presence of edema of the spinal cord; edema causes trauma to motor and sensory nerves.
    1, 3, 4 These are symptoms of autonomic dysreflexia.
244. Comprehension, planning, physiologic (b)
    1 Autonomic dysreflexia is common in such patients and is characterized by a sudden elevation in blood pressure, headache, chills, and pallor. Elevating the head of the bed 45 degrees or helping the patient to sit up usually remedies the situation automatically.
    2, 3, 4 These actions would not resolve the situation.
245. Knowledge, implementation, physiologic (a)
    2 Decadron prevents and alleviates spinal cord edema. It is administered by local injection, and it has a rapid onset and long duration.
    1 This drug is a systemic corticosteroid.
    3, 4 These drugs are diuretics.
246. Knowledge, planning, health (a)
    1 Cranberry juice promotes acidic urine and cuts down on stone formation.
    2, 3 These can possibly lead to stone formation as a result of acids found in these foods.
    4 Milk can possibly lead to stone formation as a result of calcium found in this food.

247. Comprehension, planning, environment (b)
    2 Addiction to narcotics can develop in a short time. Other measures must first be tried to alleviate pain caused by long-term problems.
    1, 3, 4 These are not relevant to the question asked.
248. Comprehension, assessment, physiologic (c)
    4 The traumatic episode produces psychotic-type behavior.
    1 It is a misconception that mental illness occurs.
    2 This is a violent jarring or shaking of the brain caused by a sudden change in momentum of the head.
    3 Negative symptomatology *is* related to the extent of organic damage.
249. Knowledge, planning, environment (b)
    3 This is the correct definition of an omphalocele.
    1 This is a displacement of some of the abdominal organs through an opening in the diaphragm into the chest cavity.
    2 This is a displacement of part of the intestine through an incomplete closure at the fetal end of the umbilical cord.
    4 This defines a condition in which the esophagus ends in a blind pouch and the lower end of the esophagus attaches to the trachea.
250. Comprehension, implementation, psychosocial (a)
    3 Parent child bonding can be impeded by separation of the ill neonate from the parents. The bonding process can be encouraged by allowing the parents to touch, hold, and talk to their infant. The infant receiving proper stimulation will thrive more quickly than one deprived of such stimulation.
    1 There is also the need to touch and hold as stated above.
    2 The nurse should explain the process, but the parents should start as soon as possible.
    4 This is an inappropriate nursing action; allowing parents to verbalize feelings will facilitate the parent-child relationship.
251. Comprehension, implementation, physiologic (b)
    1 Projectile vomiting is the result of increased intracranial pressure; the infant should be fed small frequent meals to decrease the possibility of aspiration of the feeding. The hydrocephalic head must be supported to prevent trauma to the neck from the weight of the head.
    2, 3 These are inappropriate means of feeding this infant.
    4 This is not usually necessary.
252. Comprehension, planning, physiologic (b)
    3 The postoperative position of the head is on the nonoperative side to prevent fluid and brain shift, which would traumatize the operative area of the brain.
    1 Incorrect position; this would traumatize the operative area of the brain.
    2, 4 These are not appropriate for the situation.
253. Application, implementation, psychosocial (b)
    3 The head circumference provides data to determine change over a period of time.
    1, 2 These responses may cause great concern for the mother.
    4 This is an inappropriate and nasty response by the nurse.
254. Comprehension, assessment, environment (a)
    3 Minor movements such as twitching of eyelids or face, lip smacking, and slight hand movements are commonly observed in absence (petit mal) seizures.
    1 This is common to the tonic phase of the tonic-clonic (grand mal) seizure.
    2 This is common to the clonic phase of the tonic-clonic (grand mal) seizure.
    4 This can occur during the clonic phase of the tonic-clonic (grand mal) seizure as a result of muscle relaxation; there may also be incontinence of feces.

255. Knowledge, planning, physiologic (b)
  4 Phenytoin, more commonly known as Dilantin, is classified as an anticonvulsant.
  1 Tagamet is used in treatment of gastritis. It is the trade name for a histamine H_2 receptor antagonist (cimetidine).
  2 Hydroxyzine is a short-acting central nervous system depressant. It is a minor tranquilizer known as Vistaril.
  3 Compazine is a trade name for a phenothiazine, prochlorperazine, used as an antiemetic and antipsychotic.

256. Comprehension, evaluation, physiologic (b)
  3 This is a common side effect of this medication.
  1 No photosensitivity is noted with phenytoin.
  2 Iron discolors teeth.
  4 The medication may cause drowsiness.

257. Comprehension, assessment, psychosocial (b)
  2 Giving the mother the opportunity to expand upon her concerns can clarify misconceptions. Frequently patients think that the probes to the scalp will give them shocks. She obviously has a lack of knowledge about an electroencephalogram. The nurse can tell her that the procedure is not painful and is noninvasive.
  1 This is a prying and assuming answer. The mother did not state where she got her information or even if it is false. It also calls for a yes or no answer.
  3 This calls for a yes or no answer and does not permit an opportunity for the mother to discuss her concerns.
  4 This reply is true but does nothing to assist the mother in calming her concerns. The mother has made up her mind and unless she has more information concerning the test, she is not going to consent to the EEG.

258. Application, implementation, physiologic (b)
  3 Pillows are used for patient safety.
  1 The patient should not be moved during the seizure.
  2, 4 These should not be attempted during the seizure.

259. Comprehension, evaluation, psychosocial (c)
  2 The goal is to allow him to be as independent as possible in those areas in which independence can be achieved.
  1 This does not allow for individuality and growth.
  3 This is an inappropriate response; a study does not assist in the development of family relationships.
  4 This does not encourage him to grow and develop to his full potential; it may hinder his move to become independent.

260. Comprehension, planning, health (b)
  1 These programs will ensure that educational and social needs will be met, including emotional aspects related to those needs.
  2 This is not a specific enough response.
  3 This is not the most inclusive plan for overall management of care.
  4 The focus needs to be goal-oriented.

261. Comprehension, planning, environment (b)
  1 Seizures for whatever reason are a major nursing concern and occur whenever there is damage to the motor centers of the brain.
  2, 3 Muscle tone can either be increased or decreased, depending on the nature and distribution of neuromuscular dysfunction.
  4 While sensory impairments, hearing loss, and/or abnormalities of vision are important, they are not life-threatening.

262. Knowledge, planning, physiologic (a)
  2 Cerebral palsy is trauma to the motor centers of the brain.
  1 It is not caused by premature birth alone; a variety of prenatal, perinatal, and postnatal factors contribute to the cause of this condition.
  3 Genetics play no part in cerebral damage.
  4 Erythroblastosis fetalis is a type of hemolytic anemia that occurs in newborns as a result of maternal-fetal blood group incompatibility, specifically involving the Rh factor and the ABO blood groups.

263. Application, implementation, environment (b)
  3 The flow of formula should be well-paced with no pressure and with a water flush to prevent clogging.
  1 Forced pressure can cause damage.
  2 Discarding the formula decreases the amount of nourishment and fluid received.
  4 Gastrostomy tubes are permanently in place.

264. Application, implementation, environment (b)
  3 The young child is placed in a sitting position with the neck flexed to separate the spinous processes and thus ease insertion of the needle. While in this position the child must be observed for breathing difficulties from poor lung expansion.
  1, 4 Inappropriate nursing actions; incorrect position.
  2 Inappropriate nursing action; this is not a routine part of the procedure.

265. Comprehension, planning, physiologic (b)
  1 These are the most common symptoms of the disease, including severe headache and pain.
  2 Dyspnea and high blood pressure are not common to the disease.
  3, 4 Red, raised rash is not common to the disease.

266. Application, implementation, environment (a)
  4 Direct pressure applied for 1 to 2 minutes will control the bleeding.
  1 This is not an immediate action.
  2, 3 These are not relevant to the situation.

267. Comprehension, planning, environment (b)
  2 Bacterial infections treated with antibiotics for 24 hours are not considered communicable.
  1, 4 These are incorrect and not necessary; see response No. 2.
  3 This is only one of the primary concerns.

268. Comprehension, assessment, physiologic (b)
  3 Periodic comparative observations are made to note differences in vital signs, neurologic status, and renal function; accurate intake and output measurements are essential to determine fluid replacement needs and to detect cerebral edema.
  1 These are general observations that are routine when caring for an infant with an IV infusion.
  2, 4 These are abnormal signs and should be reported; however, these are not specific only to the care of this infant.

269. Application, implementation, environment (a)
  1 Maintenance and care of the IV site are of primary importance in caring for the child with meningitis who receives medication intravenously. The long-term fluid and antibiotic therapy increases the child's susceptibility to phlebitis and fluid infiltration at the site.
  2 This is an incorrect procedure; see above response.
  3, 4 These are not necessary.

270. Application, implementation, environment (b)
    4 Time and description of the seizure are important.
    1 This is true, but only after the seizure has passed.
    2 Protection is important, but restraint could lead to severe injury.
    3 This could lead to injury of the child's mouth, especially after the seizure has started; this action is no longer recommended.
271. Comprehension, planning, physiologic (b)
    4 Cool humidified air helps to relieve the respiratory distress; syrup of ipecac may be ordered to induce vomiting, which often produces some relief of respiratory distress.
    1 Antibiotics are not used for croup; this disease is usually of viral origin; cool humidified air is used.
    2 Sedatives may produce increased respiratory distress.
    3 Antiemetics are not ordered for croup.
272. Comprehension, assessment, environment (c)
    1 Exocrine glands become obstructed as a result of thick mucoprotein.
    2 Fetal lungs usually develop normally but are later damaged by the thick tenacious secretions.
    3 Untreated upper respiratory infections do not lead to cystic fibrosis. This disease is genetically inherited.
    4 Cystic fibrosis is not caused by the use of antibiotics or the suppression of the immune system.
273. Comprehension, assessment, physiologic (c)
    4 With cystic fibrosis there is a decreased amount of pancreatic enzymes; therefore the intestines cannot absorb fats or proteins well.
    1 They should be able to eat all kinds of foods.
    2 Large, foul-smelling stools are a symptom of cystic fibrosis but are not a result of antibiotic intake.
    3 Continual vomiting is not a common symptom of cystic fibrosis.
274. Knowledge, implementation, physiologic (a)
    3 Undigested food, mainly unabsorbed fats and proteins, is excreted as a result of the lack of the digestive enzymes trypsin, chymotrypsin, amylase, and lipase. The lack of these enzymes is caused by obstruction of the pancreatic ducts.
    2 The disease process causes marked impairment in the digestion and absorption of nutrients, mainly fats and proteins and to a lesser degree carbohydrates; this is not the best answer.
    1 The chloride channel defect in the sweat glands prevents reabsorption of sodium and chloride; this does not affect stools.
    4 The impaired ability to absorb fats results in a deficiency of the fat-soluble vitamins A, D, E, and K; anemia is common; this does not affect stools.
275. Application, assessment, physiologic (c)
    2 Children with cystic fibrosis do not absorb the fat-soluble vitamins A, D, E, and K. The failure to absorb vitamin K leads to easily acquired bruises.
    1 There is no connection between a neurologic deficit and cystic fibrosis.
    3 There is no indication that the child has inadequate play supervision.
    4 Most children do not normally fall down and bruise easily.
276. Comprehension, assessment, physiologic (b)
    3 Intrinsic factors would be from internal causes, often triggered by respiratory infections.
    1 Injury to the nose is extrinsic, caused by external factors.
    2 Pollen from flowers is extrinsic, caused by external factors.
    4 Allergens in the environment are extrinsic, caused by external factors.

277. Comprehension, planning, physiologic (b)
    3 The head of the bed should be elevated, not kept flat, to facilitate breathing.
    1, 2, 4 These are common in the management and care of a child with asthma.
278. Application, evaluation, physiologic (c)
    2 Intercostal muscle retractions are considered accessory muscle use.
    1 Complaints of breathlessness indicate the problem is not being resolved.
    3 Increased respiratory rate indicates the problem may be worsening.
    4 Nasal flaring is another indicator of increased respiratory difficulty.
279. Application, planning, physiologic (b)
    2 Asthma is an obstructed airway disease caused by hypersensitivity to such agents as foods, animal fur, and pollens.
    1 Pneumonia is an acute inflammation of the lungs.
    3 Cystic fibrosis is a hereditary disease that affects the mucus-producing glands of the body.
    4 This is hay fever; it does not affect the bronchial tubes.
280. Application, implementation, environment (b)
    3 DD = 40 mg
    DH = 160 mg
    V = 1 tsp (5 ml)
    $$\frac{DD}{DH} = \frac{40}{160} \times 5\ ml = \tfrac{1}{4} \times 5\ ml = 1.25\ ml = \tfrac{1}{4}\ tsp$$
    1, 2, 4 These are not the correct dose.
281. Application, implementation, physiologic (c)
    1 This is done to prevent trauma to membranes as a result of suction from the catheter.
    2 Only the inner cannula is removed.
    3 The nurse should withdraw the catheter in a circular motion, rotating the catheter between thumb and forefinger to prevent unnecessary hypoxia.
    4 To prevent accidental dislodgment of tracheostomy, the ties are removed while someone holds the tube in place. Ties are removed only when cleansing, not when suctioning.
282. Knowledge, assessment, physiologic (a)
    2 This is a classical symptom of asthma and is caused by the trapping of air in the alveoli.
    1 Noisy and hoarse inspirations are commonly seen in croup.
    3, 4 These are not common symptoms of asthma.
283. Knowledge, implementation, physiologic (a)
    1 Adrenalin relieves most cases of acute bronchospasm.
    2 Adrenalin acts as a bronchodilator.
    3 Adrenalin increases cardiac output.
    4 Adrenalin does not stimulate constriction of the respiratory muscles.
284. Application, implementation, environment (c)
    3 A 25-gauge, ⅝-inch needle is used for subcutaneous injections.
    1 A 19-gauge, 1-inch needle is used for blood infusions.
    2 A 22-gauge, 1-inch needle is used for infants and children for intramuscular injections.
    4 A 27-gauge, ½-inch needle is used for insulin injections.
285. Knowledge, planning, environment (a)
    3 Pinkeye is also known as conjunctivitis; it is caused by bacterial or viral infection, allergy, or environmental factors.
    1 Degeneration does not occur.
    2 Pinkeye does not involve the lacrimal sac.
    4 This is a cataract.

286. Knowledge, implementation, physiologic (b)
    4 Choice of treatment depends on the causative agent, which may include antibacterial agents, antibiotics, or corticosteroids.
    1 This has no effect on the conjunctiva; it constricts the pupils.
    2 This has no effect on the conjunctiva; it burns localized tears.
    3 This has no effects on conjunctivitis.

287. Comprehension, implementation, health (b)
    1 The nurse should clear away the crusting from the inner aspect of the eye outward so as not to cross-contaminate the eye with the infection.
    2 This method cross-contaminates the eye with the infected material on the cotton ball.
    3 Removal of the crusted material is necessary for the maximum effect of the antibiotic.
    4 Hydrogen peroxide should not be used in the eyes.

288. Application, implementation, health (b)
    4 Follow orders given by the physician, including the 5 days thereafter to ensure that there is no further bacterial infection.
    1, 2 These options give no consideration to the effect of the medication on the infection.
    3 This response gives no guidance to the mother.

289. Comprehension, assessment, physiologic (b)
    4 In infants and children the eustachian tube is relatively short and straight, allowing pathogens easy access from the pharynx to the middle ear.
    1 This is true only if a blow to the ear is severe enough to rupture the tympanic membrane, allowing microbes to enter the middle ear.
    2 The intact tympanic membrane keeps pathogens in the external ear from entering the middle ear.
    3 A myringotomy is a surgical incision of the tympanic membrane; the surgery is performed to relieve pressure caused by otitis media.

290. Comprehension, planning, physiologic (c)
    2 The principal complication is loss of hearing from a variety of reasons (negative middle ear pressure, effusion in the middle ear, structural damage to the tympanic membrane); the most dreaded result of the hearing loss is the effect this loss has on speech and language development as well as on cognitive abilities.
    1 This is not a complication of this condition.
    3 This is not relevant to the situation; mastoiditis, infection of the mastoid sinus, is rare but possible.
    4 This is not relevant to this situation.

291. Comprehension, implementation, environment (a)
    2 Lying on the affected side facilitates drainage of the exudate, thus decreasing pressure buildup and promoting comfort.
    1, 3 These are not the preferred positions; see above response.
    4 Positioning on the unaffected side will not facilitate drainage; discomfort is likely to increase as a result of buildup of pressure.

292. Knowledge, implementation, health (b)
    4 This is the best response. Watching the baby and assessing whether the medicine is working is standard nursing practice.
    1 Nothing in life is ever sure, and this response is falsely assuring the mother and casting doubt in her mind.
    2 This is false assurance to a new mother and adds to her anxiety level.
    3 The nurse is suggesting that the medicine may not work, and offering to call a minister could unduly alarm a new mother.

293. Knowledge, evaluation, health (b)
    1 Chicken pox involves no serious complications. Some lesions, if scratched, may become infected.
    2 Hearing is not impaired.
    3 Eyesight is not affected.
    4 The muscular system is not involved in chicken pox.

294. Knowledge, evaluation, health (c)
    1 The exact contagious stage is not completely defined, but mumps is considered contagious until all swelling is gone.
    2 No rash is involved.
    3 The fever will subside before swelling does.
    4 Mumps is considered contagious from 1 to 2 days before onset of symptoms until swelling completely disappears.

295. Comprehension, planning, environment (a)
    1 Orchitis is an inflammation of one or both of the testes, characterized by swelling and pain, often caused by mumps, syphilis, or tuberculosis; it is the most common complication of mumps in teenage and adult males.
    2 Meningitis is an infection or inflammation of the membranes covering the brain and spinal cord; this is not a common complication of mumps.
    3 Myositis is an inflammation of muscle tissue, usually of the voluntary muscles, caused by infection, trauma, or infestation by parasites; this is not a common complication of mumps.
    4 Pyelonephritis is a diffuse pyogenic (pus-producing) infection of the pelvis and parenchyma of the kidney; this is not a common complication of mumps.

296. Knowledge, planning, environment (a)
    2 HIV or human immunodeficiency virus type I is the official name for the virus.
    1 CMV is a member of a group of large species-specific herpes-type viruses that produce a wide variety of disease effects.
    3 This is a virus that is the cause of common warts of the hands and feet, as well as lesions of the mucous membranes of the oral, anal, and genital cavities.
    4 Any of the five related viruses including herpes simplex type 1 and type 2, varicella zoster virus, Epstein-Barr virus, and cytomegalovirus.

297. Knowledge, implementation, health (b)
    1 Kaposi's sarcoma is the correct answer. In the past this cancer was rare and was associated mainly with certain ethnic groups. This form of cancer now occurs in many cases of AIDS and other immune deficiencies.
    2 Malignant melanomas are the fastest rising cancers in the United States. They develop from pigmented nevi (moles) to become a dark, spreading lesion.
    3 Basal cell carcinoma usually occurs on the upper face. It usually begins as papules that erode in the center to form a bleeding and crusted crater.
    4 Squamous cell carcinoma is a slow-growing tumor of the epidermis. It is the most common type. The lesions are hard, painless, and raised nodules.

298. Application, evaluation, physiologic (b)
    3 Medication should be given early in the day so as to not keep the child awake during evening and night hours.
    1, 2, 4 These are all true statements.

299. Comprehension, implementation, physiologic (b)
2 After five thrusts the patient's mouth should be opened and checked. If the object is visualized, a finger sweep is performed to remove it. A blind finger sweep should never be performed on a child.
1 After five thrusts the mouth check should be done, followed by five more thrusts.
3 This technique would require a blind finger sweep, which could push the object back down into the trachea.
4 Blowing into the child's mouth will cause the object to be lodged further down into the trachea or bronchus. This should be used only as a last resort.

300. Comprehension, implementation, health (b)
3 Lyme disease is caused by ticks. It is important to avoid tick infested areas and to wear long pants and a long-sleeve shirt to protect skin.
1 There is no vaccine for Lyme disease.
2 Contaminated water does not transmit Lyme disease.
4 Lyme disease is treated with tetracycline, not corticosteroids.

301. Comprehension, assessment, physiologic (c)
2 Clinical signs of severe dehydration include tachycardia (rapid, thready pulse), dry skin and mucous membranes, sunken fontanel, delayed capillary filling time, poor skin elasticity, and coolness and mottling of extremities (signs of circulatory collapse).
1 Blood pressure is low, not elevated, in severe dehydration; see response No. 2.
3 Pulse is rapid and thready, not slow; see response No. 2.
4 As the body's compensatory mechanisms take over to adjust to fluid losses, circulation is compromised and blood pressure falls, eventually resulting in metabolic acidosis. The body attempts to compensate via the respiratory system; therefore, respirations are deep and rapid (Kussmaul breathing). See response No. 2.

302. Application, implementation, physiologic (b)
3 Thermoregulation remains unstable for many months. If the patient is exposed to heat, another heat stroke may occur.
1 Hats retain body heat. Instructing him to wear one would increase the risk of heat stroke.
2 Heat stroke is caused by poor heat dissipation and loss of fluids and electrolytes. Water alone will not prevent recurrence.
4 Because thermoregulatory mechanisms are unstable, it would be better to advise the patient to avoid strenuous exercise.

303. Comprehension, planning, physiologic (c)
4 Alcohol addiction is preventable; nurses can be instrumental in recognizing the symptoms and planning effective counseling for mothers and babies in these situations.
1 "Failure to thrive" babies are not usually hyperactive and have a starved look about them—sunken eyes, large head, and very thin body (they lack body fat).
2 Genetic or hereditary defects are identifiable by chromosomal and/or genetic workup and are usually identifiable through laboratory analysis and counseling.
3 Symptoms are the same as in No. 4, except that one would not find the altered facial features.

304. Knowledge, assessment, health (b)
2 This is a true statement.
1 Child abuse includes both physical and emotional abuse.
3 Child abuse has been noted on all socioeconomic levels, yet studies do indicate that it is more common in the lower socioeconomic class.
4 Studies indicate that many times, but not always, the abused child has congenital deformities, a chronic illness, or other problems that in general are more difficult for the parents to manage.

305. Application, implementation, physiologic (b)
1 The child's safety is most important, so the nurse must report her suspicions to the proper authorities.
2 This will make the parents defensive.
3 All the social worker could do is refer them to the authorities.
4 This is important, but reporting takes priority.

306. Application, implementation, environment (c)
1 Abandonment consists of leaving the patient for any reason when the patient's condition is contingent on the presence of the caregiver.
2 Malpractice is any professional misconduct or unreasonable lack of skill. Although this could also be a ramification of the described action, the abandonment charge would be more likely.
3 The borrowed servant rule involves the physician's liability when the nurse does something wrong.
4 Respondeat Superior involves the responsibility of the hospital or institution when an employee does something wrong.

307. Comprehension, evaluation, environment (b)
2 Oxygen flow cannot be changed without consulting a physician.
1 Oxygen supports combustion. Excess heat or flame can result in an explosion.
3 The oxygen-dependent infant cannot tolerate sudden periods of time without oxygen.
4 Infants are nose breathers. If nasal passages are obstructed, oxygen cannot enter the airway as easily.

308. Comprehension, implementation, physiologic (b)
1 This position will prevent purulent material from collecting on the diaphragm, which could lead to formation of an abscess.
2 It is true that this position may decrease stress on the suture line, but this is secondary to the physiological rationale.
3 Although an upright position may help prevent aspiration in case of vomiting, the primary reason for this position is to prevent abscess formation.
4 Semi-Fowler's position alone will not prevent respiratory complications; other nursing measures will be needed to encourage deep breathing.

309. Application, implementation, physiologic (a)
4 Tepid water will cool the patient by evaporation. This mimics the body's cooling mechanism of sweating.
1 Sipping ice water will only temporarily cool the buccal surfaces of the mouth. It will not affect the core temperature.
2 Cold compresses may only cool a localized area temporarily.
3 Refrigerated alcohol may induce shivering and actually cause an increase in core temperature.

310. Knowledge, planning, environment (b)
    4 The site is basically free of major blood vessels and nerves; this is a large muscle with well-defined landmarks for safe administration. It is easily accessible from a variety of positions.
    1 The deltoid muscle can be used for small amounts of fluid; it is a small muscle close to the axillary and radial nerves; it is not a preferred site.
    2 This site can be used, but it is not preferred because it is composed of thick subcutaneous fat and thus increases the possibility of injecting into subcutaneous tissue rather than into muscle. In this way it can also increase danger of sciatic nerve injury.
    3 This is the preferred intramuscular site for infants.
311. Comprehension, implementation, health (b)
    4 Using the actual equipment or a replica can eliminate anxiety and help the child understand what will happen. This can help the child become familiar with the equipment.
    1 A 5-year-old child is capable of some reasoning but can concentrate on only one aspect of a situation at a time.
    2 This should be done, but the child may not be ready for complex situations or materials.
    3 This can be done, but in this situation the child may not be at all knowledgeable of this treatment.
312. Knowledge, assessment, environment (a)
    2 By definition, vesicles are small, thin-walled, raised skin lesions containing clear fluid; a blister.
    1 Macules are usually less than 1 cm in diameter; they are circumscribed alterations with elevations or depressions.
    3 These are macules that become slightly raised.
    4 Papules are less than 1 cm in diameter; they are solid elevations with no visible fluid.
313. Application, implementation, environment (a)
    1 To adhere and to seal properly, the self-adhesive plastic bag must be applied to a clean, dry area.
    2, 3, 4 These are incorrect procedures for obtaining a urine specimen from an infant.
314. Comprehension, assessment, physiologic (b)
    1 The nurse would need to know the average respiratory rate for age to determine abnormalities.
    2 The child's developmental level is important for the nurse to know, but the nurse can monitor the respiratory rate without this knowledge.
    3 This is very important, but no bronchodilator has been ordered.
    4 This will be important for the nurse to know to avoid theophylline toxicity if the child is given this drug.
315. Knowledge, implementation, environment (a)
    3 This is the safest and most accurate method of taking a temperature in a 2-year-old child.
    1 The rectal temperature is the method of choice, although the axillary method can be used if the rectal route cannot be used; this is not the best answer.
    2 An oral temperature should never be taken in a child of this age; rectal temperature is the method of choice; this option is inappropriate because it includes an incorrect method.
    4 The temperature could be taken by this method, but it is not the most accurate and should not be used unless the rectal route is contraindicated.

316. Application, planning, physiologic (b)
    3 The patient is losing fluids and electrolytes through vomiting and diarrhea. A fluid and electrolyte imbalance is imminent if not treated quickly.
    1 Even though the patient's nutrition is altered due to the vomiting, this is not the most pressing problem.
    2 There is no indication of alteration in health maintenance.
    4 The patient has diarrhea, not incontinence.
317. Knowledge, implementation, environment (a)
    4 In infancy, this muscle is developed and is large enough to ensure a good intramuscular site.
    1 Deltoid muscles should never be used for injection sites in infancy.
    2 The ventrogluteal muscle often is not developed enough in infants to ensure a deep intramuscular injection.
    3 The dorsogluteal muscle often does not gain size until after children start walking.
318. Comprehension, planning, environment (b)
    1 Patient safety is always a high priority. The child must be still for an injection; a second person will ensure this safety measure.
    2 Antibiotic ointment on injection sites, although not harmful, is not necessary.
    3 A toy may help focus an infant's attention for a very brief period, but when the child is touched and prepared for the injection, the toy will not distract him.
    4 The name on the identification device is generally all that is required in the patient check.
319. Application, implementation, environment (a)
    2 gr 5 = 300 mg; 1 tablet is the correct dose.
    1 This dose is too low.
    3, 4 These doses are too high.
320. Application, implementation, environment (b)
    3 $\dfrac{\text{Weight in pounds (75)} \times \text{adult dose (300 mg)}}{150}$

    $75 \times 300 = \dfrac{22,500}{150} = 150$ mg

    1, 2 These doses are too low.
    4 This dose is too high.
321. Application, implementation, environment (a)
    1 $\dfrac{\text{Child's age (8)}}{\text{Age (8)} + 12} \times$ average adult dose (500 mg)

    $\dfrac{8}{20} \times 500$ mg $= \dfrac{2}{5} \times 500$ mg $= 200$ mg

    2, 3, 4 These doses are too high.
322. Application, implementation, environment (a)
    2 The patient is in the reproductive years and needs to be protected from the x-rays. A lead apron placed from the waist down will protect the reproductive organs and will not interfere with a chest x-ray.
    1 A radiation warning sign is not necessary for a chest x-ray. This is usually used for a radium implant.
    3 Amber-colored eye shields are used when the laser is in use. They are not necessary with an x-ray.
    4 The nurse should make sure everyone leaves the room, but clearing the hall is not necessary. Safety around x-rays depends on three things: time, distance, and shielding.

323. Application, implementation, environment (b)

   4 Standard precautions are to be used on all patients when there is a risk of coming in contact with blood or body fluids.

   1 Many patients will have communicable diseases that will not be diagnosed until after the nurse has been exposed to blood or body fluids.

   2 Children under the age of 2 can have hepatitis or be HIV positive.

   3 Other patients besides surgical patients can be a risk to the nurse.

324. Comprehension, planning, health (b)

   2 This allows release of extra energy and gives the child a healthy outlook.

   1, 3 Giving in reinforces the idea that tantrums get him what he wants, so it's good to continue to have them.

   4 He is not at a level where such comprehension is possible.

325. Application, implementation, psychosocial (b)

   2 After the tantrum is over, the mother will be able to deal with the child in a calm and more controlled manner.

   1 This is a bribe, it is not recommended because it will only facilitate rather than inhibit episodes of tantrums.

   3 This action does not get at the cause of the matter.

   4 Finding out what the problem may be is good advice, but not while the child is out of control. It would be impossible to deal with her effectively during a tantrum.

MENTAL HEALTH NURSING

1. Comprehension, assessment, environment (c)
   3 The context of the specific behavior is as important as the behavior itself in making the determination of mental health or mental illness.
   1 Those closest to the individual are not always objective observers.
   2 Intelligence and education are not necessarily determinants of mental well-being.
   4 Healthy behavior is often pleasing to others, but it does not have to be pleasing to be considered healthy.

2. Comprehension, assessment, environment (a)
   2 Behaviors of the mentally ill differ in the degree of response to a situation rather than the kind of response made.
   1 A degree of conformity is expected, yet it is possible for a person to be mentally healthy without conforming entirely.
   3 The more severely disturbed the individual, the more difficult the behavior is to understand; however, the behavior can be understood.
   4 This is a common misconception. Behaviors are the result of a complex interplay of biologic, psychologic, and social influences.

3. Knowledge, assessment, health (b)
   3 This is the best definition. It suggests flexibility and the ability to cope with life's changes.
   1, 2 These may be important characteristics of mental health, yet these are not the fullest definition.
   4 Although mentally healthy individuals possess positive characteristics that one hopes to find in leaders, winning power over others is not necessarily a feature of mental health.

4. Knowledge, assessment, psychosocial (a)
   3 The key to this is goal-directedness. The nurse is in a therapeutic relationship with the patient to facilitate the improvement of his well-being.
   1 There may indeed be a feeling of warmth in the nurse-patient relationship, but the statement implies a social rather than a therapeutic relationship.
   2 It is certainly possible that the nurse and the patient may enjoy and appreciate one another, yet this is not the purpose of a therapeutic relationship.
   4 In a therapeutic relationship, the nurse promotes the patient's capacity for independence.

5. Knowledge, assessment, environment (a)
   2 The nursing process is the same with mentally ill individuals as with physically ill individuals and begins with assessment.
   1 Although it is useful to let the patient know what is expected of him, the nurse must first assess his problems.
   3 This is a very important element of building rapport with the patient so that the nurse can assess his problems.
   4 This may be important to some patients, but it is not assessment.

6. Comprehension, planning, environment (a)
   3 This describes essential personal characteristics of the nurse who is successful in working with people.
   1 This is a commonly held misconception. The nurse's role does not include holding the patient to the nurse's personal value system.
   2 This is another misconception. Although personal problems can interfere with one's work while they are acute, seeking professional help and working through personal problems increases one's skill in helping others.
   4 Enforcement of societal rules is not the role of the nurse, although successful mental health care will often render many patients more capable of living productively in society.

7. Knowledge, implementation, environment (a)
   2 This is the best answer. Successful communication results in a negotiated understanding between two or more people.
   1, 3 These may be aspects of communication, but they are not a complete definition.
   4 This is true of the communication process, but there is more to the definition of communication.

8. Application, implementation, psychosocial (a)
   4 Use of reflection will help the patient identify her feelings and encourage verbalization of them.
   1, 2, 3 These responses are nontherapeutic; they do not acknowledge the patient's feelings.

9. Application, assessment, environment (c)
   1 The patient's ability to give this information correctly tells the nurse that the patient's ability to think is intact.
   2 There is no indication of her emotional status.
   3 There is no indication of what her usual style of communicating would be.
   4 There is no indication that would reveal her coping style.

10. Application, assessment, environment (c)
    3 She would not be able to perform the tasks described if her coordination were impaired.
    1, 2, 4 These assessments cannot be made from this information.

11. Application, implementation, psychosocial (b)
    2 Using a broad opening acknowledges what the patient has said and encourages her to discuss her feelings.
    1, 4 Giving reassurance blocks communication because it is not based on truth or factual information. Also, it blocks the patient's opportunity to discuss her feelings.
    3 Challenging the patient will put her on the defensive and block communication.

12. Application, implementation, psychosocial (a)
    3 Making a broad opening statement is an effective communication strategy for encouraging the patient to verbalize her feelings.
    1 Giving reassurance is inappropriate because it is not based on fact, and it blocks the patient's opportunity to discuss her feelings. Stereotypical comments communicate that the nurse does not understand the patient's feelings.
    2 Giving reassurance blocks communication.
    4 The competency of the physician is not the issue requiring focus. The patient's feelings need to be acknowledged by the nurse.

13. Application, implementation, psychosocial (b)
    2 Stating observations encourages the patient to identify and discuss his thoughts and feelings; this is therapeutic.
    1 This reinforces the patient's perceived symptoms and is nontherapeutic.
    3 This gives false reassurance and is nontherapeutic.
    4 Changing the subject diverts the communication at an important point. It also indicates that the nurse is unable or unwilling to listen to the patient.

14. Application, implementation, environment (c)
    4 The pacing and the yelling indicate that he could benefit from prn medication at this time before he becomes more out of control.
    1 This has a threatening quality that is inappropriate.
    2, 3 Patients should never be threatened.

15. Application, implementation, psychosocial (b)
    3 Stating observations will encourage his wife to further identify her feelings and thoughts.
    1 Giving directions thwarts the wife's ability to think through her feelings.
    2 Judgmental statements block communication.
    4 "Guilty" is an emotionally charged word that may cause the patient's wife to withdraw. At this point, the nurse should encourage her to verbalize her feelings and thoughts.

16. Comprehension, implementation, environment (b)
    4 Promises are never made to patients. The information may be important to the safety or health of the patient or other patients. The patient must decide whether or not to share information after being informed that the nurse cannot make promises.
    1, 2, 3 These are inappropriate, nontherapeutic responses.

17. Comprehension, intervention, environment (b)
    2 The time the nurse has contracted with the first patient is his time. Adhering to the contract indicates that the nurse views the session as important and that she means what she says.
    1 This is contracted time with the first patient only. Inviting another patient to remain indicates that the nurse does not view her time with him as important. It also indicates that the nurse didn't mean what she said when she contracted with him. This action will affect the first patient's ability to trust the nurse.
    3 No patient should be rejected. The interruption can be handled without rejecting the second patient.
    4 This response is inappropriate because it places the first patient in an uncomfortable position and violates the nurse's contract with him.

18. Application, intervention, environment (c)
    4 Sometimes patients will open up dynamic topics just as the interview time is up. Frequently this is done to manipulate or test the nurse. The nurse should, without rejecting the patient, adhere to the terms of the contract.
    1, 3 The nurse should not extend the contracted interaction time. Adhering to the contract illustrates that the nurse means what she says, and this fosters trust.
    2 Same as No. 1; also, rudeness is never appropriate.

19. Comprehension, planning, environment (b)
    3 This lets the patient know that the nurse does not want harm to come to him, and that the situation is serious and must be shared with other staff.
    1 The nurse is reacting by feeling responsible for talking the patient out of it; this is inappropriate.
    2 This is inappropriate and could be interpreted by the patient as approval of his plan.
    4 Although necessary, this is not the priority action.

20. Application, implementation, health (b)
    3 Acceptance of the patient is important, but setting a limit on inappropriate behaviors is also necessary.
    1 The chances of manipulation are increased if all staff members interact with the patient.
    2 The patient must understand that getting hurt is a possibility but not a reason to avoid others.
    4 The patient must have the chance to observe healthier behaviors and role models.

21. Comprehension, implementation, psychosocial (b)
    3 Ego ideal is one's perception of how one should be, compared to how one perceives oneself to actually be.
    1 Body image is part of identity.
    2 Role is a description of how one fits into the society, whereas body image is one's perception of one's body.
    4 See above explanations.

22. Application, intervention, environment (b)
    2 This olfactory hallucination is common in patients experiencing tumors of the frontal lobe. The nurse's observations of clinical symptoms aid the diagnostic process.
    1 It is appropriate to present reality to the patient, but the nurse must first verbally acknowledge what he has said.
    3 This is not relevant.
    4 This is optional and entirely dependent on the patient's preference; it is not the priority.

23. Application, intervention, psychosocial (a)
    2 This invites the patient to talk about her perceptions and beliefs.
    1 This cuts off her communication with the nurse.
    3 This can make the patient feel as if the nurse is invalidating her and taking sides with the other individual.
    4 This suggests to the patient that she is falsely accusing.

24. Application, intervention, psychosocial (a)
    2 This identifies a feeling and allows the patient the opportunity to express herself.
    1 Although this conveys interest, questions that begin with "Why" often invite people to become defensive.
    3 This question may sound hostile to the patient.
    4 This response invalidates the patient's experience and may damage the nurse's therapeutic relationship with her.

25. Comprehension, assessment, psychosocial (a)
    2 This is the correct observation to make about this interchange.
    1 Although this may be true, this requires the nurse to interpret the communication in a way that may not be accurate.
    3 The nurse is not able to assess this on the basis of this limited communication. The nurse may have misinterpreted.
    4 The nurse needs more information from the patient before she can make this interpretation.

26. Application, implementation, psychosocial (a)
    4 This response acknowledges the patient's feelings and provides the opportunity for him to ventilate them.
    1 This statement does not acknowledge the patient's feelings. The focus should be on the patient, not the nurse.
    2 This will likely make the patient angrier, and it does not encourage him to verbalize his anger.
    3 This does not acknowledge the patient's feelings or encourage verbalization of his anger.

27. Application, implementation, psychosocial (b)
    4 Taking the time to sit with her indicates care and concern for her as an individual.
    1 This is the nurse's need; it demonstrates that the nurse is uncomfortable with the patient's behavior.
    2 This fails to acknowledge the patient's feelings and her ability to make her own decisions.
    3 In some circumstances, this might be appropriate, but it is not supportive.

28. Application, intervention, psychosocial (a)
    1 This response invites the patient to talk about her feelings.
    2, 3 These responses are judgmental and nontherapeutic.
    4 This is nontherapeutic because it does not acknowledge the patient's feelings.

29. Application, intervention, psychosocial (b)
    3 The nurse is seeking clarification. Once communication is clarified, the nurse has a basis for understanding.
    1 This sounds angry. Even if the patient is annoying in her agitated state, the nurse does not want to sound angry with her.
    2 The patient may be angry, but the nurse cannot determine this until the patient is permitted to express herself.
    4 This response belittles the patient and is nontherapeutic.

30. Comprehension, planning, environment (b)
    1 This provides a means of developing trust.
    2 These come from within the patient and cannot be communicated.
    3 This is an ineffective approach to care.
    4 The patient is not always able to verbalize his or her difficulties.

31. Comprehension, assessment, environment (c)
    4 Her distraction, confusion, and difficulty paying attention all indicate a change in level of consciousness.
    1 There is not enough information to indicate this.
    2 There is no indication that she is frightened.
    3 There is no indication that she is cognitively impaired.

32. Knowledge, assessment, psychosocial (a)
    3 These are a few of the common street names for amphetamines, which also act as stimulants.
    1 Stimulants are natural or synthetic drugs that stimulate the central nervous system. The drugs that the patient named are classified as amphetamines.
    2 Hallucinogens have a profound psychologic effect. The most common ones are known as LSD, PCP, and mescaline.
    4 Cocaine or crack has street names of blow, coke, snow, rock, toot, and white.

33. Application, assessment, environment (b)
    3 All of these observations relate to the patient's affect.
    1 None of these observations can accurately reveal the patient's feelings.
    2 None of these observations can accurately reveal the patient's thoughts.
    4 None of these observations can assess whether the patient is oriented.

34. Knowledge, assessment, health (b)
    4 These would not necessarily have an impact on an inpatient, but they could influence a vulnerable patient attempting to function in the community.
    1, 2, 3 The nurse on the inpatient unit should always assess these factors to give appropriate care.

35. Comprehension, planning, health (b)
    3 Depending upon where, with what populations, and under what kinds of supervision the nurse practices, her role can involve many different aspects of mental health care.
    1 This is not necessarily the case, especially in the role of the practical nurse.
    2 Physicians and social workers may provide many types of service; however, they do not control nursing practice, which is defined by legal parameters.
    4 This setting can be stressful, but nursing practice is always legally defined.

36. Knowledge, assessment, psychosocial (b)
    4 This is the definition of personality.
    1 This would include orientation to time, place, and person, as well as affect, mood, thought processes, thought content, memory, and judgment.
    2 This is similar to mental status.
    3 Behaviors, thoughts, and feelings are influenced by education, but this is not a complete answer.

37. Knowledge, planning, psychosocial (a)
    1 Understanding this basic theory will support the nurse's understanding of human behavior.
    2 This is an important part of Freud's theory, but this pertains to consciousness, not personality.
    3 This is Berne's theory. It is similar to Freud's theory, but it offers more modern explanations.
    4 These are developmental phases that are integral to building personality.

38. Knowledge, planning, psychosocial (c)
    3 This is Berne's twentieth-century version of Freud's classic nineteenth-century theory.
    1, 2 These terms belong to Freud.
    4 These are Freud's developmental phases.

39. Knowledge, planning, psychosocial (c)
    4 The animal drives of the id/child give us the energy, motivation, and passion to live.
    1 This is a function of the superego/parent.
    2, 3 These are functions of the busy ego/adult.

40. Comprehension, assessment, psychosocial (c)
    2 The ego/adult makes the rational decisions. This function integrates the needs and wishes of the id/child with the responsibilities held by the superego/parent.
    1 The id/child may be interested in having fun but may not be able to make the most responsible decisions.
    3 The superego/parent may forget how important it is to have fun.
    4 The unconscious has an influence on the personality.

41. Knowledge, planning, psychosocial (c)
    2 This is the valuable work of the superego/parent.
    1 This occurs from the cooperation between the id/child and the ego/adult.
    3 This is the work of the ego/adult.
    4 This is the work of the id/child.

42. Comprehension, assessment, psychosocial (a)
    2 This ability demonstrates coping behavior as the child becomes independent.
    1 Mental illness is unrelated.
    3 This ability is not a dysfunction.
    4 This ability does not indicate autism, because autistic children usually have learning problems.

43. Knowledge, implementation, psychosocial (c)
    1 Rogers' focus was on client-centered therapy.
    2 Sullivan's focus was on interpersonal relationships.
    3 Berne's focus was on transactional analysis.
    4 Erikson's focus was on the eight stages of development.

44. Knowledge, assessment, psychosocial (b)
    2 There is evidence to suggest that the patient is in a relationship in which she is able to have her emotional needs met. Her partner is likely to be an important support for her.
    1 Homosexuality is now viewed as a healthy alternative lifestyle. Individuals may be well adjusted or poorly adjusted in their personal relationships, just as heterosexuals may be.
    3 This is a myth that has no place in a therapeutic relationship.
    4 This is another myth that is not useful for a health-care provider.

45. Comprehension, assessment, psychosocial (a)
    2 The use of defense mechanisms becomes a problem when they prove ineffective in helping the individual implement his or her roles and responsibilities.
    1, 3, 4 Defense mechanisms protect the individual against painful experiences; these would not be criteria of defense mechanism use.

46. Comprehension, assessment, psychosocial (b)
    4 She is trying to justify behavior that is not socially acceptable.
    1 This would be trying to make up for a deficit.
    2 This is used to minimize one's actions.
    3 This would be attributing one's behavior to others.

47. Comprehension, assessment, psychosocial (b)
    3 The unpleasant event is excluded from consciousness.
    1 This would be adopting attitudes opposite one's own.
    2 This is attributing behaviors to others.
    4 This is going back to a lesser stage of development.

48. Knowledge, assessment, psychosocial (b)
    3 The child is possibly trying to identify with Elvis or replace his missing dad with a new role model. In identification, one takes on a characteristic of another individual or group while retaining his or her own personal identity.
    1 Displacement is when emotions are expressed toward something other than the source of the emotion.
    2 Dissociation is separation and detachment of emotional significance.
    4 Compensation is when one tends to excel in something such as academics or music to make up for a deficiency elsewhere.

49. Comprehension, assessment, psychosocial (b)
    2 She has regressed to an earlier stage of development.
    1 This deals with excluding thoughts from consciousness.
    3 This is taking on behaviors opposite one's own.
    4 This is justifying one's behavior.

50. Comprehension, assessment, psychosocial (c)
    2 This is a functional defense that may occur on a conscious or an unconscious level.
    1 Denial is the refusal to recognize reality.
    3 Repression is the involuntary exclusion from consciousness of painful feelings, ideas, or situations.
    4 Rationalization is offering an apparently logical or socially acceptable explanation for unacceptable behaviors.

51. Comprehension, assessment, environment (a)
    4 The husband unconsciously projects his guilt onto his wife.
    1 There is always a small measure of denial of one's own feelings when these feelings are projected onto others.
    2 Repression is the involuntary exclusion from consciousness of painful feelings, ideas, or situations.
    3 Rationalization is offering an apparently logical explanation or socially acceptable explanation for unacceptable behavior.

52. Comprehension, assessment, psychosocial (c)
    3 This patient is using her intellectual abilities to process what is occurring in her life. This will work well for her. When she is ready, she will deal effectively with her feelings.
    1 There is a rational quality to her behavior. She is using her intellect to help her cope with her experience.
    2 Denial of her feelings is a part of her intellectualization.
    4 The use of fantasy creatively employs the imagination. Children use this especially well.

53. Comprehension, assessment, environment (c)
    3 This patient is displaying an extreme discrepancy between the functioning of his superego/parent and that of his id/child.
    1 The defense of reaction formation always contains a measure of denial, just as in the defense mechanism of projection.
    2 This patient may have repressed some of his feelings; however, this is not being displayed in this description.
    4 He has not necessarily regressed to an earlier level of functioning.

54. Comprehension, assessment, environment (a)
    1 The child is coping with the stress of her move by returning to an earlier developmental stage.
    2 This situation does not describe denial. A young child can use denial, however. Her true feelings may be expressed in her play.
    3 A young child who is using repression as a defense will behave more like a "brave little soldier."
    4 This situation does not describe reaction formation. A young child using reaction formation may behave as though she is older than she really is. This pseudomaturity is a sign of stress in a child.

55. Comprehension, assessment, psychosocial (a)
    2 Her anger is displaced on the unfortunate cat.
    1 This situation does not involve identification.
    3 This situation does not involve introjection. Introjection occurs in grief work. Someone may take on the values and behaviors of a lost loved one.
    4 This situation does not involve reaction formation.

56. Comprehension, assessment, psychosocial (c)
    1 Fantasy is a thinking process that involves wishful thinking, employs the creative use of imagery, and helps the individual manage painful feelings.
    2 Denial of painful feelings may be involved to some degree when a person is employing fantasy. Like fantasy, denial is a healthy defense against pain that enables the individual to cope with life. It becomes unhealthy only when it gets in the way of effective coping.
    3 Fantasy, repression, and denial are similar in that they free the person to cope with life. This situation correctly describes fantasy because of the creative use of imagery.
    4 Descriptions of defensive behaviors often overlap. This does not offer the best description of reaction formation.

57. Application, assessment, psychosocial (c)
    1 Projection is an unconscious defense mechanism in which a person attributes his or her own unacceptable traits or impulses to another.
    2 Denial is a defense mechanism in which unpleasant realities are denied and repressed from conscious awareness.
    3 Withdrawal is a term given to a person who responds to severe physical danger or stress by retreating or being apathetic, lethargic, or depressed.
    4 Compensation is a complex defense mechanism that allows a person to avoid unpleasant or painful feelings of inadequacy. This person may engage in extraordinary efforts to replace the painful feeling(s), such as becoming a perfectionist to replace weakness or failure.

58. Application, implementation, psychosocial (b)
    2 The child who is in the depression stage wants to be alone and will not communicate with the nurse.
    1 During the denial stage the child will act normally because she does not believe anything is wrong.
    3 During the anger stage the child will lash out and be difficult to care for. She will frequently display anger at the nurse or doctor.
    4 During the final stage of acceptance, the child will no longer display anger or depression. She will recognize that death is a certainty.

59. Comprehension, assessment, psychosocial (a)
    1 This patient is clearly ignoring normal feelings about major surgery.
    2 Compensation is an exaggerated presentation in an effort to protect oneself from acknowledging one's limitations.
    3 Repression is excluding from awareness unacceptable thoughts, desires, behaviors, or wishes.
    4 Suppression is conscious exclusion of specific feelings or thoughts; suppression may also occur on an unconscious level.

60. Comprehension, evaluation, psychosocial (a)
    1 The source of gratification in the oral stage is through the mouth. The child puts everything into the mouth. The smoker displays this same action when keeping a cigarette in his/her mouth.
    2 The anal stage is displayed by a need to control elimination or retention of feces. An adult displaying these characteristics would display a need to control the people and environment around him/her.
    3 The phallic stage is when the child develops intense feelings for the parent of the opposite sex.
    4 The latency stage occurs when the child participates in more socially approved activities and becomes involved in more group interaction.

61. Application, implementation, environment (a)
    2 This is the best answer. The patient requires further assessment by the physician for this concern.
    1 Although this may be true, it is not helpful to suggest this until the patient is more fully assessed.
    3 This may be true; one would naturally want to allay his anxiety. It is best to encourage him to seek further physical assessment.
    4 This is true, but the nurse should still encourage him to see his physician.

62. Knowledge, assessment, environment (a)
    3 The presence of a specific, definable threat differentiates fear from anxiety.
    1 Fear and anxiety are physiologically similar.
    2 Behavioral responses of fear and anxiety may be similar or they may differ in that in a state of fear, a person may attempt to deal with the perceived threat.
    4 Emotional responses in states of fear and anxiety may be similar.

63. Knowledge, planning, environment (a)
    1 Mild anxiety helps one to garner the energy to focus attention and interest on the material to be learned.
    2 Learning is more difficult at this higher level of anxiety because it becomes more difficult to focus one's attention.
    3 With increasing anxiety, the individual is experiencing increasing distress. This is uncomfortable and distracts the individual from learning.
    4 Panic is extremely uncomfortable and is experienced in a similar way to severe pain. Learning becomes nearly impossible.

64. Comprehension, assessment, environment (a)
    3 Anxiety is a common experience around the turning points in one's life. It has many physiologic manifestations.
    1 Phobias are irrational fears; there's nothing in the situation that indicates her symptoms are a result of irrationality.
    2 Anxiety and depression are often seen together. If she is depressed, she will express sadness and hopelessness in addition to the symptoms she has already presented.
    4 As in anxiety, fear is experienced both psychologically and physiologically. Fear occurs in response to a known stressor.

65. Knowledge, assessment, psychosocial (b)
    2 These symptoms are indicators that the anxiety has progressed beyond the functional level of alertness. Focused intellectual performance becomes more difficult.
    1 At the alertness level, there may be perception of some threat; however, there is no decrease in organization.
    3 Severe anxiety is more pronounced and includes a sense of imminent disaster. Focused intellectual performance becomes even more difficult.
    4 The panic level of anxiety is extremely uncomfortable. Actions and behavior are extremely disorganized.

66. Application, planning, psychosocial (c)
    1 A concrete, short-term solution may resolve the crisis.
    2, 3, 4 As long-term solutions, these are not indicated in a crisis situation.

67. Comprehension, assessment, environment (b)
    3 The level of anxiety this individual is experiencing is related to garnering the energy necessary to complete the project.
    1 His anxiety as presented will not interfere with the completion of his project.
    2 There is no evidence that he has something else on his mind.
    4 There is no evidence that his anxiety level will escalate.

68. Comprehension, assessment, environment (b)
    4 Panic-level anxiety in an individual who is not psychotic is differentiated by severely restricted perception and impairment of logical thought processes.
    1 In the alertness level, there is no evidence of distorted and disconnected thoughts.
    2 Apprehension does not bring about disconnected thoughts.
    3 Severe anxiety, although quite uncomfortable and distracting, does not cause distorted and disconnected thoughts.

69. Comprehension, evaluation, psychosocial (b)
    3 This is an example of Implosive therapy. This therapy must be used only by a trained therapist.
    1 Systematic relaxation is based on the idea that anxiety and relaxation cannot coexist. If the patient can be relaxed using relaxation techniques, then anxiety will decrease.
    2 In desensitization a patient is conditioned to be nonresponsive to a stimulus. When the patient feels the first sign of anxiety, relaxation is begun.
    4 Problem solving involves the patient choosing other ways in which to cope with the stress.

70. Comprehension, planning, psychosocial (b)

2 The patient will have difficulty concentrating but needs to be instructed on ways to relax.

1 The patient will not be able to concentrate for very long on a lengthy, drawn-out history. The nurse needs to cover the patient's past medical history and a brief family history. More details can be gathered later.

3 The patient does not need to be restrained. Restraints will only increase anxiety.

4 The patient cannot concentrate for long while she is anxious. The instructions should be saved for later when the patient is relaxed.

71. Application, assessment, psychosocial (b)

3 Physical symptoms are more socially acceptable.

1 It would be healthy to confront her situation.

2 There is no evidence of regression.

4 She probably believes her symptoms are real.

72. Application, evaluation, environment (a)

1 The hospital is responsible for the safety of all patients.

2 Abuse is mistreatment of the patient.

3 Neglect is the term used for failing to provide adequate care.

4 0.5 mg is a normal dose.

73. Comprehension, assessment, environment (b)

3 At the severe anxiety level, the individual should be able to follow simple instructions and think rationally, although a decrease in rational thought may be evident.

1 His symptoms are beyond the alertness level.

2 He is experiencing a degree of anxiety greater than that of apprehension.

4 Panic-level anxiety would include a total loss of rational thinking and the inability to follow even the simplest of directions.

74. Application, implementation, psychosocial (b)

4 While being supportive, the nurse should try to get the patient to relax.

1 This inappropriately supports the described symptoms.

2 Identifying the anxiety and past experiences are not therapeutic in this situation.

3 This is an unacceptable response as the patient may interpret this to indicate that she is having a heart attack now.

75. Comprehension, assessment, psychosocial (c)

2 This is an unacceptable drive pressing for conscious discharge from within.

1 It is fear that originates from a specific source; fear is contained through reasoned action.

3 A phobia directly relates to a specific danger.

4 Situations are not always known on the conscious level.

76. Application, evaluation, psychosocial (c)

3 Antianxiety drugs decrease physiologic manifestations of anxiety such as elevated levels of blood pressure, pulse, and respiration.

1 These are signs of anxiety.

2 These are paradoxic reactions that would not support evidence of positive effects of drug therapy.

4 These are signs of anxiety.

77. Comprehension, assessment, environment (b)

3 The patient's purposeless activity, intense somatic complaint, absorption with self, and focus on his unattended apartment are all characteristics of severe anxiety.

1 Pacing indicates more than mild tension-relieving behavior.

2 Although pacing and somatic complaints are characteristic of moderate anxiety, the patient's *inability to concentrate* places him in the severe category.

4 Panic-level characteristics are not described in the situation.

78. Comprehension, assessment, psychosocial (b)

4 Patients experiencing mild anxiety are alert and able to perceive connections between situations.

1 This indicates panic-level anxiety.

2, 3 These indicate moderate anxiety.

79. Comprehension, assessment, health (a)

3 Motivation is defined as the gathering of personal resources to perform a task or reach a goal. It may be derived from perceived reward or threat of punishment. It is influenced by self-esteem and hope. Motivation is a key factor in recovery from any major illness.

1 Frustration with the sick role and perception of the opportunity to live more productively may positively influence rehabilitative efforts. Excessive frustration tends to inhibit recovery.

2 Anxiety is one of several factors that influence recovery from illness. Alertness level can positively influence recovery, while higher levels of mild activity may inhibit recovery.

4 Just as in the previous factors, optimal levels of stress tend to increase motivation. Excessive stress, however, leads to exhaustion.

80. Knowledge, assessment, psychosocial (c)

2 The general adaptation syndrome, also known as GAS, is a group of similar symptoms or phenomena that occur in response to a variety of physiologic or emotional stressors.

1 Alternative lifestyle reflects a pattern of choices based on a complex set of personal interests and resources.

3 Management of frustration is a necessary skill in everyday life. Excessive levels of frustration promote stress.

4 Management of anxiety is also a skill necessary to one's everyday functioning. Excessive anxiety, however, brings about excessive levels of stress.

81. Application, implementation, psychosocial (b)

2 By eating right and getting exercise, the nurse is dealing with her stress and will be better able to cope with the stress at work.

1 The nurse needs to maintain a certain distance in order to prevent burnout. The nurse needs to be kind and compassionate to the patient but not get personally involved.

3 It is important for the nurse to realize that some things are out of her control. If the situation cannot be changed, the nurse must be able to accept the situation in the best way possible.

4 Nurses must take time out. It is important to have time for themselves and their families.

82. Comprehension, evaluation, psychosocial (b)

3 The patient is using projection, which is to blame someone else rather than take the blame for something that has occurred.

1 There is no indication that the patient really thought the nurse had done anything to cause the argument.

2 The patient has not indicated he dislikes the nurse. He is only reacting to a stressful situation.

4 Repression is to involuntarily exclude experiences or occurrences.

83. Application, assessment, psychosocial (b)

1 Utilizing support people is an excellent way to relieve stress.

2 Excessive sleeping is a coping mechanism in response to stress, but it is not very beneficial. The patient usually ends up feeling even worse.

3 Using food, alcohol, or drugs to relieve stress is a common but ineffective response.

4 This is an example of ritualistic behavior, which can lead to obsessive-compulsive behavior.

84. Comprehension, assessment, environment (c)
    4 The symptoms of posttraumatic stress disorder (PTSD) usually begin several months or years after the traumatic event. Symptoms include nightmares, depression, and anxiety.
    1 These are not symptoms of PTSD.
    2 These symptoms can occur, but they are not the primary symptoms of PTSD.
    3 These are symptoms of schizophrenia, catatonic type.

85. Knowledge, assessment, environment (b)
    2 A perceptual experience that occurs in the absence of an external stimulus is a hallucination.
    1 Ingestion of toxic chemicals such as street drugs can cause sufficient disruption of brain chemistry to produce the type of hallucinations that are caused by mental illness.
    3 Conflict does not cause hallucinations, but it may be manifested in the content of some hallucinations. For example, a psychotic person who has low self-esteem may hear a voice telling him he is worthless.
    4 Similar to conflict, frustration does not cause hallucinations. Frustration may be symbolically manifested in the content of hallucinations.

86. Comprehension, assessment, psychosocial (a)
    2 Delusions of grandeur indicates grandiose ideas.
    1 This is making up information to answer questions with no regard to the truth.
    3 No one is out to get her.
    4 Her ideas are all along one line.

87. Application, intervention, environment (a)
    2 The nurse will not be able to change the patient's delusion, but she can change the focus of his thoughts to lessen preoccupation with delusional thoughts.
    1 The nurse should not argue about the content of delusions; she should acknowledge the patient's feelings and present reality.
    3 Although the nurse cannot change the patient's delusion, she will need to build a rapport by beginning to communicate respect and concern for him.
    4 Sharing humor with patients is important at times. This is not appropriate, however, when patients are experiencing sensory perception alterations.

88. Comprehension, assessment, psychosocial (b)
    2 This is true with obsessive-compulsive behaviors.
    1 He really has no control.
    3 He is not hallucinating.
    4 Behavior modification would not necessarily be indicated here.

89. Comprehension, assessment, psychosocial (a)
    2 The patient is not oriented in time because he thinks it is 1886.
    1 The patient is not oriented in time.
    3 Although he is confused, "not oriented" better describes this patient's state.
    4 The patient may or may not be dishonest, but this is not relevant to the situation.

90. Comprehension, assessment, psychosocial (b)
    1 Scattered thoughts are indicated by rapid and frequent topic changes.
    2 Rapid speech may or may not indicate a scattered thought process.
    3, 4 These are only general indicators.

91. Knowledge, planning, psychosocial (a)
    2 Chlorpromazine is the only antipsychotic listed. It is the prototype antipsychotic drug and the least potent of the antipsychotics.
    1 This is an antianxiety agent.
    3 This drug is a mood stabilizer.
    4 This is an antidepressant.

92. Comprehension, assessment, psychosocial (b)
    3 In schizophrenia the thought process is distorted; there is nonreality in thinking.
    1 He is not minimizing or avoiding anxiety.
    2 He is not exhibiting "highs" and "lows" in behavior.
    4 He is not exhibiting suspicious or distrustful behavior.

93. Comprehension, planning, psychosocial (b)
    3 Schizophrenic individuals have difficulty making choices; therefore, choices should be simple.
    1 This choice violates the understanding of the nature of schizophrenia.
    2 Because he is paranoid, such a discussion might be easily misunderstood.
    4 There are times when a second staff member may be required. Psychiatric attendants are equally trained, and it is discriminatory to request gender-specific assistance. If help is needed, the nurse states only that she needs help.

94. Application, intervention, environment (a)
    3 The patient is in increasing distress; thus the likelihood of her responding to her command hallucinations is quite high. She requires immediate high-level suicide precautions. The psychiatrist will be able to order a medication that can diminish her distress.
    1 The patient's level of distress has become too high for her to benefit from group activities that are ordinarily helpful. Her safety is now the nurse's most pressing concern.
    2 This intervention is helpful, but it takes time and much repetition. The priority is patient safety.
    4 The priority is patient safety.

95. Comprehension, planning, psychosocial (b)
    1 Antipsychotic drugs are essential in treating psychotic and some nonpsychotic disorders. These drugs do not cure the psychoses, but they are effective in reducing psychotic symptoms.
    2 These agents are effective in treating depression.
    3 These agents are most effective in the treatment of patients with high levels of anxiety.
    4 These drugs are used effectively in treating patients with cyclical affective disorder.

96. Application, evaluation, psychosocial (c)
    4 Antipsychotic drugs are used to remove psychotic symptoms (auditory hallucinations) or reduce their intensity. Reduction in loudness of voices heard by the patient indicates a decrease in intensity.
    1 This statement indicates no change in psychotic symptoms.
    2 The fact that the patient is not hearing voices at the moment in no way indicates an absence of auditory hallucinations.
    3 This statement indicates that the patient continues to hear voices.

97. Comprehension, implementation, physiologic (b)
    3 Foods in their own containers, such as milk or juice in cartons, hard-boiled eggs, or oranges, are more likely to be eaten by this type of patient.
    1 This reinforces the delusion; it is nontherapeutic.
    2 This is unsafe; it places the patient at risk nutritionally.
    4 This is threatening and definitely nontherapeutic.

98. Knowledge, planning, health (a)
    2 Cottage and cream cheeses are the only cheeses allowed on a tyramine-restricted diet.
    1, 3 These are high in tyramine.
    4 Summer sausage and unrefrigerated fermented sausages are high in tyramine.

99. Comprehension, evaluation, environment (b)
    4 Syncope is the only central nervous system side effect listed.
    1 This is a gastrointestinal side effect.
    2 This is a respiratory system side effect.
    3 This is a cardiovascular system side effect.
100. Knowledge, implementation, environment (b)
    2 This is exactly the effect that this medication has, although the exact way in which this works is still unknown.
    1 This is untrue; antipsychotic drugs work on the neurotransmitter system in the brain.
    3 This is also untrue. Sense of reality is unchanged; it is the decrease in unwanted stimuli that allows the patient to function.
    4 This is untrue; these medications act on dopamine synthesis.
101. Knowledge, assessment, psychosocial (a)
    2 Auditory hallucinations are quite common in schizophrenia. Thought processes are highly symbolic. It is difficult to follow the logic of the patient's thoughts, which patients often describe as racing.
    1 Unstable moods are sometimes associated with schizophrenia, but this symptom is less prominent than the racing thoughts and auditory hallucinations. Delusions of grandeur may occur, but this is more commonly associated with mania.
    3 Depressive thoughts are not necessarily indicative of schizophrenia. Many patients become depressed as a result of their awareness of the impact the illness has on their lives.
    4 Many schizophrenic patients retain good judgment. Complicated legal problems are commonly associated with the antisocial personality.
102. Application, implementation, psychosocial (b)
    1 Simple, structured tasks involving interaction with only one person at a time are best while he is exhibiting psychotic symptoms.
    2 Group activity is too complex for this patient to handle while he is actively psychotic. He will feel confused and lost.
    3 Although it is true that activity and human interaction are important for him, he is unable to apply this knowledge. He needs to be led to simple interactions while he is psychotic.
    4 A nurse should never feed into the patient's hallucinations; such actions are nontherapeutic.
103. Application, implementation, psychosocial (c)
    1 A simple, structured plan will be easiest for him to understand. He can follow only simple instructions and may need reminders.
    2 This is not a good time for him to begin the emotion-filled work of exploring his feelings; he is actively psychotic.
    3 The nurse will want to observe the patient closely while he is actively psychotic. A structured schedule will help keep him in contact with reality.
    4 There's no indication in the situation that mechanical restraints are required.

104. Application, implementation, psychosocial (b)
    4 Dry mouth and blurred vision are the most common side effects of all major tranquilizers. Informing the patient of this and helping him cope with the side effects can bring about improved compliance with the medication regimen.
    1 These side effects are not commonly reported with major tranquilizers.
    2 These are not common side effects. They may indicate a hypersensitivity to the medication. Should this occur, the nurse would report it to the psychiatrist and record it in the chart.
    3 Endocrine system side effects include moderate breast enlargement and loss of libido.
105. Comprehension, evaluation, environment (c)
    2 Extrapyramidal reactions are common side effects of major tranquilizers. Although they are not life-threatening, they are acutely uncomfortable for the patient. They require rapid intervention with medications such as diphenhydramine (Benadryl), benztropine (Cogentin), or trihexyphenidyl (Artane).
    1 Many patients believe this experience represents an allergic reaction. This is not the case.
    3 Sometimes the patient's pacing and odd movements are mistaken for a worsening of her psychosis. This can be an unfortunate error and can lead to the patient's being improperly treated.
    4 Rare side effects include agranulocytosis, cholestatic jaundice, and the occasionally fatal neuroleptic malignant syndrome.
106. Knowledge, implementation, physiologic (a)
    3 Cogentin is commonly used to treat extrapyramidal reactions to major tranquilizers.
    1 Aspirin is not effective for the extrapyramidal symptoms associated with major tranquilizers.
    2 Ativan is a minor tranquilizer used to treat anxiety.
    4 Lithium is used to treat both mania and depression. It is of no benefit in treating extrapyramidal reactions.
107. Comprehension, assessment, psychosocial (b)
    3 Delusions of this type are associated with paranoid schizophrenia.
    1 Catatonic schizophrenia typically causes the individual to appear immobile, although he may have periods of extreme excitability.
    2 This patient's delusions, though unrealistic, are organized. This does not occur in disorganized schizophrenia.
    4 Fixed delusions are not a feature of undifferentiated schizophrenia.
108. Application, implementation, psychosocial (c)
    2 Immediate action is required to prevent this patient from leaving the hospital. Command hallucinations are extremely dangerous in this patient. There is a risk he will kill someone.
    1 Safety of the patient and the community is the priority.
    3 Although the nurse will always want to establish a rapport with a patient, the safety issue takes precedence.
    4 The patient is not in a frame of mind at this time to comprehend this kind of concept. He is likely to believe he has a moral imperative to kill someone. Again, safety is the priority.

109. Application, implementation, psychosocial (b)
    3 It is important to be specific and straightforward when giving medication information. This will help build trust and decrease the patient's suspicion.
    1 Many psychotropic medications have the potential for abuse and are frequently used in suicide attempts. These medications are usually prescribed in small amounts so the patient has to return often to have the prescription refilled.
    2 This is likely to increase the patient's suspicion and foster distrust. The patient is calling about his medication; this is the issue to be addressed. Further assessment should take place after the issue of concern to the patient is given attention.
    4 Degrading a patient is never appropriate.
110. Comprehension, evaluation, health (b)
    4 Phototoxicity is a common side effect of chlorpromazine (Thorazine). Patients should be taught to apply a strong sunscreen when in the sun. Clothes and hats that cover the skin are also recommended.
    1 Nasal congestion is a common side effect. A nasal decongestant spray and an increase in fluid intake generally reduce this.
    2 Gastrointestinal distress can be relieved if the medication is taken with food.
    3 Antipsychotic drugs increase the appetite, resulting in weight gain. Patients should monitor their nutritional intake to avoid gaining unnecessary pounds.
111. Comprehension, assessment, psychosocial (c)
    2 Because delusions are a protection, they can be abandoned only when the patient feels safe and secure.
    1 The patient's delusions are not funny. Joking about delusions makes the patient feel unimportant.
    3 Patients can gain insight into their delusions, but that doesn't mean they are able to alter them.
    4 The patient and nurse do not have to like each other for the nurse-patient interaction to be therapeutic.
112. Comprehension, planning, environment (b)
    3 There is conflict between the patient's right to personal freedom and the obligation of health-care providers to protect his life.
    1 Restriction of the patient's freedom without a clear clinical reason could be viewed as illegal incarceration.
    2, 4 There is a moral obligation to protect his life.
113. Comprehension, evaluation, psychosocial (b)
    3 It will take 3 to 4 weeks to see the desired effect.
    1 This is not enough time on medication.
    2 The patient hasn't been on medication long enough yet.
    4 He hasn't been on the medication long enough yet.
114. Comprehension, planning, psychosocial (b)
    3 Monoamine oxidase inhibitors are antidepressants that provide the enzyme crucial in cognitive and language difficulties.
    1, 2, 4 These provide neither the symptomatic control nor the replacement of amino acids, which are low.
115. Application, evaluation, environment (c)
    1 These antidepressants mainly affect the central nervous system.
    2, 4 These are side effects of the tricyclic antidepressant drugs.
    3 This is a side effect of trazodone hydrochloride antidepressant drugs.

116. Comprehension, implementation, environment (b)
    4 Tyramine stimulates release of the catecholamines epinephrine and norepinephrine. Foods to be avoided are aged cheeses and meats, bananas, yeast-containing products, and alcoholic beverages.
    1 Histamine is a compound found in all cells; it is released in allergic, inflammatory reactions and causes dilation of capillaries, decreased blood pressure, increased secretion of gastric juice, and constriction of smooth muscles of the bronchi and uterus.
    2 Phenylalanine is an essential amino acid necessary for normal growth and development of infants and children and for normal protein metabolism throughout life.
    3 Lysine is an essential amino acid necessary for proper growth in infants and for maintenance of nitrogen balance in adults.
117. Application, implementation, environment (b)
    1 It is important to set a limit on the patient but also to offer the support of the nurse while setting that limit.
    2 The other patient's behavior is not the issue.
    3 This is likely to cause her to escalate her behavior and to become angrier.
    4 A manic patient cannot accept this type of redirection.
118. Application, implementation, health (c)
    2 This sets a limit without providing additional stimulus to cause further escalation of behavior.
    1 Yelling for someone can have the effect of escalating his behavior.
    3 This is false reassurance; if he is out of control enough, he will most likely attempt to hurt her.
    4 This is an overreaction and will escalate the problem needlessly without correcting it.
119. Application, implementation, environment (c)
    3 These are all symptoms of lithium toxicity.
    1 She is not experiencing a dystonic reaction.
    2 These are not signs of potassium depletion.
    4 These are signs, not side effects, of toxicity.
120. Application, implementation, psychosocial (c)
    2 Because of her distractibility, she will benefit from the nurse's calm presence. It is helpful for the nurse to talk soothingly to her and to show her some relaxation exercises.
    1 Her condition renders her unable to follow these instructions.
    3 This may have to be the nurse's second choice if the nurse is unable to calm her.
    4 She cannot benefit from the stimulation of the other patients' activity. This may excite her further.
121. Knowledge, implementation, psychosocial (b)
    1 Haldol will provide sedation that will enable the patient to rest. It will also promote more organized thought processes.
    2 Over-medication with haloperidol (Haldol) will tend to over-sedate the patient and render her inactive. This has been referred to as chemical restraint.
    3 The medication does not stimulate the appetite. The side effect of dry mouth will sometimes cause the patient to crave sweets. This can lead to weight gain.
    4 The medication will alleviate anxiety, but this is not its primary purpose for a patient with this diagnosis.

122. Knowledge, implementation, psychosocial (b)
    2 Fine tremors are common side effects of lithium carbonate.
    1 Food cravings are a common side effect of drugs that have anticholinergic properties, such as antidepressants and antipsychotics.
    3 This has not been reported as a side effect of lithium.
    4 Individuals taking lithium are sensitive to the effects of heat and must be careful of their fluid intake in hot weather. Thorazine is a drug that produces sensitivity to sunlight.

123. Application, planning, psychosocial (b)
    3 Lithium levels should be drawn 8 to 14 hours after the last dose. This would be in the morning before the first dose, when the medication is ordered tid.
    1, 2 12 to 14 hours should elapse after the last administered dose before obtaining a serum lithium level.
    4 Toxicity usually appears at serum levels higher than 1.5 mEq/L. The purpose of monitoring lithium levels is to maintain the therapeutic serum range.

124. Application, assessment, health (b)
    3 This would be an indication that her status is normalizing.
    1 Her appetite is not an adequate indicator.
    2 Eating at scheduled times does not ensure her intake is adequate.
    4 This is not a reliable indicator because she may not be eating very much anyway.

125. Comprehension, assessment, psychosocial (b)
    3 This is mood instability, as seen in her mood swing from pleasantness to rage.
    1 Flight of ideas is not indicated in her behavior.
    2 Ideas of reference are not demonstrated.
    4 Looseness of association is not indicated in this behavior.

126. Comprehension, evaluation, environment (c)
    4 Muscular weakness is the only listed side effect of lithium carbonate.
    1 This is a side effect of antidepressant medications.
    2, 3 Blurred vision is considered a toxic effect of serum concentrations above 1.5 mEq/L.

127. Comprehension, implementation, psychosocial (b)
    2 This is the most appropriate and safe response regarding lithium therapy.
    1 The nurse should be able to respond to the concern being raised by the patient's husband.
    3 Although the combination of lithium and a neuroleptic drug is often used and does achieve more rapid results, it is not within the practice of nursing to suggest this.
    4 Although this is true, it does not address the issue being raised by the patient's husband.

128. Application, implementation, environment (c)
    4 Vital signs should be taken and reported to the physician along with other assessment data.
    1 There is no indication in the situation that a code should be called at this time.
    2 Desired maintenance blood levels are 0.6 to 1.2 mEq/L; moderate to severe reactions occur at levels 2 to 2.5 mEq/L; lethargy and nonresponsiveness are characteristic of toxic drug levels; the priority action is to take vital signs and notify the physician.
    3 On the basis of the situation data, vital signs should be taken and reported to the physician, along with a description of the patient's level of consciousness.

129. Comprehension, evaluation, environment (b)
    4 This response indicates the patient understands the importance of taking her medication as prescribed.
    1 Patients should be informed never to double up on dosages if they miss a dose. The nurse should explain the dangers of increased serum concentrations and give clear directions to the patient on how and when to take medications.
    2 The physician will order appropriate laboratory work.
    3 Above-normal sodium intake will raise excretion, reducing the drug's effectiveness. The patient should be cautioned to maintain a normal sodium intake and understand that any dietary modifications should be ordered by the physician.

130. Comprehension, planning, environment (c)
    2 Carbamazepine can cause aplastic anemia, leukopenia, and thrombocytopenia, all of which are life-threatening reactions. It is imperative that complete blood cell count results be monitored.
    1 Blood sugar levels are not adversely affected by carbamazepine.
    3 Although there is the possibility of gastrointestinal side effects, a gastric analysis would not be indicated for a patient receiving carbamazepine.
    4 Urine for C & S is not a laboratory test related to carbamazepine therapy.

131. Comprehension, planning, environment (b)
    3 Patient safety is always the priority.
    1, 2, 4 These are appropriate diagnoses, but the priority is dealing with the potential for violence.

132. Application, planning, psychosocial (c)
    2 Manic patients are unable to establish limits and frequently are unaware of their impaired abilities. The nurse should evaluate how much responsibility the patient can tolerate.
    1 The patient's ability to deal with stimuli is impaired, and her attention span is too short to assist in planning unit activities.
    3 The patient's ability to deal with others is impaired, making this option inappropriate.
    4 The patient's attention span is short, rendering this response inappropriate.

133. Application, implementation, health (c)
    4 This gives a point of understanding from which to proceed in dealing with the behavior.
    1 This comes after understanding the underlying cause of behavior.
    2 This is not an issue in this situation.
    3 This is an inappropriate response; rules have no meaning at this point.

134. Comprehension, assessment, psychosocial (b)
    4 Pressured is the word used to describe rapid speech patterns.
    1 The speech pattern is not unintelligible; he was understood.
    2 Disorganized may be true but irrelevant.
    3 Variable would not be true; the speech is described as rapid.

135. Application, implementation, psychosocial (a)
    3 The patient should be informed in a nonthreatening but firm manner that her behavior is unacceptable; she should be directed toward activities that encourage more appropriate behavior. This will help her attain control.
    1, 4 These are inappropriate because it is the nurse's responsibility to protect other patients from the impact of negative behavior.
    2 It is never appropriate to threaten a patient.

136. Application, assessment, environment (b)
    3 Flight of ideas is the rapid change from one idea to another without connections; this is commonly seen in mania.
    1 Confabulation is the term that describes an attempt to fill gaps in memory with "made up" information, most commonly seen in dementia.
    2 Primary process refers to a type of thinking in which everything that happens refers to that particular individual, even when there is no connection.
    4 Neologisms are "made up" words; this is usually seen in schizophrenia.

137. Knowledge, assessment, environment (b)
    4 This level is very high; the patient should be assessed immediately.
    1 This level is above therapeutic range.
    2 This level is toxic range.
    3 See No. 4.

138. Knowledge, planning, psychosocial (b)
    3 The patient's unstable mood/affect makes him prone to sudden violence until he has recovered sufficiently to think before acting.
    1 There is no evidence his family is not coping.
    2 There might be anxiety, but it is because of the threat of violence, not necessarily their inability to cope.
    4 There is potential for injury but not to self.

139. Comprehension, assessment, psychosocial (b)
    4 Lithium is a mood stabilizer effective in treating bipolar mood disorders. Cyclothymia, schizophrenia, and schizoaffective disorders have also been treated with lithium with some success.
    1 The patient is in a manic state.
    2 Lithium does not affect one's sex drive. Female manic patients tend to demonstrate flirtatious and seductive behavior as evidence of their bipolar disorder.
    3 Lithium is classified as a mood stabilizer prescribed to achieve equilibrium of mood. The patient is currently in a manic phase; it would be dangerous to increase her manic state.

140. Comprehension, assessment, psychosocial (b)
    3 This statement is typical of the self-focus and careless attitude of the patient in the manic phase of bipolar illness.
    1 This is an unlikely answer. She would not express worry or this level of reasoning in this stage of her illness.
    2 This expression of guilt is more typical of depression, not mania.
    4 This is a very rational, appropriate statement; this is not typical of an individual who is manic.

141. Application, implementation, environment (b)
    1 Individuals who are manic need food they can eat while walking around or engaging in activity so they can maintain calorie intake.
    2 Manic individuals will not spend the time to eat a large meal.
    3 Manic individuals will not respond to a quiet environment; restlessness will not allow them to eat.
    4 Extra vitamins will not be sufficient to make up for the calorie deficit from mania.

142. Application, implementation, psychosocial (b)
    1 He will appreciate the nurse's honesty. It is very difficult for him to trust anyone.
    2 He needs to maintain social interactions. Isolation leads to further distortions of reality.
    3 Making decisions for him will invite his distrust and is nontherapeutic.
    4 He needs to be kept well involved in his treatment plan.

143. Application, implementation, psychosocial (b)
    1 This response presents reality, acknowledges the patient's statement, and casts doubt on the patient's altered thought process, all of which are therapeutic.
    2, 3 This challenges the patient's thought process, which he may be compelled to defend; therefore, this would be nontherapeutic.
    4 This reinforces the patient's hallucination and is thus nontherapeutic.

144. Application, implementation, psychosocial (c)
    2 This allows him to describe what he sees so that the nurse can further discuss what he is experiencing.
    1 Denying what he sees does not help him deal with what he believes he sees.
    3 The nurse should introduce conversation gently, but there's no indication in the situation that simple statements need to be used.
    4 Changing the subject is not therapeutic.

145. Application, implementation, environment (b)
    2 The patient's visual hallucinations are symptomatic of disturbance in brain physiology. This disturbance may be the result of electrolyte imbalance or beginning infection. The physician and/or charge nurse needs this information immediately.
    1 This is an excellent intervention. Visual hallucinations are diminished in a well-lit room. This is an important comfort measure. The nurse would most certainly do this. The *priority* is notifying the physician and/or charge nurse.
    3 This is important, too. The nurse will most certainly want to do this after notifying the physician and attending to the patient's needs for comfort.
    4 This is of no particular importance at this time.

146. Knowledge, assessment, psychosocial (a)
    3 The vision is a false sensory perception.
    1 Delusion is not a fixed false belief.
    2 In this situation there is no sensory perception that is distorted or mistaken.
    4 The defense mechanism regression is a return to an earlier developmental level.

147. Knowledge, assessment, environment (a)
    3 A fixed false belief is a delusion.
    1 The patient may experience severe anxiety or panic, which he may attribute to the delusion he believes to be true.
    2 This is too extreme to be a manifestation of stress alone.
    4 There is no evidence here of perceptual experiences.

148. Comprehension, assessment, environment (c)
    2 The patient has ingested PCP. His skin is flushed and dry because the anticholinergic properties of the drug will not allow his body to perspire. The clinical picture is similar to that of cocaine ingestion.
    1 Heroin would have caused the patient to have pinpoint or constricted pupils. He would not be hallucinating, nor would he be violent.
    3 Barbiturates would produce drowsiness in addition to the dilated pupils.
    4 Marijuana produces dilated pupils and sometimes sedation. There may be hallucinations, but they are less vivid. There is a low incidence of violent behavior with marijuana use.

149. Knowledge, assessment, environment (b)
    3 A level of 0.10 mg/dl is most commonly accepted as the legal standard for intoxication; in some states 0.8 mg/dl is the legal standard.
    1 At this level, the individual is almost always quite obviously intoxicated. If he is not intoxicated, then he has excessive alcohol tolerance.
    2 This is a toxic level. Respiratory depression and coma are expected. The individual requires intensive care and may not survive.
    4 This is lower than the legal level of intoxication. This level occurs when someone has had a drink several hours before the blood sample is taken.

150. Comprehension, evaluation, environment (c)
    2 Alcohol and diazepam (Valium) are cross-tolerant and therefore cross-addicting. The combination of the alcohol and diazepam has a cumulative effect on the patient's addiction. In addition to the discomfort associated with the withdrawal, she may still be experiencing the anxiety for which she had previously required diazepam.
    1 Her motivation cannot be fairly judged. She is undergoing an acutely uncomfortable experience.
    3 It makes no difference that one was a prescription drug and the other is not. They are still cross-addicting.
    4 This is not true. She will need to consider herself a recovering alcoholic/addict. Remaining involved in a Twelve Step or AA program will facilitate her recovery.

151. Comprehension, assessment, environment (c)
    2 The withdrawal syndrome produces effects that are opposite to the effects of the medication. If not medically managed, withdrawal from Valium can produce seizures.
    1 The nurse would not expect to find stupor. She would expect the patient to be overstimulated. It is possible for the patient to become confused and disoriented during the course of the withdrawal.
    3 The patient will not be gregarious. She will be irritable and will need to limit her contact with others. She will not be euphoric.
    4 Unmanaged withdrawal can lead to seizures, coma, and death. Since the patient is hospitalized, it is likely that these complications will be prevented.

152. Application, implementation, physiologic (b)
    1 Monitoring vital signs is essential because of the nature of the physiologic stress that patients experience. They require support and encouragement because of discomfort.
    2 Attendance at group therapy sessions may be overstimulating during the withdrawal process. Group therapy becomes extremely important after the withdrawal is complete.
    3 Adherence to mental health unit rules is helpful in that it promotes safety and involvement in treatment. The staff will need to decide which rules must be enforced and which rules require flexibility.
    4 It is not productive to explore feelings in an effort to develop insight during the withdrawal period. This kind of work is an essential part of the recovery process once the withdrawal is complete.

153. Knowledge, assessment, environment (c)
    4 Mild paranoia and irritability are associated with amphetamine drug use.
    1 Her drug use interferes with her disposition and her attitude toward compliance.
    2 The history does not indicate that her drug use and anorexia have progressed to the point that she would become disoriented and her appearance disheveled. With continued untreated drug use and the accompanying malnutrition, she could experience sufficient damage to her brain to produce these effects.
    3 As above. Without medical care, she could progress to become psychotic and delusional.

154. Knowledge, assessment, environment (c)
    4 Depression, fatigue, and lethargy are common to the syndrome of withdrawal from amphetamine drugs.
    1 Chest pain, diaphoresis, and palpitations are not part of the expected withdrawal syndrome. The patient is at risk for the development of complications such as bleeding ulcer and cardiac problems. The nurse would observe, report, and record these symptoms *immediately.*
    2 The nurse would expect the patient to experience the opposite of these symptoms.
    3 These symptoms are common to withdrawal from opiate drugs.

155. Knowledge, assessment, environment (b)
    4 Profound depression that can last for some months or years is the most likely effect. This requires ongoing therapy with good medical and psychiatric management if she is to be successful in giving up the drug.
    1 This symptom is common to withdrawal from opiate drugs.
    2 This is common to intoxication with amphetamine drugs or PCP.
    3 Euphoria is not common to withdrawal syndrome.

156. Knowledge, assessment, environment (b)
    3 He will exhibit pinpoint pupils for several hours after his last use of heroin.
    1 Dilated pupils indicate the onset of the withdrawal syndrome. If the nurse does not see these symptoms but continues to see pinpoint pupils, she suspects that this patient has managed to acquire drugs while in the hospital.
    2 If this patient exhibits hostility, it is not a result of heroin intoxication. It may be a result of his psychologic response to his arrest or it may be an indication of other psychologic problems.
    4 It is unlikely that this patient would experience profound depression at this time.

157. Application, implementation, psychosocial (c)
    1 Silence gives the patient time to collect his thoughts and reflect on what has been said. When used effectively, it encourages the patient to communicate. The patient should be the one to break the silence.
    2, 3 These actions do not encourage the patient to communicate about his problem.
    4 The patient will speak when he's ready.

158. Application, implementation, environment (a)
    3 Vital signs should be closely monitored as delirium tremens is a life-threatening situation. Also, the need for medication will depend on blood pressure measurements.
    1 This is inappropriate when the patient is experiencing the discomfort of withdrawal.
    2 To prevent exhaustion and reduce agitation, sedation should be established and maintained.
    4 Although the nurse should monitor output, vital signs are the priority.

159. Comprehension, planning, physiologic (c)
    3 Hypomagnesemia is a common problem during alcohol withdrawal; serum magnesium levels should be monitored every 1 to 3 days.
    1 Antabuse interferes with alcohol metabolism; one must be alcohol-free for a minimum of 12 hours before therapy with Antabuse is initiated.
    2 Intravenous calcium is used to treat hypermagnesemia.
    4 Morphine sulfate is a narcotic analgesic. Many drug users take a variety of drugs simultaneously. It would be inappropriate to substitute one substance for another.

160. Knowledge, assessment, environment (b)
    1 Dilated pupils are a common symptom of withdrawal from heroin and other opiates.
    2 Hostility may occur, but it is not the direct result of the withdrawal syndrome.
    3 Pinpoint pupils lead the nurse to suspect that the patient has found a way to acquire more heroin while in the hospital.
    4 This patient is unlikely to experience profound depression at this time.

161. Knowledge, health, implementation (b)
    2 Pinpoint pupils are easily identified in someone who has taken any drug of the opiate class. Euphoria is common, and respiratory depression occurs with larger doses.
    1 These symptoms occur when an addicted person begins to experience withdrawal symptoms.
    3 Dilated pupils, drowsiness, and visual hallucinations occur as a result of drugs that have anticholinergic properties. Phencyclidine (PCP) and marijuana have these properties.
    4 These are the effects of ingestion of amphetamines.

162. Application, implementation, health (c)
    2 This is an opportunity to explore how her family will or will not participate in her recovery.
    1 This is true, but it does not address what her mother is asking.
    3 This is also true, but it does not address the question of the important part played by her family.
    4 This is not the case. Attendance is strongly suggested, but no program can make it a mandatory condition of discharge.

163. Knowledge, assessment, environment (a)
    4 Tactile hallucinations are common in alcohol withdrawal. The nurse should be sure to observe, report, and record this important clinical symptom.
    1 Olfactory hallucinations or those involving the sense of smell can occur in alcohol withdrawal, but they are more commonly associated with tumors on the brain and some seizure disorders.
    2 The patient is quite likely to experience visual hallucinations in addition to the tactile hallucinations he is currently experiencing.
    3 Some individuals experience auditory hallucinations during alcohol withdrawal; however, these hallucinations are most commonly seen in schizophrenia.

164. Comprehension, planning, environment (c)
    4 This therapy is designed to help regressed and disoriented patients become more aware of present reality.
    1 This is more for self-help, without a designated leader.
    2 This helps in changing problematic aspects of behavior and is not applicable for him.
    3 This is not applicable; this type of therapy is for learning and practicing relaxation techniques.

165. Comprehension, assessment, environment (c)
    1 Poor work records are characteristic because they indicate a lack of responsibility.
    2 This is characteristic of borderline personality disorder.
    3 This is characteristic of histrionic personality disorders.
    4 This is characteristic of passive-aggressive personality disorders.

166. Comprehension, planning, environment (b)
    2 Manipulative patients want limits set on their behavior. The extent should always be that which is necessary to protect the patient and others.
    1 It is inappropriate and not necessary to set limits on all behavior, because all behavior is not manipulative.
    3 The patient should not independently set limits on his behavior but rather do so with the assistance of the nurse.
    4 It is not the role of the community to set limits on patient behavior. This is the staff's responsibility.

167. Knowledge, assessment, psychosocial (b)
    3 The most reliable evidence is that personality disorders begin at the stage of separation/individuation from the mother and that the family of origin is usually dysfunctional in some way.
    1 There is no evidence at present to suggest biochemical imbalance is involved in personality disorder.
    2 There is no evidence of a gene for personality disorder.
    4 Birth complications do not cause personality disorders.

168. Application, planning, environment (c)
    4 Individuals with personality disorders have persistent and severe difficulties in personal relationships.
    1 The patient may or may not have problems with this.
    2 If the patient is a substance abuser, this may or may not be problematic, depending on how severe and how recent substance use has been.
    3 This patient may have difficulty with rules, but this will not be the primary problem.

169. Knowledge, planning, environment (a)
    4 Some substances produce no physiologic dependence but do cause powerful psychologic dependence in the user.
    1, 2 These are each only one symptom of addiction.
    3 Not all substances that are addictive produce both of these symptoms.

170. Knowledge, assessment, environment (b)
    2 Alcoholic cardiomyopathy, hypertension, and atherosclerotic changes are only a few of the consequences of long-term alcohol abuse.
    1 Changes in the function of the pituitary and thyroid glands can also occur, but these changes are less common and not as serious.
    3 Poor nutrition and increased alcohol intake can cause loss of calcium from bones and can contribute to muscle atrophy, but cardiac changes are still more serious.
    4 Sterility and erectile dysfunction also are common with long-term alcohol abuse.

171. Application, implementation, health (c)
    3 Role modeling by the nurse is the best way to teach him how to maximize his mother's strengths and cope with her deficits until she improves.
    1 This gives false reassurance; it may take much longer, and there is no way to predict how much she will recover.
    2 This would deprive her of the comfort of his visits and denies him the opportunity to monitor her progress.
    4 This will not necessarily answer his questions any more completely or give him any more reassurance than talking with the nurse.

172. Comprehension, assessment, psychosocial (c)
    1 Maladaptation in interpersonal and social relationships is consistently a feature of personality disorders.
    2 Some individuals who have personality disorders often have the capacity to irritate others, yet some may be overly anxious to please everyone.
    3 This self-centeredness and inflexibility may be a part of a personality disorder, yet this description is less complete.
    4 The individual who is attention-seeking and overly anxious to entertain may represent a type of personality disorder. Similarly, the individual who is overly serious or withdrawn may represent another type of personality disorder.

173. Knowledge, assessment, psychosocial (b)
    3 Antisocial personality disorder is manifested by little respect for the law as well as little respect for the rights and needs of others.
    1 Avoidant personality disorder is manifested by a lack of interpersonal skills but a real desire to relate to others.
    2 Schizotypal personality disorder is manifested by a lack of genuine interest in relating to others.
    4 Impulsive personality disorder is manifested by an inability to control impulses, which leads to poor judgment.

174. Comprehension, assessment, psychosocial (c)
    3 It is useful to assess the patient's coping style. The understanding the nurse gains from this will facilitate her understanding of the patient's health education needs.
    1 A disruptive life-style is not an illness, but it does not promote health.
    2 A disruptive life-style may contribute to the development of a perceptual or affective disorder.
    4 Genetically inherited personality traits have some influence on personality and life-style.

175. Comprehension, planning, psychosocial (c)
    3 Personality disorders are resistant to change. Long-term therapy is needed.
    1 Medication is not helpful, but it is usually used on a short-term basis to manage specific symptoms.
    2 Group therapy is helpful but generally not highly successful.
    4 He is not likely to be having very much anxiety. He is more likely to cause anxiety in others.

176. Comprehension, assessment, psychosocial (c)
    2 The nurse may expect the patient to display restricted affect. He interprets teasing from others in a concrete and paranoid way. The nurse may need to protect him from teasing from other patients or his family.
    1 Paranoid personalities feel misjudged and mistreated by others and display jealousy, not sentimentality.
    3 He will not be self-indulgent. He is likely to be very disciplined in his drive for self-achievement.
    4 This is characteristic of histrionic personalities.

177. Knowledge, assessment, environment (a)
    4 Symptoms are usually quite unpleasant. They include headache, gastritis, fatigue, malaise, and irritability.
    1 Blood alcohol level may remain elevated in someone who has impaired liver function as a result of chronic alcoholism. This does not describe hangover.
    2 Hangover is accompanied by hypoglycemia and an increase of lactic acid in the blood.
    3 A sense of euphoria may occur after alcohol is ingested. It does not persist.

178. Knowledge, assessment, environment (b)
    3 Blackouts occur for the period of time during which the person is intoxicated. Many individuals deny that they have lost memory of the events.
    1 Social impairment occurs with alcoholism as a result of progressive brain damage.
    2 Wernicke's syndrome is a type of dementia that occurs as a result of the toxic effects of alcohol on the brain.
    4 Certainly one might want to forget events that occurred during a binge; however, this individual has not willfully forgotten. The toxic effects of alcohol have impaired his brain's ability to remember recent events.

179. Knowledge, assessment, environment (a)
    4 Sedatives and barbiturates are the second most commonly abused class of drugs. Many people believe that these drugs are not addictive because they are prescribed by physicians. A pattern in increasing tolerance that leads to increased use of the drugs tends to promote addiction. Use of even small quantities of alcohol in combination with these drugs greatly increases the likelihood of addiction.
    1 Amphetamines are less commonly used than sedatives.
    2 Cocaine is less commonly used than sedatives and is classified as a narcotic.
    3 Narcotics are less commonly used than sedatives.

180. Comprehension, planning, environment (b)
    3 Realistic consequences should always be addressed at the time limits are set. It is important that the patient know what consequences have been established so he has the opportunity to discuss his reactions and feelings.
    1 As a motivation to change his behavior, the patient should know the consequences at the time the limit is set.
    2 Again, consequences should be preestablished to be consistently enforced by all staff members.
    4 Manipulative patient behavior can be quite frustrating to staff members. Manipulative behaviors should be immediately identified and consequences enforced to motivate the patient to change his behavior.

181. Application, implementation, psychosocial (c)
    4 This is a fundamental skill that these patients lack and is at the root of many of their other problems.
    1, 2 These might not be possible until other issues are resolved.
    3 This is important but is part of the primary goal; see No. 4.

182. Comprehension, assessment, psychosocial (b)
    1 Manipulation is a characteristic style of relating in individuals with personality disorders.
    2 Projection is used by these individuals as a way of expressing unacceptable feelings.
    3, 4 These are not commonly used mechanisms by those with personality disorders.

183. Knowledge, assessment, environment (c)
    2 The woman is developing awareness of the impact the loss of her husband will have on her life. This is a very difficult period in her life. Grief is quite demanding physically. She is predisposed to the development of illnesses as a result of the effect grief has on the body.
    1 She has moved beyond the stage of shock and denial.
    3 During the phase of restitution, she will cope with her loss and begin to develop new ways of living a fulfilling life.
    4 Normal grieving is very distressing. There is no reason to suspect her grief reaction will be distorted.

184. Knowledge, assessment, psychosocial (a)
   4 Conversion reactions usually follow an event that triggers psychologic conflict. The primary gain is relief; the secondary gains are sympathy and increased attention from others.
   1 This is suppression.
   2 This is rationalization.
   3 This is projection.

185. Application, implementation, environment (c)
   4 This removes him from the distraction and stimulation of the general waiting area, increasing the likelihood that he will be compliant and have his scan done.
   1 He may never feel ready and may actually opt to leave.
   2 This will not decrease his anxiety or confusion; it may make it worse.
   3 This will not increase the likelihood that he will cooperate; it may make him angry.

186. Application, planning, environment (c)
   3 This acknowledges that the patient is probably tired and may be frightened as a result of his mental deficits. It gives him the opportunity to feel some control in the process of being evaluated and makes the nurse an ally, not an enemy.
   1 This is true, but there is nothing to be gained and it needlessly aggravates the patient to continue to question him when he is obviously unwilling to continue at this time.
   2 There is no reason to doubt the truth of what the patient says he is feeling. Doubting him may make him angry and argumentative.
   4 This might also be true, but his family's wishes are not the priority at this time.

187. Application, planning, health (c)
   4 This is the most accurate answer. Alzheimer's disease progresses at a different rate in different patients, although the end result is always the same.
   1 This is untrue. He will not recover from his deficits.
   2 This is true, although it does not really explain anything to his family.
   3 This is not necessarily true because the nurse has only seen him under stress. This can make his deficits appear more pronounced than they are.

188. Comprehension, evaluation, environment (b)
   2 The patient's short-term memory is too impaired to allow her to stick with the task of feeding herself.
   1 This is unlikely.
   3 There is no indication that the patient is delusional.
   4 The patient is at risk for becoming depressed, which is characteristic of stage I of Alzheimer's disease. Depression is probably not the cause of her not eating.

189. Application, implementation, physiologic (b)
   3 She needs support and encouragement to feed herself. The nurse should help her to maintain her independence as much as possible.
   1 This is indicated only if she is physically weak or impaired.
   2 The nutritionist will be helpful, but this measure is not the priority.
   4 This will not address her difficulty in feeding herself.

190. Knowledge, assessment, psychosocial (b)
   2 Memory losses are the most common symptom of the first stage of this disease.
   1 Gradual loss of motor function is characteristic of stage II of the disease.
   3 Loss of gross motor coordination is seen in stage II.
   4 Loss of fine motor coordination is seen in stage II.

191. Application, implementation, psychosocial (c)
   3 Contracting with the patient to take control of some of the compulsive behavior will help the patient become more conscious of the behavior. This will eventually help the patient to make other choices.
   1 This can be very helpful to most patients, but it is not the *most* appropriate nursing intervention.
   2 The nurse might discuss the patient's compulsive behavior after the patient has become more conscious of the behavior.
   4 Building assertiveness skills is helpful to most patients, but it is not the *most* appropriate response.

192. Comprehension, assessment, psychosocial (b)
   1 Perfectionism is a feature of the compulsive personality disorder. There is a tendency to see things as either all bad or all good, all right or all wrong.
   2 Decisiveness, or the ability to make decisions, is impaired by the need to make perfect decisions.
   3 Empathy is impaired by the person's tendency to be wrapped up in his own needs.
   4 The capacity to cooperate is impaired by the need to be in control and to have things done one's own way.

193. Comprehension, assessment, psychosocial (b)
   4 Compulsive personalities are preoccupied with rules, details, and conformity. Work and productivity are their priorities; perfectionism and superiority negatively affect their interpersonal relationships.
   1 This is characteristic of histrionic personalities.
   2 This is seen in borderline personalities.
   3 This describes schizotypal personalities.

194. Comprehension, assessment, psychosocial (b)
   2 People with agoraphobia fear being in crowds; they fear not being able to escape.
   1 They do not exhibit psychotic symptoms.
   3 Physical complaints are not a primary concern.
   4 Tachycardia is more likely.

195. Comprehension, planning, environment (a)
   4 Taking measures to reduce threats to her physical well-being caused by her ritual is the most appropriate nursing intervention.
   1 Preventing the ritual will increase the patient's anxiety.
   2 The patient already knows the ritual is silly; it is not appropriate to call attention to the ritual.
   3 Rushing the patient will increase her anxiety, which will increase her need to perform the ritual.

196. Comprehension, evaluation, psychosocial (b)
   2 This indicates anxiety has been reduced and adaptive substitutes have been acquired.
   1, 3, 4 These are symptoms of obsessive-compulsive disorder.

197. Comprehension, assessment, environment (c)
   2 The patient is suffering from bulimia. Self-induced vomiting is the cue.
   1 In anorexia nervosa, the individual simply avoids eating.
   3 Agoraphobia is the fear of open spaces.
   4 The narcissistic personality disorder is sometimes associated with eating disorders. There is no indication that the patient has a personality disorder.

198. Comprehension, assessment, psychosocial (b)
   2 Rituals around food and exercise are typical ways in which these patients attempt to control overwhelming anxiety.
   1 Patients with anorexia do not believe they are sick.
   3 Anorexic individuals exercise compulsively to increase calorie output.
   4 This is partly true, but it is not the primary reason.

199. Application, implementation, environment (b)
    4 Patients with anorexia must be reminded of the consequences of extreme weight loss, because they do not believe themselves to be doing anything harmful.
    1 This kind of statement is threatening to these patients because it confronts them with loss of control.
    2 These patients do not believe extreme thinness to be unattractive.
    3 A patient with anorexia will never take this seriously.
200. Knowledge, evaluation, psychosocial (a)
    3 Weight gain is a goal for anorexics.
    1 This doesn't mean she is better.
    2 This doesn't mean she eats them.
    4 This by itself doesn't indicate improvement.
201. Knowledge, implementation, psychosocial (b)
    4 The nurse is not being judgmental but is monitoring the patient's meal.
    1 The nurse cannot monitor the patient's intake if she leaves her for 15 minutes.
    2 This will not promote improved nutrition.
    3 This just makes the patient feel guilty.
202. Comprehension, planning, psychosocial (c)
    1 Individuals with anorexia worry about being liked and wanted by those around them. They believe that being as thin as possible will help to achieve this goal.
    2 This is not true. Individuals with anorexia tend to be high achievers in intellectual tasks.
    3 They worry about control over themselves, not others.
    4 Individuals with anorexia never feel safe from the threat of potential weight gain.
203. Comprehension, assessment, physiologic (a)
    2 Loss of body fat leads to cessation of menstrual flow.
    1 Anorexia may be related to other factors such as hospital admission.
    3 This gives the nurse no information to build on.
    4 The patient is trying to take the focus off of herself.
204. Comprehension, assessment, psychosocial (b)
    2 The parents of anorexics are characteristically rigid and overprotective.
    1, 4 These are characteristics of anorexia nervosa.
    3 These are characteristics of bulimia.
205. Knowledge, planning, health (a)
    2 A complex interaction between body and mind influences the health of the individual.
    1 The individual's role in his world may influence his well-being, but this does not describe the concept of holism.
    3 Although this may be a valid point of view, it is not the concept of holism.
    4 The collective life of the community does not describe the concept of holism as it pertains to individual health.
206. Comprehension, planning, health (c)
    4 In keeping with the concept of holism, these are the dimensions considered in planning care for an individual.
    1 These are management considerations, but they do not necessarily guide nursing care planning.
    2 These may also be management considerations, but they are not aspects of nursing care planning.
    3 These are treatment modalities that may be considered in the plan of care.
207. Comprehension, implementation, psychosocial (a)
    1 This is an appropriate goal.
    2 False reassurance is not helpful.
    3 Secluding the patient is not helpful.
    4 Future planning may only depress the patient more.

208. Comprehension, evaluation, environment (b)
    2 He cannot leave the hospital unless he is officially discharged.
    1 He does not lose civil rights unless he is declared incompetent.
    3 He may be competent, but he cannot leave voluntarily.
    4 He can vote unless he loses his civil rights.
209. Comprehension, evaluation, environment (b)
    2 Goals should be stated in behavioral terms.
    1, 3 It is difficult to know if the goal is achievable because there are no criteria for performance.
    4 It is not a behavioral goal; it does not meet nursing process criteria for an expected outcome (goal).
210. Knowledge, assessment, psychosocial (a)
    1 Shock and denial are common reactions to this kind of news. Denial is a useful defense mechanism in that it protects the person from emotional pain and thus frees him to deal with his affairs. Denial can become a dysfunctional defense if it interferes with his perception of reality or if it interferes with his seeking appropriate medical care.
    2 Anger that one has a fatal illness usually occurs after shock and denial.
    3 The degree to which one becomes depressed about a terminal illness varies with the individual.
    4 Acceptance is something one may or may not reach in the grieving process. It is healthier if one can achieve some acceptance. Emotional support from loved ones facilitates this.
211. Comprehension, assessment, environment (b)
    4 The woman can experience a normal grief reaction. Her emotional experience of grief may be complicated if she has been overly dependent on her mother or if she has difficulty expressing herself.
    1 This is not true. Mentally retarded people are capable of forming close, warm, satisfying relationships.
    2 There is no indication that she will abuse alcohol.
    3 It is not likely that she will become psychotically depressed.
212. Knowledge, assessment, psychosocial (b)
    3 Positive reinforcement is when the patient is rewarded for appropriate behavior.
    1 The tokens are not bribes; they are used in an attempt to modify behavior.
    2 The nurse may be modeling the appropriate behavior, but this isn't related to the tokens.
    4 The patient is being rewarded, so the reinforcement is positive.
213. Comprehension, planning, psychosocial (a)
    1 It is most important to establish a strong nurse-patient relationship.
    2 Verbal and nonverbal communication are both important.
    3 This may be a side effect if the room is tense.
    4 First the nurse must establish trust.
214. Comprehension, assessment, psychosocial (b)
    4 When a person is being assertive she considers not only her own needs but also those of the other person. The request is made in a normal tone of voice and is reasonable and specific.
    1 Aggression is considering only one's own feelings. The request is made in a loud and angry voice.
    2 Passive behavior is displayed when the person pushes her own needs aside and considers only the needs of others. In this situation the passive employee would have said nothing.
    3 The manipulator attempts to get her own way by using guilt.

215. Application, implementation, psychosocial (b)
    2 The nurse is making light of the patient's concerns. This statement would not enhance the communication between the nurse and patient.
    1 Changing the subject can occur when the nurse feels uncomfortable with the conversation. An example would be the patient discussing his upcoming death and the nurse starting to discuss the weather.
    3 In disagreeing, the nurse is not taking the time to find out what the patient is really feeling or trying to discuss. Disagreement will end the conversation quickly.
    4 Reassuring clichés are easily detected and make the patient distrust the nurse. An example would be "everything is going to be all right." Clichés do not enhance the communication between the nurse and patient.

216. Knowledge, assessment, psychosocial (b)
    2 A number of mentally ill patients are treated as outpatients.
    1 Hospital stays have decreased in length.
    3 Many mentally ill patients return home.
    4 Most are treated as outpatients.

217. Application, implementation, psychosocial (b)
    3 This patient needs a calm, quiet environment.
    1, 2 The patient needs decreased stimuli at this time.
    4 Now is not the time for this; the patient is too anxious.

218. Comprehension, assessment, physiologic (c)
    2 NMS is characterized by these symptoms.
    1 These are symptoms of encephalitis. Symptoms resemble those of meningitis, but their onset is more gradual.
    3 These are classic symptoms of meningococcal meningitis (bacterial meningitis).
    4 These are symptoms of gram-negative bacteremia.

219. Comprehension, evaluation, health (c)
    2 Salad dressings that do not contain MSG or cheese are allowed on a tyramine-restricted diet.
    1, 3, 4 Cheese pizza, sauerkraut, and sherry are forbidden foods on a tyramine-restricted diet.

220. Comprehension, planning, environment (b)
    3 It is important that the nursing staff be consistent and support one another in the care of this patient. It is neither possible nor wise to enforce all of the rules. The team must decide which rules are in the patient's best interest.
    1 This kind of behavior causes staff splitting. If the patient is allowed to choose favorites, staff cohesion is undermined and the staff is less effective in working together.
    2 The patient needs to have limits set on her behavior so that she can benefit from treatment.
    4 The staff has the responsibility of enforcing rules to bring about an effective treatment environment for the patient community.

221. Knowledge, implementation, environment (b)
    2 Benztropine (Cogentin) is prescribed specifically to counteract the side effect of dystonia, which is what this patient is experiencing.
    1, 4 These are antianxiety drugs and will not help.
    3 Chlorpromazine (Thorazine) is another antipsychotic drug that will worsen the reaction that he is having.

222. Knowledge, implementation, environment (b)
    4 The ordered dose is questionable, as the initial dose is usually 2 to 5 mg. The daily dosage range is 1 to 30 mg.
    1 This is incorrect.
    2 Haloperidol (Haldol) is available in both oral and IM form.
    3 Haloperidol is a short-acting antipsychotic drug that is often given to control acute psychotic symptoms.

223. Knowledge, evaluation, environment (b)
    2 Akathisia is the sensation of not being able to sit still.
    1 Dystonia is abnormal muscle spasms of the upper body.
    3 Tardive dyskinesia is abnormal movements of the face, lips, tongue, and lower extremities.
    4 Pseudoparkinsonism is abnormal stiffness of movement and facial expression.

224. Comprehension, planning, health (b)
    1 Family support has been shown to be an important reason why patients remain compliant with treatment.
    2 Education does not guarantee that families will always cooperate with treatment.
    3 The goal of teaching is for patients and families to understand that taking medications must be the responsibility of the patient.
    4 Teaching does not ensure the approval of the family. The family's *support* is sought, not their approval.

225. Application, planning, health (c)
    3 After 2 years of grieving, verbalizing on a daily basis, even if only for a few minutes, is realistic and necessary.
    1 She will need to verbalize or she will not be able to be discharged.
    2 This does not provide enough opportunity to resolve such a lengthy period of dysfunction.
    4 A weekly visit might have been sufficient earlier in this problem, but not at this point. Also, she will need more contact than this to build trust.

226. Comprehension, planning, health (a)
    2 Liquid medications are ordered for hospitalized patients with a history of noncompliance and for patients that the staff suspects may be "checking" or hoarding. The oral route of administration is always the preferred route. To counter noncompliance tendencies in outpatients, long-acting depot injections are recommended. Patients have the right to refuse treatment, and this includes medications.
    1, 3 These are not recommended for noncompliant patients; it is too easy to "check" and hoard.
    4 Only in a psychiatric *emergency* can medications be given without consent to prevent harm to the patient or to others. The parenteral route should be used only if it is clear that without the medication, the patient poses a danger to himself and/or others.

227. Comprehension, planning, psychosocial (c)
    4 Contracts emphasize patient responsibilities and level of participation.
    1 Contracts emphasize what the nurse will do *with* the patient rather than *for* the patient.
    2, 3 Emphasis is always on the patient's strengths, responsibility, and participation, not on what the nurse will not do.

228. Knowledge, planning, psychosocial (a)
    1 The theory is that patients fare better when they return to the community quickly with their support systems maintained.
    2 Although mental health of the community is a goal, it is impossible to ensure that an entire community is healthy.
    3 This is opposite of the optimal theory, above.
    4 Although some restructuring may occur, this is not the main goal.

229. Comprehension, implementation, environment (b)
    2 Goal-oriented activity is needed to provide structure.
    1 This is ineffective because it allows patients to lead the group.
    3 This is ineffective because the patient's functioning may be disturbed, disoriented, or disorganized.
    4 This is ineffective because repression does not allow feelings to be expressed.

230. Application, intervention, psychosocial (a)
    2 Listening allows the patient to experience himself more freely and fully and encourages him to work through his feelings.
    1, 3 These responses ignore the patient's need to express his feelings to the nurse.
    4 This insensitively ignores the patient's feelings and blocks communication.
231. Comprehension, planning, environment (b)
    3 Crisis intervention therapy, being short term, is usually from 1 to 6 weeks. A crisis is usually resolved within a 4- to 6-week period and focuses on the current problem only.
    1, 2, 4 Crisis intervention therapy is short term and lasts 1 to 6 weeks.
232. Knowledge, planning, environment (b)
    1 This is an absolutely fundamental need for the nurse to address before anything else.
    2 This is important, but it comes only after the patient's safety is ensured.
    3 This may or may not be an issue at this time, but it is not the nurse's first priority with her.
    4 She will probably do this if she feels safe and trusting.
233. Application, implementation, health (c)
    4 Men who batter their partners have learned to use violence as a way of expressing their feelings; they can be taught to behave differently.
    1 This is not necessarily true. Some men who have battered their partners in the past have stopped doing so with the appropriate interventions.
    2 This is not necessarily true, either. She may have sound reasons to hope that he can be different, and the nurse should explore those with her.
    3 This is judgmental and casts her in the role of victim, which will inhibit any chance of change taking place in the relationship.
234. Application, planning, health (c)
    2 Use of alcohol lowers inhibitions and increases the possibility that a person who would use violence will do so.
    1 This is not true. If he is a person who uses violence as a means of expression, he will do so even if not drinking.
    3 This is not true. Alcohol use decreases inhibitions and makes inappropriate behavior more likely to occur.
    4 This also is untrue. The causes of battering are many; drinking can only increase the likelihood that abuse will occur at a particular time.
235. Knowledge, assessment, psychosocial (b)
    2 Women from middle and upper socioeconomic status (SES) groups have more access to private physicians who will not reveal that their patients are being abused. Women from lower SES groups have to rely more on public clinics and emergency departments for treatment.
    1 Battering and abuse of women is a cross-class issue. One socioeconomic group is no more likely to encounter abuse from their partners than any other.
    3 The police respond equally to all complaints.
    4 There is no evidence to support this; men of all classes abuse women.
236. Knowledge, assessment, environment (a)
    3 Child abusers have a history of emotional deprivation, abuse, or neglect as a child.
    1 Child abuse occurs in all socioeconomic groups.
    2 Abusive parents tend to look to the child to fill their need for acceptance and love; these are unrealistic expectations of a child.
    4 Abusive parents are described as suspicious of others and have minimal, if any, social interaction.
237. Comprehension, assessment, environment (b)
    1 Abused children become visibly uncomfortable when they hear other children cry.
    2 Habit disorders are characteristics of emotional abuse.
    3 Poor peer relationship is indicative of sexual abuse.
    4 Emotional or mental lag is associated with emotional abuse.
238. Comprehension, planning, environment (a)
    3 Expressive therapy such as art or play therapy enables the child to communicate painful emotions nonverbally. Verbalization of feelings is more threatening.
    1 Group therapy requires verbal sharing, which is more threatening than nonverbal types of therapy.
    2 Hypnosis is helpful in identifying a source of anxiety. In this situation, sexual abuse is already the known source.
    4 This type of therapy is effective for phobic patients.
239. Knowledge, assessment, environment (b)
    2 Violence and abuse against women most often occurs for the first time or increases in frequency and severity during pregnancy.
    1 Battered women in most cases do not present themselves for treatment related to abuse.
    3 Battered women do not usually seek mental health services as a result of being abused.
    4 Only a small percentage of battered women seek or receive legal assistance in dealing with their abusers.
240. Application, implementation, psychosocial (b)
    2 This is a broad opening statement that encourages the patient to verbalize.
    1 False reassurance and stereotypic comments block communication.
    3 Giving directions denies the patient independence with problem-solving and is nontherapeutic.
    4 Questions of this nature make the patient feel defensive and create a stressful situation for the patient.
241. Knowledge, planning, psychosocial (c)
    3 Play therapy is the most common treatment for depression in a child. Children have the capacity to express deep feelings through symbols they choose in their play.
    1 Cognitive therapy is used for adults. This therapy emphasizes healthy ways of thinking about oneself and one's circumstances.
    2 Insight-oriented psychotherapy is used for adults. It is a deeper exploration of the self.
    4 Work therapy is used for adolescents and adults. It emphasizes building self-esteem through meaningful work.
242. Application, implementation, psychosocial (a)
    3 It is very pleasant to work with patients who improve and who appreciate the nurse's contribution to that improvement. Nevertheless, the nurse must maintain professional boundaries. It is not appropriate to meet the patient for lunch after she has been discharged.
    1, 4 It is not appropriate to agree to meet the patient for lunch. See No. 3.
    2 This is true, but the patient needs to be given an explanation so as not to feel rejected.
243. Application, implementation, health (c)
    1 Learning their symptoms can help patients to obtain rapid treatment and perhaps avoid hospitalization.
    2 This will not affect her vulnerability to depression.
    3 Decreasing stressors is constructive, but this does not affect the physiologic processes of depression.
    4 This does not guarantee that she will not become ill.

244. Application, implementation, physiologic (a)
   2 Restating and repeating the main idea is a technique that enhances communication.
   1 This challenges the patient, places the patient on the defensive, and blocks attempts to discuss unmet needs.
   3 Requesting an explanation can be intimidating to the patient, and it can block communication.
   4 Giving advice is not the role of the psychiatric nurse, nor is it therapeutic. It implies that the nurse knows best, and this fosters dependence.

245. Comprehension, implementation, psychosocial (b)
   1 This encourages the patient to use her own resources, which will minimize feelings of dependency and hopelessness associated with depression.
   2, 4 This ignores the patient's need and blocks communication.
   3 The nurse should not act for the patient unless absolutely necessary.

246. Application, assessment, psychosocial (b)
   2 Safety is the number one priority.
   1, 3 This is not the first priority.
   4 This is not most important.

247. Comprehension, assessment, environment (b)
   4 Patient safety is always the priority. The patient's statement that there is nothing left to be taken from her is the cue.
   1, 2, 3 These nursing diagnoses are all appropriate for the depressed patient, but the situation does not indicate that any of these problems are of immediate concern.

248. Comprehension, assessment, environment (b)
   3 Delusions of guilt or sin are common in depression. The individual may feel like a truly bad person, although this may not be true. Low self-esteem is also common in depression. Delusions of guilt and sin are similar to low self-esteem, but they are more severe.
   1 Delusions of grandeur involve the individual's perception that she is extremely important, privileged, or gifted. This kind of delusion is most likely to occur in a manic episode.
   2 Delusions of persecution include one's belief that a conspiracy exists to thwart or to kill the individual. This kind of delusion is often associated with delusions of grandeur. It is most likely to be seen in patients experiencing manic or paranoid episodes.
   4 Flight of ideas is seen in manic or highly agitated patients. The individual's thoughts move rapidly though logically from one subject to another. There is a quality of distractibility often associated with euphoria.

249. Knowledge, planning, psychosocial (b)
   3 Ego ideal is one's perception of how one should be, compared to how one perceives oneself to actually be.
   1 Body image is one part of identity.
   2 Role is a description of how one fits into the society, while body image is one's perception of one's body.
   4 See above descriptions.

250. Comprehension, implementation, environment (b)
   4 Although the time period varies from state to state, written notice to be discharged is required of voluntary psychiatric admissions.
   1, 3 Informal admissions (no formal or written application for admission) may leave a psychiatric facility by signing against medical advice (AMA).
   2 Voluntary admissions do not require court-ordered releases.

251. Comprehension, planning, environment (b)
   2 Constipation is a common side effect of tricyclic antidepressant drugs. Severe constipation requires immediate medical attention.
   1, 4 These are not common side effects of Pamelor.
   3 The change in her mood will be gradual over a period of 1 to 3 weeks.

252. Application, implementation, environment (c)
   2 The nurse must evaluate his suicidal intent. It may be that this suicide gesture has resolved nothing for him. He may leave the hospital only to make a more lethal gesture later.
   1 Provoking guilt in the patient will not promote his mental health.
   3 This is an accusational remark that will damage the nurse's relationship with the patient.
   4 As above. This kind of remark inhibits building professional rapport with the patient.

253. Comprehension, implementation, environment (c)
   2 One-to-one observation should begin immediately so the patient is in full view at all times.
   1 Patients who do not respond to limit-setting may need to be restrained. Restraints should be employed only when all other safety measures have failed. This is not, however, the first nursing action.
   3 Seclusion is used only when all other safety measures have failed; it would not be the first nursing action.
   4 Removing dangerous possessions is a priority and should be done by the staff member assigned to one-to-one observation.

254. Comprehension, planning, psychosocial (b)
   2 A suicidal patient may not perceive possible options, and he may need to learn new strategies for dealing with problems.
   1 It is difficult to separate gestures from realistic attempts at suicide.
   3 There is no specific requirement.
   4 Asking for reasons is not helpful.

255. Comprehension, assessment, environment (b)
   2 The patient's energy level is up, and he is more likely to take action.
   1 The patient does not have the energy.
   3, 4 Suicide is not as likely to happen now.

256. Application, assessment, psychosocial (b)
   4 This patient has five high-risk factors: sex, age, drinking, job loss, and family history of suicide.
   1, 2, 3 There are too many factors in this case for the patient to have a low risk.

257. Comprehension, planning, environment (b)
   3 Confusion is one of the major side effects. Frequent orientation is necessary during the treatment course.
   1 Electroconvulsive therapy (ECT) is not a permanent cure for depression. Maintenance treatment decreases the relapse rate.
   2 An individual who has received ECT usually completely recovers from memory loss.
   4 A decrease in symptoms of depression usually occurs after 1 to 3 weeks of treatment.

258. Comprehension, evaluation, psychosocial (b)
   4 The patient is threatening to harm herself. Keeping her safe is the nurse's highest priority.
   1, 2 These are correct, but they are not the highest priority.
   3 This may or may not be true.

259. Comprehension, assessment, environment (a)
   1 Safety comes first: what is the plan; does he have the weapon?
   2 This is not essential information.
   3 His call is a cry for help.
   4 This is not the most important thing to ask first.

260. Knowledge, planning, health (b)
   3 All community mental health centers are required by law to have in place a fully developed suicide risk detection and prevention program for all age groups.
   1 Most community mental health centers have these, but they are not legally required.
   2 Some community mental health centers offer these programs, but they are not required.
   4 These are not required to be provided by these centers.

261. Knowledge, assessment, psychosocial (b)
   2 This is the highest risk. This statement shows that the person has made a clear plan, has the means to commit the act, and has selected a time.
   1 Of all the statements, this indicates the lowest risk. If the chronic frustration continues, the risk may increase.
   3 This statement may indicate the second-highest risk. It suggests the individual may make a suicide gesture in an effort to manipulate or control the girlfriend. A suicide gesture done in an effort to manipulate can be lethal.
   4 This statement suggests relatively low immediate risk. It also suggests that the individual requires observation for an increase in suicidal intent.

262. Application, implementation, environment (a)
   3 Sharp items should be removed.
   1, 2 There is no need to deny the patient these items.
   4 Shoe laces should be removed from the shoes. There is no need to deny the patient her shoes.

263. Application, planning, health (b)
   3 Before anything is done, the rape victim must be informed of her options in regard to reporting the rape and her rights as a victim.
   1 She should not have anything done until she is informed of her rights and options.
   2 She should not shower until a decision has been made about whether physical evidence will be gathered.
   4 This should not be done until she is informed of her rights and options.

264. Application, implementation, health (b)
   2 Many times an entire family feels traumatized by an act of violence toward a loved one. Professional counseling can be useful for the entire family.
   1 This is a correct statement, but it is not the best answer.
   3 Sometimes the family may feel it is better to let the person work things out for herself. This usually results from their feeling of helplessness. The patient and her family can help one another with the guidance of a professional.
   4 Although this may sometimes be true, it does not sufficiently answer the mother's question.

265. Application, planning, psychosocial (b)
   4 Children may draw pictures to communicate their feelings.
   1 All patients deserve equal time.
   2 Distraction doesn't work in most cases.
   3 Bribery isn't usually effective when dealing with uncomfortable subjects.

266. Application, planning, psychosocial (b)
   1 This action displays caring by the nurse and will give the child comfort.
   2 The child may become frightened by too much touching. He may have a fear that he is being molested again.
   3 The child needs to have someone with him. At this point he is confused and frightened.
   4 The child will not feel comfortable discussing the incident in great detail at first. Allow time for the child to willingly discuss it.

267. Knowledge, evaluation, psychosocial (a)
   1 This is privileged communication.
   2 This refers to release from hospital, not to any relationship.
   3 There are no special malpractice laws.
   4 This is not related to the situation; this term refers to a temporary substitute for a physician who is away from the practice.

268. Comprehension, assessment, psychosocial (b)
   1 Many perceive this treatment as punishment.
   2 This may be true prior to their first treatment but after the first treatment they will understand it is not painful.
   3 It does cause temporary amnesia, but they don't realize what they have forgotten, so they can't see it as an escape.
   4 While this may be true, it is not the primary concern; the amount of current is so small that this is not possible.

269. Knowledge, implementation, psychosocial (a)
   4 This is the only accurate information and therefore the *most appropriate* response.
   1 This statement is inaccurate and does not answer the patient's question.
   2 This is an inaccurate statement and would certainly increase the patient's anxiety.
   3 The actual shock generally takes only a few seconds, but each treatment lasts approximately 15 minutes from beginning to end.

270. Knowledge, assessment, environment (a)
   3 Patients who are severely depressed and who cannot take or have not responded to medication therapy are appropriate candidates for electroconvulsive therapy (ECT). ECT has also been used for manic patients not receiving lithium and for highly suicidal patients for whom the antidepressant therapy effectiveness waiting period cannot be risked.
   1, 2, 4 Individuals with these disorders are not candidates for ECT because other more appropriate treatments are available.

271. Comprehension, planning, environment (a)
   1 The patient will be confused following the treatment and will need assistance with reorientation to his surroundings.
   2 Memory loss can persist for weeks following the course of treatment. Although this is important for the patient to know, immediately after treatment when the patient is confused is not the appropriate time for this intervention.
   3 Seizure precautions are implemented *during* the treatment. After the shock is administered, the patient experiences a grand mal seizure.
   4 The patient is NPO the morning of the treatment and voids just before treatment. Until the patient is fairly alert following the treatment, fluids would not be offered. It is appropriate to note the first voiding after treatment, but it is not necessary to monitor intake.

272. Application, assessment, psychosocial (b)
    1 Haldol decreases psychotic symptoms.
    2 A side effect is drowsiness.
    3 It does not affect blood pressure.
    4 It causes drowsiness and decreases alertness.
273. Knowledge, evaluation, environment (a)
    1 Drowsiness is the only CNS side effect listed.
    2 Dry mouth is a gastrointestinal side effect.
    3 Dizziness is a cardiovascular side effect.
    4 Urine retention is a genitourinary side effect.

274. Comprehension, planning, environment (b)
    3 In an individual in the alcoholic state, vital signs are usually elevated. Autonomic overactivity occurs, which would account for the profuse sweating.
    1 Pupils would be dilated; temperature and pulse are elevated.
    2 These are psychologic, not physiologic, manifestations.
    4 Tachycardia and diaphoresis are correct, but the blood pressure is usually elevated.
275. Knowledge, assessment, environment (a)
    1 The patient admitted himself voluntarily.
    2 He was not admitted based on a court order.
    3 He was not committed.
    4 There is no such thing as a limited admission.

CHAPTER 7

Answers and Rationales for Comprehensive Examinations

All questions have been classified by cognitive level, nursing process, patient need, and level of difficulty. These classifications are provided following the question number.

The first word signifies the cognitive level of the questions: knowledge, comprehension, or application. The second word indicates the phase of the nursing process: assessment, planning, implementation, or evaluation. The third word indicates the type of patient need and is abbreviated as follows: environment = safe, effective care environment; physiologic = physiologic integrity; psychosocial = psychosocial integrity; health = health promotion/maintenance.

The letters in parentheses indicate the difficulty of the question. The letter *a* signifies that more than 75% of students should answer the question correctly; *b* signifies that between 50% and 75% should answer correctly; and *c* signifies that between 25% and 50% should answer correctly.

Rationales for all four answer choices for each question are provided. The rationale for the correct answer is listed first, followed by the rationales for the incorrect answer choices.

COMPREHENSIVE EXAMINATION ONE: PART 1

1. Knowledge, planning, environment (a)
   4 A urine culture is done to study bacteria in the urine.
   1 It does not test kidney function.
   2 It does not check albumin.
   3 No residual urine is measured.
2. Knowledge, implementation, health (a)
   1 The National Research Council recommends an increase of a maximum of 300 calories per day during pregnancy.
   2 500 calories per day is the recommendation for lactating mothers.
   3, 4 These amounts are not usually recommended, because an undesirable weight gain could occur.
3. Knowledge, evaluation, environment (a)
   4 Stereotyping is labeling of persons into common groups.
   1 A mental set is organization of an individual's perceptions in a particular way.
   2 An ideology is a manner of thinking that is characteristic of an individual.
   3 A halo effect is a tendency to be influenced by a personal impression.

4. Knowledge, assessment, physiologic (a)
   3 When the urinary bladder is distended, the uterus is displaced to the right side.
   1 Stomach distention will not displace the uterus.
   2 The normal anatomic position of the uterus is midline.
   4 When the uterus fills with blood, it usually becomes relaxed but remains midline.
5. Knowledge, implementation, environment (a)
   3 Handwashing is the *most important* barrier against transmission of infection.
   1 Sterilization of all baby linen is impractical and not necessary.
   2 This is an appropriate action, but it is not scientifically proved to decrease the spread of infection.
   4 This is not cost effective. However, steps are taken to decrease the possibility of infection by cleansing, scrubbing, and use of disinfectants.
6. Knowledge, planning, environment (b)
   2 Anxiety, if not addressed promptly and appropriately, can increase the severity of symptoms and make treatment more difficult.
   1, 4 These are appropriate diagnoses, but they are not the first priority.
   3 There is no evidence to suggest a potential for violence.
7. Knowledge, implementation, physiologic (b)
   2 A Foley catheter, 14- to 16-gauge, with a 5 ml balloon should be used for the average adult woman.
   1 A straight catheter is not a retention catheter.
   3 An 8- to 12-Fr gauge is pediatric size.
   4 A Coude catheter is usually used for elderly men with enlarged prostate glands.
8. Comprehension, planning, psychosocial (b)
   1 Goals that are realistically established with the older adult will lead to nursing interventions most likely to achieve goals and maintain optimal functioning for the individual.
   2 The nurse will follow organizational policies and procedures, which will not conflict with including patients/residents in their plan of care. The older adult has the right to collaborate in her plan of care.
   3 This does not allow patient choices.
   4 Collaboration with all members of the health care team is instrumental in ensuring that all levels of care are being provided; however, the plan of care should always include the patient/resident to maximize outcomes.
9. Application, evaluation, environment (c)
   4 An adverse effect of the medication is urine retention; this is a serious problem and should be reported promptly.
   1, 2, 3 These are not associated with amitriptyline (Elavil) therapy.

10. Application, implementation, environment (a)
    4 An infection occurring after the patient enters the hospital is called a nosocomial infection. The source can be endogenous (within the patient) or exogenous (cross-infection).
    1 A communicable disease is one that is spread readily from one person to another.
    2 Inflammation is a defense reaction by the body to an injury or biologic agent.
    3 A carrier is a person who harbors one or more specific pathogens.

11. Knowledge, planning, physiologic (b)
    4 Bromocriptine mesylate (Parlodel) is a lactation inhibitor.
    1 Ibuprofen (Motrin) is a nonsteroidal analgesic/antiinflammatory drug.
    2 Docusate sodium (Colace) is a fecal softener.
    3 Pitocin is an oxytocic drug.

12. Application, implementation, environment (b)
    1 $$\text{gtt/min} = \frac{1000 \text{ ml} \times 15}{600 \text{ minutes}} = \frac{15,000}{600} = 25 \text{ gtt/min}$$
    2 Time must be in minutes, not hours.
    3 The nurse must use the proper formula.
    4 The nurse must guard against errors.

13. Application, evaluation, physiologic (b)
    4 This is an early side effect of niacin.
    1, 2, 3 These are not associated with adverse reactions of niacin.

14. Comprehension, assessment, physiologic (a)
    2 Eating small, frequent, nongreasy foods aids in the digestive process and helps eliminate digestive problems.
    1 Eating one large meal each day promotes delayed digestion and absorption.
    3 Sodium bicarbonate is an alkaline substance that may alter the pH level of the blood.
    4 Antacids should be used with discretion because they may alter the fluid and electrolyte balance.

15. Application, implementation, physiologic (a)
    4 Because the patient will most likely become drowsy, the nurse should pull up the side rails as a safety measure.
    1 The gown should be changed before the medication is given.
    2 Preoperative teaching should be done before the medication is given.
    3 After the patient is given medication, she is considered no longer able to give legal consent for surgery.

16. Application, implementation, psychosocial (b)
    3 This allows the patient to make decisions regarding her care and minimize the impact of changes in her life.
    1 Individuals should not be forced to participate in activities, therapy, or treatment. Nurses should acknowledge that older adults have intrinsic worth that exceeds their limitations.
    2 The nurse must recognize that older adults are important members of the health care team and that they should play a role in decision making. Older adults have a right to make informed decisions. Threats made to an older adult are not an effective means of communication nor do they produce positive outcomes.
    4 Creativity by the nurse in terms of involving older adults in activities will produce a greater degree of positive results. Instructing someone that they "have to" do something only creates a defensive position for both the resident and the health care provider.

17. Comprehension, evaluation, psychosocial (b)
    3 The nurse offered herself as a therapeutic tool to demonstrate acceptance of the patient.
    1 Open-ended questions are those requiring the patient to give answers that are descriptive and not only one word.
    2 Although she may have demonstrated empathy in her acceptance of the patient, offering herself was the primary tool. Empathy is placing oneself in another's position.
    4 Reflection is verbalizing to the patient the feelings expressed so the patient will be encouraged to elaborate.

18. Application, implementation, environment (b)
    4 A soft (boggy) uterus must be massaged immediately to prevent postpartum hemorrhage; other options lose time and may allow for greater blood loss.
    1, 2, 3 These lose time; they may allow for greater blood loss.

19. Comprehension, planning, physiologic (b)
    2 Patient safety is always a high priority, especially when equipment and patients with loose ego boundaries are involved.
    1 This would be the second concern. The patient's desire to participate is a sign of progress; however, the activity would be structured to provide safety.
    3 Unit rules in a milieu are a concern, but safety of milieu community members is a main reason for the rules.
    4 This concern area would be lowest in priority. Each patient would be dealt with individually and would confront his or her own concerns.

20. Application, implementation, physiologic (b)
    4 Tomato juice is high in salt.
    1, 2, 3 All of these are low in sodium.

21. Comprehension, assessment, psychosocial (b)
    2 Ambivalence and inability to make decisions is a key component of schizophrenia.
    1 Apathy is a lack of concern regarding an idea.
    3 Paranoia is fear or illogical delusions.
    4 Ambivalence in combination with schizophrenia becomes more than a simple defensive mechanism for dealing with stress. It contributes to the misperception of reality.

22. Comprehension, planning, physiologic (b)
    2 This is important nursing care for spinal cord injury.
    1 This is nursing care for rheumatoid arthritis.
    3 This is nursing care for a herniated intervertebral disk.
    4 This is nursing care for gouty arthritis.

23. Application, planning, physiologic (b)
    4 Because of loose ego boundaries and an inability to realistically express themselves, patients with delusions that manifest as physical symptoms should frequently be assessed. It could be a rash or other skin problem, or the patient could grab, scratch, and impair her own skin.
    1, 2, 3 These actions by the nurse are supportive of the patient's delusions and hallucinations.

24. Application, planning, psychosocial (c)
    2 Having guilt over the lifestyle changes that could have been made are a significant part of the healing process.
    1 Cardiac rehabilitation increases the ability to endure increased activity levels.
    3 Sexual activity should be refrained from until the physician allows the increased activity.
    4 Lifestyle changes will lead to examination of activity levels, weight, smoking, hormones, and many things.

25. Knowledge, assessment, physiologic (a)
    4 Impetigo, caused by *Streptococcus* or *Staphylococcus* bacteria, is a highly contagious inflammatory disorder. Common in children, it can be seen at all ages.
    1 This is an atopic dermatitis that may be the result of an allergic reaction or irritant.
    2 Pediculosis is an infestation of lice.
    3 Hives, which are an allergic reaction on the skin, are a result of an allergy to food or drugs.
26. Application, evaluation, physiologic (b)
    2 The use of alcohol while taking metronidazole can cause severe gastrointestinal distress.
    1 The medication should be taken as ordered for the best results.
    3 It is recommended that partners be treated.
    4 The use of dairy products should not cause any problems with this medication.
27. Comprehension, implementation, psychosocial (a)
    3 This response acknowledges the patient's feelings and allows the patient to express her concerns.
    1, 2 These responses discount the patient's concerns and feelings.
    4 Use of direct questioning is a nontherapeutic response.
28. Comprehension, assessment, health (b)
    2 The average incubation period is 10 to 21 days.
    1 This is the incubation period for diphtheria.
    3 This is the incubation period for encephalitis.
    4 This is the incubation period for mumps.
29. Knowledge, assessment, physiologic (b)
    2 Thrombophlebitis occurs most commonly in the deep veins in the legs.
    1 Thrombophlebitis can occur in superficial peripheral veins, for example after an IV infusion, but this is not the most common incidence.
    3 Exercise during pregnancy is health-promoting and does not normally cause a condition like thrombophlebitis.
    4 Thrombophlebitis does not occur in arteries.
30. Application, evaluation, psychosocial (c)
    2 Patients with obsessive-compulsive behaviors must first learn to substitute other behaviors for the compulsive ones so they can learn other coping mechanisms.
    1 Not using the behaviors as often in the hospital could merely mean the anxiety has been lessened.
    3 This may be an unrealistic expectation and is beyond the stage of identifying feelings.
    4 This does not express dealing with feelings and issues in a realistic manner.
31. Application, evaluation, psychosocial (c)
    1 This best describes precisely what the patient said.
    2, 3 Technical terms could be misinterpreted.
    4 This is not correct; the situation described is an example of seeing, not hearing, voices.
32. Application, implementation, physiologic (c)
    1 Absence of a pulse may indicate the fracture has interrupted blood flow to the hand.
    2 Abrasions are superficial injuries.
    3 Circulation is a higher priority than pain.
    4 This pulse may be normal considering the history and injuries of this patient.
33. Comprehension, planning, physiologic (c)
    1 This is an appropriate nursing diagnosis related to seizure disorders; anxiety is related to self-concept.
    2 This is the nursing diagnosis for degenerative diseases.
    3 This is the nursing diagnosis for Parkinson's disease.
    4 This is the nursing diagnosis for patients with Alzheimer's disease.

34. Application, implementation, physiologic (b)
    2 With any respiratory distress, clearance and airway patency must be established.
    1 The nurse must stabilize the neonate, then notify the charge nurse.
    3 This nursing action may not be sufficient to establish airway patency.
    4 Oxygen given under pressure increases the likelihood of further obstruction; the mucus should be removed first.
35. Application, planning, physiologic (b)
    1 The sciatic nerve crosses the inner lower quadrant of the buttocks.
    2 The vagal nerve is located in the chest and abdomen.
    3 The trigeminal nerve affects facial functioning.
    4 The radial nerve is in the lower forearm.
36. Comprehension, planning, environment (b)
    2 With reduced blood flow, sodium and water are retained in the body and contribute to generalized edema and increased cardiac workload. Symptoms are exaggerated when pulmonary edema develops.
    1 Diuretics are administered in the morning to prevent nocturia.
    3 The dietary regimen varies with patients; all do not need to reduce food intake.
    4 The diet may be limited in sodium and possibly in fluid.
37. Application, planning, physiologic (b)
    2 The nurse should ascertain that the patient is not pregnant. These medications are not recommended for women in the first trimester of pregnancy.
    1 These medications do not usually affect the hemoglobin levels, although the white blood cells may be affected.
    3 There is no relationship between eggs and these medications.
    4 There is no relationship between the patient's normal diet and these medications.
38. Knowledge, planning, physiologic (b)
    2 It is important to prevent injuries, especially falls.
    1 This will not repair existing damage.
    3 This is important, but not as important as preventing injury.
    4 This is not related to goals for patients with osteoporosis.
39. Knowledge, assessment, physiologic (a)
    2 The pain is a cramping pain in the legs and is not usually related to activity.
    1 This is pain (cramping in legs) usually associated with exercises.
    3 This is pain on dorsiflexion of the foot that is significant with thrombophlebitis.
    4 This is a term to describe redness of lower extremities when in a dependent position.
40. Knowledge, assessment, environment (a)
    1 In the first trimester, the fetus is developing through a rapid process of cellular growth that allows basic organs and systems to be formed. Because of this process, the fetus is more susceptible to genetic mutation and/or malformation.
    2, 3 During the second trimester, the fetus is already formed; therefore, malformations are less likely to occur.
    4 The last half of pregnancy includes the second and third trimester.
41. Knowledge, implementation, environment (b)
    4 These agents are used to treat patients with thought disorders.
    1 These are used to treat depression.
    2 These agents are used to treat depression and enuresis.
    3 These agents are used to help induce sleep.

42. Application, evaluation, health (b)
    2 Patients with active genital herpes (lesions present or developing) should not engage in sexual activity. Sexual relations at this time can easily transmit the virus to the partner.
    1 Condoms should always be worn as a part of safe-sex practice.
    3 The diaphragm does not protect against any type of sexually transmitted disease.
    4 The patient should have regular Pap smear tests because there is a relationship between genital herpes and an increased risk of cervical cancer.

43. Application, planning, psychosocial (c)
    2 This allows the patient input into decisions about her care.
    1 This doesn't allow for the patient's individual needs.
    3 This is not an important factor at this time.
    4 The patient is the primary focus at this point.

44. Application, assessment, physiologic (b)
    4 A 2-cm spot of blood on the dressing is not uncommon after surgery. The spot should be marked and assessed for evidence of further bleeding.
    1 The team leader or physician need only be notified if there is evidence of an abnormal amount of bleeding.
    2 The first surgical dressing is usually removed by the physician unless there is an unusual reason not to do so.
    3 Reinforcing the dressing for a very small spot makes further assessment difficult.

45. Knowledge, assessment, physiologic (b)
    3 Multiple sclerosis (MS) is a common degenerative neurologic disease. The cause is unknown. Because of the wide distribution of areas of degeneration, the variety of signs and symptoms is greater than in other neurologic diseases.
    1 These are signs and symptoms of Parkinson's disease.
    2 These are signs and symptoms of cerebral vascular accident (CVA), or stroke.
    4 These are signs and symptoms of leukemia.

46. Knowledge, assessment, health (a)
    1 AIDS is the acronym for acquired immunodeficiency syndrome. The virus causing AIDS is known as human immunodeficiency virus (HIV). HIV attacks both the immune and nervous systems.
    2 This is the definition of systemic lupus erythematosus, an autoimmune disorder.
    3 This is the definition of multiple myeloma, an immunodeficiency disease.
    4 This defines a condition known as atopic dermatitis.

47. Application, implementation, health (c)
    4 If she is a danger to herself and/or others because she is delusional, she can be committed to the hospital even if she does not want to stay there.
    1 Her roommate cannot take responsibility for the patient's welfare.
    2 Her parents cannot legally sign her out of the hospital if the psychiatrist determines that she needs to stay.
    3 She cannot be detained in the emergency room; she must either be allowed to leave or be committed to the hospital as an inpatient.

48. Application, evaluation, physiologic (b)
    3 Antabuse causes extreme illness (vomiting, headache, flushing) when a patient has *any* alcohol, including that found in over-the-counter cough syrups.
    1 Any alcohol will affect a patient receiving Antabuse.
    2 Antabuse has no effect on desire for alcohol, except through negative reinforcement.
    4 Although metabolism of alcohol is affected, Antabuse causes the alcohol to have an exaggerated effect.

49. Application, implementation, environment (b)
    4 Information to include relevant to medication teaching is the name of the medication (trade and/or generic names), the time when medications should be taken, whether the medication should be taken with or without meals, any precautions to take when preparing the medication, how much medication to take, the reason the person is receiving each medication, the most common side effects, what action to take if side effects occur, what to do if the person forgets to take a dose of the medication, and what to do if the person experiences nausea or vomiting and is unable to take oral medication.
    1 Medications should be taken on a regular schedule; there are times when a patient needs to call the physician when an unpleasant side effect occurs. An allergic reaction requires emergency intervention. Medications should not be doubled without a physician's order.
    2 Medications should be taken as prescribed; some medications are to be taken with food, others are taken without food. An adequate amount of liquid to ensure safe swallowing is 8 ounces.
    3 Medications should not be shared with other individuals and it is very important the patients know the names and purposes of medications prescribed.

50. Knowledge, planning, physiologic (a)
    4 A pneumothorax is a collection of air between the chest wall and the lung. The chest tube will release air from the pleural cavity.
    1 In this situation, the chest tube is inserted to remove air, not to instill medication.
    2 Following chest surgeries, a chest tube is often used to drain secretions.
    3 With a hemothorax, a chest tube would drain blood.

51. Comprehension, assessment, health (b)
    4 A 1-month-old infant is usually able to lift his head and turn it from side to side while in a prone position.
    1 Smiling and laughing are expected at 2 to 3 months of age.
    2, 3 Holding a rattle and rolling from his back to his side are characteristics of the infant at around 4 months of age.

52. Knowledge, assessment, physiologic (c)
    3 The infant's red blood cells are excessively high at birth, but are soon destroyed naturally by the body.
    1 Physiologic jaundice does not indicate mother/baby blood incompatibility.
    2 There is no damage to the liver.
    4 This does not cause physiologic jaundice.

53. Application, implementation, psychosocial (a)
    1 This response allows the nurse to further explore the patient's feelings before deciding on further action.
    2, 3 This response negates the patient's feelings and is nontherapeutic.
    4 This action may be appropriate after the patient further explains her feelings and the nurse determines that medical assistance is needed.

54. Knowledge, assessment, physiologic (a)
    1 Fluids, fresh fruit, vegetables, and fiber increase peristalsis and promote bowel regularity.
    2 Use of a Fleet enema may induce labor.
    3 Good posture promotes well-being, but it does not necessarily aid in bowel elimination.
    4 Suppositories are not recommended unless ordered by a physician.

55. Application, implementation, physiologic (a)
    1 The blue pigtail should be irrigated with air; this does not require disconnection of the sump to the suction apparatus.
    2 Water should never be introduced into the pigtail.
    3 Unless absolutely necessary, the suction does not have to be disconnected for irrigation if the pigtail is used. Disconnecting the suction would require additional time for the pressure to build up once the suction is reconnected.
    4 Saline, not water, is recommended by most physicians for irrigation.

56. Comprehension, implementation, physiologic (b)
    3 Lanoxin strengthens cardiac force and efficiency.
    1 Inderal is used to control irregular heartbeats and elevated blood pressure.
    2 Aspirin suppresses platelet coagulation; it is used for angina pectoris.
    4 Atropine increases heart rate; it is used for cardiac dysrhythmias.

57. Comprehension, assessment, health (b)
    3 Usually an infant of 4 months is not able to sit without support.
    1, 2, 4 Usually 4-month-old infants demonstrate these.

58. Application, evaluation, psychosocial (c)
    2 Denial is the number one defense mechanism used by substance abusers. If he is not discussing his abuse, he probably has not confronted the problem yet.
    1 Manipulation is also a common coping mechanism used by individuals addicted to alcohol, but this is more an example of avoidance and denial than an attempt to get drugs or rewards through manipulating the nursing staff.
    3 Limit setting is appropriate for acting out and other behaviors, but the nurse cannot limit-set with an individual who uses a psychologic defense mechanism.
    4 Verbalization of feelings will only occur after patients have accepted the fact that that the problem exists.

59. Comprehension, implementation, psychosocial (a)
    1 Seeking clarification is taking a patient's broad statement and working to clarify the statements to get more information.
    2 Encouraging comparison is the process of getting patients to compare this feeling or time to similar instances to gain insight.
    3 Summarizing is restating briefly the overall meaning of the interaction.
    4 Focusing is helping to keep the patient dealing with the subject.

60. Application, implementation, psychosocial (a)
    2 The nurse lets the patient express all her feelings and gives her reassurance.
    1 This is not the best time to teach the patient.
    3 The patient is concerned about her condition and needs to be reassured.
    4 By avoiding the subject, the patient might think that the nurse does not care.

61. Application, implementation, physiologic (c)
    3 Acyclovir will help resolve the lesions in 2 to 6 weeks.
    1 There is no known cure for herpes infections. Acyclovir will only treat the symptoms.
    2 The patient should not decrease her fluid intake. This may lead to a urinary tract infection.
    4 Soaking in warm water may help the patient by easing the discomfort of the lesions.

62. Application, implementation, physiologic (a)
    3 The drainage bag should be lower than the level of the bladder to prevent urinary stasis and backflow of urine.
    1 Extra loops of hanging tubing will contribute to urinary stasis.
    2 To prevent bacterial contamination, the drainage system should never be taken apart.
    4 The catheter should be taped to the abdomen for the adult male patient. This prevents pulling of the catheter.

63. Application, implementation, environment (a)
    2 Convert grams to milligrams
    0.2 g = 200 mg
    $$\frac{\text{Desired}}{\text{Have}} \times \text{Quantity}$$
    $$\frac{200 \text{ mg}}{50 \text{ mg}} \times 1 = 4 \text{ capsules daily} = 1 \text{ capsule/dose}$$
    1 This is an incorrect calculation; dose is too low.
    3, 4 These are incorrect calculations; doses are too high.

64. Comprehension, assessment, physiologic (b)
    2 In addition to the stated signs and symptoms, poor skin turgor also indicates dehydration.
    1 These signs and symptoms are the exact opposite of those in No. 2 and are not symptomatic of dehydration.
    3 These are signs and symptoms of failure to thrive.
    4 These are symptoms of celiac disease.

65. Comprehension, planning, physiologic (b)
    1 The ventrogluteal site is a safe and less painful location for an intramuscular injection.
    2 The syringe should be held at a 90-degree angle.
    3 The site should be marked with the use of the nurse's fingers and palm.
    4 A 1½-inch needle is the most common for an average-size adult. A ⅝-inch needle is not likely to reach the muscle.

66. Knowledge, planning, health (b)
    4 Although other selections may be true, this selection enables the nurse to design a plan that will ultimately promote the change to a healthful behavior.
    1 This fact could be incorporated in the patient teaching; however, it is not the prime consideration in promoting healthy behaviors.
    2 This is inappropriate because it challenges the patient's sense of being and does not promote a therapeutic relationship.
    3 This fact should be included in promoting healthful behaviors, but it is not the correct answer given the other selections.

67. Comprehension, assessment, health (c)
    4 The causes of acute diarrhea may vary; many causes are considered infectious. *Escherichia coli* is an example of a common causative organism.
    1, 2, 3 These may be the causes of *chronic* diarrhea.

68. Application, planning, health (b)
    2 Young adolescents often seek independence from the family and hold viewpoints that are different from those of the parents.
    1 Seeking assistance from a qualified source does not necessarily mean that the adolescent is becoming disrespectful.
    3 Seeking independence from the family normally begins in early adolescence (ages 11 to 14 for females and ages 13 to 15 for males).
    4 There is no indication that professional therapy is needed. Most adolescents do not need professional therapy at this stage of development.

69. Comprehension, assessment, health (c)
    1 During the toddler period, growth is slower than in infancy; gross motor coordination increases. Toddlers gain about 5 to 10 lb (2 to 4.5 kg) each year and 3 inches (7.5 cm) in height per year.
    2 Expected growth is 5 to 10 lb each year and 3 inches in height.
    3 Just the opposite is true.
    4 This is characteristic of a 3- to 5-year-old child.

70. Application, evaluation, physiologic (b)
    3 The dressing should not be damp with serosanguinous drainage. This may be an indication of wound dehiscence.
    1 This is a good indication of a well-hydrated patient.
    2 This is an expected reaction to incisional pain on the third postoperative day.
    4 This is a normal response for a recovering patient.

71. Application, implementation, physiologic (b)
    3 The answer is 31 gtt/min (125 × 15 = 1875; 1875 ÷ 60 = 31.2)
    1 15 is the ratio of drops per milliliter.
    2, 4 These are incorrect calculations.

72. Application, implementation, physiologic (a)
    2 The nurse should check the incision for possible dehiscence.
    1 This gives the patient the notion that he caused the problem or had some control over it.
    3 This response ignores the patient's concerns and provides false assurance.
    4 This is not a priority action in this situation.

73. Comprehension, assessment, physiologic (c)
    2 Although reflexes are present, the nervous system is not highly developed at birth.
    1 This is a conducive environment for the infant.
    3 Newborns usually have good muscle tone.
    4 This is not necessarily the cause.

74. Comprehension, planning, health (a)
    3 Acceptance by peers, as well as peer relationships, is important to young adolescents.
    1 Dressing in the same manner as the peer group is normal for this age-group.
    2 This is not considered narcissistic but a normal part of development.
    4 There is no evidence of promiscuity.

75. Comprehension, assessment, environment (b)
    2 This is common in abused children. Other indicators may include unexplained scars, bruises, and injuries; signs of physical neglect, such as malnourishment; and the parents' inconsistent emotional reaction in regard to the extent of the child's injury.
    1 This is not a sign of abuse.
    3 Abused children are often suspicious and shy.
    4 This is not typical in an abusive environment.

76. Knowledge, assessment, psychologic (a)
    3 Separation anxiety is common in children this age and may be exaggerated during times of illness.
    1 Temper tantrums may occur in children this age, but the description given does not suggest an outburst usually seen in tantrums.
    2 Neither the nurse nor the mother did anything that would support loss of self-image in this situation.
    4 Although the child is dependent on his mother for support at this time, a dependent coping mode is usually identified in an older child who refuses to perform independent activities.

77. Comprehension, assessment, health (b)
    4 Usually at this time muscle coordination increases and teeth erupt. The infant is resistant to being held close while feeding.
    1, 2, 3 The infant may also demonstrate other signs, but these are not necessarily signs that he is ready for weaning.

78. Application, implementation, health (b)
    1 During the first year or so after menarche, periods are often irregular because initial menstrual periods are anovulatory.
    2 Irregular menses during the first year after menarche are considered normal.
    3 This response ignores the adolescent's concern.
    4 The nurse should instruct the adolescent about normal menstrual concerns and should encourage her to communicate with her parents if possible.

79. Comprehension, assessment, health (b)
    1 This is developing and demonstrating autonomy in addition to maintaining a sense of security and control.
    2 These are characteristics of infants 6 to 7 months of age.
    3 These are characteristics of infants 8 to 9 months of age.
    4 These are characteristics of preschoolers (3 to 5 years of age).

80. Knowledge, implementation, environment (a)
    2 Examining the perineum would be the initial action to adequately validate the complaint of the patient.
    1 This may be appropriate if ordered, but assessment is imperative for collection of baseline data.
    3 Heat enables healing; however, initial assessment is done first.
    4 Assessment must take place before reporting findings to the nurse in charge.

81. Application, implementation, physiologic (b)
    4 An explanation of the need to prevent decubitus will help the family to understand and cooperate with the plan; it also recognizes their concern for her need to rest.
    1 This option ignores the family's concerns and could evoke anger, especially if the family is fearful of her deteriorating condition.
    2 The nurse could choose to wait another hour if concern was not high for the patient developing a decubitus; however, an explanation to the family would be best.
    3 This is also ignoring the family's concern. The nurse can independently explain the purpose of the treatment.

82. Comprehension, evaluation, physiologic (b)
    3 Skin that is cool to the touch and even slightly swollen is an indication that the IV is infiltrated.
    1 A backflow of blood when the IV bag is lowered is an indication that the IV is patent.
    2 There can be many reasons why the IV is dripping too slowly; for example, the roller clamp may be too tight, or the IV bag is hanging too low.
    4 The connection needs to be tightened; the IV may be patent.

83. Knowledge, implementation, environment (b)
    2 Medications that are to be given subcutaneously should not be injected into the muscle.
    1 The medication should be injected below the surface layer of the skin.
    3 This technique will not prevent tracking.
    4 The Z-track technique prevents medications that stain from tracking.

84. Comprehension, implementation, environment (b)
    4 The vastus lateralis site would be the best choice because this area is not burned and is usually a large muscle in males.
    1 The deltoid site would not be a good choice for an irritating medication such as hydroxyzine (Vistaril), which should be given by the Z-track method.
    2 The dorsogluteal site would involve burned skin, and absorption of the medication could be hindered.
    3 The ventrogluteal site could be chosen if the skin were not severely burned, but a midaxillary site would probably involve this area.
85. Comprehension, assessment, health (b)
    3 These are the typical signs and symptoms that appear following the incubation period (2 to 3 weeks) and about 24 to 36 hours before the rash. It is also important to remember that aspirin should never be given with chicken pox because it has been implicated in development of Reye's syndrome. Because the child has a slight fever, only Tylenol should be given.
    1 These are clinical signs and symptoms of rubeola (regular measles).
    2 These are symptoms of German measles (rubella).
    4 These are clinical symptoms of mumps.
86. Knowledge, planning, physiologic (c)
    4 This is a noninvasive test that measures the amplitude of the pulsations over an artery.
    1 This makes echoes from sound waves used to study movements and dimensions of the cardiac structure.
    2 This is a test designed to detect cardiac ischemia during exercise or exertion.
    3 This is a tracing of the electrical impulses of the heart.
87. Comprehension, planning, physiologic (b)
    3 Pain is related to loss of skeletal integrity and soft tissue trauma. Impaired physical mobility is related to neuromuscular/skeletal impairment, pain, and discomfort. Altered peripheral tissue perfusion is related to vascular injury or interruption of arterial/venous flow, secondary to edema.
    1 This is a nursing diagnosis for the patient with Ménière's disease.
    2 This is a nursing diagnosis for hypoglycemia.
    4 This is a nursing diagnosis for amputation of the leg, above or below the knee.
88. Comprehension, assessment, physiologic (a)
    1 Leg pain not associated with activity (intermittent claudication) is typical with Buerger's disease.
    2 This is an indication of phlebitis.
    3 This is an indication of varicose veins.
    4 This is an indication of thrombophlebitis.
89. Application, implementation, physiologic (b)
    4 Isolation should be implemented because chicken pox is spread indirectly through articles freshly soiled by discharges from the skin or mucous membrane of infected persons.
    1 This is the nursing intervention for rubeola (regular measles).
    2 This is the nursing intervention for mumps.
    3 This is the nursing intervention for pertussis (whooping cough).
90. Knowledge, evaluation, health (b)
    1 Literature documents that the medicine should be held if the heart rate is 60/min or below. A heart rate of 50/min may be acceptable to her physician; orders should be written to cover the nurse.
    2 A heart rate of 50/min is too low to safely assume that the beta blocker should be continued.
    3 Beta blockers should not be abruptly discontinued; 1 week without the medication could cause serious consequences.
    4 Beta blockers should not be abruptly discontinued.
91. Knowledge, implementation, health (a)
    3 The postpartum follow-up visit takes place at 6 weeks, at which time the physician assesses healing and the process of involution. Sexual intercourse may be resumed when involution and healing are complete.
    1, 2 The healing process may be interrupted and/or an increased risk for infection may occur if sexual relations are resumed too soon.
    4 The healing and involution process is usually complete in 6 weeks; therefore there is no need to wait 12 weeks.
92. Comprehension, assessment, health (b)
    4 This is a result of the 2 year old's inquisitive, assertive behavior that helps him learn by touch, taste, and sight.
    1 These are the most common accidents for infants 7 to 12 months of age.
    2 These are the most common accidents for newborns.
    3 These are the most common accidents for infants 1 to 6 months of age.
93. Knowledge, evaluation, physiologic (a)
    1 Quality indicators emphasize the need for quality patient care. QI provides a means of monitoring and evaluating the quality and appropriateness of care.
    2 The diagnosis related groups (DRGs) set standards for reimbursement to the hospital by the insurance companies and Medicare and Medicaid.
    3 Risk management is used to identify and address potential economic loss.
    4 The infection control committee is in charge of identifying infections and their causes.
94. Application, implementation, environment (a)
    2 $\dfrac{0.25 \text{ mg}}{0.125} \times 1 \text{ tab} = 2$
    1 This is an incorrect calculation; the dose is too low.
    3, 4 These are incorrect calculations; the doses are too high.
95. Comprehension, assessment, physiologic (b)
    4 Red blood cell count in newborns is very high (range 5 to 7 million). Red blood cells are destroyed soon after birth.
    1, 2 These are not the cause for bright red skin.
    3 This is not common in infants; in anemia, the skin is pale.
96. Knowledge, assessment, physiologic (a)
    2 The use of antibiotics can alter the normal flora of the vaginal area and urethra, leading to the invasion of the fungal organism *Candida*.
    1 Yogurt has no relationship to a fungal infection.
    3 Normal use of deodorant soaps should not cause fungal infection.
    4 The use of scented toilet paper is not recommended for women who have repeated urinary tract infections, but by itself this does not cause a fungal infection.

97. Comprehension, implementation, psychosocial (a)
    1 In this option, the nurse is correcting a misconception and supporting the patient's desire to breast-feed.
    2 This response is not therapeutic; it discourages the patient's choice.
    3 This reply does not address the patient's feelings about breast-feeding.
    4 This is an example of advice-giving, which is nontherapeutic.
98. Comprehension, implementation, environment (b)
    3 This response validates the feelings of the patient.
    1 This does not address the reality of the patient.
    2 This reinforces the patient's delusional thinking.
    4 This response gives false assurance; the patient has no reason to believe this.
99. Comprehension, implementation, physiologic (c)
    1 The temperature would be 102.6° F (39.2° C), and the Tylenol should be given as ordered.
    2 The nurse could be held liable for any consequences that may occur if the orders were clear and were not followed.
    3 The nurse could have made an error in calculation, but she would be held accountable for the error.
    4 A rectal or axillary temperature is usually preferred in pediatric patients unless the child is old enough to safely follow instructions for an oral temperature.
100. Knowledge, assessment, physiologic (b)
    3 Increased vaginal discharge is common.
    1 Minor swelling is expected, but reporting excessive swelling of hands, feet, ankles, and face is a must.
    2 Early morning vomiting during the first 3 months is normal, but persistent vomiting at any time during pregnancy is serious.
    4 This is abnormal; the nurse must report to the physician.
101. Application, evaluation, health (c)
    4 Methenamine will make the urine a blue or blue-green color.
    1 Nitrofurantoin, not methenamine, will make the urine a red-orange color.
    2 A patient with an infection or bladder inflammation should increase the amount of fluids taken.
    3 Urine that appears pink or bloody should be reported to the physician because it is not caused by the medication.
102. Application, planning, health (b)
    4 Restraints should be loosened every 2 hours for range of motion exercises and to ensure that circulation is not being hindered. This also allows for repositioning of the patient.
    1 There is not enough information to suggest that the restraints could be left off all day.
    2 The patient should be turned more frequently than every 6 to 8 hours to prevent decubitus formation.
    3 As written, this option is too vague to offer safe care. A few hours could be any number.
103. Application, assessment, physiologic (b)
    1 The nurse should notify the team leader or physician because the patient's potassium level is below the normal range (3.5 to 5 mEq/L) and may affect the administration of anesthesia.
    2 This is not a priority action.
    3 The team leader or physician should be notified.
    4 Although orange juice does contain potassium, the priority is to notify the team leader or physician to get the physician's decision on the correct source of potassium, if any, to be administered.

104. Application, implementation, environment (a)
    2 8 oz = 240 ml $\dfrac{2880 \text{ ml}}{240 \text{ ml}} = 12$
    1, 3, 4 These are incorrect calculations.
105. Application, implementation, health (c)
    2 Obtaining some history is essential to quickly and safely treat this patient.
    1 This does not address the safety needs of this patient.
    3 Although she is an adult, she may not be competent or legally responsible at this time.
    4 Her confidentiality is not violated by obtaining a health history from her family, because she is incoherent.
106. Application, planning, physiologic (b)
    3 The patient should be NPO for 10 to 12 hours beforehand; food may stimulate the gallbladder to contract and expel the contrast media.
    1 If an oral contrast medium is used, an IV is not usually needed.
    2 The area does not need to be prepped or shaved for an x-ray examination.
    4 The patient should be NPO for 10 to 12 hours before the test.
107. Application, implementation, health (b)
    2 Tub bathing or showering is a good hygiene practice. Soap and water ensure cleanliness.
    1 Either tub bathing or showering should be encouraged.
    3 This is an old wives' tale.
    4 Fresh water and soap will not contaminate or bring bacteria to the perineal area.
108. Knowledge, evaluation, environment (c)
    4 A living will allows the patient to decide that extraordinary measures will not be taken.
    1 The intent of a living will is to allow the patient, not the family, to decide what measures will be taken.
    2 This is a legal (probated) will; it does not take the place of a living will.
    3 A living will states what should not be done in the event of a terminal illness.
109. Application, implementation, physiologic (b)
    2 The patient's head should be turned to the side to prevent aspiration.
    1 This is not the priority measure; it can be done after the patient is in the bed.
    3 He can be safely placed in bed after he stops vomiting.
    4 This is not a priority measure. After he is safely in bed, the ordered medication can be given. If this does not help the patient, the physician may need to be notified.
110. Comprehension, evaluation, physiologic (a)
    2 The medicine was absorbed systemically to affect the heart (palpitations) and the central nervous system (feeling faint). The nurse should have worn gloves during application.
    1 A local effect would have been manifested on or around the hands in the form of burning, a rash, or irritation to the skin.
    3 An additive effect involves the complementary effect of one drug given with another drug.
    4 A teratogenic effect involves congenital anomalies when a fetus is exposed to drugs during pregnancy.

111. Application, implementation, physiologic (a)

3 Respiratory distress must be treated immediately as per the physician's orders.

1 If the chemotherapy is ordered to be resumed, it can be done after her immediate needs are met.

2 Pain relief should be accomplished after treating the respiratory problems.

4 Orienting the patient is a normal admission procedure, but it is not a priority in this situation.

112. Comprehension, planning, environment (b)

2 When determining an individual's ability to perform any task or meet a need, an individual's whole self must be evaluated. Once norms and deficits have been identified, an appropriate plan of care can be developed whether in the home or in an institutionalized setting.

1 These are important to consider, but the statement is asking for an identification of assessment data to determine rehabilitative limits.

3 These are related to assessing environmental concerns, not the individual's ability for rehabilitation/restoration.

4 These are appropriate for consideration; however, the type of dwelling structure should be assessed under environmental concerns.

113. Knowledge, assessment, psychosocial (b)

3 Altered family processes are evident in the family's behavior. Assistance with coping behaviors can be facilitated by the nurse.

1 When a nursing diagnosis is written, the relational statement should be something that the nurse can change. This is not true of this statement.

2 The nurse cannot change or cure the patient's illness.

4 This is an inappropriate nursing diagnosis; this is not evident.

114. Application, planning, physiologic (b)

2 The patient is considered at risk for a pulmonary embolism.

1 The patient will need to be on bed rest, with exercises contraindicated at this time.

3 Reducing fluid intake will decrease the plasma fluid, increasing the patient's risk of an embolism

4 The affected leg should be elevated to promote venous return.

115. Application, planning, environment (c)

3 For the safety of the patients, things such as sharp objects or anything that could be used to harm themselves or others must be removed.

1 This is an inaccurate answer, and it gives false assurance.

2 This is an inaccurate answer, and it could frighten the patient.

4 This is not the reason some of her possessions might be sent home; they might also be kept on the unit for her.

116. Application, planning, physiologic (c)

3 Patients who have an order for suicide precautions have strictly limited and highly supervised activities until the immediate danger is over.

1 Occupational therapy allows tools, strings, and other items that are easily used to harm oneself. All therapies are limited until the immediate danger is over.

2 The patient's anxiety should initially be treated with therapeutic nursing communication and removal from the anxiety-producing area.

4 Outdoor activities are a privilege after suicide precautions are removed. There is opportunity for self-harm or for the patient to leave the therapeutic environment.

117. Knowledge, assessment, physiologic (a)

3 A "burning" or painful sensation when voiding accompanied by frequency of urination are the most common symptoms of a urinary tract infection, specifically cystitis.

1 Most patients do not feel faint. Another cause for this symptom should be investigated.

2 The inability to void is a possible symptom of a urinary tract infection (UTI); however, because this occurs only when she is away from home, the possibility of the "bashful bladder syndrome" should be investigated.

4 This is not a common symptom. Another cause should be investigated.

118. Comprehension, assessment, physiologic (b)

4 Morphine slows respiration.

1 This is important, but breathing is more important.

2, 3 This is not affected as much as respiration.

119. Comprehension, implementation, psychosocial (a)

4 The use of therapeutic communication techniques helps identify the reason for her behavior.

1 This ignores the patient's needs.

2 This is inappropriate; there are no data given to support any history of mental illness.

3 This response ignores the patient's needs and is a nontherapeutic nursing action; emotional responses such as this are within nursing's domain for appropriate action.

120. Knowledge, assessment, psychosocial (b)

3 Thinking that others are looking at or judging one in a harmful or negative way is a common thought disorder of many forms of psychosis.

1 The thought-about aliens are not connected in any way to anything else.

2 This is a general term that does not describe the specific symptoms that the patient is experiencing.

4 This term describes a physical symptom.

121. Application, implementation, psychosocial (a)

2 This is the statement recommended by Dr. E. Kübler-Ross. It is important for the patient to know that the nurse will try to help the patient. This response does not negate the patient's sense of hope.

1 This relates a false sense of hope.

3 This relates a false sense of hope and gives the patient a sense of doubt about the adequacy of her health-care providers.

4 This does not recognize the patient's concerns or feelings.

122. Application, implementation, environment (b)

2 Extrapyramidal symptoms are both the most common and most serious side effects of antipsychotic medications; they are controlled with antiparkinsonian drugs.

1 Weight gain is a common side effect of antipsychotic drugs. Calorie intake should be monitored, not encouraged.

3 Antipsychotic drugs do not cause or contribute to potassium excess.

4 Antipsychotic drugs can cause drowsiness and lethargy; usually these patients require extra rest, not exercise.

123. Application, assessment, psychosocial (a)

4 The patient in the stage of depression may be nonverbal while realizing she is going to die and feeling a severe sense of loss.

1 During denial, the patient does not believe the diagnosis is correct. This is not evident in this situation.

2 During the stage of anger, the patient usually verbalizes anger with a sense of helplessness.

3 During bargaining, the patient is usually trying to bargain her way out of the situation. This is not evident in this situation.

124. Comprehension, planning, physiologic (a)
    4 Because smoking constricts blood vessels, it should be avoided; cold temperatures aggravate the symptoms.
    1, 2 These do not relate to Buerger's disease.
    3 This would not be sufficient to provide warmth, which is recommended for patients with Buerger's disease.

125. Comprehension, evaluation, physiologic (c)
    2 The placenta is located near the cervical os. As the cervix prepares for labor, separation occurs, resulting in painless bleeding.
    1 Abdominal pain is more often noted with abruptio placentae.
    3 Uterine tenderness is more often noted with abruptio placentae.
    4 Tetanic contractions are also common with abruptio placentae.

COMPREHENSIVE EXAMINATION ONE: PART 2

126. Comprehension, planning, psychosocial (c)
    1 Most states require an autopsy when a child's death is unexplained.
    2 SIDS is 4 to 5 times more common among siblings, but no genetic link has been found, so genetic testing would be of no benefit.
    3 Hospice assists the patient and the family of the patient who is near death. There would be no reason for a hospice referral since the infant is dead.
    4 There would be no reason for blood tests.

127. Knowledge, implementation, physiologic (a)
    4 The drying of the cast is a gradual process. Keeping the cast uncovered will facilitate the process; covering the cast prolongs the drying process. The patient should also be repositioned (unless restricted) so that all sides of the cast are exposed to the air.
    1 The cast should dry naturally. Application of heat (lamps, fans) can cause the cast to dry unevenly. The strength of the cast will be affected.
    2 The cast should be handled with the palms of the hands. Fingertips could leave an indentation that might create a pressure area.
    3 Casts are "windowed" only in emergency situations.

128. Comprehension, evaluation, environment (b)
    3 The Centers for Disease Control and Prevention (CDC) recommends that blood and body fluid precautions (standard precautions) be consistently used for *all* patients.
    1, 2, 4 These options do not reflect CDC recommendations.

129. Knowledge, evaluation, environment (a)
    3 Kaposi's sarcoma is a malignant opportunistic cancer occurring in AIDS. The lesions may have the appearance of bruises or moles and are often described as purplish-red or dark purple.
    1 Tuberculosis is a bacterial infection commonly occurring in the lungs.
    2 Herpes simplex is a skin disease producing small blisters.
    4 *Pneumocystis carinii* pneumonia is a respiratory disease that is seen in many patients with AIDS. The infection is usually fatal without treatment.

130. Comprehension, assessment, psychosocial (c)
    4 An individual with an antisocial personality has a history of difficulties with personal relationships. This person does not profit from experience or punishment; he has no real loyalties to any individuals, groups, or codes; and he uses the defense mechanism of rationalization. Those with personality disorders have difficulty handling change.
    1, 2, 3 These are other types of personality disorders.

131. Comprehension, implementation, psychosocial (b)
    4 The current goal of community treatment is to return the individual to the home environment as soon as possible and to provide a support system within the community. This facilitates treatment and return to as near-normal functioning as possible.
    1 The goal is to return the patient home as quickly as possible. The development of support systems and change of attitude are *not* the most recent changes.
    2, 3 These are not recent developments; they were used in very early treatment of mental illness.

132. Application, implementation, physiologic (b)
    2 Relaxation techniques can enable the patient to fall asleep.
    1 Sleeping medications interfere with REM sleep and can cause more sleep disturbances.
    3 Strenuous exercise will make it difficult to fall asleep. Regular exercise can help sleep disturbances when done earlier in the day.
    4 Warm milk can actually cause more sleep problems. The high fat content of the milk will make digestion active throughout the night and can disturb sleep.

133. Knowledge, implementation, environment (a)
    4 To maintain effective traction, the weights should hang free. The weights should not rest on the floor or touch the bed. The ropes holding the weights should also hang free of any obstruction.
    1 The patient should be encouraged to move and continue ROM exercises of the unaffected joints as permitted. The patient can use the trapeze to help. Immobilization can lead to skin breakdown.
    2 The amount of weight ordered must be maintained for the traction to be effective. The weights hold the fractured bone in place.
    3 Skeletal traction is applied by the physician. The nurse should have a baseline measurement of the amount of protrusion of the pin. If there is a change, the nurse should notify the physician.

134. Application, assessment, physiologic (c)
    3 The peak action of NPH (intermediate-acting) insulin is 4 to 12 hours after administration.
    1, 2, 4 These are incorrect times for peak action of intermediate-acting insulin.

135. Application, assessment, environment (b)
    3 Previous injuries may be documented in older medical records or x-ray examinations.
    1 This action is not necessary.
    2 This action is not usually necessary and may frighten the child.
    4 This is not an appropriate action.

136. Comprehension, implementation, environment (b)
    3 Bending a joint toward the body is known as flexion.
    1 Hyperextension bends the joint away from the midline.
    2 Extension is the normal, unbent position.
    4 Supination turns the palm upward.

137. Application, implementation, environment (a)

3 $150 \text{ mg} \times \dfrac{5 \text{ ml}}{125 \text{ mg}} = 6$

1, 2 These are incorrect calculations; the doses are too low.

4 This is an incorrect calculation; the dose is too high.

138. Application, planning, health (b)

4 The injection should be given after the child is no longer ill. The measles, mumps, rubella (MMR) can be given after 15 months of age.

1 The MMR should not be administered during times of illness or fever.

2 Reye's syndrome could occur as a result of aspirin administration given during febrile conditions.

3 Injections can be postponed but should never be skipped entirely. A second MMR is now required for entry into school.

139. Application, planning, environment (b)

3 The antibiotic must be maintained at a therapeutic blood level and should be taken as ordered without skipping a dose, until completed.

1 Even though the child may begin to feel better and the signs and symptoms decrease, the antibiotic should be continued for the prescribed time.

2 A therapeutic blood level cannot be reached with long periods between doses.

4 The antibiotic may aid in reducing the temperature before the disease process is completely resolved.

140. Comprehension, evaluation, physiologic (b)

2 It is important to note if swelling has compromised circulation.

1 Fractured wrists rarely cause respiratory trouble such as emboli.

3 Range of motion should be normal to the fingers following wrist fractures.

4 The legibility of her signature is not a priority at this time.

141. Application, planning, environment (c)

1 Isolation is needed with respiratory precautions. The nurse should wear a high-efficiency mask and wash her hands carefully.

2 Isolation is needed. The nurse need normally wear only a mask. Only if there is a possibility of gross contamination of the nurse's clothing are a gown and gloves necessary.

3, 4 Isolation is necessary, with the patient remaining in her room. The nurse should wear a mask.

142. Application, implementation, health (b)

3 This is a reassuring statement. It correctly informs the patient that the stoma has no nerve endings in the inner luminal lining and therefore the patient cannot perceive pain in that location.

1 This is reassuring, but it does not inform the patient that the stoma has no pain receptors.

2 Dressing or pouch changes should not cause the patient pain.

4 This response ignores the patient's concern and instead focuses on the nurse.

143. Knowledge, implementation, health (a)

2 These are the signs and symptoms of mononucleosis.

1 These are symptoms of AIDS.

3 These are symptoms of juvenile-onset diabetes mellitus.

4 These are potential signs of substance abuse.

144. Application, implementation, environment (c)

4 Autonomy is acting independently within the boundaries of practice.

1 Independence means being free from the influence or control of others; however, the professional term for this concept is autonomy.

2 Accountability is defined as being answerable for one's own actions.

3 Responsibility refers to the carrying out of duties within the practice of nursing.

145. Comprehension, assessment, environment (b)

4 The human immunodeficiency virus (HIV) test is used to detect HIV, which is the virus that causes acquired immunodeficiency syndrome (AIDS). A positive HIV test documents the exposure of the patient to HIV.

1 The test indicates exposure to HIV.

2 AIDS wasting syndrome is a series of clinical findings that are suggestive of immunodeficiency and are characteristic of AIDS.

3 The definite diagnosis of AIDS is inclusive of the whole syndrome and usually indicates the presence of opportunistic diseases.

146. Comprehension, planning, psychosocial (b)

1 Nurses who see the elderly as helpless, passive, dependent, and incapable of decision making generally see little potential for improvement. When nurses have a positive attitude and view the elderly as capable, willing participants in their plan of care, the outcome is very different.

2 A negative attitude leads to low expectations, ignoring patient preferences, and indifference in observing physical signs of deterioration. Negativity produces poor outcomes.

3 A negative viewpoint held by many in this country, this statement is inaccurate.

4 Nurses should follow the physician's orders in a positive manner consistent with providing optimal care to patients; this will result in optimal performance.

147. Application, implementation, health (b)

2 Most patients with tuberculosis have anorexia, nausea, and weight loss accompanying the disease. Good nutrition is essential to healing.

1 There is no reason why the patient cannot cook at home.

3 If the patient prefers "fast foods," these will need to be included to an extent in the diet instruction. This statement is an assumption.

4 The medication needed for treatment will most likely make her anorexia, nausea, and weight loss worse.

148. Application, assessment, environment (b)

2 Diarrhea is the frequent passage of loose, liquid stools. It indicates a disturbance in intestinal motility and absorption that could interfere with fluid and electrolyte balance.

1 The frequency varies; although the color is usually green, foods can affect the color.

3 Amounts vary with individuals; the color can be affected by foods.

4 Frequency and amounts vary with individuals.

149. Comprehension, assessment, physiologic (c)

1 Because of the estrogen factor, women typically have heart attacks 10 years later than men.

2 One half of the population dying from heart disease are women.

3 Men have a higher mortality rate for heart disease.

4 Four times as many women die from heart disease as from breast cancer.

150. Application, evaluation, health (b)
    2 Foods such as cabbage, cucumbers, and radishes produce more gas, causing more odor from the colostomy.
    1 Citrus fruits are helpful in the healing process. Acetic acid is vitamin C.
    3 Foods high in iron help in the healing process. Oatmeal and cream of wheat help keep the stool soft, which is normal for a transverse colostomy.
    4 Juices such as apple and cranberry help keep the stool soft and reduce the amount of odor from the stool.

151. Knowledge, implementation, health (a)
    1 A neonate instinctively knows his own hunger needs. The neonate will eventually establish a pattern of regularity on the basis of his need.
    2, 3 These options violate the accepted standard of demand feeding.
    4 This selection does not allow for the infant's need from hunger.

152. Application, planning, psychosocial (c)
    1 Poor impulse control may be demonstrated through drinking, overeating, and substance abuse. Other characteristics include attempts to manipulate others, periodic over-dependency on others, and inappropriate behavior for the situation.
    2 Characteristics include severe anxiety, physical manifestations of anxiety, and attacks occurring suddenly and without reason. Onset is frequently in the late twenties.
    3 This disorder is known as schizophrenia and is characterized by inappropriate emotional responses; displays of incoherent, bizarre behavior; and trouble relating to others.
    4 Mood swings with one or more manic episodes, possibly alternating with episodes of depression, are characteristic.

153. Comprehension, planning, psychosocial (a)
    3 This selection focuses on the specific needs (love and belonging) of a toddler who has a new sibling.
    1 This suggestion is unrealistic and impractical.
    2 Ignoring jealous behavior will *not* diminish this normal response and in fact may exacerbate the jealous reactions.
    4 The children need to be together to develop a bond that leads to a healthy relationship.

154. Application, planning, health (c)
    1 After beginning the medication therapy, compliant patients are not contagious after about 3 weeks and may return to work. Follow-up therapy includes sputum cultures and is necessary for 1 year.
    2 While therapy may be completed at home, it is not necessary to remain away from work for the entire year.
    3 Patients are no longer sent to a tuberculosis hospital or sanitorium.
    4 Patients are contagious during the first 3 weeks of therapy and should remain away from work no matter how they feel.

155. Knowledge, planning, physiologic (a)
    1 Demerol is a narcotic analgesic.
    2 Nausea and vomiting are a side effects of Demerol.
    3 It does not affect urine output.
    4 It does not dissolve stones.

156. Knowledge, assessment, psychosocial (c)
    4 With rationalization, the person denies actual thoughts and justifies his actions by giving untrue, but seemingly acceptable, reasons for his behavior.
    1 Reaction formation takes place when the conscious behavior is completely opposite to the unconscious process.
    2 Compensation is when an individual makes up for a "deficiency" in one area by excelling in or emphasizing another area.
    3 In conversion, emotional conflicts are turned into a physical symptom, which provides the individual with some sort of benefit (secondary gain).

157. Comprehension, assessment, physiologic (c)
    1 A positive response is the development of an indurated area measuring 10 mm or more around the intradermal injection site on the forearm.
    2 A rash on both forearms indicates another clinical problem.
    3 The test is administered on the inner aspect of the forearm, not the deltoid muscle.
    4 A productive cough is usually present with tuberculosis, but it is not made worse by testing.

158. Knowledge, planning, physiologic (a)
    2 At birth, the clamping procedure eliminates blood and oxygen supply to the cord area; because of this procedure, the umbilical cord normally falls off between the seventh and tenth day.
    1 At days three and four, the cord is still firmly attached at the umbilicus.
    3, 4 If the cord is still attached after 10 days, the area should be assessed for moisture and/or infection. If these are present, the mother should be instructed to notify the physician.

159. Application, planning, physiologic (b)
    2 The relaxation of skeletal muscles from these agents could result in severe respiratory depression, even apnea leading to death if respirations are not assisted.
    1 The central nervous system is not altered; the patient should be aware of surroundings.
    3 Although prolonged lack of oxygen because of respiratory difficulty could result in this diagnosis, the priority choice is altered respiratory function.
    4 These drugs do not produce sedation or loss of consciousness; the patient still feels pain.

160. Application, assessment, physiologic (b)
    1 These are symptoms of cardiogenic shock.
    2 Symptoms of pulmonary edema include severe dyspnea, coughing, orthopnea, and production of frothy, pink-tinged sputum.
    3 Symptoms of pulmonary embolism usually include onset of shortness of breath, with or without pleuritic chest pain.
    4 Symptoms of right-sided failure are pitting edema, distended neck veins, fatigue, and increase in the size of the abdomen.

161. Comprehension, assessment, environment (c)
    3 The laboratory results are lower than normal. The average range is: hematocrit, adult female, 38% to 47%; hemoglobin, adult female, 12 to 16 g/dl.
    1 The values are not higher than normal.
    2 The values are not within the normal range.
    4 While the values are below the normal range, they are not considered life threatening. Tissue perfusion can still occur.

162. Knowledge, assessment, physiologic (a)
    3 Breech presentation could be buttocks, feet, or knees first.
    1 The long axis of the body indicates a transverse lie, which means that the fetus is lying crosswise in the uterus; normal delivery is impossible.
    2 In the shoulder position, the scapula is presenting.
    4 The vertex position is a cephalic (head) presentation.

163. Application, evaluation, health (b)
    2 The patient should be weighing himself every day at about the same time, in the same type of clothing, and on the same scale set at zero every morning. Assessment of accurate weighing could determine a false weight gain.
    1 Unless other signs and symptoms of distress are apparent, the 10-lb weight gain may be managed by adjusting the medication and may not require hospitalization.
    3 Seeing the physician would be sound advice if other signs and symptoms were present. The first step, however, would be to assess that the 10-lb weight gain is accurate.
    4 A decrease in fluids without accurate assessment of the weight gain could lead to serious problems.

164. Comprehension, planning, environment (b)
    2 Most causes of acute diarrhea are considered infectious; to rest the bowel, nothing is offered by mouth.
    1 This may be offered *after* frequency of stools has decreased.
    3 This is the intervention for pyloric stenosis.
    4 This is the intervention for hyperthermia.

165. Comprehension, planning, physiologic (a)
    4 Respiratory difficulties are life threatening and therefore take the highest priority in responding to a neonate's needs.
    1 Skin eruptions may be normal or abnormal, but they are not life threatening.
    2 Frequent crying may indicate an underlying problem, but given the selections, respiratory difficulties take priority.
    3 Cyanotic hands and feet are expected in the neonate because the circulation of the blood in the baby at birth is not at the same development throughout the body.

166. Knowledge, implementation, environment (a)
    3 The right patient. The nurse falsely assumed that the patient in bed 2 was the right patient. Nurses must always adhere to the five rights of medication administration: the right patient, the right medication, the right amount, the right dose, and the right route. Documentation must also be included in the rights of medication administration.
    1, 2, 4 These were all verified by the nurse.

167. Comprehension, planning, physiologic (b)
    3 Retinal detachment is a serious complication that may occur as a result of the intricate surgery of a cataract extraction.
    1 Refractive errors are not a complication of cataract extraction and may even be corrected by this type of surgery.
    2 This is an inflammation of the conjunctiva and would not be a complication of cataract extraction.
    4 Optic atrophy relates to atrophy of the optic nerve; it is unrelated to complications of cataract surgery.

168. Application, implementation, psychosocial (b)
    3 By asking the patient if he would like to see the stoma, the nurse can evaluate his readiness to begin learning about his care.
    1 Showing the patient the stoma if he is not ready to see it does not provide care appropriate to his stage of grieving.
    2 This action ignores the patient's feelings and does not help him move through the grieving process.
    4 Discussing home care is inappropriate when the patient is not ready to learn.

169. Knowledge, planning, environment (c)
    3 Streptokinase and alteplase (Activase) are both tissue plasminogen activators, which dissolve clot formation.
    1 Nitroglycerin is an antianginal vasodilator.
    2 Inderal is used for hypertension.
    4 Heparin is an anticoagulant.

170. Comprehension, assessment, environment (a)
    1 With the sudden change in the frequency and character of the stool, there is a rapid loss of fluid that results in acid-base imbalance and dehydration.
    2, 3, 4 These are not usually findings in diarrhea.

171. Knowledge, assessment, physiologic (a)
    2 Milia are plugged sebaceous glands usually found on the nose and cheeks of neonates.
    1 Vernix caseosa is a grayish-white, cheeselike body of creamy substance found on the infant at birth; it protects the skin of the fetus in the uterus.
    3 Lanugo is soft, fine hair found on the baby at birth.
    4 Mongolian spots are darkened pigmented areas found on the lower back or buttocks; they are usually found on dark-complexioned neonates.

172. Application, planning, environment (c)
    4 Depressed patients are difficult to relate to because of their feelings of hopelessness and apathy. The lack of success by the nursing assistants may lead to withdrawal or feelings of anger toward the patient.
    1 Depressed patients are not necessarily lazy.
    2 Poor personal grooming may be a factor; however, this can be easily managed.
    3 Depressed patients are typically dependent on others.

173. Comprehension, implementation, physiologic (b)
    3 A pacifier satisfies a baby's sucking needs.
    1, 2 These may help, but they won't satisfy the baby's sucking needs.
    4 Infants with diarrhea are usually kept in isolation initially because they may have a communicable disease.

174. Comprehension, planning, physiologic (b)
    3 Edema occurs following trauma and immediately following cast application. Elevation of the extremity best controls the situation. Controlling edema also helps alleviate neurovascular compromise.
    1 Following cast application, there is some swelling. Cast application to an extremity is done primarily for immobilization.
    2 Medication therapy is not considered the most effective way to control edema.
    4 Heat should not be applied to the cast because damage may result.

175. Comprehension, assessment, environment (c)
    2 Elavil is an antidepressant with sedative effects. It usually takes 2 to 4 weeks to achieve favorable results.
    1, 3, 4 These are incorrect. Although the sedative effect may be apparent before the antidepressant effect is noted, an adequate therapeutic effect may take as long as 30 days to develop.

176. Application, implementation, environment (b)
    3 Increased fluids are needed because there is a potential fluid volume deficit related to decreased oral intake and because it is necessary to liquefy secretions and aid in their expectoration. A cool-air humidifier helps to moisten mucous membranes and prevent further irritation. Adequate rest and nutrition are primary measures to encourage healing.
    1 This is the intervention for otitis media.
    2 This is the intervention for meningitis.
    4 This is the intervention for asthma.
177. Application, planning, psychosocial (b)
    4 This provides an opportunity for the patient to express his concerns and frustrations and helps reduce feelings of loneliness.
    1 This does not address immediate problems; it ignores his feelings and actual behavior (crying).
    2, 3 These measures ignore feelings and actual behavior.
178. Application, planning, environment (b)
    3 Patients with low hematocrit and hemoglobin values may become light-headed and faint during ambulation.
    1 Ability to take oral fluids normally should not be affected.
    2 Adequate medication for pain control should be administered.
    4 Laboratory values are not low enough to grossly interfere with renal function. The patient should be able to void.
179. Comprehension, planning, physiologic (c)
    1 Presentations other than cephalic, or those in which the presenting part is not fully engaged, predispose the patient to the complication of a prolapsed cord.
    2 No hemorrhage is usually involved with rupture of the membranes.
    3 This is a very rapid delivery, usually without sterile preparation.
    4 A nuchal cord is an abnormal but common condition in which the umbilical cord is wrapped around the neck of the fetus in utero or of the baby as it is delivered.
180. Comprehension, implementation, psychosocial (a)
    3 This is the most accurate decription of an EEG.
    1 Patients are placed in a cylindrical tube for an MRI, not an electroencephalogram.
    2, 4 Radiopaque substances are not used to evaluate brain wave activity.
181. Application, evaluation, environment (a)
    4 Intramuscular injections should be avoided in patients receiving anticoagulants.
    1 Warfarin (Coumadin) is affected by food, so it should be given before meals.
    2 Prothrombin time levels are collected daily at the onset of therapy and weekly thereafter to monitor therapeutic levels at the desired prothrombin time.
    3 If the patient is near discharge, the nurse would begin to ambulate him to ensure his activity at home would be safe. After 7 to 14 days, the thrombus would dissolve and the patient would need to resume activity to prevent further thrombus formation.
182. Knowledge, planning, physiologic (a)
    1 These preparations might prevent gonorrheal infection of the eyes, which can lead to blindness.
    2 Syphilis can cause deformities in the fetus.
    3 Oxygen pressure (Po_2) of arterial blood is measured. If Po_2 is greater than 100 mm Hg, retrolental fibroplasia, which results in blindness, occurs.
    4 This is not an occurrence.

183. Application, implementation, health (a)
    4 Because of the patient's hematocrit and hemoglobin levels, the nurse should emphasize leafy green vegetables as a good source of iron.
    1 Citrus fruits are excellent sources of vitamin C and should be included in the diet, but in this situation the sources of nutritional iron should be emphasized.
    2, 3 These foods are not good sources of iron.
184. Application, evaluation, health (c)
    1 The patient is at increased risk for infections; therefore he should have someone else clean the cat's litter pan.
    2, 3 This is not appropriate teaching.
    4 AIDS is not transmitted by just being in contact with others. This is not appropriate teaching.
185. Application, evaluation, health (b)
    3 Iron preparations such as ferrous sulfate are often taken with meals to prevent gastric irritation.
    1 Iron preparations taken on an empty stomach may be more completely absorbed but can cause gastric irritation and distress.
    2 Laxatives may promote inadequate absorption of nutrients. If the patient becomes constipated, the nurse should recommend an increase in the amount of roughage in the diet.
    4 Liquids will not provide the bulk needed to prevent gastric distress.
186. Knowledge, implementation, physiologic (a)
    3 Fatigue is an approved NANDA nursing diagnosis treatable by the licensed nurse.
    1, 2, 4 These are regarded as medical diagnoses warranting collaborative interventions.
187. Application, implementation, environment (a)
    3 Postoperatively the patient should lie flat or in low-Fowler's position on the unoperated side to avoid undue strain on the operative area.
    1 Turning and deep breathing may be permitted, but coughing is contraindicated because of the danger of complications such as bleeding or retinal detachment.
    2, 4 These positions are contraindicated immediately following surgery.
188. Comprehension, implementation, physiologic (b)
    1 The residual amount of feeding should not be more than half of the amount being given. In this case 240 ml or less should have been aspirated. The residual amount indicates that the patient is not absorbing the feeding as fast as it is being given. The physician should be notified.
    2 Continuing the feeding could result in distention and aspiration pneumonia.
    3 If the patient has not tolerated 480 ml, it is doubtful that more will be tolerated in one feeding.
    4 Even half of the amount could result in aspiration and should be held.
189. Application, planning, physiologic (b)
    3 This patient is at risk for seizures, delusions, and neurologic impairment.
    1 Intake and output is not a factor of high priority; reporting it every 2 hours would be significant only if it were markedly abnormal.
    2 Neurologic checks every hour would waste time on nonessential tasks and take away from the quiet restful environment this patient needs.
    4 Sedation is a medical order that is physician-dependent. Although sedation is likely, it is not an independent nursing action.

190. Comprehension, assessment, physiologic (b)
 3 Any time there is concern about a pulse counted in 15 seconds, the nurse should check the apical pulse for 1 full minute. The apical pulse is more accurate than a radial pulse.
 1 Even for 1 full minute, the radial pulse can be misleading if ectopic beats or an irregular rhythm exist.
 2 An apical pulse taken for 15 seconds is not as accurate as a pulse taken for a full minute.
 4 The radial pulse could be erroneous in both arms if the rhythm is irregular or the pulse is weak.
191. Comprehension, evaluation, environment (b)
 2 Glucotrol frequently interacts with many other medications and must be mentioned every time a new drug is prescribed.
 1 Many factors influence blood sugar; one drug cannot keep levels stable at all times.
 3 This drug should be taken before breakfast; if it causes gastrointestinal upset, it should be taken with meals.
 4 Although drowsiness may be a side effect, it is not normal to frequently feel drowsy. This should be reported to the patient's physician.
192. Comprehension, planning, environment (a)
 2 This statement is correct; the outcome is patient-centered and measurable, and it includes a time frame.
 1 This statement is incorrect; it is neither patient-centered nor measurable.
 3, 4 These choices are inappropriate; they do not contain outcome terminology.
193. Comprehension, implementation, psychosocial (a)
 3 Obtaining drugs and taking them is a full-time job for an addict. The person needs to learn new skills and interests.
 1, 2, 4 It may be true that the addict fears authorities, avoids family and friends, and possibly has a false sense of security, but these are not the main reasons a new life-style is necessary.
194. Application, implementation, psychosocial (b)
 4 It is important to set limits and present reality to support this patient as she deals with the emotional stress, powerlessness, and physical illness that may be precipitating her manic episode.
 1 Emphasizing the diet plan supports the exaggerated thoughts.
 2 This requires a physician's intervention.
 3 It is unrealistic to expect a manic patient to remain in bed.
195. Knowledge, planning, environment (a)
 4 The angle of entry for the injection should be almost parallel to the skin.
 1 This angle would be appropriate for an intramuscular injection.
 2 This angle of entry would be appropriate for an intramuscular injection on a thin or frail person.
 3 This angle of entry would be appropriate for a subcutaneous injection.
196. Comprehension, evaluation, physiologic (a)
 3 This is considered a normal range. A 30 beat/min deviation from the baseline may be used to determine conditions.
 1, 2 Below 120 beats/min is considered to be bradycardia.
 4 Above 160 beats/min is considered to be tachycardia.

197. Knowledge, evaluation, health (b)
 2 Malaise, soreness, and a raised red area at the site of injection is common after most immunizations. Instruction to the mother is that this may remain for several days.
 1 Two of these symptoms are severe and would warrant referral to the physician.
 3 These symptoms are not common and would warrant referral to the physician.
 4 Although immunizations can cause low-grade fever and malaise, welts and high-grade fever are unexpected reactions and require further assessment.
198. Knowledge, implementation, environment (a)
 3 Good handwashing is the single most effective way to help prevent the spread of infections and should be practiced before and after all contact with a patient.
 1 Sterile gloves are not always needed for procedures and treatment.
 2 Isolation gowns are an effective way to decrease contamination, but they are not always necessary.
 4 Unless providing wound care or a special procedure, the family should not need gloves.
199. Application, planning, health (b)
 4 Use of oral contraceptives and antibiotics together may cause the contraceptives to be ineffective in preventing pregnancy. The patient should use additional protection.
 1 Antibiotics should always be taken until completed, unless otherwise instructed by the physician.
 2 Erythromycin can be irritating to the stomach and is better tolerated with food.
 3 Erythromycin is a relatively safe drug. Allergies should always be assessed; however, any questionable allergy warrants further investigation.
200. Comprehension, implementation, health (c)
 3 A person may experience flashbacks, which are defined as the spontaneous recurrence of the drug experience without using the drug. There may be changes in thought content, perception, subjective emotional experience, and judgment. Physically, there may be increased pulse rate, sweating, and tremors.
 1 LSD is not physically addictive.
 2 These are withdrawal signs of barbiturates; there are not any specific withdrawal symptoms for LSD.
 4 These are characteristics of amphetamine intoxication.
201. Application, implementation, physiologic (b)
 3 Trendelenburg's position places the head lower than the feet. Increasing the intravenous fluids could raise the blood pressure until the physician is notified.
 1 Low-Fowler's position requires the head to be raised about 20 inches and could drop the blood pressure further.
 2 Semi-Fowler's position requires the head to be raised 45 degrees and could increase both blood pressure and dizziness.
 4 Reverse Trendelenburg's position is placing the feet lower than the head with the bed flat; this position could lower the blood pressure.
202. Comprehension, planning, physiologic (c)
 4 The nurse uses the logrolling technique to keep the body in alignment and to lessen strain on the vertebral column.
 1 The nurse should assist the patient in turning.
 2 To ensure alignment, pillows are used between the legs when the patient is in the side-lying position.
 3 The nurse will encourage, not limit, range-of-motion exercises.

203. Comprehension, planning, environment (b)
    4 Aerosolization is the normal route for the spread of *Mycobacterium* tuberculosis.
    1 Repeated close contact is usually needed for transmission of tuberculosis.
    2 Feces is not the route of transmission for tuberculosis.
    3 These common tests do not transmit tuberculosis.

204. Comprehension, assessment, physiologic (c)
    3 Hallucinogens have a profound psychologic effect on people, often described as a process of amplification. This effect is called a "trip." A negative experience is referred to as a "bad trip," during which the individual feels the reaction to the drug will never end and a panic reaction ensues.
    1 These are symptoms or effects of central nervous system depressants.
    2 These are physical effects of marijuana.
    4 These are symptoms of withdrawal from inhalants.

205. Application, implementation, environment (b)
    3 Potassium often burns at the infusion site and is not tolerated at fast rates. A slower rate may be tolerated better, but an order from the physician would be needed.
    1 The IV site may not be irritated yet, and the IV may not need to be restarted.
    2 This option does not provide adequate protection for the nurse, and it requires a physician's order.
    4 High concentrations of potassium can lead to thrombophlebitis and can cause extreme discomfort if administered too fast.

206. Knowledge, planning, physiologic (a)
    1 A magnesium preparation is the treatment of choice for convulsions in pregnancy. This controls convulsions by blocking neuromuscular transmission.
    2 A low potassium level could result in similar symptoms, but potassium is not the recommended electrolyte for these conditions.
    3 Sodium would increase the fluid retention that usually occurs in eclampsia.
    4 Calcium may be needed for replacement in pregnancy, but it will not aid in eclampsia.

207. Application, planning, physiologic (b)
    2 The unconscious patient frequently does not have a blink reflex. The eyelids may not close completely. If the eyes are not kept moist, corneal ulcerations will form.
    1 The unconscious patient should not be fed until she is conscious enough to have a good swallowing reflex. The patient could easily choke while being fed. Usually a feeding tube is inserted to allow for nutrition.
    3 The patient should be placed in a sitting position every day, but 8 hours is too long for the patient to sit up. Sitting up this long could cause pressure sores on the coccyx.
    4 A back rub would be a good way to supply tactile stimulus to the patient and also to help prevent pressure sores, but four times per shift may not be feasible.

208. Comprehension, assessment, psychosocial (c)
    4 Numbness is a characteristic of posttraumatic stress disorder, as evidenced by the individual's lack of affect when speaking of the event.
    1, 2 These may be part of the syndrome, but they are not shown in this situation.
    3 Reliving is not described in this situation.

209. Application, evaluation, psychosocial (b)
    3 Patients who have planned a time with little chance of discovery, use lethal methods, and act on that plan are very serious about their identified solution of suicide.
    1 The patient's suicide plan could not be analyzed with the information given.
    2 She planned a time when her husband was away; therefore she did not intend to be rescued.
    4 Sleeping pills are a lethal tool and are often used because they are considered painless.

210. Application, planning, psychosocial (b)
    4 Eating is a social event, and the patient is more likely to eat smaller portions at a sitting.
    1 This doesn't mean he will eat them.
    2 He needs to eat.
    3 He needs socialization.

211. Application, evaluation, psychosocial (b)
    1 These are examples of the environmental factors affecting eating behaviors.
    2 These are examples of the biologic factors affecting eating.
    3 These are examples of the sociocultural factors affecting eating.
    4 These are examples of the psychologic factors affecting eating.

212. Application, implementation, health (b)
    2 Child protection services must be notified. This is required by the Federal Child Abuse Prevention and Treatment Act of 1974.
    1 This may be done; however, the priority is notification of child protection services.
    3 This may be recommended by child protection services or the court.
    4 This is not appropriate at this time; however, the mother should be told that child protection services will be notified.

213. Comprehension, planning, physiologic (a)
    4 This is the intervention for *heat exhaustion.*
    1 This is the intervention for frostbite.
    2 This is the intervention for insulin reaction.
    3 This is the intervention for heatstroke.

214. Comprehension, assessment, environment (b)
    1 Fractures occurring during infancy or toddlerhood are commonly a result of abuse or trauma. Fractures are not normally sustained by the infant while in a crib.
    2 Whether the child is crying or not, at 18 months of age it would be difficult to get accurate information from her in the emergency room.
    3 This is not a priority at this time.
    4 This is not a priority at this time. If her immunizations are up to date, a tetanus immunization is not needed.

215. Knowledge, implementation, environment (c)
    2 This is the correct procedure for Leopold's maneuver.
    1 Homans' sign is pain in the calf with dorsiflexion of the foot; it is indicative of thrombophlebitis or thrombosis.
    3 Chadwick's sign is a bluish coloration of the vagina in early pregnancy.
    4 Ritgen's maneuver assists in delivery of the fetal head.

216. Knowledge, planning, physiologic (c)
    1 Menstruation does not usually occur, but ovulation may; thus pregnancy is possible.
    2 Ovulation may occur.
    3 She does not have to stop breast-feeding.
    4 The uterus still returns to normal in 3 to 4 weeks.

217. Comprehension, evaluation, physiologic (c)
    1 The pH of amniotic fluid is 7.5, or alkaline.
    2 The pH of amniotic fluid is always alkaline, never acid.
    3, 4 These do not verify rupture of membranes.

218. Comprehension, assessment, physiologic (b)

2 By definition, stress is a specific response by the body to a stimulus that disturbs normal functioning.

1 This defines defense mechanisms.

3 This is the definition of anxiety.

4 This describes frustration.

219. Application, implementation, physiologic (b)

1 The secretions are scant because the patient has been NPO and the peristaltic action is diminished from the surgery and anesthetic.

2 The physician should be called immediately only in emergency situations.

3 While patency is an important consideration, irrigation is implemented with caution in gastric surgeries; if implemented, this is done with only small amounts of solution and by physician's orders.

4 High suction is always contraindicated in any situation unless specifically ordered by a physician.

220. Application, assessment, physiologic (b)

3 It is important to establish baseline values so changes may be assessed.

1 This is true, but it is not the primary reason.

2 It is a policy in some institutions, but this is not the primary reason.

4 The care plan is important, but to evaluate patient needs, the baseline values are necessary.

221. Application, implementation, psychosocial (b)

1 The family may need the time with the deceased family member so they can cope with the death.

2 The grieving process may not begin until the realization that the death of their loved one really has occurred. This may require a viewing of the body.

3 Waiting may only increase the grieving and create suspicion in the family that something is being hidden.

4 Friends may be helpful during a crisis, but often families need private time with the deceased.

222. Comprehension, assessment, environment (c)

4 Vitamin B_{12} stimulates the intrinsic factor, which is needed for red blood cell formation.

1 Vitamin B_{12} does not relieve distention.

2 Vitamin B_{12} aids in blood cell formation and neural function.

3 Vitamin B_{12} does not directly stimulate appetite.

223. Comprehension, assessment, health (b)

3 A breast-feeding mother should always check with her physician concerning medications that may be passed to the infant through the breast milk.

1 The medicine may be detrimental to the infant the first time it is taken; the side effects for the infant could be severe.

2 Even half of an adult dose could be harmful to the infant.

4 Although textbooks state pregnancy classifications for drugs, there is no guarantee that a drug will not affect the infant.

224. Application, implementation, environment (c)

2 This is a truthful statement and does not make a judgment. It lets the patient know the nurse understands what he is experiencing.

1 This gives false assurance.

3 With this response the nurse is making a moral judgment.

4 This is too technical and may be misinterpreted.

225. Knowledge, evaluation, physiologic (b)

4 This occurs with dilation of the cervix.

1 This refers to the relation of the presenting part to the mother's birth canal.

2 This is not applicable.

3 This describes Braxton-Hicks contractions.

226. Knowledge, evaluation, environment (b)

1 There are no scientific studies that prove that LSD increases creativity.

2, 3, 4 These are common side effects of LSD.

227. Application, assessment, environment (c)

3 This question allows the patient to describe the pain experience.

1, 2, 4 These questions can be answered with a "yes" or "no" and would not provide the information needed about the pain experience.

228. Application, planning, environment (b)

4 Because of his age and medical conditions, epinephrine would not be recommended because it can increase the blood pressure and raise the blood sugar.

1 Betadine is used before surgery on unbroken skin.

2 Benzoin spray is a demulcent and protectant.

3 Epinephrine is combined with lidocaine to slow the absorption and prolong the effect of the local anesthetic. A prolonged increase in blood pressure would not be suggested for this patient; see No. 4.

229. Comprehension, assessment, environment (c)

2 Hallucinogens primarily affect changes in thought content, perception, and subjective emotional experience. Other hallucinogens include mescaline, psilocybin and psilocin, and morning glory seeds (heavenly blue, pearly gates, flying saucers).

1 Bennies and speed are amphetamines; hash is marijuana.

3 These refer to heroin, which is a narcotic.

4 Rainbows are barbiturates, and M refers to morphine.

230. Application, implementation, health (b)

3 Skipping doses can alter the therapeutic blood level necessary to keep the patient free of seizures.

1 This response does not emphasize the need to avoid skipping doses.

2 This response is not inappropriate; it should, however, be followed with instruction on the proper way to take the medication as prescribed.

4 Organizing the medication by each day does not stress the need not to miss a dose.

231. Comprehension, implementation, health (b)

4 Stress is individualized. How stress is perceived by an individual determines whether the stress produces anxiety in the individual.

1 Health factors do affect individual stress.

2 The nurse should help patients develop *adaptive* patterns.

3 Any type of changes in situations or events can contribute to stress.

232. Application, evaluation, psychosocial (c)

4 Tertiary prevention begins early in the period of recovery from an illness. It involves actions such as taking medication as ordered, active and passive exercises, and moving and positioning to prevent complications from inactivity.

1 Immunizations are an example of primary prevention. In primary prevention the goal is to prevent occurrence of disease.

2 Flu vaccines are also an example of primary prevention.

3 Breast self-examinations are an example of secondary prevention, which consists of screening methods to find problems early.

233. Knowledge, planning, physiologic (a)

3 Ulcerative colitis is the inflammation and ulceration of the colon and rectum.

1, 2 These are incorrect definitions.

4 Constipation does not usually occur in ulcerative colitis.

234. Knowledge, implementation, environment (c)
    1 A myelogram aids in the diagnosis of a herniated inter-vertebral disk. Medication is injected into the lumbar sub-arachnoid space.
    2 This describes electromyography (EMG).
    3 This describes an electroencephalogram (EEG).
    4 This describes computerized tomography (CT).

235. Knowledge, evaluation, environment (a)
    3 After the age of 35, a mother has an increased risk (1 in 400) of having a baby with Down syndrome.
    1 Pitocin is not related to the development of Down syn-drome. Down syndrome is a genetic anomaly.
    2 A prolonged labor, even with possible fetal anoxia, does not cause Down syndrome.
    4 Multiparity by itself does not cause a genetic anomaly.

236. Knowledge, assessment, environment (a)
    1 By definition, mental illness may be exhibited by behav-ior that is conspicuous, threatening, and disruptive of re-lationships or that deviates significantly from behavior that is considered socially acceptable.
    2, 3, 4 These are signs of mentally *healthy* individuals.

237. Comprehension, implementation, physiologic (b)
    2 The Sims' position allows easy access to the rectum.
    1 Lithotomy is the position for a pelvic examination or child bearing.
    3 Dorsal recumbent has the patient positioned on the back.
    4 Right lateral means the fluid from the enema will run up into the sigmoid colon.

238. Knowledge, implementation, physiologic (b)
    3 The apical pulse should be taken for 1 full minute and the medication withheld if the rate is below 60.
    1 A cardiac monitor is not usually needed for the stable pa-tient.
    2 The radial pulse is not accurate because there may be a pulse deficit.
    4 Because the patient is oriented, there is no need to check his mouth.

239. Application, evaluation, physiologic (c)
    3 Pulmonary therapy should not be done immediately be-fore or after meals because of the fatigue and loss of ap-petite that may occur.
    1 Therapy done before meals may make her too tired to eat, or she may lose her appetite from coughing up the thick secretions.
    2 Therapy should be done routinely as a pulmonary pro-phylaxis.
    4 Therapy must be done on a routine basis.

240. Application, implementation, physiologic (c)
    1 Morphine is an opiate receptor that affects the central nervous system, causing more relaxed respirations.
    2 The causative factor is not removed when administering oxygen.
    3 The causative factor is not removed when talking to her alone.
    4 This is contraindicated because it increases circulating blood to heart and lungs, which can increase the respira-tory rate.

241. Application, assessment, physiologic (c)
    3 The presence of large, bulky, foul-smelling stools is an-other symptom of cystic fibrosis.
    1 This is not related to the child's problem.
    2 This is not priority information.
    4 This is important, but it is not a priority at this time.

242. Application, implementation, psychosocial (b)
    2 Babies with Down syndrome may appear hypotonic (floppy). This may lead the mother to believe that the baby does not like to be held or cuddled. The nurse should role-model mothering and assist the mother to hold the baby.
    1 To promote mother-infant bonding, the baby should not be kept in the nursery unless absolutely necessary.
    3 Leaving the mother and baby alone does not facilitate bonding or grieving.
    4 The infant does not need to be in Isolette unless there are additional physical problems. The patient should be allowed to handle the baby's care, if possible.

243. Knowledge, planning, environment (a)
    2 Sympathomimetic drugs include Adrenalin, which is usu-ally given in cases of allergic reaction.
    1 Ganglionic agents are usually recommended in antihy-pertensive crisis.
    3 Parasympathetic blocking agents include mydriatic, cy-cloplegic, and antispasmodic drugs.
    4 Neuromuscular blocking agents are used for relaxation of muscles and spasms.

244. Application, implementation, psychosocial (a)
    1 This response acknowledges the patient's fears and keeps the discussion open.
    2 This statement negates the patient's feeling of fear.
    3 This statement concurs with the patient's fear.
    4 This statement changes the topic and ignores the patient's fear.

245. Knowledge, assessment, physiologic (b)
    1 The sodium and chloride content of sweat is increased to five times above average when cystic fibrosis is pres-ent.
    2 This is usually a normal finding.
    3 This is expected among preschool children.
    4 This may be a normal finding among preschool children.

246. Application, implementation, psychosocial (b)
    3 This response acknowledges the patient's feelings and leads to further discussion.
    1 This response does not adequately acknowledge the pa-tient's feelings and closes the discussion.
    2 This response ignores the patient's feelings and leads her to believe that something was wrong with the fetus.
    4 Physiologically, this response is correct, but it ignores the patient's feeling of loss in this pregnancy.

247. Knowledge, assessment, physiologic (a)
    3 Amphetamines are drugs that stimulate the central ner-vous system (CNS) and result in insomnia, tremors, and excitability.
    1 Alcohol, a CNS depressant, produces sleep and sedation.
    2 Antihistamines usually produce drowsiness, although they can produce CNS excitation in children. They usu-ally do not produce tremors.
    4 Sympathomimetic drugs can produce anxiety, but they lessen fatigue.

248. Application, implementation, environment (a)
    3 Foul odor may indicate an infection requiring antibiotics.
    1 Foul odor is not normal.
    2 This is not likely, unless the physician specifically or-ders it.
    4 Counting pads does not take care of the problem.

249. Application, assessment, physiologic (a)

    4 Clotting time is partial thromboplastin time; this is used to evaluate heparin therapy.

    1 The nurse needs to evaluate clotting.

    2 This is not essential information in relation to the anticoagulant.

    3 This is used to cvaluate Coumadin therapy.

250. Knowledge, assessment, physiologic (a)

    2 Other symptoms may include anorexia, irritability, and an occasional cough.

    1 These are symptoms of gastrocntcritis.

    3 These are symptoms of acute otitis media.

    4 These are symptoms of intussusception.

COMPREHENSIVE EXAMINATION TWO: PART 1

1. Application, assessment, physiologic (a)
   3 If an infection is present, tonsil surgery is postponed until infection subsides.
   1 This is not necessarily needed.
   2 Hemorrhage could occur after, not before, surgery.
   4 This is not accurate information.

2. Application, implementation, health (c)
   4 This acknowledges that the mother feels upset and disappointed in her ability to protect her daughter.
   1 This is a falsely reassuring answer. It does not address the reality of what the mother is feeling.
   2 This gives false reassurance. The nurse cannot know at this time how much of an effect the abuse will have.
   3 This is also not the case. The child will be upset over what has occurred whether or not her mother shows that she is upset.

3. Application, planning, environment (b)
   2 Narcan is used to reverse respiratory depression caused by narcotics.
   1 Adrenalin is the fight or flight hormone.
   3 Benadryl is an antihistamine and antiemetic.
   4 Antivert is for dizziness.

4. Application, implementation, physiologic (b)
   4 Further footdrop can be prevented by proper positioning of the feet. Podus boots are helpful in maintaining this proper alignment.
   1 This should be done regardless of footdrop, but it will not guarantee that the footdrop will not worsen.
   2 This may help and is an appropriate choice, but it should not limit the nurse in independent measures as explained in the correct response.
   3 This option may help, but the footdrop will worsen if the foot is not properly positioned between exercises.

5. Application, evaluation, health (b)
   4 Gingival hyperplasia often occurs. The nurse should stress oral hygiene on an ongoing basis as part of discharge planning and teaching.
   1 The medication is given on a prescribed basis, and serum blood levels can be done to determine the best dose.
   2 Alcohol should not be taken because it decreases the effect of the medication.
   3 The patient should have an available supply, but it is not necessary to keep it with him at all times. It should be taken only as prescribed by a physician.

6. Comprehension, assessment, physiologic (b)
   4 Bleeding may not be visible on the front of the dressing because it will drain down by gravity to the back of the patient's neck.
   1 Just a visual inspection of the dressing for dried blood is not thorough enough.
   2 Changes in hemoglobin and hematocrit could reflect more than bleeding.
   3 Checking the wound in this manner places the patient at risk for infection.

7. Comprehension, implementation, physiologic (b)
   2 Fluids will allow softer stools, and exercise promotes peristalsis.
   1 Analgesia often slows peristalsis.
   3 Rest will slow peristalsis. Calories have no effect on stools.
   4 Laxatives will aid with elimination, but they should be used only after nursing measures of increased fiber, fluids, and activity. Laxatives require a physician's order. Sitz baths do not promote elimination.

8. Comprehension, implementation, health (b)
   2 Most obstetricians do this as a routine for patients over 35 years of age; it helps to identify high-risk mothers and possible fetal problems.
   1 This would not be evident during early stages of pregnancy.
   3 Nothing in her medical history would necessitate doing this test; heterozygote testing is for unrecognized genetic problems.
   4 This test is usually done during the last trimester.

9. Knowledge, implementation, physiologic (a)
   3 The Moro or startle reflex is elicited by a loud noise or sudden movement.
   1 The grasp reflex is elicited by placing a finger in the ulnar side of the infant's palm.
   2 Babinski's reflex or grasp reflex is elicited by stimulating the outer sole of the foot.
   4 Tonic neck reflex is elicited when the infant's head is quickly turned to one side.

10. Comprehension, assessment, psychosocial (c)
    2 Diuretic drugs are more likely to cause electrolyte imbalances, which can lead to delirium.
    1 Antibiotics can cause gastrointestinal disturbance, which can disrupt electrolyte balance. No. 2, however, is the more likely problem.
    3 This could have caused disruption at the time, but it is most likely not contributing to the present problem.
    4 This is not an abnormally great weight loss.

11. Comprehension, evaluation, physiologic (c)
    2 Postoperative edema, intubation for surgery, and surgery can all cause damage to the laryngeal nerve, with resulting vocal changes. The voice should be assessed for tone and quality. Having the patient speak when vital signs are checked in the postoperative period is an important part of nursing care.
    1 Hemorrhage is evaluated through such assessments as vital signs, skin color, and dressing checks.
    3, 4 Assessing the patient's ability to speak after a thyroidectomy is related to concerns about laryngeal edema or damage; it is not a measure of lower airway problems or level of consciousness. Airway obstruction problems would result in such symptoms as stridor and cyanosis.

12. Application, implementation, health (c)
    4 The diabetic patient may not feel pressure points from tight-fitting socks/stockings. Feet with arterial insufficiency are prone to necrosis and infection. To avoid pressure points, stockings with seams or mended socks should not be used.
    1 The toenails should be cut straight across because cutting the toenails in a curved fashion could lead to ingrown nails.
    2 Alcohol will dry the skin; this places the skin at risk for damage.
    3 Heating pads should not be used. The diabetic patient may experience burns because discomfort may not be felt.

13. Comprehension, assessment, environment (b)
    3 The history she has given indicates a recent onset of symptoms and also identifies possible reasons for the crisis.
    1 She does not have the changes in function that would indicate depression; nor is there indication of a prior history of depression.
    2 The situation does not present signs and symptoms of an anxiety neurosis.
    4 There is no indication in the situation that the patient has schizophrenia.

14. Comprehension, assessment, physiologic (b)
    2 An Apgar score of 4 to 7 indicates a mild to moderately depressed newborn.
    1 An Apgar score of 8 to 10 indicates a vigorous newborn.
    3 An assessment of 0 is given when respiration is initiated or absent. Respiratory efforts are usually affected when the Apgar score is 4 or less.
    4 The respiratory rate of a newborn is faster; if there are no problems, it is usually between 30 and 45.

15. Knowledge, implementation, environment (a)
    4 Cleansing from front to back with an individual wipe and voiding a small amount in the toilet before collecting the sample cleanses the meatus of microorganisms.
    1 The word "void" may not be understood by the patient; in addition, the wipes are not provided for cleansing the hands.
    2 This explanation does not offer enough instruction on the cleansing.
    3 Although this would not violate the technique for collection of the specimen, it is inconvenient for the patient.

16. Knowledge, assessment, health (a)
    3 Morning sickness is the appropriate term for nausea and vomiting during pregnancy, occurring usually during the first trimester.
    1 Pernicious vomiting is a term used to designate vomiting occasionally occurring in pregnancy that becomes so prolonged and excessive as to threaten the mother's life.
    2 Vomitus marinus refers to seasickness.
    4 Hyperemesis gravidarum is another term for pernicious vomiting.

17. Application, evaluation, health (b)
    4 Regularly scheduled meals are part of the overall treatment plan. The timing of the meals and allowed snacks helps prevent problems such as hypoglycemia and hyperglycemia.
    1 Desserts can be included in the diet as part of the daily caloric requirements. Desserts are not restricted to fresh fruit.
    2 Food may need to be increased during periods of heavy exercise.
    3 The exchange system allows for substitutions and flexibility in the diet. So-called "dietetic" foods do not have to be used. Often, these foods are high in sodium and can be more costly.

18. Knowledge, assessment, health (b)
    1 This is a condition occurring in the latter months of pregnancy. It is characterized by acute elevation of blood pressure, edema, and proteinuria, but without convulsions or coma as seen in eclampsia.
    2 This is a condition occurring in the second half of pregnancy and sometimes in the puerperium. It is characterized by acute elevation of blood pressure, proteinuria, edema, sodium retention, convulsions and sometimes coma.
    3 This is excessive tension or pressure exerted by body fluids; also known as high blood pressure.
    4 This is a condition of exalted strength or tone of the body.

19. Knowledge, assessment, health (c)
    3 Human chorionic gonadatropin (HCG), originating in chorionic tissue, is excreted in the urine during early stages of pregnancy. It is also secreted by choriocarcinomas.
    1 The adrenocorticotropic hormone is excreted by the pituitary gland and stimulates the cortex of the adrenal gland.
    2 The follicle-stimulating hormone is excreted by the pituitary gland and stimulates the follicle to produce estrogen in the female.
    4 The thyroid-stimulating hormone stimulates the thyroid to produce thyroid hormone.

20. Knowledge, implementation, psychosocial (a)
    4 Newborns usually need 18 to 20 hours of sleep daily.
    1 Infants need more than brief naps.
    2 Newborns are not likely to stay awake all night.
    3 After 1 month, infants usually sleep 15 to 18 hours a day.

21. Application, assessment, environment (b)
    1 Orientation to time is an important indicator of the general level of confusion or orientation.
    2 This is more appropriate to assess mood.
    3 This is more appropriate to assess short-term memory.
    4 This is more appropriate to assess judgment.

22. Comprehension, evaluation, physiologic (b)
    1 Thyroid hormone replacement therapy helps restore a normal metabolic rate but also places stress on the cardiovascular system. The patient should be monitored for signs of heart failure or chest pain. The patient should be taught to take his pulse and to report chest pain or shortness of breath.
    2, 3 Constipation and decreased activity are associated with hypothyroidism.
    4 Sore throat and fever are side effects of certain antithyroid medications.

23. Comprehension, planning, environment (b)
    4 She is definitely at risk for harm if she is not closely supervised.
    1, 2, 3 These are true, but they are not the highest priority.

24. Comprehension, implementation, physiologic (c)
    4 The halo fixation device provides for spinal stabilization and the promotion of further healing without the use of a special bed.
    1 Pins are used to insert the traction apparatus, and pin site care is provided to prevent infection at the pin sites.
    2 The use of the halo apparatus provides for greater mobility, but the patient will still have limited head motion and will need assistance with mobilization.
    3 Traction weights are not used with this type of spinal immobilization.

25. Comprehension, assessment, environment (b)
    2 The first changes usually associated with chronic glaucoma are associated with peripheral visual ability. Patients may complain of bumping into things or stumbling.
    1 Eye pain can be associated with acute closed-angle glaucoma, burns, or corneal injuries.
    3 Tearing and redness after reading may indicate a refraction disorder.
    4 A decreased ability to focus on near objects is indicative of a refraction disorder.

26. Application, implementation, physiologic (b)
    3 Medication should be placed in the conjunctival sac, not on the cornea. The eye should not be touched with the dropper or the tip of the tube.
    1 Pressure should not be applied to the eye because corneal damage could occur.
    2 The eye should be gently closed for 2 to 3 minutes to spread the medication.
    4 Excess fluid or encrusted secretions should be cleaned by wiping from the inner to the outer canthus. Cleaning from outer to inner canthus could spread infection.

27. Application, implementation, physiologic (c)
    1 Diuretics are considered high-risk drugs in the elderly and should be used with caution because of reduced total body water and decreased renal function.
    2 Side effects are common.
    3 Diuretics and digoxin are frequently prescribed in the treatment of congestive heart failure and must be carefully monitored for therapeutic effectiveness.
    4 The elderly have decreased body weight and renal reserves.

28. Application, implementation, environment (b)
    3 Clorox is a caustic agent and should not be vomited. Because of the child's age and the unknown amount of Clorox, a physician should assess the child's condition.
    1, 2 The syrup of ipecac will cause vomiting, which is contraindicated in this situation.
    4 The first part of the answer is correct, but because the child is so young and the amount is unknown, a panic-stricken mother cannot adequately assess the child.

29. Knowledge, assessment, physiologic (a)
    3 Females usually complete puberty by 14 years of age.
    1 Females are slightly ahead of males in physical development.
    2 Males usually begin pubertal changes at 14 years of age.
    4 Females experience puberty slightly ahead of males.

30. Comprehension, implementation, environment (b)
    1 Changing damp gowns and bedding protects the child from chilling.
    2 This does not directly aid in promoting safety or comfort.
    3 The child needs freedom to move in the crib.
    4 The child should be positioned for maximal lung expansion, for example in high-Fowler's position.

31. Knowledge, assessment, physiologic (c)
    3 This is correct; the eustachian tube is shorter, wider, and straighter in an infant.
    1, 4 These are not true. See the correct response in No. 3.
    2 This is not relevant to the situation.

32. Comprehension, assessment, physiologic (c)
    4 Air passages are smaller in children, and when these passages swell, respiratory distress occurs.
    1 The infant's diet is not necessarily a factor at this time.
    2 This is not true.
    3 Infants can be given antibiotic drugs if necessary.

33. Knowledge, evaluation, environment (a)
    3 Both food and insulin may need to be adjusted when an exercise program is started. The best way to determine the needs is to have the patient check his blood sugar level before and after exercise.
    1 The effects of insulin may be potentiated by exercise; therefore, exercise may cause the blood sugar to drop.
    2 Fruit or juice may be necessary to prevent hypoglycemia.
    4 Planned exercise is important and should be part of the diabetic individual's treatment program. Insulin-dependent diabetic individuals can participate in an exercise program.

34. Knowledge, evaluation, physiologic (a)
    3 Daily weights reflect water retention (1 kg = 1 L water) and can be used to estimate fluid retention.
    1 Intake and output records are important, but weight is the most accurate indicator.
    2 Blood urea nitrogen (BUN) levels measure the amount of urea nitrogen in the blood. BUN levels and their relationship to serum creatinine concentration are useful in evaluating fluid volume status. Fluid volume deficit would be indicated by a BUN out of proportion to the serum creatinine level.
    4 Skin turgor refers to the elasticity of the skin. A test for skin turgor is not the most accurate method of evaluating fluid status.

35. Comprehension, implementation, environment (b)
    4 Patients with delirium are extremely disoriented and need to be frequently reoriented to help them feel safe.
    1 This is impractical with a patient in delirium.
    2 She is unlikely to be able to read or use them.
    3 She is unlikely to be able to understand or follow verbal instructions.

36. Application, assessment, physiologic (b)
    1 Functional incontinence results when patients are physically unable to make use of toileting facilities.
    2 Overdistension of the bladder causes overflow incontinence.
    3 Increases in intraabdominal pressure cause stress incontinence.
    4 Urge incontinence results from a delayed sensation of a full bladder.

37. Knowledge, evaluation, physiologic (a)
    3 Pilocarpine is used in the treatment of glaucoma because intraocular pressure is lowered, thus increasing the outflow of aqueous humor.
    1 Pilocarpine creates miosis (constriction) of the pupil.
    2, 4 These are not the actions of the drug.

38. Comprehension, evaluation, physiologic (c)
    3 When the lung has re-expanded, no fluctuation of fluid in the long tube of the water-seal bottle will occur. If there is an absence of complications, the lung usually reexpands in 2 to 3 days.
    1 Fluctuation in the water-seal chamber indicates that the lung has not re-expanded.
    2 With a pneumothorax, the chest tube releases air from the pleural cavity.
    4 Continuous bubbling usually indicates an air leak.

39. Knowledge, assessment, environment (a)
    2 The brachial artery is located on the inner aspect of the antecubital fossa.
    1 The radial artery is where the pulse is normally taken.
    3 The correct location is the inner aspect of the antecubital fossa.
    4 This is not an exact location.

40. Application, implementation, environment (b)
    3 $\dfrac{500 \text{ ml}}{50 \text{ ml}} = 10$ hours.
    1, 2, 3 These are incorrect calculations.

41. Comprehension, evaluation, physiologic (b)
    3 When myocardial cells are injured, intracellular enzymes are released. CK-MB (formerly called CPK) is the most specific enzyme indicating myocardial injury. CK-MB rises within 4 to 8 hours of the infarction.
    1 This is indicative of injury, not infection.
    2 The myocardial infarct location is noted on the ECG.
    4 The CK-MB is specific for the myocardium, not the kidneys.

42. Comprehension, implementation, physiologic (b)
    3 Most physicians will allow showers eventually, but the patient must be able to stand on his own without complications.
    1 The nurse should be with the patient the first time the shower is taken, but the first postoperative day is too soon for a shower.
    2 This response allows the patient to freely ambulate on his own, and he may not know when to limit activity.
    4 Most physicians allow showers before suture removal. The nurse can coordinate the time of the dressing change and the shower when ordered.

43. Comprehension, implementation, physiologic (b)
    2 This response is a prudent nursing measure because the patient will be more cooperative when pain is well-managed.
    1 Although dangling will increase lung expansion, it does not help or eliminate the pain.
    3 Explanations do not necessarily promote patient cooperation.
    4 This does not help the patient to cooperate with the nursing intervention; also, the nurse is ignoring the responsibility to the patient.

44. Application, assessment, physiologic (b)
    3 The complaints suggest a fecal impaction, which should be ruled out before administration of medicine or other treatments.
    1 A laxative could cause severe cramping if a fecal impaction is present.
    2 An antidiarrheal medication could worsen an impaction.
    4 The patient's physical condition should be the priority concern.

45. Application, implementation, environment (b)
    3 $\dfrac{\text{Desired}}{\text{Have}} \times \text{Quantity} =$
    $\dfrac{1200 \text{ mg}}{100 \text{ mg}} \times 1 \text{ tab} =$
    $12 \times 1 \text{ tab} = 12 \text{ tablets} =$
    4 tablets three times a day (tid)
    1, 2 These are incorrect calculations, the doses are too low.
    4 This is an incorrect calculation; the dose is too high.

46. Comprehension, implementation, health (c)
    2 A person can stop using alcohol and be in recovery, but this does not mean that the underlying illness has disappeared. Alcohol dependence is a chronic illness, even if the person is not currently using the substance.
    1 Her underlying illness is still present.
    3 This response does not answer the mother's question.
    4 Her illness is present whether or not she has any permanent physical changes.

47. Knowledge, planning, health (a)
    2 The long-term goals of nursing care in the elderly, regardless of living arrangements, is to promote a health maintenance plan that allows for maximal physical, psychosocial, and spiritual health.
    1 Maintaining physiologic integrity is important, and it should be defined by the individual. The goal of nursing care is health maintenance and optimal physical, psychosocial, and spiritual health.
    3 Physical functioning in the elderly is important regardless of where the individual resides. Physical functioning is only one component and does not address the whole person.
    4 Care planning should be accomplished in collaboration with the individual and significant others.

48. Comprehension, implementation, environment (b)
    1 Drowsiness and dizziness may occur and should decrease after a few weeks. If the side effects do not subside, the physician may need to adjust the medication. Driving is contraindicated in the presence of these side effects.
    2 Absorption is enhanced by administration with meals.
    3 Abrupt withdrawal of medication can precipitate seizures.
    4 Photosensitivity may occur; the patient requires protection with sunscreen and proper clothing.

49. Application, planning, environment (b)
    2 There is the possibility of aspiration of formula and air in stomach.
    1 There is still the possibility of aspiration, a dangerous result of bottle-feeding.
    3 The mother needs rest. Sitting and holding the baby allows for rest, enjoyment, and bonding.
    4 Holding the baby provides cuddling and close contact.

50. Knowledge, planning, psychosocial (a)
    3 This is factual and supportive, truthful information.
    1 This response ignores the patient's question and is nontherapeutic.
    2 This response fails to identify the patient's emotional need.
    4 This response is patronizing, devalues the patient's feeling, and is nontherapeutic.

51. Knowledge, implementation, health (a)
    3 Activity eases false labor; it will not affect true labor.
    1 False labor often begins in the lower abdomen.
    2 False labor is characterized by irregular contractions that do not increase in duration or intensity.
    4 Breathing techniques control pain, not contractions.

52. Application, evaluation, psychosocial (b)
    3 Regression is a coping mechanism to deal with stressful situations. The child is probably experiencing separation anxiety from his parents and home. The child reacts by reverting back to a behavior that occurred when he felt loved and cared for.
    1 It is a normal reaction for a child to become frightened in the hospital. This is not a sign of being spoiled.
    2 The child is having a normal reaction to a stressful situation.
    4 The child is not displaying manipulative behavior. Manipulating involves using guilt to get his way.

53. Knowledge, assessment, environment (a)
    4 The clinical findings of hyperthyroid disease result from thyroid hormone excess. Heat intolerance is often a common complaint.
    1, 2, 3 These findings are associated with hypothyroid function (insufficient thyroid hormone).

54. Application, evaluation, physiologic (c)
    3 Complaints of tingling or numbness in the fingertips are associated with hypocalcemia.
    1, 2, 4 These complaints are not associated with tetany.

55. Knowledge, evaluation, physiologic (a)
    4 A decreased supply of oxygen to the brain can cause confusion, impaired judgment, and altered levels of consciousness.
    1 Tachycardia, not bradycardia, is associated with hypoxia.
    2 Retention of carbon dioxide can cause a red or ruddy skin color.
    3 Auscultation of breath sounds provides information about airflow through the tracheobronchial tree.

56. Application, planning, health (c)
    1 The "morning after" pill is the only known therapy currently prescribed to prevent a pregnancy after unprotected intercourse.
    2 This is untrue. If she were ovulating at the time of the rape, she could become pregnant.
    3 This is only true if she elects not to use hormonal therapy.
    4 Spermicidal douche will not prevent pregnancy after unprotected intercourse, especially since several hours have elapsed since the rape.
57. Knowledge, planning, environment (c)
    3 It is mandatory that all cases of suspected or actual child abuse be reported to child protection authorities immediately. The nurse has a legal as well as an ethical obligation to do so.
    1 This is important and should occur as part of treating this family, but it is not the first priority.
    2 This should not be done until child protection authorities are contacted.
    4 This should not be done until child protection authorities are notified; it should not be done by the family.
58. Knowledge, planning, environment (b)
    2 The nurse should position the patient slightly on the side to facilitate drainage. Flexing her knees eliminates use of pillows; it does not hamper breathing.
    1 The prone position increases the chance of aspiration.
    3, 4 These positions do not facilitate drainage after a tonsillectomy and adenoidectomy.
59. Knowledge, planning, environment (b)
    1 Drugs such as Valium are highly addictive and should be prescribed only when absolutely necessary.
    2 This is true, but it is not the most important reason they are not usually prescribed to treat anxiety symptoms.
    3 This can occur in individuals who are physically and/or psychologically dependent on them.
    4 This is not necessarily true; antianxiety drugs can be very effective in treating symptoms such as muscle tension and gastrointestinal complaints.
60. Application, evaluation, health (c)
    2 This indicates that her sense of reality is intact and that she understands the need for support and reinforcement of the gains she made during hospitalization.
    1 This indicates that she is still not accepting that she has a chronic illness and will need to take medication on a permanent basis.
    3 This indicates that she is still thinking in a manic grandiose way.
    4 This also could indicate that she is not accepting realistic limits.
61. Application, evaluation, psychosocial (c)
    4 After a stroke, both the individual and the family are at risk for coping problems related to the various physical and mental changes as a result of the stroke. Emotional lability is often a part of the problem.
    1 The data do not support a nursing diagnosis of severe anxiety.
    2 The data do not support the nursing diagnosis of a deficit related to diversional activity.
    3 The data do not support an alteration in terms of sensory-perceptual abilities.

62. Comprehension, implementation, psychosocial (b)
    4 Thrombolytic agents, such as streptokinase and urokinase, dissolve clots, decreasing and preventing extension of the existing clot.
    1 Thrombolytic agents do not "thin" the blood as was once thought.
    2 This is a description of products such as aspirin with anticoagulant properties.
    3 This is a description of the action of an anticoagulant.
63. Application, planning, psychosocial (c)
    1 A psychologic problem may be of higher priority than a physical one. The patient's fear of dying needs to be dealt with to lower his anxiety.
    2 The anxiety is probably a result of the fear of dying. If the fear is causing the problem of anxiety, then fear should be priority.
    3 Although impaired gas exchange is of concern because of his chest trauma, it is not life threatening at this time.
    4 This choice is not the best because resolving both the fear and anxiety first may subsequently reduce the shortness of breath.
64. Application, implementation, environment (a)
    4 The patient is lying on her back with her legs in stirrups. This enables the physician to examine the genitals and do a pelvic examination.
    1 The patient is lying on her back with her legs straight; all body parts are in appropriate alignment; the physician is unable to examine the genitals and do a pelvic examination with the patient in this position.
    2 Supine position is the same as the horizontal recumbent position.
    3 This dorsal recumbent position has the patient lie on her back with knees flexed. Although this position may be used, it is not the *preferred* position for a pelvic examination.
65. Comprehension, implementation, environment (b)
    1 The recommended site for subcutaneous administration of heparin is the abdomen; injection sites should be rotated to avoid bruising.
    2 Rubbing the site after administration of subcutaneous heparin can increase the risk of bleeding and bruising.
    3 The intramuscular route is not recommended due to risk of hematoma.
    4 IV heparin should be on an infusion pump or other volume-controlled unit for accuracy and safety.
66. Knowledge, planning, psychosocial (a)
    3 These are all symptoms characteristic of a personality disorder.
    1 This is not an accepted psychiatric diagnosis.
    2 This does not cover all the symptoms mentioned.
    4 Substance abuse is one of the symptoms in this case; it is not the diagnosis.
67. Application, implementation, environment (c)
    2 $\dfrac{\text{Desired}}{\text{Have}} \times \text{Quantity}$
    $\dfrac{8,000 \text{ U}}{10,000 \text{ U}} \times 1 \text{ ml} = 0.8 \text{ ml.}$
    1, 3, 4 These are incorrect calculations.
68. Knowledge, assessment, physiologic (b)
    1 Hemorrhage is the single most common complication because bleeding is concealed.
    2 This is not a complication.
    3 This is not relative to this condition.
    4 It might hurt to talk, but there is no loss of speech.

69. Application, assessment, environment (b)
    1 The change in condition could be related to other reasons, but it may be drug related.
    2 Further evaluation by the physician is needed to determine the cause of central nervous system (CNS) changes.
    3 The signs and symptoms are indicative of CNS depression; they would worsen with additional medication.
    4 Close observation would be needed for the next few hours whether or not the medication were administered.
70. Application, implementation, environment (b)
    3 $1/6$ gr. $= 10$ mg $\dfrac{10 \text{ mg}}{15 \text{ mg}} = 0.66$
    (round to 0.7).
    1, 4 This is too much.
    2 This is not enough.
71. Comprehension, planning, environment (b)
    2 In this situation, turning the patient to decrease further breakdown and to aid in increasing circulation does not require a physician's order.
    1 Whirlpool baths require a physician's order.
    3 Penicillin is a medication that requires a physician's order.
    4 Hydrogen peroxide and povidone iodine (Betadine) are treatments requiring a physician's order.
72. Application, planning, psychosocial (b)
    2 Safety of the students is the most important priority. In cases of alleged abuse by teachers, teachers are usually put on leave until the situation is resolved.
    1 This is important, but not as important as ensuring safety and protection from further abuse.
    3 This is important, but it will be easier if she believes that adults around her can protect her from further abuse.
    4 This is not the responsibility of the nurse.
73. Comprehension, implementation, physiologic (b)
    2 Following a cesarean section and general anesthesia, peristalsis is slowed. The nurse acknowledges the patient's request and provides an explanation that is therapeutic.
    1 This reply avoids the patient's emotional need.
    3 This is a nontherapeutic response; it does not acknowledge the patient's emotional need.
    4 This response neither directly answers the question posed by the patient, nor is it factually correct; IV fluids do not quench the thirst drive.
74. Application, assessment, psychosocial (c)
    4 Children who are abused most often feel guilty about what has occurred and feel responsible for not stopping the abuser.
    1 Many times children are not certain about this, which is one reason the abuse is often not immediately revealed.
    2 This might be true, but rituals are patterns of behavior, not emotions.
    3 This might also be true, but rationalization is not a defense likely to be employed by a child.
75. Comprehension, implementation, environment (a)
    2 A 24-hour specimen begins with the patient emptying his bladder and then discarding that specimen. The nurse notes the time the bladder was emptied and instructs the patient to save each urine specimen. The urine collection procedure is ended 24 hours after the patient first emptied his bladder. The patient voids at this time, and this last urine collection is added to the sample.
    1, 3, 4 These are not accurate 24-hour urine collection procedures.

76. Knowledge, planning, environment (b)
    4 The most important concern of the nurse in this phase is preventing physical harm while the substance is withdrawn from the patient's body.
    1, 2 These are important goals, but only after detoxification.
    3 This is important but secondary to physiologic safety factors.
77. Application, implementation, environment (c)
    2 Two cans q4h would equal 12 cans in 24 hours, 2880 calories, and less than 3000 milliliters.
    1 One and a half (1.5) cans would result in 9 cans in 24 hours and only 2160 calories.
    3 This would be over the amount of calories and milliliters ordered by the physician.
    4 There are six 4-hour periods in 24 hours; this could cause confusion in the number of cans needed.
78. Comprehension, assessment, physiologic (c)
    3 Frequent swallowing, restlessness, spitting up bright-red blood, and increased respirations and pulse are indications of excessive bleeding.
    1 Flushed face is not indicative of excessive bleeding. Loss of consciousness may result but would not be an early sign of excessive bleeding.
    2 Tarry stools are indicative of bleeding at this time.
    4 These signs do not indicate bleeding.
79. Knowledge, assessment, physiologic (b)
    2 Croup is spasmodic laryngitis.
    1 Croup is not an infection of the pharynx.
    3 Croup is characterized by spasms of the larynx, not the trachea.
    4 Croup does not affect lung tissue.
80. Application, implementation, physiologic (b)
    2 Clear liquids and Gatorade are less irritating than natural juices.
    1 Natural juices are irritating to the throat.
    3 Cool drinks are more soothing to the throat.
    4 Milk products are not used initially because they coat the mouth and throat, causing the child to clear her throat more often. This could initiate bleeding.
81. Comprehension, evaluation, health (b)
    3 Oral iron preparations may cause constipation and dark-colored (black) stools.
    1 Because side effects include gastrointestinal upset, the medication may be taken with meals.
    2 Liquid iron preparations may stain the teeth.
    4 Vitamin C aids in the absorption of iron.
82. Application, planning, physiologic (b)
    4 $\dfrac{\text{Desired}}{\text{Have}} \times \text{Quantity} = \dfrac{250 \text{ mg}}{125 \text{ mg}} \times 5 \text{ ml} =$
    $2 \times 5 \text{ ml} = 10 \text{ ml}$
    1, 2, 3 These are insufficient quantities.
83. Knowledge, planning, health (a)
    3 These foods contain high levels of tyramine, which could cause hypertension. Compliance in taking the medication is necessary; it should not be abruptly stopped.
    1 Bananas and yogurt contain moderate amounts of tyramine and should be consumed only occasionally. The medicine is usually not ordered prn.
    2 Seasonings and milk are not on the listed foods containing tyramine and therefore present no harm.
    4 Colas and fruit are not on the listed foods containing tyramine; however, the last part of the answer is correct.

84. Comprehension, assessment, environment (b)
    1 The anemia associated with chronic renal failure reflects hypoproliferative activity of the bone marrow. The main cause is decreased production of erythropoietin by the kidney.
    2 Hypertension usually occurs and is probably a result of sodium retention and increased extracellular fluid volume.
    3 Hyperkalemia, not hypokalemia, is one of the most serious electrolyte problems seen in chronic renal failure.
    4 Weight gain as a result of fluid retention frequently occurs.

85. Comprehension, assessment, physiologic (b)
    1 Elevated serum glucose levels, dehydration, and nausea and vomiting are some of the clinical findings associated with hyperglycemia.
    2, 3, 4 All are clinical findings associated with hypoglycemia.

86. Application, implementation, physiologic (c)
    1 The access should be palpated to check and document the presence of adequate blood flow.
    2 There will be some swelling in the extremity after the procedure; it is necessary to keep the extremity elevated.
    3 Blood pressure should not be taken in the arm with the access, nor should blood be withdrawn from that arm.
    4 The only restriction is the avoidance of tight clothing around the access because this may decrease blood flow and cause clotting.

87. Comprehension, evaluation, environment (a)
    4 The normal range for the systolic pressure is 120 to 140; the normal diastolic range is 60 to 90. A diastolic pressure above 90 may be indicative of hypertension.
    1, 2 Both the systolic and diastolic pressure values are within the average range.
    3 Although both the systolic and diastolic pressures are slightly low, this is not considered abnormal.

88. Knowledge, implementation, environment (a)
    3 To provide a safe distance that does not endanger skin integrity, the heat lamp should be applied at a distance of 1½ to 2 feet.
    1 Heat lamps do not need to be warmed up. The warmth begins as soon as the lamp is turned on.
    2 The strongest wattage to be used for heat applications is 40 watts.
    4 To protect the skin from damage, heat lamps should be used for no more than 20 minutes.

89. Knowledge, implementation, environment (a)
    4 He needs a quiet environment within normal limits.
    1 There is no need for sedation every 4 hours.
    2 A dark room would frighten him and make him anxious.
    3 He needs rest, and so does his mother.

90. Knowledge, assessment, psychosocial (b)
    2 This is absolutely essential. She may be in danger of serious illness or death from her severe weight loss.
    1, 3 These are important, but they are not the nurse's *first* priority.
    4 This should be done in cooperation with her physician after her physical status is assessed.

91. Comprehension, planning, physiologic (b)
    3 NPH, an intermediate-acting insulin, is used as part of insulin-maintenance therapy.
    1 Regular insulin (short-acting) is used as part of "sliding scale" coverage; it may be used as supplemental doses when patients are medically unstable.
    2 Acute hypoglycemia is treated with glucose, not with insulin.
    4 Regular (fast-acting) insulin, not an intermediate-acting insulin, is needed in treating acute ketoacidosis. Regular insulin is usually given intravenously.

92. Comprehension, implementation, physiologic (b)
    2 Lowering protein intake decreases metabolic end products such as urea. Sodium is restricted, depending on the degree of edema and hypertension. Potassium is usually restricted because of the problems with hyperkalemia.
    1 Fluids are usually restricted so that the patient does not have excess weight gain between dialysis treatments.
    3 Protein and sodium are usually decreased.
    4 Sufficient calories are needed from fat to maintain body weight.

93. Knowledge, planning, physiologic (b)
    4 Safety and physiologic integrity are always the most appropriate short-term goals.
    1 This is a long-term goal.
    2 Alteration of body image is a very long-term goal.
    3 This is important, especially to help reinforce the gains that the patient needs to make in treatment, but it is a long-term goal.

94. Comprehension, assessment, environment (b)
    2 This is descriptive of hemodialysis.
    1 This is descriptive of continuous arteriovenous hemofiltration.
    3 This is descriptive of peritoneal dialysis.
    4 This is descriptive of continuous ambulatory peritoneal dialysis.

95. Comprehension, implementation, physiologic (b)
    3 Inhalation anesthetic drugs are eliminated by the lungs; proper aeration of the alveoli aids in the elimination of these gases after surgery.
    1 Age may determine the use of a spirometer, but the device is not standard for all patients. The condition of the lungs, length of the surgery, and anticipated recovery also determine the use of an incentive spirometer.
    2 Although partially correct, this is not the best explanation for the patient who does not feel he needs the treatment.
    4 Secretions will not necessarily be loosened by a spirometer.

96. Knowledge, assessment, psychosocial (b)
    2 Delirium is characterized by sudden onset of symptoms with no prior deficits.
    1 This is more suggestive of normal aging or dementia.
    3 This reflects a bias about the elderly; people do not necessarily present with delirium just because they get older. There is no indication of the patient's age in this situation.
    4 The symptom of depression is more similar to that of dementia, not delirium.

97. Application, planning, health (a)
    4 These are signs of inflammation and should be clarified with patients even though many may know the signs already.
    1 Although swelling may be of concern, coolness is not a sign of infection.
    2 Some soreness and bruising is expected around the site; the patient should know the difference between pain and soreness.
    3 This explanation is too vague and assumes that the patient knows what to look for.
98. Comprehension, evaluation, health (b)
    2 Constrictive clothing should be avoided over the area. The skin is more sensitive in the treatment area and is subject to injury.
    1 Creams, lotions, and deodorants should not be used on the area. After the first 2 weeks of treatment, the skin usually becomes red and dry. Changes in the skin are common during therapy.
    3, 4 The skin is already dry; use of an astringent or alcohol on the area will only make the skin more dry.
99. Comprehension, implementation, psychosocial (b)
    2 Acknowledging her concerns will allow the mother to further communicate her fear.
    1 This statement does not offer assurance and would probably hinder further conversation.
    3 The nurse should be sincere and listen carefully to what the patient is saying without belittling her feelings.
    4 This action would convey to the patient that either the nurse is not listening or she does not care.
100. Knowledge, planning, environment (b)
    4 Verbalization of concerns will decrease the need to have somatic and other types of symptoms.
    1 This could be an appropriate long-term goal, but it is not the immediate primary focus.
    2 This will be a consequence of helping the patient to verbalize, which is the priority.
    3 This may not be necessary, and it is not appropriate as an immediate goal.
101. Comprehension, assessment, physiologic (b)
    2 A thrill should be palpated over the vascular access if the vascular access is patent. The vascular access could have clotted off if the thrill is absent.
    1 Blood pressure measurement should not be taken under any circumstances in the arm with the vascular access.
    3 Soreness would not be an immediate concern after surgery.
    4 Although concern for HIV infection may need to be addressed, it is not an immediate concern.
102. Application, evaluation, health (b)
    4 Sublingual nitroglycerin should be taken at the *earliest* sign of chest discomfort. The patient should sit down, place one tablet under his tongue, and allow it to dissolve.
    1 A patient may be taught to dissolve one tablet under the tongue 5 minutes before participating in an activity that the patient knows causes chest discomfort. However, taking the medication at the *earliest* sign of chest discomfort is the most appropriate patient response in the beginning stage of patient teaching.
    2, 3 Sublingual nitroglycerin is for use when chest discomfort occurs.
103. Application, evaluation, health (b)
    3 The stoma should be cleaned with a clean wash cloth. The use of soaps should be avoided because they irritate the skin around the stoma.
    1 This is a healthful practice that should be done. This statement indicates patient understanding of discharge teachings.
    2 The stoma should be assessed daily for any sign of infection. This statement indicates patient understanding of discharge teachings.
    4 Foreign material (hairs) could lead to inhalation. This statement indicates patient understanding of discharge teachings.
104. Comprehension, planning, physiologic (b)
    2 A low-stimulus, quiet environment should be provided. Fatigue, dyspnea, tachycardia, and constant activity place the patient at risk for congestive heart failure.
    1 The hyperthyroid patient will need a high-calorie diet and between-meal feedings. Most hyperthyroid patients experience weight loss even with an increased appetite.
    3 Skin is usually warm and moist with increased perspiration. Frequent hygiene measures (e.g., baths, change of clothing and bed linens) should be encouraged.
    4 The room is usually kept cool because the patient typically has heat intolerance.
105. Application, assessment, psychosocial (c)
    2 Current coping is most strongly determined by how the patient has coped with stress in the past.
    1 This could serve to moderate the immediate crisis, but it will not be the final determination of what the patient will do to get himself to his precrisis level.
    3 This may not be what is necessary to decrease feelings of inadequacy or of being overwhelmed.
    4 Therapy promotes long-term change, but it is not a good predictor of how a patient will react to or resolve a crisis.
106. Application, planning, health (a)
    3 The removal of nits from the hair shaft is essential and may be easier if the comb is fine-toothed and dipped in vinegar.
    1 The shampoo is usually recommended for 8 to 10 minutes.
    2 A repeat of the shampoo is recommended in 7 to 10 days.
    4 All bed linen and clothing should be washed in hot water, using bleach if possible.
107. Knowledge, assessment, environment (a)
    2 Bulging or protrusion of the eyeballs occurs, and orbit and lid muscle function is altered with hyperthyroidism. The patient also appears to be staring because blinking is reduced. These eye changes are referred to as exophthalmos.
    1, 3, 4 These findings are associated with problems of visual acuity and inflammation.
108. Application, planning, health (c)
    3 Urinary stones frequently develop in spinal cord–injured patients. The need for increasing the intake of fluids should be emphasized.
    1 Fluids are primarily given to combat the formation of calculi.
    2 Because of immobility, the patient is at increased risk for pulmonary problems, but the primary concern is renal calculi.
    4 Spinal shock occurs after the acute injury.

109. Application, implementation, environment (b)
  2 A portable chest x-ray examination should be done in the room to prevent disease transmission to others in the hospital.
  1 Because the patient is coughing frequently, the mask is needed; disease transmission during a trip to the radiology department is high.
  3 The infection control nurse could be contacted, but she will probably suggest either notifying the physician or option No. 2.
  4 Although the technicians should be protected, the risk of contamination during a trip to the radiology department is high.
110. Knowledge, assessment, physiologic (a)
  2 Bradycardia, or slowing of the heart rate, occurs in spinal shock. Vasoconstrictive responses are blocked, blood pressure drops, and heart rate slows.
  1 Hypotension, not hypertension, is associated with spinal shock.
  3 Muscle flaccidity, not spasticity, is associated with spinal shock.
  4 Seizures do not occur in spinal shock.
111. Application, implementation, physiologic (b)
  2 The wound should be irrigated with the flow of liquid from the least contaminated to the most contaminated area, best facilitated by a dangling position.
  1 Lying flat would soil the linen and possibly cross-contaminate the wound during irrigation.
  3, 4 These positions could result in the liquid flowing from the most contaminated area (ulcer) to the least contaminated area (laceration).
112. Comprehension, assessment, environment (a)
  3 Following rupture of membranes (ROM), a prolapsed cord may occur, causing fetal distress. Initially the nurse must check fetal well-being.
  4 This will be done routinely q15min.
  1 If the fetus is fully engaged, there is less chance of cord pressure occurring, but fetal heart tones are a better indication of fetal well-being.
  2 Labor may accelerate following membrane rupture.
113. Knowledge, implementation, environment (a)
  2 Diabetic individuals are prone to infections and heal poorly. Clean footwear assists in preventing infections. The nails should be trimmed carefully to avoid cutting the surrounding skin or producing ingrown nails.
  1 Diabetic individuals should assess the feet daily for cuts and irritations. Vascular changes associated with diabetes contribute to poor healing.
  3 Improper footwear and nail-trimming can lead to serious complications for the diabetic as described in Nos. 1 and 2.
  4 Diabetic individuals should assess their feet daily.
114. Application, planning, physiologic (b)
  2 Vaginal examinations may precipitate acute bleeding. The physician will determine if delivery will be by cesarean section. Labor progression will be determined by monitoring contractions.
  1 Ultrasound is a possibility but requires a physician's order.
  3 This situation does not indicate active bleeding. Also, women in active labor do not wear pads.
  4 There is no information related to blood loss in this situation; type and cross match require a physician's order.

115. Comprehension, evaluation, physiologic (c)
  4 Signs of respiratory distress and tachycardia are associated with circulatory overload.
  1 Febrile reactions include chills, fever, and headache. These usually occur 1 to 1½ hours after the start of the transfusion.
  2 Allergic reactions usually occur within the first 30 minutes and are associated with hives, itching, facial edema, and wheezing.
  3 An acute hemolytic reaction usually occurs immediately and is associated with a burning sensation along the vein, chest pain, low back pain, abrupt fever, and chills.
116. Comprehension, assessment, environment (c)
  1 Following the acute injury at the cervical level, the patient will have a loss of reflexes below the level of injury.
  2 Deep-tendon reflexes will be absent, not hyperactive, following the acute injury.
  3 Paralysis, not sensory loss, is noted below the injury.
  4 Temperature sensation (sensory) is lost below the level of the injury.
117. Application, implementation, environment (c)
  2 $\dfrac{100 \text{ ml} \times 10}{x} = 33$
  $33x = 1000$
  $x = 30 \text{ min.}$
  1, 3, 4 These are incorrect calculations.
118. Application, implementation, psychosocial (c)
  3 The clinical picture of acute spinal injury changes as edema develops or subsides or if complications occur. Telling the parents that at this time "it is too early to know" provides them with feedback and gives an honest answer to their questions.
  1 It is too early after the injury to know the full extent of function impairment.
  2, 4 These responses give false reassurance and are nontherapeutic.
119. Knowledge, assessment, environment (a)
  1 A gush of blood or transient increase in bleeding is a sign of placental separation.
  2 The umbilical cord lengthens with placental separation.
  3 The uterus tightens just before placental separation.
  4 Placental separation decreases cord pulsation.
120. Knowledge, planning, environment (a)
  2 Following the fracture, skeletal traction is used to immobilize the cervical region at the level of the injuries. Pain and muscle spasms are reduced, and the injured vertebrae are aligned into position.
  1 Even with cervical tongs in place, the patient will not have *normal* head and neck movement. The patient must be moved as a unit to prevent movement of the spine. The patient may be placed on a special bed (e.g., the Kinetic Rotorest bed) to facilitate turning.
  3 This type of traction is used to support the injured cervical vertebrae.
  4 Traction addresses the fracture, but it is not used to prevent the development of spinal shock. Spinal shock usually occurs with spinal cord injuries and may last from days to months.

121. Application, implementation, physiologic (b)
    2 Most often hypotension in labor is a result of uterine pressure decreasing venous return.
    1 This position counteracts the normal direction and pressure on the diaphragm.
    3 If there were a continued decline in hemodynamic status this would be appropriate.
    4 This would be appropriate routine monitoring if blood pressure and pulse declined further, but immediately turning the patient will promote placental perfusion and increase venous return. This may be all that is needed.

122. Knowledge, assessment, physiologic (a)
    2 Phenylalanine is found in the blood of infants with phenylketonuria (PKU).
    1 Tyrosine results when phenylalanine is properly digested.
    3 Phenylpyruvic acid is a derivative of phenylalanine and is found in the urine of a child with PKU.
    4 Phenylalanine hydroxylase is an enzyme that converts phenylalanine to tyrosine.

123. Knowledge, assessment, physiologic (a)
    3 Interference with proper nervous system development in the child with phenylketonuria (PKU) results in mental retardation in most affected infants. This is a result of phenylalanine accumulating in the blood.
    1, 2 PKU does not affect these organs directly.
    4 PKU does not cause seizures.

124. Knowledge, assessment, physiologic (a)
    4 A potential side effect is agranulocytosis. The occurrence of a sore throat and fever should be reported immediately.
    1 Tachycardia often occurs in the hyperthyroid patient and is not abnormal for this condition.
    2 Body weight should be monitored, but some weight gain may occur as the metabolic rate is adjusted.
    3 A metallic taste is associated with iodine preparations (Lugol's solution, saturated solution of potassium iodide [SSKI]) used in the treatment of hyperthyroidism.

125. Knowledge, planning, health (a)
    3 Animal and vegetable proteins should be controlled in the diet. Protein contains phenylalanine.
    1, 2, 4 A low-protein diet is prescribed for a patient with phenlketonuria (PKU); these substances are not modified.

COMPREHENSIVE EXAMINATION TWO: PART 2

126. Application, planning, environment (b)
    3 Many developmentalists have suggested that adolescents have not reached a cognitive level at which they can fully understand what will happen as a result of their actions.
    1 This is not necessarily true.
    2 Not all adolescents need to do this.
    4 Adolescents as a group are more likely to be trusting of health-care providers than of other adults.

127. Application, implementation, physiologic (b)
    3 With decreased protection from the leukocytes, the defense against infection is greatly reduced. Prevention of infections is crucial to the patient's survival.
    1 Bleeding precautions are associated with thrombocytopenia (decreased platelets).
    2 Rest is important but not specific to leukopenia.
    4 Antiemetics are used to manage nausea and vomiting.

128. Knowledge, implementation, environment (b)
    2 Mumps involves swelling and pain in the parotid glands.
    1 Measles is a communicable disease involving runny eyes and nose, followed by rash.
    3 Scarlet fever does not affect the parotid glands.
    4 Chicken pox involves skin eruptions.

129. Comprehension, implementation, environment (c)
    2 Vital signs are necessary to determine if the nitrate can be given without harmful effects to the patient; sublingual (SL) nitrate is fast acting.
    1 A transdermal patch is usually not used for chest pain; it is used for prevention of chest pain.
    3 This is unsafe practice. The blood pressure could have been too low before the first dose, and another type of medication may be needed.
    4 Taking a *detailed* history would be unsafe in the presence of chest pain. The nurse can quickly secure enough history about the chest pain to appropriately intervene.

130. Comprehension, planning, health (b)
    4 Emptying the breast with each feeding promotes the supply-and-demand principle. By emptying the breast, a new supply of milk will be available for the next feeding.
    1 An exercise regimen promotes well-being but does not ensure an adequate supply of milk.
    2 Adequate oral fluid intake is important; however, it does not have to be milk. The supply-and-demand principle supersedes the adequate fluid intake.
    3 Protein itself does not ensure an adequate milk supply.

131. Knowledge, planning, physiologic (b)
    3 Excessive coughing exhausts the child, so care must include comfort and rest.
    1 The child is not severely ill, but complications can occur.
    2 This condition does not necessarily require hospitalization.
    4 Careful medical attention is required.

132. Application, implementation, physiologic (c)
    2 A regular voiding schedule helps prevent overdistention of the bladder. The schedule can be started with offering the urinal or toileting the patient every 2 hours and then gradually increasing the time span.
    1 An adequate fluid intake is important to help ensure an ample urine supply. Fluids should be taken at regular intervals during the day and should be limited in the evening hours.
    3 Checking for residual urine is an invasive procedure and places the patient at risk for infection.
    4 Adult diapers are not part of a retraining program and do not support the patient psychologically.

133. Application, implementation, health (b)
    3 This answers their question and also provides an opening to obtain support and information from the family.
    1 This is an inaccurate answer; the patient cannot get better simply because she wants to.
    2 This is a closed answer and does not engage the family.
    4 This may or may not be true, but it gives the family false assurance and is nontherapeutic.

134. Comprehension, implementation, physiologic (b)
    2 The patient should sit upright for meals and for 30 minutes after meals to decrease aspiration risk.
    1 Sitting up for meals should be encouraged.
    3 Swallowing with the head slightly flexed facilitates the swallowing process and reduces aspiration risk.
    4 Weakness is on the right side, so the patient should be encouraged to place food in the unaffected (left) side of the mouth.

135. Comprehension, planning, physiologic (a)
    4 Meperidine (Demerol) is relatively safe, and 50 mg is an acceptable dose.
    1 The dose is within normal limits.
    2 The infant will not require naloxone (Narcan) if meperidine is given during the active stage of labor.
    3 The oral route is the slowest acting.

136. Knowledge, assessment, physiologic (a)
    1 Cyanosis develops as the child grows, and stenosis becomes more severe; the infant is called a "blue baby." The squatting position improves oxygenation.
    2 Pink tetralogy is seen when infundibular stenosis is minimal and no cyanosis develops. Clubbing of the fingers is the result of inadequate oxygen supply that causes cyanosis.
    3 Retarded growth is usually seen in patent ductus arteriosus.
    4 These symptoms occur in coarctation of the aorta.

137. Comprehension, assessment, physiologic (b)
    2 A baseline heart rate is needed to determine any adverse reactions that may occur during administration of the drug. Adverse reactions include palpitations and increased heart rate.
    1 Temperature should not be indicative of any adverse reaction to the drug.
    3 The sputum specimen is not altered by the use of metaproterenol (Alupent).
    4 Blood specimens are not altered by the use of metaproterenol.

138. Application, implementation, health (b)
    3 It is important that the nurse give him an explanation about why she is not available to date him. This reinforces the limits of their therapeutic relationship.
    1 This is nontherapeutic; it does not provide an opportunity for patient teaching.
    2 This is a rejection of the patient and is not therapeutic.
    4 It is not appropriate for the nurse to be upset by this question because it is normal for patients to test the limits of the therapeutic relationship.

139. Comprehension, planning, environment (b)
    2 Limited fluid intake can lead to serious fluid and electrolyte imbalances and requires careful monitoring.
    1 The patient may or may not be anxious in relation to the environment.
    3 This might be true; but it is not the highest priority.
    4 This is a priority, but it is not the highest.

140. Knowledge, assessment, physiologic (a)
    2 Abruptio placentae symptoms include severe pain, tense boardlike abdomen, fetal distress, and often concealed bleeding.
    1 Bleeding would only occur with a partial separation and apparent hemorrhage. It is not the norm for all abruptio placentae patients.
    3 Most often the abdomen is boardlike; individual contractions are not apparent.
    4 These are symptoms of placenta previa.

141. Application, implementation, environment (c)
    1 This offers the presence of the nurse to help the patient feel safe and decreases the potential for violence.
    2 Secluding a patient who is hearing voices provides no therapeutic benefit.
    3, 4 These do not acknowledge what the patient is feeling, nor do they address the potential for violence.

142. Knowledge, assessment, psychosocial (b)
    2 Rape is an act of violence and aggression expressed through sexual means; the object is the expression of violent, not sexual feelings.
    1 A common misconception is that the rapist is physically frustrated. This is untrue; many acts of rape are committed by men who are sexually dysfunctional.
    3 This is also untrue; the only dominance involved is that of aggressor/assailant over victim.
    4 This is another misconception, that the rapist is someone who has questions about his or her sexuality and uses the rape for reassurance.

143. Comprehension, planning, health (b)
    4 The juice will disguise the flavor, and sucking on a straw will prevent the iron from staining the teeth.
    1 The child may refuse the milk with the iron and even later on, without the iron, which could be detrimental to growth and development; iron also binds with calcium, which decreases overall absorption of iron.
    2 Administration with a dropper is not appropriate; the iron could come in contact with the teeth.
    3 Even on a cookie, the iron may come in contact with the teeth.

144. Comprehension, implementation, physiologic (b)
    2 This allows any accumulated secretions to drain from his mouth.
    1 If activity has ceased, this is not an appropriate first action.
    3 If activity has ceased, this is not an appropriate first action. When a patient is on seizure precautions, vital signs should be checked at regular intervals because hyperthermia may bring about seizure activity.
    4 Oxygen may be needed during a seizure if the patient is hypoxic.

145. Comprehension, assessment, physiologic (c)
    3 The Glasgow Coma Scale provides information about the patient's level of consciousness. The areas assessed are the patient's ability to speak, obey commands, and open the eyes.
    1 Emotional reactions are not part of the Coma Scale assessment.
    2 Intellectual functioning is not part of the Coma Scale assessment.
    4 These areas of neurologic assessment are important, but the Coma Scale assesses level of consciousness only.

146. Comprehension, assessment, health (a)
    2 A DPT booster is recommended for children between 4 and 6 years of age.
    1 He should have received them as an infant, followed by a booster before starting school.
    3 No chicken pox vaccine that offers active immunization is currently available, although those who are susceptible and at risk for severe disease may be passively protected.
    4 This is not required.

147. Application, assessment, physiologic (b)
    4 A rebound effect can occur 15 minutes after Narcan is given. Although vital signs should increase immediately after the medicine is given, a drop in respirations to the original rate may occur in 15 to 20 minutes.
    1 An increase in blood pressure can occur with too-rapid reversal. The antagonist (naloxone) will also antagonize beneficial analgesic effects, and pain will return. Increased blood pressure is an observable sign of acute pain.
    2 The pulse may stay the same or rise slightly after Narcan is given, especially if the pain returns.
    3 An increase in respirations would be expected immediately after administration of Narcan.

148. Application, evaluation, health (c)
    4 Because of the characteristically small nose and nasal passages and decreased muscle tone that can inhibit respiratory efforts, the baby will be more inclined to upper respiratory infections (URIs) than will other newborns.
    1 Overfeeding will lead to obesity, a common problem of Down syndrome children.
    2 The baby should be dressed in the same manner as other babies.
    3 The baby should be treated the same as other babies in regard to visitors. Normal socialization should be encouraged.

149. Knowledge, assessment, psychosocial (b)
    3 Rape is a crime that victimizes persons of all ages and ethnic/racial groups; it is committed by the same cross section of the population.
    1 It is a common misconception that rape is a crime committed by members of a lower socioeconomic class.
    2 It is a common prejudice that blacks commit or are the victims of more rapes than whites.
    4 It is also a common prejudice that persons of color or urban dwellers are more likely to rape or be raped.

150. Knowledge, assessment, psychosocial (b)
    2 This is the most common reaction immediately following an attack, especially rape. Most victims report later that they felt numb and removed from any feelings about the experience immediately afterward.
    1 This is unlikely because the experience of being raped produces profound shock.
    3 An unfortunate and false assumption sometimes made about women who are raped is that they wanted to have sex with their assailant.
    4 This is possible, but it is not the most likely explanation.

151. Comprehension, assessment, physiologic (c)
    1 These are average vital signs for a 2 year old.
    2 These are average vital signs for a newborn.
    3 These are average vital signs for a 12 year old.
    4 These are average vital signs for a 6 year old.

152. Comprehension, evaluation, physiologic (b)
    4 Elevation of the feet will aid in increasing the blood pressure; another dose of nitroglycerin would only lower the blood pressure further.
    1 The priority is to increase the patient's blood pressure and notify the physician.
    2 Although both of these actions should be initiated, the nurse could first try to elevate the blood pressure by measures that do not require a physician's order.
    3 The first part of the answer is correct, but the administration of another dose of nitroglycerin is contraindicated because of the blood pressure reading.

153. Application, implementation, physiologic (c)
    1 Clear drainage from the nose or ear often indicates the occurrence of a CSF (cerebrospinal fluid) leak. The patient may also complain of a "postnasal drip." The physician should be notified because meningitis could develop.
    2 Because of the danger of meningitis, the physician should be notified.
    3 This type of drainage is not normal mucus drainage. The drainage will be clear to pale-colored and may be seen as a "halo" around sanguineous or serosanguineous drainage.
    4 This is not the appropriate action; reinforcing the dressing and waiting until the physician arrives leaves the patient at risk for infection.

154. Application, implementation, environment (b)
    2 This allows the nurse and patient to establish a working relationship and gives the patient support and reinforcement.
    1 Ignoring these symptoms could be dangerous and may communicate a lack of caring to the patient.
    3 She is unable to set limits for herself and needs the nurse to do so for her until she is healthier.
    4 This is punitive and nontherapeutic; it does not help the goal of encouraging the patient to participate as much as she is able.

155. Comprehension, implementation, environment (c)
    4 Neither the patient nor any of his belongings are radioactive when external radiation therapy is used. Patients should be informed of this information before the therapy commences.
    1 External radiation is directed at a specific target area that is carefully identified and outlined (by purple marks).
    2, 3 The patient is not radioactive at any time during the treatment.

156. Application, evaluation, environment (c)
    2 Tachycardia is often a side effect of theophylline and may require monitoring and further evaluation. The licensed practical nurse is expected to know the effects of medications administered.
    1, 3 Bronchodilation and improved breathing patterns are the expected outcomes of theophylline preparations.
    4 Theophylline breaks down to a stimulant in the body; tachycardia is a common side effect.

157. Knowledge, assessment, physiologic (b)
    2 The presence of inner epicanthal folds and small ears, sometimes low-set, are characteristics of Down syndrome.
    1 Blue hands and feet (acrocyanosis) and irregular respirations are normal immediately after birth.
    3 The normal head circumference is 2 to 3 cm (1 inch) larger than the chest circumference at birth. If the baby has a considerable amount of molding, the circumferences may be equal for a few days after birth.
    4 This is normal infant posture (the fetal position).

158. Comprehension, assessment, physiologic (b)
    4 Excretion may be hindered by the ineffective action of the kidneys, thereby affecting the half-life of a drug. The kidneys are the main organs involved in excretion, thus causing a higher dose of the medication to circulate over a longer period of time.
    1 Absorption is involved with the process from the time the drug enters the body and the bloodstream.
    2 Distribution is involved with the transportation of the drug through the body.
    3 Metabolism is the way the body inactivates the drug; it primarily involves the liver.

159. Comprehension, evaluation, physiologic (c)
    4 Pituitary function disturbances in the form of diabetes insipidus (DI) can occur after intracranial surgery. DI is manifested by polyuria and urine that is low in specific gravity.
    1 The increase in temperature may be related to infection or an increase in intracranial pressure.
    2 Sluggish pupils are more likely related to changes in neurologic status, such as an increase in intracranial pressure.
    3 Clear drainage on the dressing often indicates the occurrence of a cerebrospinal fluid leak.

160. Knowledge, implementation, environment (a)
    2 Checking the breast in both the supine and erect positions allows one to examine the breasts and the chest area. In the supine position, the breasts "flatten," making them easier to examine.
    1 The breasts should be examined 7 to 10 days after menses. Breasts have a tendency to become swollen and lumpy before the start of the menstrual period.
    3 The examination should be done monthly, preferably on the same day.
    4 Women should use the flat part of the fingers for the examination.

161. Application, planning, psychosocial (b)
    3 Women facing possible loss of a child have great amounts of grief (anticipatory) and stress.
    1 With a threatened abortion, care will be aimed at preserving the fetus, not in removal of retained tissue.
    2 If the patient was bleeding heavily, fluid replacement would be a priority. At this time electrolyte replacement may not be necessary.
    4 Oxytocin would be used only in an incomplete abortion.

162. Application, intervention, physiologic (b)
    4 The most common reason for postpartum bleeding is a relaxed fundus. Massage will cause the muscles to tighten and will constrict blood vessels.
    1 This action would be taken second to check the extent of fluid loss. The first action should be to stop the cause.
    2 This is not a primary intervention for a conscious patient.
    3 A patient at risk for blood loss and shock should not be given PO fluids until her status is assessed and found stable.

163. Application, implementation, psychosocial (c)
    4 It is not possible to determine the extent of disability, retardation, or learning ability immediately after birth. Specialists will make this determination over a period of time.
    1 Genetic counseling can normally determine the source of the problem, but it cannot predict the extent of disability.
    2 The nurse should not predict the extent of disability or lead the mother to believe something that may not be true.
    3 The nurse cannot predict the extent of disability.

164. Application, implementation, psychosocial (b)
    3 This response allows the patient the opportunity to express her feelings about the surgery.
    1 The patient may not know the answer to this "why" question. Not knowing what to answer may increase her anxiety.
    2 This statement ignores the patient's concerns about surgery and her fear of dying.
    4 This offers false assurance, does not address the patient's concerns, and is nontherapeutic.

165. Knowledge, assessment, environment (a)
    4 Rubella, German measles, and 3-day measles are the same.
    1 This is not German measles.
    2 Roseola is another communicable disease.
    3 Scarlet fever is another communicable disease that has no immunization.

166. Comprehension, assessment, physiologic (c)
    3 The clumping of malformed cells obstructs blood vessels and destroys red blood cells.
    1 No infection is involved.
    2 This is not relative to the situation at this time.
    4 White blood cells are not involved.

167. Knowledge, evaluation, physiologic (b)
    1 Drug tolerance is a condition of cellular adaptation to a substance so that increasingly larger doses are necessary to obtain the desired effect.
    2 An additive effect is the increased effect of combining two drugs with similar actions.
    3 An idiosyncratic reaction is an unusual reaction the first time the drug is taken.
    4 Effects of psychologic dependence occur when the user desires the drug during withdrawal.

168. Comprehension, planning, physiologic (b)
    2 Diphtheria and tetanus should be updated every 10 years.
    1 Polio does not need revaccination if the normal childhood vaccines were given.
    3 It is not necessary to repeat pertussis past the childhood vaccines.
    4 Polio and pertussis should be given before the child is 6 years old.

169. Application, implementation, physiologic (b)
    4 Fertilization occurs in the outer one third of the fallopian tubes.
    1 The uterus is the site of implantation.
    2 The corpus luteum is a yellowish mass formed in the graafian follicle after the egg has been released from the ovary.
    3 The vagina is the female organ of copulation.

170. Application, implementation, environment (b)
    4 The nurse must let the patient define exactly what she needs the most—when and how.
    1 This is important, but it is not the nurse's first priority.
    2 This may or may not be necessary and is not the highest priority.
    3 This is very important, but she is probably not able to use this information at this time.

171. Knowledge, assessment, environment (a)
    1 With biopsy, a small amount of breast tissue is removed for examination under a microscope. Actual malignant cells can be seen and identified.
    2 Ultrasonography is useful in distinguishing between cystic and solid tumor bodies.
    3, 4 These are radiographic examinations. No direct tissue is examined. Mammography, the radiographic examination of the breast, is a useful screening device for detection of breast tumors.

172. Application, planning, environment (c)
    4 The main purpose for taking interferon with Tylenol is to limit flu-like symptoms associated with this drug therapy.
    1 Nausea and vomiting are side effects of interferon treatment, but Tylenol would not help these problems.
    2 Tylenol would help any fever associated with this drug therapy, but the main reason for taking Tylenol is to treat the flu-like symptoms.
    3 Sore throat is not a common side effect of interferon.

173. Knowledge, assessment, physiologic (a)
    2 Anorexia, nausea, and vomiting are symptoms of digitalis toxicity.
    1 Back pain is not an adverse reaction to digitalis.
    3 Weight gain should be monitored during digitalis therapy and may indicate that the medicine is not working well, but weight gain does not imply toxicity.
    4 Although fatigue can be an adverse reaction, signs and symptoms of digitalis toxicity are more prominent.

174. Comprehension, implementation, physiologic (a)
    3 The greatest risk of hemorrhage occurs within a few hours of delivery; the uterus must remain firm to control bleeding.
    1 Keeping the environment comfortable is desired but not essential.
    2 Offering sips of water is appropriate, but the concern for hemorrhage is greater than fluid deficit in the early post-delivery period.
    4 Taking the temperature is an appropriate measure, but assessing the uterus takes precedence.
175. Comprehension, assessment, psychosocial (b)
    4 Erickson theorized that the greatest challenge of adolescence is the formation of a unique identity.
    1 This is the task of the toddler stage.
    2 This is the task of the preschool stage.
    3 This is the task of young adulthood.
176. Comprehension, planning, physiologic (c)
    3 Immediately after surgery, it would be important to assess the patient's respiratory status because of her history of smoking.
    1 This is not a priority since the situation does not identify this as a problem.
    2 The patient may have difficulty ambulating the first time because of pain, but this would not be the immediate postoperative concern.
    4 Her weight needs to be addressed in the care plan, but this would not be the immediate concern.
177. Application, planning, health (c)
    2 This is the least threatening and most structured way for a patient to both obtain social skills and have increased social interaction with those likely to be receptive to him.
    1 This is probably not realistic and may be setting the individual up for failure.
    3 This may be too complex a task for the patient; it would not necessarily provide opportunities for socialization.
    4 This is a potentially helpful means for greater social contact for this patient, but it does not provide assistance for him to develop social skills.
178. Comprehension, assessment, psychosocial (b)
    2 Anorexic individuals have a disturbance in the way they experience their body shape, size, or weight. The patient clearly states her disturbance over the size of her hands and feet.
    1, 3, 4 These are appropriate nursing diagnoses for the patient with anorexia nervosa. The situation, however, does not indicate these as priority diagnoses for this patient.
179. Knowledge, planning, physiologic (a)
    3 Individuals with hypothyroidism have a decreased tolerance to cold. A warm environment should be provided.
    1, 2 These interventions are appropriate for the patient with hyperthyroidism.
    4 If hypoglycemia is evident, serum glucose levels would be the most accurate indicator.
180. Knowledge, implementation, physiologic (a)
    3 The nurse should remain with the patient until seizure activity has stopped. During this time the nurse can protect the patient from injury as well as observe the seizure activity.
    1 Inserting an object *during* the seizure can cause teeth damage. Tongue blades are no longer recommended in this situation.
    2 The patient should not be left alone.
    4 Resistance against the restraints can cause injury.

181. Knowledge, assessment, psychosocial (b)
    1 The symptoms described here are the diagnostic criteria for major depression.
    2 There is nothing in this patient's history to indicate a personality disorder.
    3 She could be using substances, but this is not the most likely diagnosis.
    4 There is no evidence of a formal thought disorder.
182. Application, assessment, physiologic (c)
    1 The nurse should carefully assess the baby's heart sounds because cardiac anomalies are commonly found with Down syndrome.
    2 Cognitive (learning) deficits cannot be assessed immediately after birth.
    3 Visual impairments should be evaluated later by a pediatric ophthalmologist.
    4 Hearing impairments should be evaluated by a pediatric physician specialist.
183. Application, planning, health (c)
    4 Giving patients long-acting injectable forms of antipsychotic drugs has been shown to increase compliance because the patient is not responsible for medicating himself and the number of appointments to the outpatient mental health clinic for medications is reduced.
    1 This might increase the chances he would get his medication, but it would not further other important goals such as maintaining or increasing his independence.
    2 This would remove the responsibility from the patient and place it onto his health providers.
    3 This might increase his compliance only if the timing of his medications is the reason for noncompliance.
184. Application, implementation, physiologic (b)
    3 Noting what and when the last medication was given is important; the nurse should not give pain medication earlier than ordered unless the physician orders it.
    1 Vital signs may not be the same as during the preoperative period, but they are still within a safe range.
    2 Respirations of 18 are within normal limits; oxygen does not interfere with narcotic administration.
    4 Other measures can be effective and safe in controlling pain, but they do not always work.
185. Application, assessment, health (c)
    3 The most important role of the nurse is to assist the patient in regaining his or her psychologic balance despite current stressful circumstances.
    1 This may or may not be the case, depending on the individual patient's support system.
    2 This must be done by the patient himself; the nurse can only assist in the process.
    4 Her primary responsibility is to the patient.
186. Knowledge, assessment, physiologic (a)
    4 Clinical findings associated with hypothyroidism include edema of the face and eyelids.
    1, 2, 3 These symptoms are associated with hyperthyroidism.
187. Knowledge, assessment, physiologic (b)
    2 Nursing interventions for this condition include keeping the omphalocele covered with gauze and moistened with normal saline until surgery can be performed.
    1 This is where the upper esophagus ends in a blind pouch.
    3 This is a distention of the lower colon caused by lack of nerve cells in the wall of the colon.
    4 This is a narrowing of the distal end of the stomach.

188. Comprehension, assessment, physiologic (c)

    2 The cell life cycle is disrupted with the use of chemotherapeutic drugs. Cells most vulnerable are those that are actively dividing or about to divide. As a result, both normal and malignant cells are affected and/or destroyed.

    1 Both single and combination chemotherapeutic agents may cause numerous side effects.

    3 Chemotherapeutic drugs may be given by many routes, all of which produce numerous side effects.

    4 Chemotherapeutic drugs must be given more than once because only a fraction of cells are dividing at one time. Side effects are also related to dose strength. As doses are increased, major toxicities are more likely.

189. Knowledge, implementation, physiologic (a)

    4 Human chorionic gonadotropin stimulates ovulation for women trying to become pregnant.

    1 Rho-gam is given after pregnancy to Rh-negative mothers delivering Rh-positive babies.

    2 Ergot alkaloids are used to treat postpartum hemorrhage.

    3 Androgens are male hormones used for replacement therapy and to relieve postpartum breast engorgement.

190. Application, assessment, environment (c)

    2 This is true. *All 50 states require this to be reported.*

    1 This statement is only partially true. The nurse can report directly to proper authorities as well as to the physician.

    3 This is untrue. Laws *do grant immunity* from civil suits to those who are required to report child abuse.

    4 This is untrue. This is *not* considered legal privileged communication. All states require notification.

191. Comprehension, planning, physiologic (b)

    4 Circulation is decreased in the right arm (operative arm) because the axillary lymph nodes have been removed. An invasive procedure (drawing blood) increases risk of infection. Lymphedema may also occur in the operative arm.

    1 Movement is encouraged, not limited. Arm exercises help the patient retain the use of the arm.

    2 Elevation of the right arm will aid in decreasing edema.

    3 The patient should be encouraged to use her right arm.

192. Application, implementation, environment (b)

    3 With the head lower than the body, the drops will flow by gravity into the swollen nasal passages.

    1 Sitting up does not promote flow by gravity.

    2 The infant's head should remain lower than the body for 2 to 3 minutes.

    4 This is not the preferred position.

193. Application, implementation, environment (b)

    1 $\frac{3}{4} \text{ gr} \times \frac{60 \text{ mg}}{1 \text{ gr}} \times \frac{1 \text{ ml}}{30 \text{ mg}} = \frac{3/4 \times 2}{1}$

    $= 1.5 \text{ ml per dose}$

    2, 3, 4 These calculations are incorrect; the amounts are too high.

194. Comprehension, assessment, physiologic (b)

    1 Changes in level of consciousness (e.g., drowsiness) occur because of reduced oxygen supply to the cortex. The level of consciousness is a sensitive indicator of the patient's neurologic status.

    2, 3, 4 These signs of increased intracranial pressure often do not appear until the intracranial pressure has been elevated for some time.

195. Comprehension, implementation, physiologic (b)

    4 Massaging the calf could result in dislodging part of the clot and is contraindicated.

    1 A bed bath should not produce any harm to the patient as long as excessive rubbing to the left leg does not occur.

    2, 3 Turning the patient will not produce any harmful effects, but proper alignment should be maintained on the weak side.

196. Comprehension, planning, environment (b)

    4 This combination would allow for two meals on days, one meal at evening and fluid for medications at night.

    1 Most patients do not need 400 ml of fluid on the night shift.

    2 This does not allow for two meals on the 7 to 3 shift or any fluids at night.

    3 This does not equal 1400 ml of fluid for 24 hours.

197. Application, planning, psychosocial (b)

    2 Allowing the patient time to communicate her feelings and ventilate her frustrations will help the nurse to determine appropriate nursing interventions and will let the patient know the nurse cares.

    1 Medical intervention is premature at this time; nursing interventions should be tried before calling the physician.

    3 At age 25, a fresh makeover with her own personal gown may help; however, a depilitary might require handling and rubbing of the leg.

    4 The family could play an important part in the patient's recovery at this time, but she may not respond to them either.

198. Application, implementation, environment (c)

    4 Periocular edema often occurs on the side of the incision. This may cause the eye to be swollen. It will typically subside in a few days.

    1 This is not the most appropriate action. The physician does not need to be notified.

    2 Keeping the head of the bed elevated to 30 degrees and not in a flat position will facilitate drainage of fluid.

    3 This action is not the most appropriate choice. The glasses may be another source of discomfort because the area around the eyes is already swollen. Light, cool compresses over the eyes will help reduce the edema.

199. Comprehension, implementation, physiologic (a)

    1 Any tissue passed vaginally must be examined to determine if products of conception were expelled.

    2 The position of the patient is not a priority unless she is hemorrhaging.

    3 Providing a quiet environment is conducive to well-being; however, it is not the priority.

    4 Fluids may be held in this situation, given the possibility of a dilation and curettage (D&C) in the future.

200. Application, implementation, environment (b)

    2 $0.5 \text{ gr} \times \frac{60 \text{ mg}}{1 \text{ g}} \times \frac{7.4 \text{ ml}}{30 \text{ mg}} \times \frac{1 \text{ tsp}}{5 \text{ ml}} = \frac{7.4}{5}$

    $= 1.48 \text{ tsp}$

    1 This is an incorrect calculation; dose is too low.

    3, 4 These are incorrect calculations; doses are too high.

201. Knowledge, implementation, physiologic (a)

    3 Gentle pressure on the infant's chin breaks the suction, decreasing trauma to the nipple.

    1 Pressure to the infant's lips would not comfortably release the suction and could potentially injure the infant or harm the nipple.

    2, 4 The nose and forehead have no anatomic relationship to the lips and the reflex of sucking.

202. Comprehension, assessment, physiologic (b)
    4 Any unusual vaginal discharge requires immediate evaluation because it may be amniotic fluid.
    1 Quickening may not yet have occurred.
    2 Dependent swelling is not unusual.
    3 Weight gain over 2 lb/week is significant.

203. Knowledge, assessment, physiologic (a)
    2 The Croupette is used for smaller patients and provides cool moist air and oxygen to facilitate breathing.
    1 Aerosol therapy is inappropriate for a 16 month old and does not deliver cool, moist air and oxygen.
    3 This does not provide cool moist air.
    4 Air provided should be cool and moist, not warm and moist.

204. Comprehension, implementation, physiologic (b)
    2 As sodium leaves the body, so does potassium.
    1 Urinary output will be increased.
    3 This is not important.
    4 This is not required.

205. Application, evaluation, health (c)
    1 Asking the mother for feedback is the best way for the nurse to determine if the instructions were understood.
    2 Providing opportunity for feedback fosters communication and will enable the nurse to immediately modify her teaching plan, if appropriate. To instruct the mother to call with any questions blocks communication.
    3 Interpreting all medical terms should have been done in teaching. Feedback from the mother will still be necessary to determine if the medical terms were understood.
    4 Checking for the presence of communication barriers should have been done in the assessment phase before teaching.

206. Application, planning, health (b)
    2 The goal in crisis intervention is to assist the patient to return to at least her precrisis level of function.
    1, 4 The situation does not identify the nature of the situational crisis.
    3 This would occur as a result of a return to her precrisis level of function.

207. Comprehension, planning, health (a)
    2 Using Nägele's rule, take the first day of the last menstrual period (October 4), count back 3 months (July 4), and add 7 days (July 11).
    1, 3, 4 These are incorrect calculations.

208. Application, planning, environment (c)
    4 The intervention should state how often and by whom, as well as the characteristics of the sputum to be assessed.
    1 This is within the nurse's realm and does not require a physician's order.
    2 The intervention is appropriate, but it gives little direction for others using the plan.
    3 It is an appropriate but poorly written intervention.

209. Application, assessment, environment (b)
    1 Some bleeding can happen later, but most postpartum hemorrhage occurs during the first hour as a result of atony of the uterus or vaginal lacerations.
    2, 3 Bleeding is usually a result of retention of placental tissue.
    4 Most bleeding will occur within the first hour following delivery; see No. 1.

210. Application, implementation, environment (c)
    2 $\dfrac{30 \text{ gtt}}{1 \text{ min}} \times \dfrac{1 \text{ ml}}{60 \text{ gtt}} \times \dfrac{1 \text{ g}}{500 \text{ cc}} \times \dfrac{1000 \text{ mg}}{1 \text{ g}} = \dfrac{2}{2} = 1$
    1 This is an incorrect calculation; dose is too low.
    3, 4 These are incorrect calculations, doses are too high.

211. Knowledge, implementation, physiologic (a)
    1 Tinctures are alcohol or water and alcohol solutions that can produce reactions when mixed with Antabuse.
    2 Oral solutions usually contain only water and the medication particles; they should not interfere with Antabuse.
    3 Enteric-coated tablets are protected by a coating from dissolving in the stomach; they should not interfere with Antabuse.
    4 Sustained-release tablets allow slow distribution over time and will not interact with Antabuse.

212. Comprehension, evaluation, physiologic (c)
    3 With increased blood volume, both become lower: Hgb 12 to 16 g/dl blood; Hct 37% to 47%.
    1, 2, 4 Both decrease; see No. 3.

213. Application, planning, physiologic (b)
    2 Supportive therapy, such as blood transfusion, pain relief, and fluids, is necessary.
    1 This is not treatment for sickle cell crisis or sickle cell anemia.
    3 Fluids are appropriate in this situation.
    4 Passive range-of-motion exercises are performed to promote circulation.

214. Knowledge, assessment, physiologic (a)
    3 Appendicitis is the inflammation of the cecum and is not related to hernia formation.
    1 Congenital defects may allow for hernia formation.
    2 Obesity increases muscular weakness, with the possibility of herniation.
    4 A weakened muscular wall will increase the likelihood of hernia formation.

215. Comprehension, planning, health (b)
    1 The suggested diet for patients with diverticulitis is low-fat, no fried foods, and moderate fiber intake.
    2 This selection includes foods that are fried and high in fat.
    3 This selection includes foods with high fat content.
    4 Strawberry yogurt may be appropriate if it is low fat, but the chocolate chip cookies are not.

216. Comprehension, evaluation, health (b)
    4 Cigarettes can retard fetal growth. Research indicates that smoking may complicate a pregnancy.
    1, 2 These are true statements.
    3 There is no safe limit of alcohol for a fetus. The patient should eliminate alcohol intake.

217. Comprehension, implementation, physiologic (a)
    3 A nursing judgment requires that equipment and additional assessment data be obtained before initiating any other actions.
    1 This action is contraindicated in abdominal surgery patients without the order of the physician.
    2 This action would require additional assessment and is beyond the scope of practice for the licensed practical nurse in this situation.
    4 This action may be taken, but it is not the initial approach in this situation.

218. Comprehension, planning, health (b)
    3 The patient has symptoms of preeclampsia. Bed rest and decreased salt intake will help to reduce the symptoms.
    1 Bed rest is appropriate, but decreasing caloric intake would not be therapeutic in preeclampsia.
    2 These would be contraindicated.
    4 Reducing the salt intake is appropriate, but moderate exercise is contraindicated.

219. Knowledge, assessment, physiologic (b)
    1 Breast changes are a subjective, presumptive sign of pregnancy.
    2 Goodell's sign is a softening of the cervix, an objective probable sign of pregnancy.
    3 Positive urine pregnancy test is an objective probable sign of pregnancy.
    4 Chadwick's sign is an objective probable sign of pregnancy.
220. Comprehension, assessment, environment (b)
    2 This is peripheral cyanosis, a blue color of hands and feet in most infants at birth that may persist for 7 to 10 days.
    1, 3 These conditions even in adults are usually noted in the hands. These options were too general even though warming, in adults, induces vasodilation, and the blue discoloration becomes mottled with red.
    4 The most probable substance with which a newborn may be covered is vernix caseosa, which is a white cheesy substance that is not usually confined to the extremities.
221. Knowledge, evaluation, physiologic (a)
    3 Buccal tablets are to dissolve next to the cheek.
    1 A troche can dissolve anywhere in the mouth.
    2 Often tablets that dissolve should not be followed with water.
    4 This is sublingual administration.
222. Knowledge, assessment, physiologic (a)
    1 Down syndrome is the most common chromosomal abnormality of a generalized syndrome and is caused by the presence of an extra chromosome 21 in the G group or, in a small percentage of cases, by the translocation of chromosomes 14 or 15 in the D group and chromosomes 21 or 22.
    2 Patau's syndrome (trisomy 13) has an extra chromosome at the number 13 position.
    3 Turner's syndrome (XO) or (45 XO), appearing in females, is characterized by the absence (missing) of one X chromosome.
    4 Klinefelter's syndrome (XXY), a syndrome of gonadal defects appearing in males, is characterized by an extra X chromosome.
223. Comprehension, evaluation, health (a)
    3 The pancreas either decreases the amount of insulin production or fails to produce insulin, causing the glucose level to elevate in the blood.
    1 This may cause a temporary increase of blood glucose, but it does not cause diabetes mellitus.
    2 Eating less would cause a decrease of blood glucose. Eating or avoiding certain foods does not cause diabetes mellitus.
    4 This produces insulin shock.
224. Knowledge, assessment, physiologic (a)
    4 Otitis media is a common complication of an upper respiratory tract infection in young children.
    1, 2, 3 These conditions can accompany otitis media, but they are not the most common complications.
225. Comprehension, evaluation, physiologic (c)
    1 Miotic drugs cause constriction of the pupils, which helps to facilitate the drainage of the aqueous humor.
    2 Mydriatic drugs cause dilation of the pupils, which would further hinder the circulation of the aqueous humor.
    3 Diaphoresis is the term for excessive perspiration.
    4 Diuresis is the term for increased urinary output.

226. Application, evaluation, health (b)
    1 Diets high in purines should be restricted because purines break down into uric acid.
    2, 3, 4 These nutrients do not apply to gout.
227. Knowledge, implementation, health (a)
    1 For children under 3 years of age, the ear is drawn down and back; the patient is 5 months old.
    2, 3 For older children and adults, the ear is pulled up and back.
    4 For infants the ear is pulled down and back.
228. Comprehension, evaluation, physiologic (a)
    4 Pernicious anemia results from the lack of the intrinsic factor found in the lining of the stomach. This is a chronic condition and must be treated with injections of vitamin B_{12}.
    1 Whole blood is usually given to patients with hemorrhagic anemia because of the loss of a large quantity of blood.
    2 Packed cells may be given when only the cells of blood need to be replaced, such as in sickle cell anemia.
    3 Injections of Imferon are usually administered to patients with severe iron-deficiency anemia.
229. Knowledge, implementation, physiologic (a)
    4 The child will most likely be able to sit alone using her hands for support by 6½ to 7½ months.
    1 In motor sequence, walking with assistance starts between 11 and 12 months of age.
    2 In motor development, the child can feed herself with a spoon and will have some spills at 15 months of age.
    3 In motor sequence, standing holding onto furniture or pulling self up starts about 9 to 11 months of age.
230. Comprehension, evaluation, environment (c)
    4 A hemolytic reaction is a result of incompatible blood, which may result in decreased urine output and hematuria.
    1 This is an allergic reaction.
    2 This is a pyogenic reaction as a result of contaminated blood.
    3 This is not a result of a hemolytic reaction. Hypertension makes this statement incorrect. Hypotension occurs.
231. Application, planning, health (b)
    4 A rehabilitative focus does not wait until problems occur. It is a proactive approach to nursing care planning that deals with prevention of problems.
    1 This approach may be appropriate but is not the best response relevant to rehabilitative care planning.
    2 This approach may be appropriate and selected as one component of the care plan; however, addressing actual and potential problems is a more comprehensive approach.
    3 This is not the most complete response.
232. Comprehension, evaluation, environment (b)
    3 When a patient is given incompatible blood, the red blood cells react by clumping, or agglutinating.
    1 Achromia refers to the absence or loss of normal skin pigment.
    2 Agnosia is the total or partial loss of the ability to recognize familiar objects or persons through sensory stimuli as a result of organic brain syndrome.
    4 Anticoagulation refers to the prevention or delaying of coagulation (clotting) of the blood.

233. Knowledge, implementation, physiologic (a)
   1 Keeping a child in an upright position helps ease the motion of the diaphragm in breathing.
   2 Oxygen may not be needed; also, the child has not been examined by a physician to give this order.
   3 This child is in respiratory distress and is having difficulty breathing, so this would not be the first thing to do in this situation. The physician has not seen the child to give an order for aerosol treatment.
   4 The nurse should monitor the respiratory rate more frequently, but this would not be the nurse's first intervention.

234. Comprehension, evaluation, environment (b)
   1 Any pain, dyspnea, change in blood pressure, or dysrhythmia that is precipitated by an activity could indicate the patient's inability to tolerate activities.
   2 This does not necessitate stopping rehabilitation, because the patient must be taught to understand risk factors regarding health.
   3 This does not necessitate stopping rehabilitation, because the patient must be taught dietary modifications.
   4 The patient must be instructed about prescribed medications.

235. Knowledge, implementation, health (b)
   3 Both of these foods contain tyramine, which causes hypertension in combination with an monoamine oxidase (MAO) inhibitor.
   1 This is necessary with lithium, not with MAO inhibitors.
   2 This is a side effect of lithium, not of MAO inhibitors.
   4 This is a symptom of lithium toxicity, not of MAO inhibitors.

236. Knowledge, evaluation, physiologic (b)
   2 Nitrates dilate central vessels; this causes an increase in cranial pressure, resulting in headaches.
   1 Nitrates may reduce, not increase, blood pressure.
   3 Nitrates do not directly affect the pulse rate.
   4 Nitrates do not cause drowsiness.

237. Application, implementation, environment (c)
   3 Patients are disoriented after electroconvulsive therapy (ECT) and require orientation as they begin to awaken.
   1 Patients are not alert enough after ECT to take fluids.
   2 Patients should be allowed to rest and sleep as they recover from anesthesia.
   4 Patients are not alert enough after ECT to eat.

238. Application, evaluation, health (a)
   4 Weighing a patient daily is an accurate measurement for fluid increases and/or decreases.
   1 Daily weighing is only one factor in the assessment of medication change.
   2 Daily weighing is not indicated when weight reduction is the goal.
   3 This is an inappropriate response; the patient's diagnosis should be discussed with her by her physician.

239. Application, implementation, health (c)
   2 Once a person has an episode of major depression, his or her chances of having another one are increased.
   1 This is false assurance, which is nontherapeutic.
   3 This could be true, but it is not necessarily the case.
   4 This is false assurance, which is nontherapeutic. She could become depressed again despite these treatments.

240. Comprehension, implementation, health (a)
   2 This is a good example of modeling. By observing someone who is successful in his or her life change, the patient becomes motivated to succeed.
   1 This is an example of imagery. It can help motivate the patient and relieve stress.
   3, 4 These are examples of operant conditioning. They are based on the belief that all behaviors are determined by their consequences. If positive reinforcement occurs, then the behavior will probably be repeated. If negative reinforcement occurs, then the behavior will not be repeated.

241. Comprehension, evaluation, physiologic (b)
   1 Absorption is decreased when diarrhea occurs. The drug is passed through the intestine too quickly for proper absorption to occur.
   2 Drug elimination involves primarily the kidney.
   3 Drug metabolism involves primarily the liver.
   4 Drug distribution would be altered by blood flow within the vessels.

242. Knowledge, assessment, physiologic (a)
   3 With a perforation of an ulcer, the abdominal cavity fills with fluid or blood, leading to distention.
   1 Clay-colored stools indicate a lack of bile, which may be associated with gallbladder dysfunction.
   2 Coffee-ground emesis is indicative of an upper gastrointestinal bleed, possibly related to ulcer pathology; this is not a sign of perforation.
   4 Distention after eating is usually related to the type of foods ingested or to decreased peristalsis.

243. Application, evaluation, environment (b)
   3 It is important for the nurse to always follow facility policy and procedure for reporting errors or omissions. The Quality Assurance committee should be made aware of such incidents to determine if a problem does exist.
   1 The physician is not next in authority on the unit and would probably defer to the supervising nurse.
   2 Confrontation is not the responsibility of the staff nurse; it could result in unpleasant working conditions.
   4 This is unnecessary and inappropriate; facility policy and procedures must be followed.

244. Knowledge, planning, physiologic (a)
   4 Beverages containing caffeine are avoided by patients with peptic ulcer disease because caffeine stimulates gastric secretions; this increases gastric mucosal irritation.
   1 Caffeine physiologically stimulates the central nervous system; it does not depress it.
   2 Caffeine does not specifically alter the fluid electrolyte balance.
   3 The use of caffeine products actually *increases* rather than delays the production of gastric secretions.

245. Application, evaluation, environment (b)
   4 This is actual and factual data that does not imply the nurse's opinion or dissatisfaction.
   1 This is labeling the patient instead of describing what was measurable about his behavior.
   2 Although it is important to note in the chart, this is too vague as written.
   3 The first part is an opinion and labels the patient.

246. Knowledge, assessment, physiologic (a)
   4 An elevated white blood cell count is indicative of an inflammatory process.
   1 Red blood cell elevation is correlated with diseases of the blood-forming organs, such as polycythemia.
   2 An elevated hemoglobin level may indicate dehydration, pulmonary obstructive disease, or congestive heart failure and is not necessarily an inflammatory process.
   3 Serum lipase is usually elevated in biliary disease.

247. Knowledge, evaluation, health (a)
    2 A tetanus booster is recommended every 10 years; the patient should make a notation of the date it was received.
    1 Within 3 years, the booster should be sufficient for any major injuries.
    3 A tetanus injection offers active immunity but does not offer protection for life.
    4 If the patient suffers another accident and cannot remember the date, the physician may elect to order another booster.

248. Application, implementation, physiologic (b)
    3 Nitro-Bid has a vasodilating effect and may cause orthostatic hypotension. For safety, the medication is administered when the patient is in a recumbent position.
    1 Although the dose may be calculated by the patient's weight, the physician orders the amount of medication to be administered.
    2 Nitrate levels are not usually obtained when taking nitroglycerin derivatives.
    4 Nitro-Bid does not affect the ECG pattern.

249. Comprehension, evaluation, physiologic (b)
    4 Illness weakens the body's ability to fight infection. An elderly individual may have a lowered defense because of age. Hospitalized patients are also at higher risk of developing nosocomial infections.
    1 Terminal illness can cause an individual to be more susceptible to infection, but the home environment may not be as risky as the hospital.
    2 If a nursing student follows hospital policy and uses proper protocol, the student is at no greater risk of infection than are other health personnel.
    3 Although a laceration can become infected as a result of a break in the skin barrier, proper cleaning at home will allow for healthy recovery.

250. Application, evaluation, physiologic (b)
    3 Any difficulty breathing (dyspnea, wheezing, SOB, orthopnea) can be signs of a blood reaction and should be immediately reported. The blood transfusion should be stopped at once.
    1 Blood is often slightly cooler than vascular temperature. If chilling occurs, blankets are provided. Blood should be warmed. Significant chilling can be an adverse reaction.
    2 Voiding is a normal occurrence, especially with the IV fluid administration.
    4 Blood is normally given very slowly for the first 15 minutes. If the patient is not considered high risk for circulatory overload, the rate can then be increased.